GUIDE TO THERAPEUTIC ONCOLOGY

GUIDE TO THERAPEUTIC ONCOLOGY

Editors:

PATRICK R. BERGEVIN, M.D.
Chief of Oncology, Coney Island Hospital;
Co-Director, Division of Oncology,
Maimonides Medical Center;
Assistant Professor of Medicine,
Downstate Medical Center, Brooklyn, New York

JOHANNES BLOM, M.D.
Chief, Oncology Section, Hematology-Oncology Service,
Walter Reed Army Medical Center;
Associate Professor of Medicine,
Uniformed Services University of the Health Sciences;
Clinical Associate Professor, Department of Medicine,
Georgetown University Medical Center,
Washington, D.C.

DOUGLASS C. TORMEY, M.D., PH.D.
Associate Professor of Human Oncology and Medicine,
University of Wisconsin Medical Center,
Madison, Wisconsin

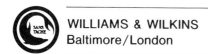

WILLIAMS & WILKINS
Baltimore/London

Made in the United States of America

Library of Congress Cataloging in Publication Data

Main entry under title:
Guide to therapeutic oncology.
    Includes index.
    1. Cancer. 2. Oncology. I. Title: Therapeutic oncology. II. Bergevin, Patrick R.
III. Blom, Johannes. IV. Tormey, Douglass C. [DNLM: 1. Neoplasms—Therapy.
QZ266 G946]
RC270.8.G84   616.9'92   79-10850
ISBN 0-683-00599-5

Composed and printed at the
Waverly Press, Inc.
Mt. Royal and Guilford Aves.
Baltimore, Md 21202, U.S.A.

Preface

Oncology has become a rapidly developing discipline encompassing many specialties of medicine. The management of patients with suspected malignancies requires a sophisticated approach to diagnosing and evaluating stage and extent of disease in order to provide the best available treatment program. Many of the management decisions are best made by a team of medical oncologists, surgeons, radiotherapists, pathologists, psychosocial, and nursing personnel. In the near future, this team may include immunologists.

This *Guide to Therapeutic Oncology* is intended to be a concise reference for the natural history, diagnostic evaluation, and available treatment modalities for various tumors. It is designed for use by students, house staff, oncologic trainees, and nurses, as well as the practicing physician. The extensive bibliography should serve as a ready reference for those who desire detailed source information.

- The introduction provides an overview of the various disciplines involved in the treatment of the cancer patient.

- The role of the surgeon as a primary physician and as a "technician" on the physician team is indicated very frankly.

- General radiotherapeutic and chemotherapeutic principles are discussed with insight into tumor cell kinetics and basic therapeutic concepts.

- The importance of documenting drug side effects is stressed, along with general therapeutic complications and drug dosage guidelines.

- Explanation of the design and purpose of clinical trials will serve as a guide to orderly evaluation of patients for those physicians not involved in clinical investigation.

- Chemotherapeutic agents are classified by derivation or mechanism of action and by cycle specificity.

- The commonly used standard and investigational drugs are discussed with attention to biochemistry, pharmacology, side effects, and administration.

v

PREFACE

- The growing evidence of coagulation abnormalities in patients with malignant disease warrants a separate section.

- Hematologic and solid tumors are presented individually and the literature is surveyed with emphasis on a rational approach to therapy.

- Where appropriate, diagnostic and staging procedures, pathology, and other pertinent information are discussed.

Contributors

ALTER, AARON, M.D. (*deceased*), Former Director Division of Hematology, Maimonides Medical Center, Brooklyn, NY
Associate Professor of Medicine, Downstate Medical Center, Brooklyn, NY

BERGEVIN, PATRICK R., M.D., Chief of Oncology, Coney Island Hospital, Brooklyn, NY
Co-Director, Division of Oncology, Maimonides Medical Center, Brooklyn, NY
Assistant Professor of Medicine, Downstate Medical Center, Brooklyn, NY

BLOM, JOHANNES, M.D., Chief, Oncology Section, Hematology-Oncology Service, Walter Reed Army Medical Center, Washington, DC
Associate Professor of Medicine, Uniformed Services University of the Health Sciences, Bethesda, MD
Clinical Associate Professor, Department of Medicine, Georgetown University Medical Center, Washington, DC

CANELLOS, GEORGE P., M.D., F.A.C.P., Chief of Medicine, Sidney Farber Cancer Institute, Boston, MA
Associate Professor of Medicine, Harvard Medical School, Boston, MA
Senior Associate in Medicine, Peter Bent Brigham Hospital, Boston, MA

CHABNER, BRUCE A., M.D., B.A., Chief, Clinical Pharmacology Branch, Division of Cancer Treatment, NCI, NIH, Bethesda, MD

COHEN, PHILIP, M.D., B.A., Associate Professor of Medicine, Division of Hematology and Oncology, The George Washington University Medical Center, Washington, DC
Chairman, Cancer Committee, George Washington University Medical Center, Washington, DC

COHEN, STEPHEN C., M.D., Clinical Associate Professor of Department of Medicine, University of Texas Health Science Center of San Antonio, San Antonio, TX

COMIS, ROBERT L., M.D., B.S., Assistant Professor of Medicine, Chief, Section of Oncology, State University of New York, Upstate Medical Center, Syracuse, NY
Assistant Attending Physician, State University Hospital, Syracuse, NY

COX, JAMES D., M.D., Professor and Director of Therapeutic Radiology, The Medical College of Wisconsin, Milwaukee, WI
Director, Therapeutic Radiology, Milwaukee Regional Medical Center, Milwaukee, WI

DEGENSHEIN, GEORGE A., M.D., F.A.C.S., Director of Surgery, Maimonides Medical Center, Brooklyn, NY
Clinical Professor of Surgery, State University of New York, Downstate Medical Center, Clinical Associate Dean, Brooklyn, NY

FREILICH, ROGER E., D.M.D., Staff Oral Surgeon, St. Mary's Hospital and Community Hospital of the Palm Beaches, West Palm Beach, FL
Assistant Oral Surgeon (*Former*), Coney Island Hospital, Brooklyn, NY

GOLITZ, LOREN E., M.D., Assistant Professor of Dermatology and Pathology, University of Colorado Medical Center, Denver, CO
Chief of Dermatology, Denver General Hospital, Denver, CO

HANSEN, HEINE, H., M.D., Chief, Chemotherapy Department R, Radium Center, Finsen Institute, 49 Strandboulevarden, DK-2100 Copenhagen, Denmark

KIMBALL, DANIEL B., JR., M.D., Assistant Chief, Department of Medicine, Walter Reed Army Medical Center, Washington, DC
Associate Professor, Department of Medicine, Uniformed Services University of the Health Sciences, Bethesda, MD
Consultant in Hematology/Medical Oncology to Surgeon General, United States Army

MACDONALD, JOHN S., M.D., Associate Professor of Medicine, Vincent T. Lombardi Cancer Research Center, Georgetown University Medical Center, Washington, DC

MCCAULEY, JAMES J., M.D., Medical Oncologist and Hematologist and Staff Member, Department of Medicine, Community Memorial Hospital, Toms River, NJ

MILLER, CHARLES F., M.D., Chief, Hematology-Oncology Division, Tripler Army Medical Center, Honolulu, HI
Staff, Hematology-Oncology Service, Walter Reed Army Medical Center, Washington, DC
Assistant Professor of Medicine, Uniformed Services University of the Health Sciences, Bethesda, MD
Assistant Professor of Medicine, Georgetown University Medical Center, Washington, DC

MISKOFF, RICHARD A., M.D., A.B., Internal Medicine, Hematology-Oncology, Woodbridge, NJ
Assisting Attending Physician, John F. Kennedy Medical Center, Edison, NJ

NATHANSON, LARRY, M.D., F.A.C.P., Chief, Medical Oncology Service, New England Medical Center, Professor of Medicine, Tufts University School of Medicine, Boston, MA

NAWABI, ISMAT U. M.D., Acting Director, Division of Hematology, Maimonides Medical Center, Brooklyn, NY

Assistant Professor, Department of Medicine, State University of New York, Downstate Medical Center, Brooklyn, NY

PARK, ROBERT C., M.D., B.S., Chief, Department of OB-GYN, Walter Reed Army Medical Center, Washington, DC

Professor, Department of OB-GYN, Uniformed Services University of the Health Sciences, Bethesda, MD

PETTY, WILLIAM M., JR., M.D., B.A., Associate Professor of Obstetrics and Gynecology, University of Oregon Health Sciences Center, Portland, OR

RUYMANN, FREDERICK B., M.D., B.A., Chief, Pediatric Hematology-Oncology Service, Walter Reed Army Medical Center, Washington, DC

Assistant Chief, Department of Pediatrics, Walter Reed Army Medical Center, Washington, DC

Associate Professor of Pediatrics, Uniformed Services University of the Health Sciences, Bethesda, MD

SCHEIN, PHILIP S., M.D., Chief, Division of Medical Oncology, Professor of Medicine and Pharmacology, Vincent T. Lombardi Cancer Research Center, Georgetown University School of Medicine, Washington, DC

SCIALLA, SALVATORE J., M.D., B.S., B.PH., Assistant Chief Hematology-Oncology Service, Walter Reed Army Medical Center, Washington, DC

Acting Director Coagulation Research Laboratory, Walter Reed Institute of Research, Washington, DC

Assistant Professor, Hematology-Oncology Division, Department of Medicine, Uniformed Services University of the Health Sciences, Bethesda, MD

Clinical Instructor, Department of Medicine, School of Medicine, Georgetown University Medical Center, Washington, DC

Lecturer in Hematology-Oncology, George Washington University School of Medicine, Washington, DC

TORMEY, DOUGLASS C., M.D., PH.D., Associate Professor Human Oncology and Medicine, University of Wisconsin Medical Center., Madison, WI

WASHINGTON, ALEXANDER W., JR., B.S., M.D., Assistant Chief of Medicine, Hematology-Oncology, U.S. Public Health Service Hospital, New Orleans, LA

WEISBERG, JEFFREY I., D.O., Chief, Hematology-Oncology, USPHS Hospital, Staten Island, NY

Clinical Assistant Professor, Department of Medicine, State University of New York at Downstate Medical Center, Brooklyn, NY

Diplomates of American Boards of Internal Medicine, Hematology and Medical Oncology, TAMARAC-FT. Lauderdale, FL

Contents

I. General Principles

II. Chemotherapy

CONTENTS

III. Neoplastic Diseases

IV. Additional Topics on Cancer

I
General Principles

Chapter 1

Current Concepts of Cancer Therapy: An Overview

JAMES J. McCAULEY, M.D.

Cancer represents the total of many diverse diseases occurring in any of the tissues or organ systems. While no single definition of the malignant neoplastic process is universally agreed upon, all such diseases have in common the characteristic of an abnormal and uncontrolled proliferation of transformed or altered tissues at one or more primary points within the host, and frequently at one or more metastatic sites. Many morphologic criteria have been applied to such cancerous processes, but the *malignancy* of a neoplasm is more often defined in terms of its behavior, that is, by its ability to invade normal surrounding host tissues and metastasize to distant sites by way of the lymphatic and vascular channels. As the process of neoplastic growth, invasion and metastasis proceeds the tumor often exerts systemic *paraneoplastic* effects on the host which contribute directly or indirectly to that tumor's morbidity and mortality for the host (Hall, 1974).

Until recently our view of the malignant process was a relatively static one based on tumor morphology and on the anatomic extent of the process within the patient, and the therapeutic approach was based on a somewhat outdated and incomplete concept of tumor biology and the mechanisms of tumor spread and host containment. This view theorized that the cancer began in a single site, growing locally and remaining confined to regional lymphatics and only later metastasizing to more distant sites. Although we now know it to be incomplete and in many ways inaccurate, given this biologic conception of cancer, certain philosophies and techniques of surgical management evolved around the turn of the last century, which until recently remained virtually unchallenged and unchanged. A prominent example may be seen in the historical evolution of the classical Halstead radical mastectomy in the manage-

ment of breast cancer (Fisher, 1977a, b). Similar thinking was involved in
the development and refinement of the radical surgical extirpative procedures for cancers of the lung, pancreas, and other organs. These
procedures were designed with curative intent in appropriately selected
patients. However, as many of our surgical colleagues would now agree,
in spite of improvements in supportive measures and refinements in
surgical technique, the primary surgical management of many malignant
diseases has long since reached a plateau in terms of therapeutic yield
and efficacy. The stage of the disease at the time of presentation is a
prime factor in the resectability of that disease, especially when curative
(as opposed to palliative) resection is the therapeutic goal. Thus, many
lesions present at a point too far advanced to be technically, beneficially,
or curatively resectable. However, even in many "early" (i.e., small and
apparently localized) solid tumors, the duration of postoperative periods
free from disease relapse and overall survival figures have been disappointing. In many such cases the relapses have not occurred locally
(especially if postoperative radiotherapy had been employed adjuvant to
surgery), but at more distant sites. Such a natural course in many
surgically treated "local" malignancies has become more understandable
as a result of the recent concept of subclinical systemic disease (foci of
micrometastases) at the time of presentation. The early empirical use of
adjuvant programs of chemotherapy failed to alter the disease course in
such patients because of a lack of knowledge of tumor biology and of the
necessary therapeutic design requirements; such early chemotherapy
trials were of inadequate dose and duration, often employed only a single
cytotoxic agent, and were prompted by discovery of circulating tumor
cells in cancer patients at the perioperative period (Fisher et al., 1968,
1975). In the present era of cancer chemotherapy, however, many advances have been made in both the theoretical design and the efficacy of
this treatment modality. The substantial advances in our understanding
of tumor biology and the cell kinetics of both normal and neoplastic cells,
together with the development of many newer chemotherapeutic agents,
has resulted in programs of primary or adjuvant chemotherapy which
now play important roles in the control or cure of many cancers. For
these reasons the view of the role (but not the more selective applicability)
of surgery in the management of malignancy is being reshaped and re-
examined (Crile, 1978; DeVita, 1978; Fisher, 1977a). If, as many surgeons
now do, one accepts the concept of systemic micrometastases at the time
of tumor presentation, then the therapeutic necessity for some form of
systemic treatment becomes apparent (Schabel, 1975; Sugarbaker et al.,
1977). Indeed, it is now felt that 60% of all patients with cancer (with the
exception of nonmelanomatous skin cancer) already have systemic dis-

ease (clinical or subclinical metastases) at the time of diagnosis (Frei, 1972). The concept of a combined modality approach to many malignancies is therefore currently accepted. Each of the major anticancer therapeutic disciplines, formerly separate and compartmentalized, now often joins hands with the others in the treatment of a particular malignancy. The exact therapy indicated in a particular disease will depend on the stage of that disease in the patient, our knowledge of its natural course, and the efficacy of the various therapeutic modalities. Surgery alone may still be the therapy of choice, and with true curative potential, in certain early and truly localized cancers (e.g., nonmelanomatous skin cancers, stage one malignant melanoma, pathologically proven stage one breast carcinoma, etc.).

In other cancers, which are characteristically widespread or aggressive at presentation, chemotherapy may be the primary modality of choice, as in the hematologic malignancies, small cell carcinoma of the lung (Abeloff et al., 1976; Johnson et al., 1976) or female choriocarcinoma (Lewis, 1976). Indeed, in the case of the hematologic malignancies, a certain percentage are now considered to be curable (i.e., life expectancy with treatment approaches the normal life span) in some of the disease types. Prominent examples include childhood acute lymphocytic leukemia (Henderson, 1974), Hodgkin's disease (DeVita et al., 1972), and certain histologic subtypes of the malignant lymphomas (e.g., Burkitt's lymphoma (Ziegler, 1977) and diffuse histiocytic lymphoma (DeVita et al., 1975)).

In certain of the solid tumors, particularly the childhood solid tumors, chemotherapy regimens used as adjuvants to extirpative surgery or radiotherapy have played an important role in the long term survival or cure of disease. Examples include Wilms' tumor (D'Angio et al., 1976), Ewing's sarcoma (Rosen et al., 1978), osteosarcoma (Carter and Friedman, 1978), rhabdomyosarcoma (Maurer et al., 1977), and retinoblastoma (Lemerle et al., 1978).

Since patients with even a single malignant disease are comprised of heterogeneous subsets, not all of which will respond favorably or equally well to a given therapeutic regimen, a constant goal in the design and analysis of prospective studies is the discovery or selection of such prognostic subsets of patients and the identification of the corresponding responsible variables. Once such prognostic subsets are defined (e.g., stage of disease, immune status of the host, and performance status), therapeutic variations may then be designed specifically for them. The single most important prognostic indicator is generally the stage of the disease, since often (but not always) the prognosis for survival and for therapeutic response is worse in the more advanced stages.

TREATMENT—THE OTHER EDGE OF THE SWORD: IMMEDIATE AND LONG
TERM TOXICITY

In spite of the very real theoretical and clinical therapeutic advances
that have been made with antitumor chemotherapy, there is growing
concern about the corresponding host toxicity associated with its use. In
addition, some combination chemotherapy regimens are being combined
in the treatment of certain cancers (especially Hodgkin's disease) with
radiotherapy, whose toxic and carcinogenic potential is well known. As
was the intention of the designers of such increasingly toxic and complex
anticancer regimens, the remission durations and survival of many patients with malignancy are becoming progressively longer. Alarmingly,
however, the incidence of immediate and especially of long term associated complications is also increasing as these patients, in disease-free
remission or even "cured," live long enough to express these potential
longer term toxic effects. These delayed toxicities are often dramatic and
shattering in their impact on the patient: Many patients are now at
increased risk to develop late second malignancies, and damage to the
germ cells of the patient may compromise or ablate his or her fertility or
exert damaging effects on any offspring (Bender and Young, 1978). This
effect on the gene pool may not be limited to the first generation, but
may be transmitted or expressed in succeeding generations as well. Since
the incidence, determination, and analysis of such long term effects as
these may take years or decades in the individual and generations in
families, no firm conclusions as to the cause-effect relations of toxic
therapy to such effects is yet possible. It is heavily incumbent on clinicians
and other investigators to therefore carefully monitor clinical trials and
all other data which may shed light on these issues and aid in the
determination of realistic risk-versus-benefit ratios for such types of
therapy. The individual with a cancer which he is informed may terminate
his life in weeks or months or years will frequently and understandably
opt for such therapeutic regimens on the chance that his life may be
extended or that he may be cured. However, it may some day be
incumbent upon the investigator or therapist to inform the patient of the
possiblity or even likelihood of second malignancies and compromised
fertility and childbearing potential, and to offer genetic counseling.

The data with regard to the long term toxic effects on the patient
treated with various anticancer modalities have recently been summarized by several workers (Arseneau et al., 1974; Cadman, 1977; Harris,
1976; Hersh, 1974). We now know that various single agents, and especially the alkylating agents, are associated with the late occurrence of
second malignancies (Gonzales, 1977; Haque et al., 1976; Penn, 1976).
Combination chemotherapy regimens, such as those currently employed
in the treatment of Hodgkin's disease, are also associated with reports of

second cancers (Sahakian et al., 1974), now that such patients are surviving long enough for such potential effects to be expressed. Radiotherapy has also long been known for its late carcinogenic potential as a result of such studies as those dealing with (1) the survivors of the nuclear bombings of Hiroshima and Nagasaki (Ishimaru, 1971; Parker et al., 1974) and (2) the delayed incidence of thyroid and other cancers in children and adults who in former years had received radiotherapy to the head and neck for a number of conditions (Favus et al., 1976; Schneider et al., 1978). Now that the treatment of Hodgkin's disease sometimes utilizes combined modality regimens which incorporate both radiotherapy and combination chemotherapy, either simultaneously or sequentially, increased survival and even cure is one result. Unfortunately, there also appears in this subset of patients to be a 10- to 30-fold increase in the incidence of second malignancies with such combined modality regimens, compared with only a 3-fold increase for either modality alone (Arseneau et al., 1972).

These statistics indicate a definite trend toward second cancers in patients receiving one toxic modality of therapy and an even higher incidence in patients who receive two such modalities. Yet for a number of reasons one cannot conclude from these statistical associations alone that such therapy is the cause of the second malignancies. *First*, untreated patients with one cancer are known to have a higher incidence of second malignancy than the general population (Moertel and Hagedorn, 1957). *Second*, with the more effective chemotherapy and other anticancer modalities now available many cancer patients are surviving for longer periods, and this additional survival may allow increased opportunity for the expression of such a potential for second cancers. *Third*, as will be detailed further below, an acquired immunodeficiency syndrome seen in many cancer patients may be contributory to the potential for further cancers in patients with a history of malignancy.

On the other hand, there are cogent considerations which cause some investigators to feel that there is an increased risk for second malignancies following chemotherapy and/or radiotherapy. They further feel that such therapy occasions this increased risk and may directly or indirectly cause additional cancers. Such feelings are based on a consideration of the immunosuppressive and carcinogenic effects of these forms of therapy. Attention has been focused on the possible role of congenital or acquired immunodeficiency in the etiology of cancer, since there is a manyfold increase in malignant diseases in such patients compared to the general population. Congenital immunodeficiency states in which there appears to be a true increase in the incidence of malignancies, especially of the lymphomatous variety, include Bloom syndrome, ataxia telangiectasia, Wiskott-Aldrich syndrome, and common variable immunodeficiency

(Louie and Schwartz, 1978). A marked increase in the incidence of lymphoma and skin cancer is also observed in patients with the acquired or iatrogenic immunodeficiency seen in renal transplant recipients. Cancer in such immunodeficient or immunosuppressed patients has been theorized to be due to a deficiency in host immune surveillance mechanisms which allows the evolution and unimpeded growth of malignant clones of cells. However, this simplistic view of the role of immunodeficiency states in the etiology of malignant tumors is now becoming less acceptable, in part because of the restricted spectrum of cancers seen in such conditions. Some workers are therefore proposing modifications of the immune surveillance theory in the case of cancer in immune deficiency, or totally different theories. Nevertheless, it is accepted that the intact and properly regulated immune mechanisms of the host constitute a barrier to the growth of malignant clones of cells, and it is therefore probable that each human being thereby averts countless clinical malignancies during his or her lifetime. Spontaneous regression of proven cancers have also been documented in the medical literature, and the immune response of the host has been theorized to be a major factor in such a course. It is also known that the function and the efficiency of the immune system declines with age, in inverse proportion to the increase in the incidence of cancer with age, a point which would seem to support a role for the immune system in the prevention and control of malignancy.

All of this background is meant by way of prologue and context to the fact that chemotherapy and radiotherapy are known to be immunosuppressive (Harris et al., 1976; Penn, 1978) and might therefore have the effect of altering host immune resistance to the development and growth of additional malignancies. (It might be parenthetically added that surgery and even trauma are known to have immunosuppressive effects (Park et al., 1971; Slode et al., 1975).) However, a note of caution concerning the interpretation of these data should be injected here, for there is current evidence which strongly implicates tumor biologic mechanisms in the etiology of the acquired immune deficiency syndrome commonly associated with malignancy (Roubanian and Talal, 1978). This brings us back to the point mentioned above, that patients with cancer, even untreated, have an increased incidence of second malignancies. Host *tumor*-associated immunosuppression may well be a major factor in such a continuing malignant diathesis, and such an effect might express itself clinically long after remission or cure of the first cancer had been effected by therapy. Therefore, to imply a causative role to the immunosuppressive effect of antitumor therapy *alone* may be unjustified. However, the *added* effect of immunosuppressive chemotherapy or radiotherapy may well *further* increase the chances of the cancer patient developing a second malignancy.

In an effort to offset or minimize the toxicity of combination chemo-therapy, certain therapeutic strategies are employed where possible to maximize tumor cell kill while at the same time minimizing toxicity to host tissues:

1. Most agents used in combination regimens have been previously shown to have activity against the specific tumor against which the therapy is directed. Exceptions, however, are made in the case of rela-tively inactive agents which may be of value in kinetic manipulation of the tumor within the combination, or which may allow favorable modi-fication of the pharmacology of the other anticancer agents.

2. Cytotoxic agents are combined for simultaneous or sequential use according to their additive or synergistic effects on tumor cell kinetics or biochemistry.

3. Combination regimens, where possible, are designed such that the component drugs have differing but complimentary biochemical sites of action, while also having nonoverlapping host tissue toxicities.

4. Exploitable differences between tumor and host cellular kinetics and biochemistry are sought as bases for shifting the narrow therapeutic index in favor of the host and to the detriment of the tumor. One such strategy is based on an analysis of kinetics of growing masses of tumor cells: As tumor mass increases the initial exponential kinetic growth pattern changes and the kinetic profile of the component tumor cells becomes more heterogeneous as many of the cells leave the proliferating cell cycle to enter a resting phase. The proportional growth fraction of the tumor therefore decreases as its mass increases. Since most cytotoxic agents operate by first order kinetics (that is, they kill a constant fraction of cells rather than a constant number) and exert their effect primarily on cells in the proliferating cycle, such altered tumor cell kinetics are a major factor in the resistance of tumors to chemotherapy. However, this same kinetic characteristic may also be turned to the advantage of the oncologist, as tumors may be manipulated in various ways which recruit resting cells back into the proliferating cycle, thereby exposing them to elimination by chemotherapy. This ability to manipulate tumor cell kinetics is therefore an exploitable advantage. The elimination of masses of tumor cells by surgical removal or by cytotoxic chemotherapy or radiotherapy should in theory result in the entry of increasing numbers of tumor cells into the proliferating cycle in proportion to the reduction of tumor mass. Also, the cyclic and intermittent use of the various single and combination chemotherapy regimens not only promotes recruitment of resting tumor cells into the proliferating cycle, but at the same time allows the recovery and regeneration of host tissues.

5. Cytotoxic agents may be specifically chosen for their ability to reach special sites of tumor origin or sequestration. Thus, for example, the

lipid-soluble nitrosoureas and procarbazine may be chosen for brain tumors by virtue of their ability to cross the blood-brain barrier.

Specialized techniques for the administration of chemotherapy have also been developed to shift the therapeutic ratio of tumor host toxicity in favor of the host, or to manage tumor foci not readily treatable by more conventional systemic techniques of chemotherapy:

1. Local intra-arterial infusions of cytotoxic agents may be utilized in an effort to selectively kill tumor cells within the infusion field with much less of an effect systemically on host tissues outside of the region of the tumor. Continuous infusions by this technique are particularly useful, since a set dose of antitumor drug may be delivered more selectively to the tumor over longer periods, while the effect on host tissues is much less because of systemic dilution and because of detoxification by host tissues and organs (liver, kidneys). Slower and more prolonged infusions at decreased drug per volume of infusate are less toxic to the host (as opposed to pulse infusions at higher concentrations), but the tumor mass still receives the full toxic effect of such infusions.

2. Special techniques have been developed for the chemotherapy of malignant disease in closed spaces or other sequestered areas which may provide sanctuaries for tumor cells from conventional systemic forms of chemotherapy. Examples include the use of intrathecal routes of administration for meningeal foci of leukemia, lymphoma, and various solid tumors; and the local instillation of antitumor agents directly into closed serosal spaces (pleural, pericardial, peritoneal, etc.) for malignant effusions or other disease foci in these areas.

3. Selective postchemotherapy "rescue" techniques allow the use of larger systemic doses of cytotoxic chemotherapy in a manner which increases tumor cell kill while protecting or "rescuing" sensitive host tissues. The postchemotherapy interval prior to rescue is designed to maximize tumor cell kill prior to the point at which host tissues must be preserved from severe damage by a specific antidote. A classical example of this technique is the use of high dose methotrexate with citrovorum rescue in the treatment of acute leukemia, osteogenic sarcoma, and other malignancies (Bertino, 1977).

Finally, various supportive measures and newer therapeutic techniques have been developed in recent years which rescue patients from many of the complications which accompany the toxic effects of chemotherapy, or which actually increase the tolerance of certain patients for chemotherapy. Examples of important currently available supportive measures include the restoration of blood cellular elements in patients made cytopenic by chemotherapy, thereby preventing or participating in the management of such complications as leukopenia and infection, anemia, and thrombocytopenic bleeding. In addition, the mortality rate of infections in patients undergoing therapy for cancer has also decreased as a result of the continuing availability of newer and more effective antibiotics.

NEWER FORMS OF THERAPY: NUTRITIONAL THERAPY AND IMMUNOTHERAPY

Nutritional Therapy

Frequently cancer patients display abnormalities in the state of their nutrition, their nutritional processes, and their metabolism (Berg, 1976). Such abnormalities frequently correlate with the stage of malignant disease in the patient and may decrease or be eliminated with appropriate local or systemic anticancer therapy. Many different mechanisms may contribute to the decreased intake of food, improper absorption or utilization of nutrients, weight loss and a cachectic state. *First,* the anxiety associated with the knowledge of their diagnosis, and the toxic side effects of various forms of therapy may singly or in combination alter taste or desire for food, produce anorexia, or cause nausea, vomiting, or diarrhea. *Second,* certain tumors of the alimentary tract, such as those of the oropharynx, esophagus, stomach, or small intestines, may mechanically affect the intake or absorption of nutrients because of dysphagia or obstruction. *Third,* various gastrointestinal (GI) tumors may interfere with alimentation and absorption functionally. Thus certain GI tract tumors may be associated with malabsorption or protein-losing enteropathy (Waldman et al., 1974) and functional pancreatic islet cell tumors, and carcinoid tumors of the GI tract may be associated with malabsorption, diarrhea, ulcer disease, or hypoglycemia (Schein et al., 1975). The latter tumors, mediate such effects by the ectopic production of hormones such as gastrin, insulin, and serotonin. *Fourth,* weight loss may result from a hypercatabolic state due to infections, or tumor effect.

Finally, after a process of exclusion of other causes, a *fifth* cause of nutritional malfunction in the cancer patients is the frequently seen paraneoplastic syndrome of *malignant cachexia,* or the cachexia of cancer (Costa, 1977). This syndrome is relentlessly progressive in the untreated cancer patient (and frequently in patients receiving therapy), and is more characteristically associated with advanced disease. The syndrome expresses itself clinically by cachexia, or a state of marked and progressive weight loss due to an often rapid loss in muscle and adipose mass. Biochemically and physiologically it is characterized by a generalized catabolic state, negative nitrogen balance, depletion of protein, fat and carbohydrate tissue stores, abnormalities and tissue compartmental shifts in fluids and electrolyes, and impaired host nutrition and nutritive processes. The syndrome may also be accompanied by a hypermetabolic state relative to the state of nutrition of the host (which is often poor), and frequently is associated clinically with anorexia, or changes in the desire for food. The prognostic and therapeutic implications of this paraneoplastic state are poor, since it not only correlates with advanced disease, but also because it is associated with (and is a factor in) a poor overall state of health and performance. Such patients have an increased susceptibility to infections and a decreased tolerance for most conventional forms of antitumor therapy. For these reasons their responses to such forms of therapy are usually poor and of short duration. However, because the syndrome is reversible with appropriate and effective antitumor therapy, it is felt to be mediated by the distant effect of tumor hormones or other tumor products.

Various of the heterogeneous tumor biologic mechanisms responsible singly and in combination for this malignant syndrome are now being appreciated and analyzed. Thus, with regard to the anorexia which frequently is characteristic of malignant cachexia, various workers have postulated a number of mechanisms. Theologides (1976), for instance, has postulated that tumor-produced peptides, oligonucleotides, and other small intermediary metabolites may play a role. Such small molecules would circulate systemically and might easily enter cells at strategic locations. Thus their anorectic effects may be mediated by a direct effect, for instance, on the hypothalamic regulatory centers and other satiety and hunger centers of the central nervous system, or on peripheral neuroendocrine cells or receptors. Along a similar line, Nakahara and Fukuoka have postulated the existence of a tumor substance or group of substances which they have termed "toxohormone" (Nakahara, 1967). This tumor product has now been isolated and partially purified, and is thought to be a protein (Ohnuma, 1974).

The work of DeWys and Walters (1975) suggests that taste changes in cancer patients may also play a role in anorexia or other changes in the desire for food. Their qualitative and biochemical studies of patients with cancer suggest that quantitative changes in taste sensitivity may underly the qualitative alterations of taste which contribute in part to the anorexia of malignant cachexia. In this regard they have demonstrated a correlation between patient-reported general decrease in taste sensation and an elevated threshold for sweet (sucrose) dietary items, and a correlation between patient aversion for meat and a decreased taste threshold for bitter (urea). Such taste abnormalities have been reversed with programs of parenteral nutrition, implying that some nutritional deficit underlies them. The specific biochemical components which might lead to these changes in taste are not known with certainty but deficiencies in such minerals as zinc and copper have also been correlated with impairment of taste (Russ and DeWys, 1978). One might postulate either tumor consumption of such essential trace elements or malabsorption as possible etiologies of these deficiencies. Certainly, in the malnourished state that many of the patients with malignant cachexia exhibit, abnormal bowel function and malabsorption might occur. The confirmation of such theories awaits further data.

Many other pathologic tumor effects aside from the anorectic ones discussed to this point are implicated in the pathogenesis of malignant cachexia and its associated metabolic abnormalities. Thus numerous additional tumor biologic mechanisms and products are thought to mediate such cancer-associated abnormalities as fat depletion, protein depletion and hypoalbuminemia, abnormal glucose utilization and hypoglycemia, and disorders of fluids and electrolytes (Cahill, 1974; Costa, 1977; Gordon, 1974; Waterhouse, 1974).

Finally, as already indicated, a very important component in the genesis of anorexia and other contributory aspects of poor nutrition in the cancer patient is the iatrogenic one which results from the effects of such forms of treatment as surgery (Shils, 1977b), radiotherapy and chemotherapy (Shils, 1968).

The patient with malignancy may die of his state of malnutrition even in the absence of the destruction or obstruction by cancer of vital organs. However, nutritional support or therapy may reverse malnutrition and cachexia in a certain percentage of these patients, permitting their salvage and increased survival when used as an adjuvant to surgery, radiotherapy, or chemotherapy (Copeland and Dudrick, 1975). In addition to improving or restoring host nutrition to the point where patients may tolerate more morbid and toxic therapies, nutritional therapy may have additional benefits. Thus, some studies indicate that adjuvant nutritional therapy and support prior to and concomitant with chemotherapy and/or radiotherapy results in decreased host GI or hematologic toxicity (Copeland et al., 1975; Issell et al., 1978; Signori and Signori, 1978). Some investigators have expressed an aversion to the concept of adjuvant nutritional therapy on the basis that it might enhance tumor growth (Cameron and Pavlet, 1976; Terpeka and Waterhouse, 1956). Other workers feel that this would be a very unlikely turn of events, and that, on the contrary, such nutritional supplementation would allow more tumor cells to leave the resting state, enter the proliferating cell cycle, and thereby become sensitive to the effect of cytotoxic antitumor agents (Copeland and Dudrick, 1975) (Shils, 1977a). There is some experimental animal and neoplastic tissue culture data to support such a tumor cell recruitment theory. There is also evidence which links the catabolic and malnourished state of the patient with malignant cachexia etiologically to the immunosuppressed state which is often seen in such patients (Gertner et al., 1978). Some workers claim that nutritional therapy has had an immunorestorative effect in such patients (Law et al., 1973). This may indeed be a factor in the immunosuppression of the cancer patient, but the mechanisms by which tumors escape host immune surveillance and suppress host immunity are far more complex.

The ideal and most physiologic manner in which to implement nutritional therapy in the cancer patient is by way of the patient's own alimentary tract. This might be accomplished in the patient with an intact and functional GI tract by oral or nasogastric feeding of specialized diet and nutrients (DeWys and Herbst, 1977; Shils, 1977a). However, in the case of the patient with an obstructed GI tract, or one with enteropathic or malabsorptive syndromes, such alimentative forms of nutrition would be ineffective. In such cases, some form of total parenteral nutrition, such as intravenous hyperalimentation is necessary. The technical and nutritive details of such alimentary and hyperalimentary forms of nutritional support in the cancer patient have recently been reviewed (Dudrick et al., 1977; Ota et al., 1978). The parenteral forms of nutrition are not without their complications, however, and this form of nutritional therapy should be instituted and maintained by those experienced in both technique and complications.

Various steroid preparations have also been incorporated by some workers into the overall scheme of their therapy. Corticosteroids have thus been used to improve the overall feeling of well being of the cancer patient and perhaps increase the motivation for food intake. However, the glycemic and other complications often seen with such drugs may negate any such potential attractions. The use of androgenic anabolic steroids have received attention also in the attempt to reverse the catabolic state seen in many cancer patients, but their usefulness and the nature of their effect remains to be demonstrated (Brodsky, 1973).

Immunotherapy

Several considerations concerning immunity and cancer lead to the conclusion that there is both a need for and great promise in an immunotherapeutic approach to the management of malignant disease. *First,* the immune status per se of the patient with cancer has some prognostic importance, as in general the course and prognosis for response to conventional therapies is better in immunocompetent patients and worse in immunocompromised or immunoincompetent patients (Hersh et al., 1976; Konio and Leventhal, 1976; Krown et al., 1978). In addition once the therapy of the cancer has begun, immunosuppressant forms of therapy such as radiotherapy and chemotherapy may themselves alter the immune status of the host (even the trauma of surgery is known to adversely affect immune function). Some workers also claim that host antitumor immunocompetence may be reflected microscopically in the immunomorphology (or lack of it) of pathologic sections of resected tumor specimens. Thus, histologic evidence of antitumor immunity in the form of tumor infiltration by immune cellular elements (lymphocytes and plasma cells) and macrophages or other reticuloendothelial cells, as well as regional lymph node hyper-reactivity and sinus histiocytosis, and perivascular round cell infiltrates in the region of the tumor, are interpreted by some workers as correlates for improved disease prognosis and predictors of a favorable response to therapy (Black et al., 1971; Pihl et al., 1977; Wartman, 1959).

Second, numerous tumors have been found to produce substances which are specific to the tumor (of nonhost origin) and which are also immunogenic, as evidenced by the presence in host sera of specific antibodies unbound or complexed to their antigens in the form of immune complexes (Barlow and Bhattacharya, 1975; Frost et al., 1976; Herberman et al., 1976; Leventhal et al., 1978; MacDonald, 1976; Primack, 1974). Such tumor-specific antigens are able to elicit both T and B cell host immune responses. This antigenic specificity of tumor cell surface markers or tumor cell products constitutes another exploitable difference between the tissues of the tumor and those of the host, and has been utilized in the design and implementation of specific forms of antitumor immunotherapy.

Third, there is the previously mentioned susceptibility to malignancy with various congenital or acquired immunodeficiency states. Such an association would seem to imply that a failure in host immune function is responsible for the development of cancer in such patients, as expressed in the immune surveillance concept popularized by Burnet (1971). So simplistic an etiologic concept, however, is belied by the restricted range of the types of malignancy seen in such patients. In contrast to the wide range of tumors which develop in the general population, patients with immunodeficiency states are prone to develop predominantly leukemias or lymphoproliferative malignancies. The precise pathogenetic mechanisms which give rise to these tumors in immunodeficiency states is not known, but there is speculation concerning the role of distorted or abnormal immune regulatory mechanisms which might allow or stimulate evolution of malignant clones of immunocytes or myeloid elements.

Fourth, as more has been learned about the function of the normal immune system and its functional and regulatory mechanisms, such observations have been applied to the studies of the immune responses of the cancer patient, and much has been learned thereby of the immunobiology of tumor-host relations. Studies in animals and man have at least partially delineated the various elements involved in the immune response of the host to the tumor. Tumor immunologic nonidentity is implied by the previously mentioned concept of a host immune response to tumor-specific antigens. Thus, at the immune effector level, various forms of antitumor immune cytotoxicity are observed, including both humoral and cell-mediated types: (1) Cell-mediated immunity is effected by specifically and nonspecifically activated lymphocytes (predominantly T cells) and macrophages (monocytes, histiocytes, and other phagocytic cells of the reticuloendothelial system). The activation of these immune effector cells results in the lysis of tumor cells and may occur independent of humoral immune modulation in some instances. In other instances the participation of antibody (antibody-dependent cell-mediated cytotoxicity) or complement (complement-dependent cell-mediated cytotoxicity) may be required. In the latter instances, antibody or complement must bind to specific receptors on the surface membrane of the T cells or macrophages before they can be activated. (2) Humoral mechanisms include both antibody and complement-mediated cytotoxicity.

The correct implementation of these final stages of antitumor immune activity requires the presence of an intact and properly regulated host immune system. If this system is compromised prior to the neoplastic event, that very deficit may contribute to the genesis of the cancer. On the other hand, once neoplasia has occurred, the immune integrity of the host may be damaged or compromised because of tumor biologic mechanisms, as we shall see below. The genetic loci which control the phenotypic expression of the immune identity of the individual are now becoming clear, as are the gene products at the cellular level which define the idiotype of the individual and establish cells as "self" elements (Paul and Benecerraf, 1977). Among the more important of such cellular membrane markers are the HLA antigenic markers, although the determinants of self-identity are now known to be more complex (Katz, 1977; Zuckerman and Douglass, 1976). Normal mechanisms of immune tolerance of "self" and intolerance for all other (or "nonself") substances mediate a necessary discrimination in the function of the immune system and in the attack on any foreign antigens, as in the case of infections and neoplasms. The fact that there is an immune response by the host to the tumor implies some antigenic transformation during the time of carcinogenesis or malignant transformation, a conclusion supported by the discovery of tumor-specific antigens in many malignancies. Another necessary aspect of the regulation of the immune functions is the appropriate limitation of the immune response once initiated, so that at the proper time it is deactivated. Thus, not only are normal immune effector elements required in the immune response, but also normally functioning modulating or regulating elements, such as the recently identified "suppressor" and "helper" T cells. Such regulated and discriminant function is necessary if the host is to be safe from attack by its own immune system. Any breakdown of self/ nonself discriminant function anywhere along the chain of command from the genome to the effector elements may result in autoimmune disease, immunodeficiency, neoplasia, and other diseases (Friou, 1974).

And yet, in the face of apparently adequate immune function, vast numbers of malignant tumors occur in nature. Environmental carcinogens that are in some manner capable of generating such tumors in the face of immunity are one explanation. A more likely explanation, however, is that our present state of knowledge of this extremely complex biologic system is woefully inadequate to understand this apparent contradiction. Our present means of in vivo and in vitro evaluation of this system is very likely equally crude, but provide working yardsticks which do produce measurements of prognostic and immune functional usefulness. Another explanation for malignant disease in animals and man is the correlation between the incidence of malignancy and the decline in function of host immunity with increasing age. This is probably a factor in the poorer prognosis that older patients have with regard to the natural history of their malignancies and their response to therapy.

Finally, aside from the above considerations, there is the apparent paradox that many tumors, which in vitro demonstrate marked sensitivity to humoral and cellular immune attack, still grow, metastasize, and kill the host in vivo. In this regard, there is now increasing evidence that biologic mechanisms of the tumor itself play an active role in mediating its escape from host immune surveillance. This is often reflected clinically and biometrically in host immunodeficiency or immunoincompetence. Thus the clinical state of the patient, disease complications, and standard assessments of immune competence and response may suggest either a specific deficiency in antitumor immunity or a more generalized and tumor-nonspecific acquired immunodeficiency state. Such host immune deficits, and more specifically the more generalized state of nonspecific immune deficiency, constitute an often-observed paraneoplastic syndrome, which generally correlates with the stage of the disease (Browder and Chretien, 1977; Koperszytych et al., 1976). This acquired immunodeficiency of cancer is usually not seen in the early stages of malignancy, but develops and progresses as the stage of the disease advances, is characterized almost exclusively by deficiencies in cell-mediated immunity, and constitutes a major factor in the increased incidence and morbidity of infectious complications commonly seen in patients with the later stages of cancer (it will be recalled that the two leading causes of death in malignancy are infection and malnutrition). This acquired paraneoplastic state also is a major negative prognostic indicator and contributes to the overall poor prognosis and poor response to therapy in advanced malignant disease. And yet, such immune deficits, especially if mild, are reversible with response of the tumor to therapy, a fact which supports the concept that they represent a systemic effect of the tumor.

Much detailed information has recently been obtained about the specific tumor biologic mechanisms which mediate these defects in host immunity: (1) Modulation of tumor surface antigenic structure may occur in response to host immunologic attack. This may involve redistribution of surface antigens by dispersal and capping or endocytosis. In addition, tumors may manufacture substances which effectively mask immunogenic antigens from host immune attack. (2) Tumor cells may have rapid turnover and shedding of cell surface antigens, with a consequent overload or exhaustion of the host immune response because of excess free or complexed tumor antigens (Nicholson and Poste, 1976). Such antigen shedding may tie up or consume tumor-specific antibodies unbound in the serum or on the surface of sensitized immune cells, thereby inactivating antibody-mediated and antibody-dependent cell-mediated antitumor immune mechanisms. These and other tumor biologic mechanisms relate to the concept of "serum blocking factor," a nonspecific term which describes the inhibition of immune function by sera from cancer patients (Baldwin and Price, 1976; Yonemoto et al., 1978). Such serum blocking activity is now known to be mediated by various heterogeneous tumor mechanisms and substances. Thus, soluble tumor antigens, tumor antigens complexed with specific antibody, and prostaglandins of tumor cell origin are known to inhibit immune function both in vivo and in vitro. In addition, the tumor may stimulate the host production of "enhancing antibody," or antibody which enhances rather than inhibits tumor cell growth and function (Harris and Copeland, 1974). Also, the presence in the serum of tumor products which may mask tumor antigenic sites and thereby shield tumor cells from immune attack has been demonstrated. Further evidence of the tumor origin of these and other serum blocking factors is the fact that the titer of such serum activity diminishes and disappears with effective treatment of the tumor (surgical resection or debulking, chemotherapy, etc.) Some investigators have also utilized plasmapheresis to remove or decrease serum blocking activity, with resultant improvement in both the tumor-specific and general immune status of the patient (Israel et al., 1977). Such an approach might therefore also be reasonably expected to improve the response to conventional therapies. (3) Tumor cells may produce various substances (enzymes, prostaglandins, etc.) which subvert or damage humoral or cell-mediated host immune mechanisms (Harvey et al., 1978). The ectopic production of human chorionic gonadotropin by trophoblastic and nontrophoblastic tumors, for instance, has been reported to have a depressive effect on host lymphoid cells (Lange et al., 1976). Likewise, tumor cell prostaglandins have been implicated in T cell depression (Plescia et al., 1976). Tumor cells may also be able to negatively influence host antitumor immunity by influencing the host's T cell modulators; thus, tumors may be responsible for the elaboration of clones of suppressor T cells which switch off antitumor immune attack, or the suppression of key host helper T cells important in specific or nonspecific antitumor attack. In another ploy, certain tumors are also able to stimulate increased activation of plasminogen to plasmin, the fibrinolytic enzyme, resulting in the cleavage and inactivation of antitumor antibodies (and thereby subverting anti-body-mediated and antibody-dependent cell-mediated cytotoxicity) (Na-thanson and Kempner, 1978). (4) With progressive tumor growth, there is often the evolution of heterogeneous subgroups of cells in terms of their immunologic determinents, cell kinetics, membrane receptors, and cell functions. Some such subgroups will survive by virtue of their capacity to resist one or another form of antitumor attack (host immune attack, therapeutic attack by such modalities as chemotherapy, hormonal ma-nipulation, immunotherapy, etc.) (5) The rapidity of growth and spread of some tumors, as reflected in their growth fraction or tendency to early metastasis, may allow the malignancy to "outrun" host immune responses and establish an early and irreversible advantage which the host may never overcome.

To place such anti-immune tumor biology in proper perspective, it should again be emphasized that the appearance and magnitude of such deficits in host immunity generally correlate with increasing stages of cancer, and that defects in cell-mediated immunity predominate.

A number of different immunotherapeutic approaches to malignant disease have been designed and implemented in experimental and care-fully monitored clinical trials. Such approaches represent a spectrum of immunostimulative and immunorestorative forms of manipulation of the host immune system designed to augment both general and specific (antitumor) immune function in patients with cancer (Terry and Wind-horst, 1977). Such therapy is of potential value especially in cancer patients with the acquired paraneoplastic immunodeficiency syndrome described previously, but also in patients with relatively intact and competent immune function. Such immune modulation is now being used not only to stimulate antitumor immunity but also to increase host tolerance to the more toxic conventional forms of cancer treatment. Immunotherapy here has an advantage in that it is a relatively nontoxic form of therapy for the host and will therefore not augment significantly the toxicity of surgery, radiotherapy, or chemotherapy. On the contrary, there are data from immunotherapy studies which suggest that patients receiving chemoimmunotherapy may have diminished tissue toxicity from the chemotherapy, allowing them to tolerate more of such cytotoxic treatment than would otherwise be possible. Thus, patients with ad-vanced disease, immunoincompetence, and low tolerance for toxic ther-apy have occasionally had their immunity and their tolerance for such therapy improved by immunotherapy, and patients with standard tolerance have had that tolerance increased by immunotherapy, allowing them to receive higher than normal amounts of chemotherapy with little or no increase in toxicity. Such a situation is analogous to that described earlier for nutritional therapy as an adjuvant to other forms of anticancer treatment. Thus both nutritional and immunomodulative forms of therapy have supportive, restorative, and toxicity-reducing roles, as well as primary therapeutic roles in the management of the cancer patient. The various specific approaches to immunotherapy have recently been reviewed (Hersh et al., 1977). The implementation of these diverse forms of immunotherapy is placed in a more proper perspective by the mention of certain guidelines in their use:

1. Immunotherapy may be of benefit in any patient with cancer, even those assessed as having adequate immune responses, in whom additional immune augmentation may favorably affect their disease course or their response to other forms of therapy. However, immunorestorative and immunostimulative therapy are particularly suggested in those cancer patients with absent or subnormal immunocompetence, as their correlated poor prognosis for therapeutic response to other modalities may be favorably altered by such immunotherapy. In addition, it should be recalled that immunotherapy may also reduce host toxicity from conventional forms of therapy, thereby perhaps allowing even more aggressive chemotherapy or radiotherapy.

2. The various immunotherapeutic approaches may be employed separately, as they have been in many trials, but may be additive or synergistic in their effects on augmentation of host immunity if employed in combinations or in sequence (Shibata et al., 1976). In combining forms of immunotherapy, as in combination chemotherapy, the goal is increased tumor damage. In another sense, however, immunotherapy is designed to stimulate in the host immune system an awareness of the tumor if such an awareness is lacking; and if that awareness is present but ineffective because of tumor subversive mechanisms, immunotherapy should be specifically designed to minimize or eliminate such interference as well as to further augment host antitumor immunity. At the present stage of our knowledge, the most appropriate approach or combination of approaches to the immunotherapy of an individual cancer patient would seem to be that based on a careful assessment and delineation of tumor-host immunobiology in that particular person. Such an assessment would involve not only a thorough baseline delineation of the in vivo and in vitro immune capabilities of the patient, but also a careful delineation of the immune biology of the tumor (including any subversive anti-immune mechanisms) so that appropriate and correlated specific and nonspecific countermeasures might be planned. Such a pretherapy tumor-host immunologic workup and assessment might, for instance, dictate the simul-

taneous or sequential use of (a) immunorestorative therapy with levamisole to reactivate and replenish immune cellular elements, and plasmapheresis to reduce or remove serum blocking factor; (b) BCG to nonspecifically stimulate host immunity, and (c) active and specific immunotherapy with tumor-specific antigens or enzyme-modified autologous tumor cells. In following the effects of such immunotherapy programs as this or those of any other design, sequential repetition of the baseline patient and tumor immune profiles is essential in defining and quantifying the effects of the therapy.

3. Experience and research in the immunotherapy of animal and human tumors has emphasized the importance of minimal tumor burden as a factor predictive for response to such therapy (Fahey et al., 1976; Mathé et al., 1976). As in the case of chemotherapy before it, the cellular kinetic data of tumor immunotherapy are now being defined. In the patient with advanced disease, the sheer mass of tumor, combined with the effect of tumor anti-immune mechanisms, is overwhelming to the host immune system, and the chance of a good response to immunotherapy is less than in patients with minimal tumor load. The optimal candidates for immunotherapy are patients who have had their tumor mass substantially reduced by other antitumor modalities. One example consists of the postoperative use of immunotherapy or chemoimmunotherapy in various solid tumors. Such therapy, by definition, includes cases with clinical disease limited only to locoregional spread, the surgical removal of which would leave only micrometastatic tumor deposits remaining, a situation similar to the setting for the use of adjuvant chemotherapy. Such immunotherapy treatment regimens have been designed and implemented for trials in such "solid" tumors as cancers of the breast, lung, colon, and bladder, and osteosarcoma. Another example is represented by the postinduction use of immunotherapy in certain patients with the acute and chronic leukemias. Only after the intensive induction phase of chemotherapy has removed all evidence of disease (complete remission) or substantially reduced it (partial remission) is immunotherapy instituted in the maintenance phase of therapy, usually concomitantly with chemotherapy regimens designed to maintain such remissions and prevent relapse. (In addition, there have been immunotherapy protocols implemented where immunotherapy is begun in the induction phase of such hematologic malignancies).

4. At the present time, immunotherapy is designed predominantly to augment cell-mediated immunity, and there are cogent reasons for this: First, the acquired immunodeficiency seen in cancer patients is almost exclusively limited to defects in cell-mediated immunity. Secondly, antibodies are known under certain circumstances to enhance rather than inhibit tumor growth (so-called "enhancing" antibodies). Therefore, until

more is learned of the intricacies and control mechanisms involved in the interaction of the humoral and cellular forms of immunity, most immunotherapists prefer to selectively augment host cell-mediated immunity and minimize any possible augmentation of host antibody production.

5. It should also be noted that some of the more successful therapeutic designs have utilized immunostimulants applied locoregionally with respect to foci of tumor growth (i.e., intralesionally, proximate to local groups of lymph nodes, etc.), and perhaps such local immunotherapy should be emphasized in the design of future trials (Arai and Wallace, 1978; McKneally et al., 1972; Yamamura, 1977; Zbar, 1978).

In conclusion, immunotherapy is still an empirical discipline, and in the early and hesitant stages in terms of history, theory, design, implementation, and efficacy, a stage perhaps comparable to that of chemotherapy 25 years ago. As has been pointed out by others (Terry, 1977) this is predictable given the enormity of the attempt to define and integrate two such diverse and extremely complex areas of biology as immune function and neoplastic disease. Before immunotherapy can have a solid basis much more must be learned of the biology of immunity, and specifically of the immunobiologic mechanisms operative in vivo in the patient with malignancy. However, there is a general feeling of optimism concerning the future of this anticancer treatment modality.

CONCLUDING REMARKS

This brief overview of the management of the patient with cancer has emphasized the value of several of the individual anticancer therapeutic modalities, while also stressing the fact that the overall plan of therapy in the individual patient with a malignant disease must often be the product of a multidisciplinary approach. Experience has shown that it is the *first* therapeutic attempt at the elimination of a malignancy which is the only one likely to lead to a cure or even to long term survival. It follows then that only careful investigation and definition of the stage of the disease and the tumor-host relationship in the individual patient will allow the most rational and effective therapeutic management of that patient.

REFERENCES

Abeloff, M. D., Ettinger, D. S., et al. Management of small cell carcinoma of the lung; therapy, staging and biochemical markers. Cancer, *38:* 1394–1401, 1976.

Arai, K., and Wallace, H. W. Effect of local immunotherapy upon tumor at a distal site. Proc. Am. Assoc. Cancer Res., *19:* 120, 1978.

Arseneau, J. C., Canellos, G. P., et al. Recently recognized complications of cancer chemotherapy. Ann. N.Y. Acad. Sci., *230:* 481–488, 1974.

Arseneau, J. C., Sponzo, R. W., and Levin, D. L. Nonlymphomatous malignant tumors complicating Hodgkin's disease. N. Engl. J. Med., *287:* 1119–1122, 1972.

Baldwin, R. W., and Price, M. R. Tumor antigens and tumor-host relationships. Ann. Rev. Intern. Med., *27:* 151–161, 1976.

Barlow, J. J., and Bhattacharya, M. Tumor markers in ovarian cancer; tumor-associated antigens. Semin. Oncol., *2:* 203–210, 1975.

Bender, R. A., and Young, R. C. Effects of cancer treatment on individual and generational genetics. Semin. Oncol., *5:* 47–56, 1978.

Berg, J. W. Nutrition and cancer. Semin. Oncol., *3:* 17–23, 1976.

Bertino, J. R. "Rescue" techniques in cancer chemotherapy; use of leucovorin and other rescue agents after methotrexate treatment. Semin. Oncol., *4:* 203–216, 1977.

Black, M. M., Freeman, C., et al. Prognostic significance of microscopic structure of gastric carcinomas and their regional lymph nodes. Cancer, *27:* 703–711, 1971.

Brodsky, I. The role of androgens and anabolic steroids in the treatment of cancer. Semin. Drug Treat., *3:* 1–11, 1973.

Browder, J. P., and Chretien, P. B. Immune reactivity in head and neck squamous carcinoma and relevance to design of immunotherapy trials. Semin. Oncol., *4:* 431–439, 1977.

Burnet, F. M. Implications of immunological surveillance for cancer therapy. Isr. J. Med. Sci., *7:* 9–16, 1971.

Cadman, E. Toxicity of chemotherapeutic agents. *In* Cancer—A Comprehensive Treatise, Vol. 5: Chemotherapy, edited by F. F. Becker, pp. 59–112. Plenum Press, New York, 1977.

Cahill, G. F., Jr. Hyperglycemia. Ann. N.Y. Acad. Sci., *230:* 161–167, 1974.

Cameron, I. L., and Pavlet, W. A. Stimulation of growth of a transplantable hepatoma in rats by parenteral nutrition. J. Natl. Cancer Inst., *56:* 597–601, 1976.

Carter, S. K., and Friedman, M. Osteogenic sarcoma: treatment overview and some comments on the interpretation of clinical trial data. Cancer Treat. Rep., *62:* 199–204, 1978.

Copeland, E. M., III, and Dudrick, S. J. Cancer: nutritional concepts. Semin. Oncol., *2:* 329–335, 1975.

Copeland, E. M., III, MacFayden, B. V., et al. Intravenous hyperalimentation as an adjunct to cancer chemotherapy. Am. J. Surg., *129:* 167–173, 1975.

Costa, G. Cachexia, the metabolic component of neoplastic diseases. Cancer Res., *23:* 2327–2335, 1977.

Crile, G, Jr. Changing attitudes toward the treatment of cancer. Cleve. Clin. Q., *44:* 49–56, 1978.

D'Angio, G. J., Evans, E. E., et al. The treatment of Wilms' tumor; results of the national Wilms' tumor study. Cancer, *38:* 633–646, 1976.

DeVita, V. T. The evolution of therapeutic research in cancer. N. Engl. J. Med., *298:* 907–910, 1978.

DeVita, V. T., Canellos, G. P., and Moxley, J. M., III A decade of combination chemotherapy of advanced Hodgkin's disease. Cancer, *30:* 1495–1504, 1972.

DeVita, V. T., Chabner, B., et al. Advanced diffuse histiocytic lymphoma, a potentially curable disease; results with combination chemotherapy. Lancet, *1:* 248–250, 1975.

DeWys, W. D., and Herbst, S. H. Oral feeding in the nutritional management of the cancer patient. Cancer Res., *37:* 2429–2431, 1977.

DeWys, W. D., and Walters, K. Abnormalities of taste sensation in cancer patients. Cancer, *36:* 1888–1896, 1975.

Dudrick S. J., MacFayden, B. V., et al. Parenteral nutrition techniques in cancer patients. Cancer Res., *37:* 2240–2450, 1977.

Fahey, J. L., Brosman, S., et al. Immunotherapy and human tumor immunology. Ann. Intern. Med., *84:* 454–465, 1976.

Favus, M. J., Schneider, A. B., et al. Thyroid cancer occurring as a late consequence of head and neck radiation. N. Engl J. Med., *294:* 1019–1025, 1976.

Fisher, B. The changing role of surgery in the treatment of cancer. *In* Cancer—A Comprehensive Treatise; Vol. 6. Radiotherapy, Surgery and Immunotherapy, edited by F. F. Becker, pp. 401–424. Plenum Press, New York, 1977a.

Fisher, B. Surgery of primary breast cancer. *In* Breast Cancer—Advances in Research and Treatment; Vol. 1. Current Approaches to Therapy, edited by W. L. McGuire, pp. 1–42. Plenum Medical Book Co., New York, 1977b.

Fisher, B., Ravadin, R. G., et al. Surgical adjuvant chemotherapy in cancer of the breast. Ann. Surg., *168:* 337–356, 1968.

Fisher, B., Slack, N., et al. Ten year followup results of patients with carcinoma of the breast in a cooperative trial evaluating surgical adjuvant chemotherapy. Surg. Gynecol. Obstet., *140:* 528–534, 1975.

Frei, E., III Combination cancer therapy. Cancer Res., *32:* 2593–2607, 1972.

Friedman, H., Specter, S., et al. Tumor-associated immunosuppressive factors. Ann. N.Y. Acad. Sci., *276:* 417–431, 1976.

Friou, G. J. Current knowledge and concepts of the relationship of malignancy, autoimmunity, and immunologic disease. Ann. N.Y. Acad. Sci., *230:* 23–53, 1974.

Frost, P., Rose, N. R., and Choe, B. Immunology of prostatic carcinoma—an overview. Semin. Oncol., *3:* 107–114, 1976.

Gertner, M. H., Mullen, J. L., et al. Evaluation of nutrition and immunocompetence in cancer and noncancer patients. Proc. Am. Soc. Clin. Oncol., *19:* 344, 1978.

Gonzales, F. Acute leukemia in multiple myeloma. Ann. Intern. Med., *86:* 440–443, 1977.

Gordon, G. S. Hyper- and hypocalcemia: pathogenesis and treatment. Ann. N.Y. Acad. Sci., *230:* 168–180, 1974.

Hall, T. C. (Ed.) Paraneoplastic syndromes. Ann. N.Y. Acad. Sci., *230:* 1–577, 1974.

Haque, T., Lutcher, C., et al. Chemotherapy-associated acute myelogenous leukemia and ovarian carcinoma. Am. J. Med. Sci., *272:* 225–228, 1976.

Harris, C. C. The carcinogenicity of anticancer drugs; a hazard in man. Cancer, *37:* 1014–1023, 1976.

Harris, J., and Copeland, D. Impaired immunoresponsiveness in tumor patients. Ann. N.Y. Acad. Sci., *230:* 56–85, 1974.

Harris, J., Senger, D., et al. The effect of immunosuppressive chemotherapy on immune function in patients with malignant disease. Cancer, *37:* 1058–1069, 1976.

Harvey, H. A., Lipton, A., et al. Inhibition of in vitro lymphocyte function by alpha-1 glycoprotein, tumor-related glycopeptide, and fibrinogen degradation products. Proc. Am. Assoc. Cancer Res., *19:* 24, 1978.

Henderson, E. S. Acute lymphoblastic leukemia. *In* Cancer Medicine, edited by J. F. Holland and E. Frei, III, pp. 1173–1199. Lea & Febiger, Philadelphia, 1974.

Herberman, R. B., Campbell, D. A., et al. Immunogenicity of tumor antigens. Ann. N.Y. Acad. Sci., *276:* 26–45, 1976.

Hersh, E. M. Modification of host defense mechanisms. *In* Cancer Medicine, edited by J. F. Holland and E. Frei, III, pp. 681–698. Lea & Febiger, Philadelphia, 1974.

Hersh, E. M., Gutterman, J. U., et al. Immunocompetence, immunodeficiency, and prognosis in cancer. Ann. N.Y. Acad. Sci., *276:* 386–407, 1976.

Hersh, E. M., Mavligit, G. M., and Gutterman, J. U. Immunotherapy of cancer. *In* Cancer—A Comprehensive Treatise; Vol. 6. Radiotherapy, Surgery and Immunotherapy, edited by F. F. Becker, pp. 425–532. New York: Plenum Press, 1977.

Ishimaru, T. Leukemia in atomic bomb survivors; Hiroshima and Nagasaki. Radiat. Res. *45:* 216, 1971.

Israel, L., Edelstein, R., et al. Plasmapheresis in patients with disseminated cancer; clinical results and correlation with changes in serum protein. The concept of "nonspecific blocking factors." Cancer, *40:* 3146–3154, 1977.

Issell, B. F., Valdivieso, M., et al. Protection of Chemotherapy Toxicities by Intravenous Hyperalimentation. Proc. Am. Assoc. Cancer Res., *19:* 149, 1978.

Johnson, R. E., Brereton, H. D., and Kent, C. H. Small cell carcinoma of the lung; attempts to remedy causes of past therapeutic failures. Lancet, *1:* 289–291, 1976.

Katz, D. H. Genetic controls and cellular interactions in antibody formation. Hosp. Pract., *12:* 85–99, 1977.

Konior, G. S. and Leventhal, B. G. Immunocompetence and prognosis in acute leukemia. Semin. Oncol., *3:* 283–288, 1976.

Koperszytych, S., Rezkallah, M. T., et al. Cell-mediated immunity in patients with carcinoma; correlation between clinical stage and immunocompetence. Cancer, *38:* 1149–1154, 1976.

Krown, S. E., Pinsky, C. M., et al. Immune reactivity and prognosis in patients with breast cancer. Proc. Am. Soc. Clin. Oncol., *19:* 351, 1978.

Lange, P. H., Hakala, T. R., and Fraley, E. E. Suppression of antitumor lymphocyte-mediated cytotoxicity by human chorionic gonadotropins. J. Urol., *115:* 95–98, 1976.

Law, D. K., Dudrick, S. J., and Abdou, N. I. Immunocompetence of patients with protein-calorie malnutrition; the effects of nutritional repletion. Ann. Intern. Med., *79:* 545–550, 1973.

Lemerle, J., Bloch-Michael, R, et al. Chemotherapy as primary treatment in children with bilateral retinoblastoma. Proc. Am. Soc. Clin. Oncol., *17:* 416, 1978.

Leventhal, B. G., Mirro, J., and Konior Yarbro, G. S. Immune reactivity to tumor antigens in leukemia and lymphoma. Semin. Hematol., *15:* 157–180, 1978.

Lewis, J. J. Current status of treatment of gestational trophoblastic disease. Cancer, *38:* 620–626, 1976.

Louie, S., and Schwartz, R. S. Immunodeficiency and the pathogenesis of lymphoma and leukemia. Semin. Hematol., *15:* 117–138, 1978.

MacDonald, J. S. The immunobiology of colorectal cancer. Semin. Oncol., *3:* 421–432, 1976.

Mathé, G., Schwartzenberg, I., et al. Experimental and clinical immunopharmacology data applicable to cancer chemotherapy. Ann. N.Y. Acad. Sci., *277:* 467–484, 1976.

Maurer, H. M., Moon, T., et al. The intergroup rhabdomyosarcoma study; a preliminary report., Cancer, *40:* 2015–2026, 1977.

McKneally, M. F., Maver, C. M., and Kausel, H. W. Regional immunotherapy of lung cancer using postoperative intrapleural BCG. *In* Immunotherapy of Cancer: Present Status of Trials in Man, edited by W. D. Terry and D. Windhorst, pp. 161–172. Raven Press, New York, 1977.

Moertel, C. G., and Hagedorn, A. G. Leukemia or lymphoma and coexistent primary malignant lesions; a review of the literature and study of 120 cases. Blood, *12:* 788–803, 1957.

Nakahara, W. Toxohormone. *In* Methods in Cancer Research, edited by H. Bush, Vol. 2, pp. 203–237. Academic Press, New York, 1967.

Nathanson, S. D., and Kempner, D. Blocking of specific binding to tumor antigens by fibrinolysin-cleaved antibody. Proc. Am. Assoc. Cancer Res., *19:* 133, 1978.

Nicholson, G. L., and Poste, G. The cancer cell; dynamic aspects and modifications in cell-surface organization. N. Engl. J. Med., *295:* 197–203, 253–258, 1976.

Ohnuma, T. Hepatic catalase. *In* Cancer Medicine, edited by J. E. Holland and E. Frei III, pp. 1044–1046. Lea & Febiger, Philadelphia, 1974.

Ota, D. M., Imbembo, A. L., and Zuidema, G. D. Total parenteral nutrition. Surgery, *83:* 503–520, 1978.

Park, S. K., Brody, J. I., et al. Immunosuppressive effect of surgery. Lancet, *1:* 53–55, 1971.

Parker, L. N., Belsky, J. L., et al. Thyroid carcinoma after exposure to atomic radiation; a continuing survey of a fixed population, Hiroshima and Nagasaki, 1958–1971. Ann. Intern. Med., *80:* 600–604, 1974.

Paul, W. E., and Benecerraf, B. Functional specificity of thymus-dependent lymphocytes. Science, *195:* 1293–1300, 1977.

Penn, I. Second malignant neoplasms associated with immunosuppressive medications.

Cancer, *37*: 1024–1032, 1976.

Penn, I. Malignancies associated with immunosuppressive or cytotoxic therapy. Surgery, *83*: 492–502, 1978.

Pihl, E., Malahy, M. A., et al. Immunomorphological features of prognostic significance in Dukes' B colorectal carcinoma. Cancer Res., *37*: 4145–4149, 1977.

Plescia, O. J., Grinwich, K., and Plescia, A. M. Subversive activity of syngeneic tumor cells as an escape mechanism from immune surveillance and the role of prostaglandins. Ann. N.Y. Acad. Sci., *276*: 455–466, 1976.

Primack, A. The production of markers by bronchogenic carcinoma. Semin. Oncol., *1*: 235–244, 1974.

Rosen, G., Caparros, B., et al. Curability of Ewing's sarcoma and considerations for future therapeutic trials. Cancer, *41*: 888–899, 1978.

Roubanian, J. R., and Talal, N. Neoplasia, autoimmunity and the immune response. Adv. Intern. Med., *24*: 435–450, 1978.

Russ, J. E., and DeWys, W. D. Correction of the taste abnormality of malignancy with intravenous hyperalimentation. Arch. Intern. Med., *138*: 799–800, 1978.

Sahakian, G. J., Al-Mondhiry, H., et al. Acute leukemia in Hodgkin's disease. Cancer, *33*: 1369–1375, 1974.

Schabel F. M., Jr. Concepts for the treatment of micrometastases. Cancer, *35*: 15–24, 1975.

Schein, P. S., Macdonald, J. S., et al. Nutritional complications of cancer and its treatment. Semin. Oncol., *2*: 337–347, 1975.

Schneider, A. B., Favus, M. J., et al. Incidence, prevalance and characteristics of radiation-induced thyroid tumors. Am. J. Med., *64*: 243–252, 1978.

Shibata, H. R., Jerry, L. M., et al. Immunotherapy of human malignant melanoma with irradiated tumor cells, oral BCG and levamisole. Ann. N.Y. Acad. Sci., *277*: 355–367, 1976.

Shils, M. E. Enteral nutrition by tube. Cancer Res., *37*: 2432–2439, 1977a.

Shils, M. E. Effects on nutrition of surgery of the liver, pancreas and genitourinary tract. Cancer Res., *37*: 2387–2394, 1977b.

Shils, M. E. Nutrition in neoplastic diseases. *In* Modern Nutrition in Health and Disease, edited by M. G. Wohl and R. S. Goodhart, Ed. 4, pp. 1012–1024. Lea & Febiger, Philadelphia, 1968.

Signori, O. R., and Signori, E. E. Short-term additional parenteral nutrition by I.V. hyperalimentation as an adjunct to chemotherapy. Proc. Am. Soc. Clin. Oncol., *19*: 311, 1978.

Slode, M. S., Simmons, R. L., et al. Immunosuppression after major surgery in normal patients. Surgery, *78*: 363–372, 1975.

Sugarbaker, E. V., Ketcham, A. S., and Zubrod, G.F. Interdisciplinary cancer therapy; adjuvant therapy. Curr. Probl. Surg., *14*: 1–69, 1977.

Terpeka, A. R., and Waterhouse, C. Metabolic observations during the forced feeding of patients with cancer. Am. J. Med., *20*: 225–238, 1956.

Terry, W. D. Concluding remarks. *In* Immunotherapy of Cancer: Present Status of Trials in Man, edited by W.D. Terry and D. Windhorst, pp. 664–669. Raven Press, New York, 1977.

Terry, W. D., and Windhorst, D. (Eds.) Immunotherapy of Cancer: Present Status of Trials in Man. Raven Press, New York, 1977.

Theologides, A. Anorexia-producing intermediary metabolites. Am. J. Clin. Nutr., *29*: 552–558, 1976.

Waldmann, T. A., Broder, S., and Strobar, W. Protein-losing enteropathies in malignancy. Ann. N.Y. Acad. Sci., *230*: 306–317, 1974.

Wartman, W. B. Sinus cell hyperplasia of lymph nodes regional to adenocarcinomas of the breast and colon. Br. J. Cancer, *13*: 389–397, 1959.

Waterhouse, C. How tumors affect host metabolism. Ann. N.Y. Acad. Sci., *230*: 86–93, 1974.

Yamamura, Y. Immunotherapy of lung cancer with oil-attached wall skeleton of BCG. *In* Immunotherapy of Cancer: Present Status of Trials in Man, edited by W. D. Terry and D. Windhorst, pp. 173–180. Raven Press, New York, 1977.

Yonemoto, R. H., Fujisawa, T., and Waldman, S. R. Effect of serum blocking factors in leukocyte adherence inhibition in breast cancer patients; specificity and correlation with tumor burden. Cancer, *41:* 1289–1297, 1978.

Zbar, B. Immunotherapy of bilateral lymph node metastasis by intralesional or paralesional injection of M. bovis (BCG). Proc. Am. Assoc. Cancer Res., *19:* 87, 1978.

Ziegler, J. L. Burkitt's lymphoma. Med. Clin. North Am., *61:* 1073–1082, 1977.

Zuckerman, S. H., and Douglas, S. D. Membrane receptors and genetics of cells involved in the immune response. N.Y. State J. Med., *76:* 1085–1098, 1976.

Chapter 2

Principles of Oncologic Surgery

GEORGE A. DEGENSHEIN, M.D., F.A.C.S.

The role of the surgeon in the management of malignant disease is a changing one. Until the turn of the century, surgery was virtually the only effective method available to treat cancer. The introduction of radiotherapy led to a competition of modalities with specific areas ultimately identified as best treated by one or the other method or a combination of both. Some areas of controversy still exist. The introduction of chemotherapy and immunotherapy have now placed the surgeon in proper perspective as a member of a cooperative team to manage cancer. He can no longer walk away from an operating table where he has encountered either local or advanced disease and make the final judgment that no more can be done. Many patients in the past have been abandoned in this manner. Thus, it becomes necessary for the surgeon to understand the capabilities of the other disciplines. He may be required to place a clip for identification of areas to irradiate; he may have to reduce bulk of tumor; he may have to fix ovaries out of the area to be irradiated in Hodgkin's disease in young women; he may have to place a perfusion catheter and he may have to consider a course of irradiation to make a tumor operable.

The surgeon makes his best contribution in "early" cases when the disease has not disseminated beyond the local area, knowing full well that cells may be seeded elsewhere. Surgeons of experience learn that host resistance is often a determining factor and are cautious in using the term cure. Except for diagnostic biopsy, justifiable palliation or ablative therapy, surgery in cases of advanced malignancy is seldom indicated. To do a splendid radical mastectomy on an inflammatory carcinoma of the breast is a triumph of technique over reason; other management should be tried. The proper management of cancer has become multidisciplinary and must continue so in the best interest of the patient.

SURGICAL ASPECTS OF DIAGNOSIS

Numerous sophisticated and noninvasive techniques have been developed for the diagnosis of cancer and hopefully many more will come. Nevertheless, the most informative diagnostic procedure remains the biopsy. The cell type, the degree of tissue activity, the presence of lymphatic or vascular invasion, and other information available on direct section are extremely important in guiding the management of each case. With few exceptions, tumors should be biopsied unless the risk of the procedure exceeds the need for the tissue.

Methods of Biopsy

SURFACE BIOPSY FOR MATERIAL FOR CYTOLOGIC STUDY

Direct Smears and Washings. These have been effective for the cervix, mucosal lesions, or ulcerated tumors. Duodenal washings are gaining in popularity and may provide evidence of pancreatic carcinoma. Bronchial and other cavity washings may also be diagnostic.

Brushings and Scrapings. These may be effective during endoscopy when forceps biopsy may increase the hazard. Scrapings may be sufficient in Paget's disease and may also be judicious in cases highly suspicious of malignant melanoma where adequate excisional biopsy would require skin graft or leave a serious cosmetic defect.

Needle Aspiration. Needle aspiration of tumors can be diagnostic especially where there is central necrosis of the tumor. Aspiration of benign cysts is well known and has been used in breasts, kidneys and subcutaneous masses. Suction aspiration of nipples has been reported as effective in providing material for cytologic study.

The success of the above methods varies with the expertise of the provider of the material and the dedication of the pathologist to careful cytologic examination. A negative result should never be taken as positive proof that a malignancy does not exist.

NEEDLE BIOPSY

This method varies from needle aspiration in that it is meant to deliver a distinct segment of tissue for paraffin section examination. The Vim-Silverman and Menghini needles have been used traditionally for liver biopsy and other newer needles for biopsy of tumors are now available.

The technique is to insert the needle, under local skin infiltration, into the suspected tissue, project the inner stylet and then advance the outer needle so that the rim actually cuts through a circle of tissue which is entrapped in the inner segment. Needle biopsy is suitable for large soft tissue tumors, thyroid tissue where cyst or inflammatory disease is suspected, and other accessible tumors. This method is gaining popularity with breast cancer. It is performed as an office or hospital preoperative procedure and should be reserved for cases where the clinical diagnosis of cancer is most likely and definitive surgery is already scheduled. In that way, when positive, the surgeon can prepare the patient emotionally for surgery. The obvious additional dividend is avoiding the delay in the operating room while a frozen section is being done. Transcutaneous and transbronchial needle biopsy of pulmonary lesions is somewhat controversial but may be diagnostic especially in coin lesions (Gibbon et al., 1969). The transcutaneous method is performed under fluoroscopic control and is ordinarily performed with a spinal type of needle. The findings of an oat cell carcinoma may alter the need for thoracotomy.

Complications with needle biopsy are uncommon if the surgeon remains alert to aneurysms and major vessel variations. Again, a negative biopsy does not rule out carcinoma.

INCISIONAL BIOPSY

Incisional biopsy is practiced most frequently during endoscopy where lesions are incompletely removed by biopsy forceps. Where feasible, especially in the rectum and colon, polyps should be removed completely so that a full tissue examination can be done. A few random bites from a large villus adenoma can hardly rule out carcinoma if the specimens are benign. Laparoscopy has been well developed by the gynecologist where tissue from pelvic lesions is available.

Scalpel incisional biopsy is used where a lesion is large and excision may lead to unwarranted cosmetic defects if the lesion is benign. It is also used where the tumor tissue is heavily infiltrated into deeper structures—especially in the neck. Excisional biopsy of a Virchow node could be damaging to neurovascular structures below. Incisional biopsy is justified in cases of obvious advanced malignancy for tissue diagnosis to aid in the choice of management. Where possible an adequate disc-shaped or pie-cut segment should be removed, involving the core as well as the outer edge of the tumor. The inclusion of a bit of normal adjacent tissue when available is helpful to the pathologist. It is important to place the incision so that it can be easily included well within the margins of the possibly subsequently resected specimen since suture line recurrence is not rare.

EXCISIONAL BIOPSY

The most desirable biopsy is excisional biopsy since it provides a total specimen for pathological review and, done properly, reduces spread of tumor cells to a minimum. If the lesion is benign, excision is curative and in some instances of malignancy such as basal cell carcinoma it can be a definitive procedure.

Technique. For lesions on the skin, a diamond-shaped area of the skin should be infiltrated with a small amount of diluted local anesthetic well away from the lesion. An elliptical incision is made around the lesion. The margin around the lesion has been a great source of controversy; some arguing the need for 5 times the diameter of the lesion in suspected melanoma and others presenting evidence that only 3 mm are necessary. The surgeon must make this judgment based on his degree of suspicion keeping two prime factors in mind. The excised area must be compatible with primary closure of the wound and must be cosmetically acceptable, otherwise scrape or incisional biopsy should be considered. One thing is certain; the biopsy should be three dimensional and the depth of tissue, where safe, should equal the lateral margins. A great aid for operating on skin lesions is the use of a 2½ times magnified jeweler's loop especially for lesions on the face so that margins of tumor can be well identified. One piece specimens are the rule, but, where fragmented, the surgeon must tag the appropriate edges with sutures for the pathologist to be able to report excision line with involvement or freedom from tumor.

For subcutaneous lesions, the same procedure is used and where practical the skin above should be included. For lymph nodes, an entire untraumatized node or chain of nodes should be removed without disruption of the specimen.

In deeper areas, the surgeon must be concerned with tumor spread and should dissect into the nearest normal tissue plane around the tumor. At least a full centimeter of uninvolved tissue should be obtained and the tumor must not be grasped or penetrated by any instrument. The recent work on dissemination of tumor by merely handling it is noteworthy, and no-touch techniques have been developed (Turnbull, 1975). These techniques are merely another reflection of the need for gentle surgery in every circumstance. Cauterization has been used traditionally to seal areas from spread and other tools are in the research laboratories, but nothing will change the need for the surgeon to follow the Hippocratic dictum: "Primum non nocere." First do no harm.

Pancreatic biopsy deserves a special note. It has a distinct morbidity and, on occasion, a mortality. The introduction of intraoperative transduodenal biopsy with a needle into the adjacent pancreatic tumor area has lowered the morbidity but the basic problem with direct pancreatic biopsy is that the information received from the tissue obtained is unreliable. Multiple biopsies in a single case have been reported as pancreatitis only to find a carcinoma missed by the biopsy in the finally resected or postmortem specimen. The delay on the operating table and the poor correlation do not justify biopsy except in unusual circumstances. An adjacent node, of course, should be sent for section. In the hands of the experienced oncologic surgeon, the diagnosis of pancreatic carcinoma is made on the gross evaluation at the operating table with a false positive incidence of approximately 5% in good hands. The false negative rate with biopsy is considerably higher. Duodenal washings and sonography may be of value preoperatively.

The development of mammography has led to a special problem in breast biopsy. A significant number of cases without a palpable mass are being identified by microcalcification or other mammographic evidence of malignancy. Blind biopsy may miss the area involved and leave the malignancy behind. There is also a tendency to do wide excisions to assure that the suspicious area is in the specimen, so that the pathologist is at a loss to choose the exact site for frozen section or even paraffin sections from a substantial segment of breast. This problem requires a cooperative effort on the part of the radiologist, the pathologist, and the surgeon. A needle with hypaque or methylene blue may be placed at the site of the suspicious area with mammographic control. Other markers are in use. The patient is then taken to the operating room where the tissue is excised. The specimen is then sliced, layed out in a regular pattern, and x-rayed to identify the area of calcification to ascertain that it has been removed. The pathologist can then pick up that small slice of tissue with the calcifications for section. The time delay is unfortunate, but necessary. Small radiographic units for the operating room are now being made for this purpose and administrative expedition of notification and transport procedures can substantially reduce the time lag.

Sister Mary Joseph's sign is worthy of comment. This palpable firm umbilical node can be excised for biopsy as an office procedure and when positive is diagnostic of intra-abdominal carcinoma with liver metastases which is not curable with extirpative surgery. In those instances hospitalization and laparotomy can be avoided and the patient can be considered for other forms of treatment.

EXPLORATORY SURGERY

With the development of improved radiography, angiography, sonography, endoscopy, nuclear scans, and a host of biochemical tests, the need for exploratory surgery has fallen off. Nevertheless, there is a limited but essential place for exploration not only for diagnosis, but sometimes for determination of curability, palliability, and more recently for staging.

Neurosurgery

The neurosurgeon does have the occasion to explore for diagnosis but since he works primarily with space occupying lesions, the diagnostic surgical procedure must also be definitive where possible and is rarely done for biopsy alone. A tumor of the brain or spinal cord may behave in a malignant manner despite benign pathology; a subdural hematoma or a meningioma may be as fatal as an astrocytoma. Exploration is generally essential for management.

Head and Neck Surgery

The head and neck is a confined space and the number of critical structures may make excisional biopsy dangerous or limit the margins of excision. Diagnosis in the orifices involved in this area can usually be made by endoscopic or direct biopsies to provide evidence for the need for radical surgery. Exploration of cold nodules of the thyroid continues to be indicated and lobectomy should be done to provide the excisional biopsy specimen. Parotid tumors require excisional biopsy of the lobe if possible. The integrity of the facial nerve must be considered if the deep lobe is involved in a malignancy.

Thoracic Surgery

The need for exploratory thoracotomy has been sharply reduced with the advent of an impressive battery of diagnostic examinations. Despite this, there are a number of cases where thoracotomy is necessary for coin lesions and also for cases of positive cytology where a specific lesion cannot be localized. The development of mediastinoscopy has been important in curtailing the number of exploratory thoracotomies, since the finding of positive nodes makes the case incurable with surgery with the possible exception of some cases of squamous cell carcinoma (Gibbons et al., 1969). It is apparent that exploratory thoracotomy should never be carried out until the pulmonary and medical status of the patient is carefully evaluated so that in the event that exploration led to a resection, this would be well tolerated.

One caution is worthy of discussion. In the early days of thoracic surgery a chest x-ray was taken and, if a suspicious lesion was found, thoracotomy was performed. Today, the availability of cytology, bronchoscopy, bronchography, angiography, transcutaneous and transbronchial needle biopsy, pleural biopsy, scalene node biopsy, mediastinoscopy, and other procedures may make the diagnostic workup an ordeal almost equal to a thoracotomy. It is important for the pulmonary physician or surgeon to utilize only those procedures most likely to provide results and avoid the others. Only the rare case should require all of the procedures available.

Abdominal Surgery

Planned and thorough exploration of the abdomen should be carried out in almost every instance of elective abdominal surgery not involving a purulent process. Every time an elective cholecystectomy or a gastrectomy or other major abdominal procedure is performed, a formal exploration should be carried out before the pertinent pathology is approached. Such an examination takes little time and may on occasion lead to the discovery of an unanticipated malignancy (Degenshein, 1969). Many surgeons have operated for malignancy in the abdomen on cases which were explored less than a year before for other pathology and the current tumor was not identified.

The term "exploratory laparotomy" justifiably fell into disfavor when it was used to avoid a recorded preoperative diagnosis on the part of the surgeon so that his diagnostic acumen could not be judged when comparing it to the postoperative. The exploratory laparotomy germane to malignant disease has other implications. Nonsurgical diagnostic procedures still leave open questions as to malignancy, especially in the gastrointestinal tract, although colonoscopy has made a significant contribution. Pancreatic carcinoma is sometimes inaccessible to definite preoperative diagnosis. The surgeon is called on occasion to explore a patient with an unexplained fever who has been examined exhaustively without positive findings. In such cases, lymphoma is the most frequent single diagnosis made after exploratory laparotomy.

Cancer, since it represents a host of diseases, will be no easier to classify than infection, but whatever subclassifications can be arrived at should be used internationally. Although individual gross and pathological classifications exist for specific tumors such as Haagensen's Columbia classification for breast cancer or FIGO (International Federation of Gynecologists and Obstetricians) for ovarian cancer, there is a need for a universal language so that we can compare results from various major centers in the world. The best available system that exists today is the TNM classification which provides the basic information that the clinician needs to identify the best modality for treatment, but even that system has deficiencies. In Hodgkin's disease, for example, current therapy varies with whether disease exists on both sides of the diaphragm; whether symptoms are present and the extent of the invasion. Thus a Stage II is treated differently from a Stage IV. Here again, in Hodgkin's disease, the surgeon is a member of a multidisciplinary team where the extent of the disease must be known to decide whether the patient will have radiation or chemotherapy or on occasion a combination of both.

The "mini lap" has come into use for exploratory surgery and may be justified when a radical procedure such as amputation or hemipelvectomy is considered. Peritoneoscopy and liver scans may be unreliable to identify liver metastases. A small subcostal or right upper quadrant incision is made and the liver and adjacent structures examined for metastasis. If negative, the major procedure can be carried out; if positive, the radical surgery is unwarranted.

Genitourinary Surgery

Prostatic cancer is usually diagnosed by needle or open perineal biopsy. Exploration may on occasion be necessary for kidney tumors but these are well identified by radiographic and angiographic techniques.

Gynecologic Surgery

Laparoscopy is usually diagnostic for intra-abdominal malignancies, but exploratory laparotomy may be necessary to determine resectability of uterine or ovarian malignancies.

Endocrine Surgery

Exploration is often necessary in parathyroid tumors, adrenal tumors, pancreatic endocrine tumors, carcinoids with liver involvement, and others. Here, again, the exploration usually leads to a definitive procedure based on frozen section biopsies.

Orthopaedic Surgery

Bone tumors seldom require exploration except for a biopsy.

SURGICAL THERAPY

The development of oncologic surgery as a specialty has mixed implications. It is expected that the oncologic surgeon is technically more capable of carrying out radical procedures than the general surgeon. The realistic fact remains that few general surgeons can do a sufficient number of pancreaticoduodenectomies or pelvic exenterations or "commandos" or hemipelvectomies to maintain expertise in these areas. In spite of this, most malignancies continue to be treated by general surgeons who certainly are competent in many areas. Regionalization of centers to treat the more complex cases is justified, but slow in development. The prime common requisite for any surgeon who operates for malignancy is that he has a continuous exposure to the latest developments in radiotherapy, chemotherapy, and now immunotherapy. More than half of the cancers are treated today with radiation or chemotherapy whether in combination with surgery or with each other. The surgeon may be fully aware of the current attitudes of the other disciplines in repetitive cases, but for the less usual case preoperative consultation or presentation to a group may be rewarding for the patient. It is also important for the radiotherapist or chemotherapist to witness the pathology in the operating room in many instances.

Preoperative Preparation

Before even coming to a decision as to the type and extent of surgery, a complete medical and psychological evaluation is necessary. Adequate preoperative preparation based on a proper evaluation is necessary to maintain acceptable morbidity and mortality. In intestinal obstructions especially, there must be careful replenishment of the static fluid debt. Adequate decompression may convert a multistaged operative procedure to a single one. Oral toilet must be checked; respiratory status can be improved; anemia and electrolyte disturbances require correction. In jaundice and in debilitating conditions, coagulation defects must be identified and overcome. Reassurance of the patient and psychological preparation for the trip to the operating room, the anesthesia, the recovery room, the postoperative period, and a justification for the number of tubes to exit from the patient's body, cannot be overemphasized.

Technical Aspects of Cancer Surgery

There is good evidence that cancer treated adequately at the initial procedure has significantly higher survival rates than if inadequate procedures are performed and then redone properly even if only a short time later.

The critical decision for the surgeon to make at the operating table is whether to attempt curative surgery or whether only palliation is appropriate. In general, when disease is localized to a single organ and has only adjacent or lymph node spread, curative surgery should be carried out. The key to curative surgery is the total but gentle removal of the involved organ with its regional lymph node area where feasible. This requires a detailed knowledge of the anatomy of the part, especially the vascular and lymphatic supply. The work of Turnbull (1975) and others has made surgeons aware of the marked dissemination of viable tumor cells into the venous drainage during rough handling of the tumor itself. Recent evidence in immunology tells us that the body defenses may handle such a shower of cells, but, if the burden is too large, it may outstrip the immunologic defenses. Rough surgery does disseminate viable tumor cells into the systemic circulation. The vasculature should be ligated first at the appropriate point and the margins of resection should be wide.

It is beyond the scope of this chapter to go into details of operative technique but a discussion of the extent of the procedures for the more frequent malignancies is justified since recently many of the traditional procedures have come under fire.

Lung Cancer

Segmental resection or lobectomy is reserved for noninfiltrative small carcinomas which do not encroach upon the main bronchus. Larger or invasive lesions usually require pneumonectomy. Little controversy exists because the extent of the resection is often based on mechanical needs.

Oat cell carcinoma is incurable by surgery in the great majority of cases and is usually subjected to radiation and chemotherapy.

Of all cases subjected to curative surgery on the basis of the preoperative workup, the 5–7 year survival is about 30%.

Breast

The controversy is well known and based on an ignorance of history. Lumpectomy and partial mastectomy were practiced by superb surgeons at the turn of the century and Halsted (1907) proclaimed that his chiefs never thought they cured a single case. If and when we can know with certainty that a lesion is confined to a local area, then perhaps a lesser procedure should be considered, but the finding by Robbins (1974) of multicentric foci in more than 50% of the breasts removed make even that a discouraging choice. At least 17% of cases with lesions less than 1 cm have axillary nodes involved. A woman with a 2-cm localized lesion picked up on routine screening (Gilbertson, 1974) has a 90% chance for a 5-year survival with a radical mastectomy; even if the figure fell only to 80% with a partial resection that still represents 10 dead women. The modified radical has become more popular recently and is a reasonable compromise. Leaving the pectoral muscles allows for a more desirable cosmetic effect and curtails some of the incidence of edema of the arm. It should, however, be used only where the Rotter's interpectoral nodes are negative and the tumor does not reach the pectoral fascia. Done properly, this procedure allows for a full axillary dissection after division or retraction of the pectoralis minor. Crile performed partial mastectomy with or without axillary dissection at the Cleveland Clinic in only 12% of their cases from 1957 to 1970. Currently the procedure of choice at the Cleveland Clinic for potentially surgically curable breast cancer is modified radical mastectomy and is performed in 80% of the cases. (Hermann and Steiger, 1978).

There is a need for better reconstructive surgery for breast amputees which would counteract the need for performing lesser procedures. How to handle the opposite breast is also an area of controversy with an increased practice of mirror image biopsy. With good followup, a second breast carcinoma can be detected early and be treated adequately. The survival rates for metachronous bilateral mastectomy for two independent primaries is as good as that for a single carcinoma.

With the introduction of receptor site studies to determine hormone dependency of breast cancers, and the availability of chemotherapy, the prospect for recurrent breast cancer and also for hormone dependent advanced primaries, is promising. Combined oophorectomy and adrenalectomy can now be performed with more than 85% remission rate in properly selected cases with metastatic disease who are both estrogen and progesterone receptor positive (Degenshein et al., 1977). Newer antihormone drugs such as tamoxifen and aminoglutethamide are under study for endocrine manipulation and if effective may well replace ablative surgery.

Recurrent breast cancer, if a local recurrence, reflects a failure of the original procedure and may justify local reoperation if no distant spread can be found. Radiation may be effective in preventing further local recurrence.

Colon Cancer

The margins of resection for colon cancer are in little controversy. Sigmoid resections require dissection to include the area supplied by the inferior mesenteric vessels. Right or left hemicolectomy is used for right or left lesions and transverse colon tumor resection requires area supplied by the middle colic artery.

The rectum is an area of great controversy. For lesions high in the rectum, an anterior resection and reanastomosis is a satisfactory procedure. This is based on the fact that lymphatic drainage is proximal and a margin of 4 cm below a circumscribed tumor is adequate (with confirmation by frozen section). When, however, one goes below 7 or 8 cm from the dentate line, an abdominoperineal resection will usually be required. Pull-through procedures have not gained universal acceptance since they have many complications and a greater recurrence rate. Thirty-five years ago, the Mayo Clinic reported low rectal carcinomas treated by fulguration with a startlingly good statistical survival. Recent reintroduction in significant numbers by Madden and others has led to reevaluation. Deddish reported in 1974 86 cases of carcinoma of the rectum and rectosigmoid treated by fulguration with a 5-year survival of 83.5% and a 10-year survival of 72.2%. This was a highly select group of cases of superficial lesions and admittedly the results for unselected cases with more radical procedures were better, but for the poor risk patient it may become an acceptable compromise. Perhaps with the addition of radiotherapy and chemotherapy, such a method may substantially reduce the ravages of the permanent colostomy, but this is still to be proven. Newer direct and indirect radiotherapeutic measures are also being studied. The development of colonoscopy may provide us with more suitable early cases for local excision higher in the colon. Recurrent carcinoma of the colon may justify reoperation if distant spread is not established.

There has been a recent renewal of interest in the excision of solitary liver metastases from intestinal carcinoma where resection of the tumor can be done satisfactorily. Small numbers of cases are being reported after "metastastectomy" or hepatic lobectomy with a significant number of 5-year survivals. Perhaps the reduction of tumor bulk allows host defenses or chemotherapy to become more effective. In centers where the mortality and morbidity for hepatic lobectomy is acceptable, such procedures may well be indicated.

Carcinoma of the Prostate

Radical prostatectomy with node dissection has been recommended for carcinoma without evidence of systemic spread. The older age group does require special considerations regarding medical contraindications. A great problem also exists in younger men because radical prostatectomy is always associated with impotence. A recent report by Whitmore (1972) using iodine-125 implantation in prostatic cancer after node dissection claims retained potency. Further studies of this and other methods must still be carried out.

Renal Cell Carcinoma

The introduction of radical nephrectomy for renal cell carcinoma has had a statistically significant extension of survival, especially in cases which have not yet penetrated Gerota's fascia (67%—5-year survival).

Pancreatic Carcinoma

Pancreatic carcinoma is on the increase and surgical cure is almost nonexistent with the standard pancreaticoduodenectomy. Improved diagnostic techniques are providing cases a bit earlier but resectability is rarely synonymous with curability. The introduction by Fortner (1974) of total regional pancreatectomy is an attempt to do a complete resection with a dissection of the node-bearing area. In Type I, total pancreatectomy is combined with total gastrectomy, splenectomy, and duodenectomy. The retropancreatic portion of the portal vein is resected allowing for a periaortic and pericaval lymph node dissection. The middle colic vessels are resected and the superior mesenteric vein is reanastamosed to the portal vein. In Type II the celiac axis, a portion of the hepatic artery, the base of the superior mesenteric artery and the adjacent aortic wall are resected. A bifurcated dacron graft is used for reconstruction. We are fortunate to have men who are capable of carrying out such extensive procedures under good control, but, until the long term results, the morbidity and the mortality are available, these procedures must be considered experimental.

Uncommon Technical Surgical Demands

There are malignancies which are uncommon and may require extensive procedures. Even major cancer centers do not accumulate a sufficient number of cases to set definite policy. Hemicorporectomy, hemipelvectomy, pelvic exenteration, and hepatic lobectomy should not be done in every hospital, not only that the technical demands may exceed availability, but mainly because the decision to perform such extensive procedures should be made by those who have the greatest experience.

Experimental or new extended procedures must also be done under rigid control in special centers so that the value of the procedure can be carefully assessed before recommending it for general use.

Postoperative Care

Radical surgery can be justified only if top quality immediate and progressive postoperative care is available. It is a most important factor in maintaining acceptable mortality and morbidity. It starts in the preoperative period with instruction to the patient. It requires a trained nursing staff and combined medical and surgical input. A specially trained medical officer should be in constant attendance. Adequate monitoring equipment and emergency treatment vehicles are necessary. Overtreatment can be as dangerous as undertreatment.

PALLIATIVE SURGERY

All human beings must die, but how they die not infrequently comes into the domain of the surgeon. A patient may have an obstructing carcinoma of the stomach which is technically inoperable for cure. A simple gastrojejunostomy may give the patient many months of relatively comfortable life. A frequent problem is extrahepatic biliary obstruction from carcinoma of the head of the pancreas. Cholecystojejunostomy has been used traditionally with or without a Roux-en-y jejunal limb. It is often inadequate and depends on a patent cystic duct. For the past 18 years we have used lateral choledochoduodenostomy for bypass in an aged population with low morbidity and mortality and with uniformly satisfactory results for decompression of the biliary tree (Degenshein, 1974). If the tumor compresses the duodenum significantly, gastrojejunostomy may be in order to allay the need for such a decision if the patient lives long enough to develop obstruction. To do palliative surgery on a patient with extensively spread malignant disease, who, by all standards available, has a very short time to live is unjustifiable. For this decision, the surgeon must individualize each case and consider a host of factors other than survival time alone. Certainly if a foul smelling or ulcerated area can be safely excised for comfort, it should be done.

Sometimes the extent of palliative surgery may be massive. In proximal carcinomas of the stomach a thoracoabdominal esophagogastrectomy is a high price to pay for palliation. We have, on occasion, used a Heyrovski type of procedure where a simple anastomosis of a free segment of the fundus of the stomach to the esophagus can be palliative. Esophagogastric tubes may also be justified.

With the introduction of immunotherapy, reduction of tumor load may be of value in the future, but we are talking about reducing tumor mass to a rather small number of cells so that resecting half of a large ovarian carcinoma is not of great value. Patients who have partial resections for incurable carcinomas usually have a more rapid downhill course than if they were not subjected to surgery. Even Celsus made this observation 2000 years ago.

The placement of perfusion catheters may be a task for the surgeon to attempt regional or organ chemotherapy. Although many centers find this of value, the procedure has not gained universal favor. It may be that improved drugs or immunotherapeutic agents will provide an impetus to perfusion. Many other palliative procedures are available for many malignant processes and the surgeon must be guided by philosophical concerns. The key to the decision is to provide the patient with as much useful, comfortable, and productive life as medical science can offer. The relief of pain falls into the category of palliative surgery. When medication no longer is satisfactory and the patient has an expected reasonable period of survival, neurosurgical relief in the form of chordotomy or rhizotomy may be justified and can add dignity to the path to death.

RECONSTRUCTIVE SURGERY

Until a better means for controlling cancer is available, we continue to face the ravages of radical surgery. Patients lose limbs, breasts, and parts of the face. Others must have colostomies or ileostomies. Radical surgery may prolong life, but if it does not provide the patient with satisfactory cosmetics and function, it reflects an additional failure. We must, wherever possible, avoid substituting a living death for a threatened one.

The application of prostheses for amputated limbs is a well developed art. Rehabilitation centers have also developed excellent programs for restoring function. Cosmetic surgery for lesions of the face are well developed, but too often the patient is reticent to undergo more surgery than is necessary for cure. Tattoo artists to reestablish vermillion borders of the lip and speech therapists to overcome the disabilities native to oral or laryngeal surgery have done splendid work. The results with breast reconstruction have been discouraging in the past. The rising popularity of a modified radical mastectomy with less radical skin excision has led to better potential for reconstruction. A transverse mastectomy incision is preferable. At the time of mastectomy, the nipple can be removed and the subareolar tissue is sent for pathologic study to exclude evidence of residual malignancy in that area. After sterile storage at low temperature until the sections are read, the nipple area may be autotransplanted to the abdomen of the patient. Subsequently an inflatable silicone prosthesis can be placed subcutaneously or subpectorally. Ultimately, the nipple can be transplanted from the abdomen to the skin over the prosthesis. Further work is necessary to ultimately develop a satisfactory breast reconstruction, but the basis for it is available.

Colostomy has serious emotional implications. Most patients can be trained to irrigate themselves once every other day and are usually safe without a device between times. Ileostomy is a different matter. It is often done in young people who live a long period of time afterward. The Kock operation which creates a reservoir and a variable degree of continence is under trial at the present time. In our animal laboratory, we are working toward an ileal valve for continence which must still be considered experimental. In Germany, Hennig, Feustel, and others are using magnetic forces with samarium cobalt to occlude the colostomy and ileostomy openings. A circular magnet is placed about the fascia and the colostomy is drawn through it and matured. An obturator is then placed into the colostomy opening and can be removed by the patient periodically for irrigation. This work is promising, but the number of human cases is still small and evaluation must await a larger trial group.

CONCLUSIONS

Despite the improved results of surgery with early detection, the ultimate solution to malignancy must come from prophylaxis or systemic treatment. Until that time, the surgeon must carry out those procedures traditionally known to prolong life. He must be slow to accept new procedures that have not yet been proven and yet must be quick to alter his techniques as soon as evidence justifies a change. He must continue to change his attitudes as knowledge from other disciplines becomes known. In this dynamic atmosphere he can be most productive until a more definitive answer for malignancy is available.

REFERENCES

Deddish, M. R. Local excision. Surg. Clin. North Am., *54*: 877–880, 1974.

Degenshein, G. A. Exploration of the abdomen. Surgery, *65*: 721–722, 1969.

Degenshein, G. A. Choledochoduodenostomy; an 18 year study of 175 consecutive cases. Surgery, *76*: 319–324, 1974.

Dengenshein, G. A., Bloom, N., Ceccarelli, F., Daluvoy, R., and Tobin, E. Estrogen and progesterone receptor site studies as guides to the management of advanced breast cancer. Dis. Breast, *3*: January–March, 1977.

Fortner, J. G. Recent advances in pancreatic cancer. Surg. Clin. North Am. *54*: 859–863, 1974.

Gibbon, J. H., Jr., Sabiston, D. C., and Spencer, F. C. Surgery of the Chest, ed. 2, pg. 359 W. B. Saunders, Philadelphia, 1969.

Gilbertson, V. A. The early detection of breast cancer. Semin. Oncol., *1*: 87–89, 1974.

Halsted, W. The results of radical surgery for cure of carcinoma of the breast. Ann. Surg., July, 1907.

Hermann, R. E., and Steiger, E. Modified radical mastectomy. Surg. Clin. North Am., *58*:

743–754, 1978.

Robbins, G. F. The rationale for the treatment of women with potentially curable breast carcinoma. Surg. Clin. North Am., *54*: 793–800, 1974.

Turnbull, R. B., Jr. Current concepts in cancer; cancer of the G.I. tract: colon, rectum, anus. The no-touch isolation technique of resection. J.A.M.A., *231*: 1181–1182, 1975.

Whitmore, W. Retropubic implantation of I-125 in the treatment of prostatic carcinoma. J. Urol., *108:* 918–920, 1972.

Chapter 3

Fundamentals of Radiation Oncology

JAMES D. COX, M.D.

Therapeutic radiology, or radiation oncology as it has come to be called in recent years, is still a young and rapidly developing clinical specialty. The full scope of the use of ionizing radiations in the curative treatment of patients with malignant disease has not yet been realized. Not only are revolutionary clinical experiences being reported, but increasingly sophisticated laboratory studies are beginning to influence clinical research. In practice, radiation oncology is an integration of tumor pathology, clinical assessment, human radiation biology, and radiologic physics. It is narrow in that it is confined to the care of patients with cancer, but broad in that it cuts across nearly every medical specialty.

HISTORICAL PERSPECTIVES

Within a year of the discovery of x-ray by Roentgen (1895), they were administered to patients with cancer in several countries. Single applications of very large doses were used at first, especially in Germany. Such treatments profoundly affected the tumor, but just as profoundly injured normal tissues. The resulting ulceration healed slowly and poorly—hardly a competitive approach to cancer operations which, while extensive, usually healed by primary intention.

Becquerel accidentally became aware of the biologic effects of radium in 1901, 5 years after discovery of the element by the Curies. He carried 200 mg of radium in a shirt pocket for some 6 hours. Cutaneous erythema occurred 2 weeks later, progressed to ulceration, and healed only after several weeks (Cantril, 1957). Soon radium salt was placed in containers and applied to the skin, placed in body orifices (intracavitary irradiation), and implanted directly into neoplasms (interstitial irradiation) with considerable success.

Probably the most important conceptual development in the history of

44

this discipline resulted from animal studies reported in 1922 by Regaud. He demonstrated that spermatogenesis could be permanently suppressed by four fractions of irradiation in a period of 10 days without damage to the scrotal skin, whereas the same effect could not be accomplished by a single massive dose even though radionecrosis of the skin resulted. Thus, repeated small applications of radiations to a rapid cell-renewal system served as a model for the irradiation of malignant tumors. Soon, cancer of the larynx was shown to be curable by such an approach (Regaud, et al., 1922). Coutard found an even more impressive increase in therapeutic ratio when daily treatments were given over a period of several weeks, an approach which came to be known as his "protracted-fractionated method." Elaboration of the concept of *fractionation*, with better measurements of dose and greater understanding of the malignant diseases to which it was applied, encompass much of the progress in radiation oncology in the past half century.

In a few centers, large quantities of radium were accumulated to produce a telecurietherapy unit, i.e., one which could treat patients with the gamma rays from radium placed at a distance rather than deposited directly within body cavities or implanted into tissues (brachycurietherapy). Clinical experience with such units suggested that there were advantages to using higher energy radiations. Between 1930 and 1950, technical advances permitted the development of high energy or supervoltage (>500 kV) x-ray generators. The advantages of supervoltage radiations over the widely available 200 kV x-rays became obvious. Increased penetration of the radiations and decreased reaction of the overlying skin ("skin sparing") permitted the delivery of doses sufficient to achieve previously unattainable control of deep seated tumors. Additional benefits of less scatter to surrounding tissues, less absorption in bone, and somewhat lesser effects on normal tissues contributed to a widened applicability of external irradiation. In the middle 1950's, cobalt-60 teletherapy units became widely available, and the impact of radiation therapy upon the overall problem of malignant disease was greatly accelerated.

Since the dose received in depth was no longer dependent upon the tolerance of the skin overlying the tumor, attention was directed to establishing more carefully the tolerance of tissues in proximity to the tumor, as well as doses required to achieve a high likelihood of eradication of the malignant process. Consquently, the expression of the *exposure* to ionizing radiations, the *roentgen* or R accepted in 1937, gave way to expression of the *absorbed dose*, the *rad*, in 1953. Since the radiation oncologist can manipulate the volume irradiated, the intensity of the irradiation per treatment, the number of treatments, and the separation between the treatments or overall time of a course of therapy, many individualized treatment regimens evolved. In recent years attempts have been made to compare these treatment regimens with regard to effects on normal tissues and to reduce them to a common mathematical expression (Ellis, 1968). Similar analyses of tumor control probabilities related to time-dose-volume relationships have proved useful for malignant epithelial tumors (Shukovsky, 1970; Shukovsky and Fletcher, 1973), but not for very radiosensitive tumors (Cox et al., 1974). Brachytherapy has also undergone an evolution since the first applications of radium at the turn of the century. It was soon recognized that protracting the dose, i.e., using low intensity sources for longer periods of time, improved the therapeutic ratio. This was characteristic of the Curie Foundation's system of intrauterine and intravaginal radium therapy for cancer of the cervix. Careful research on optimal arrangements of radium sources to achieve a homogenous dose distribution throughout a given volume, such as the Manchester System for radium usage, led to higher control rates with lesser effects to normal tissues. In the past decade, afterloading systems have been developed for intracavitary and interstitial applications of radioactive materials. With these techniques, *nonradioactive applicators* are placed, verified with roentgenograms or fluoroscopy, and then adjusted to meet strict criteria of three-dimensional distribution; the radioactive sources are inserted as the last step. Decreased exposure and, of greater importance, more satisfactory distribution of sources are considerable advantages over the direct application methods. Increased local control rates have been demonstrated with afterloading techniques (Pierquin et al., 1970, 1971).

Therapeutic radiology actually began as a separate specialty with the recognition in the 1920s that irradiation was potentially curative for patients with cancer. It developed more rapidly in Europe where three generations of physicians have devoted themselves exclusively to radiation oncology. In the United States, the development was much slower; as recently as 1959, there were only 111 physicians in the United States exclusively involved in this specialty. Since that time there has been a 10-fold increase in the number of radiation oncologists, but it is estimated that more than twice the current number will be necessary to care for the two-thirds of all cancer patients who require either curative or palliative irradiation.

PHYSICAL BASIS OF RADIATION ONCOLOGY

The electromagnetic radiations of importance to the radiation oncologist are those with a wavelength of 1 Ångstrom or less. These have the capacity to produce ionizations and excitations in biologic material. There is no difference between x-rays and gamma rays. They occupy the same range of wavelengths in the electromagnetic spectrum, have the same energy, and produce identical biological effects. The two names result from different origins of photons: x-rays (*Bremsstrahlung*) are produced as a result of deceleration of electrons in the vicinity of the nuclei of the absorbing substance while gamma rays are photons which originate within the nucleus of an unstable atom. Electrons, per se, also have a place in the armamentarium of the radiation oncologist. Other particulate radiations are being evaluated for medical usefulness. These include fast neutrons, negative pi mesons, protons, and high energy stripped nuclei (e.g., carbon and helium). None of them yet has an established place in the treatment of malignant diseases.

When x- or gamma rays enter biologic material, energy is converted into chemical damage and heat. At the energies of most x- and gamma ray sources currently in use, the primary events are the interactions of photons with electrons in the outer layers of atoms with scattering of both the photons and the electrons (Compton scattering). The scattered electrons in turn cause ionizations and excitations; most importantly, they interact with water to form highly reactive free radicals. With higher energy photons, scatter of secondary electrons is more in the forward direction, that is in the direction of the primary beam; it takes some distance for the interactions to summate and reach a maximum after which the energy of the beam dissipates by a constant fraction per unit depth. Figure 3.1 compares the distributions of energy as a function of depth. The upper left portion of this figure demonstrates the physical basis for skin sparing; the maximum dose occurs below the skin surface, unlike conventional x-rays.

The most commonly used sources for external irradiation are listed in Table 3.1. Although it is not readily apparent, there is a great deal of overlap among the teletherapy sources. For example there is little to choose between the gamma rays from cobalt-60 and 2–6-mV x-rays. The edge of the beam from x-ray generators is much sharper than that from cobalt units which can be important when irradiating close to critical structures such as the lens of the eye. However, in general, the successful treatment with any unit will not depend upon the physical characteristics of the beam so much as the manner in which it is utilized by the radiation oncologist. In this regard, the radiation therapy equipment and technical staff are for the radiation oncologist what the operating room and its staff are for the surgical oncologist.

The sources most widely employed for intracavitary or interstitial therapy are listed in Table 3.2. Again, the various brachytherapy sources have overlapping capabilities, each has specific advantages. For example, iridium-192 is the only isotope listed which can be used satisfactorily with an afterloading technique when implanting it directly into tissues. The others can be used in afterloading intracavitary applicators, however.

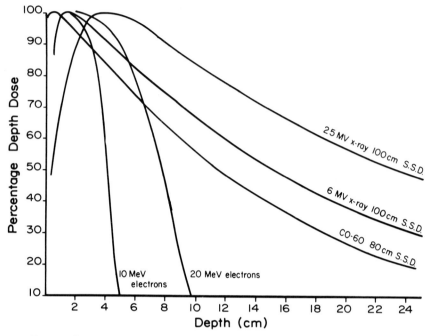

Fig. 3.1. Comparison of depth doses of commonly used supervoltage radiations.

TABLE 3.1

Teleradiotherapy Sources

Unit	Mean Energy (meV)* Photons
150–440 kVp x-ray	0.06–0.14
^{137}Cs-teletherapy	0.66
^{60}Co-teletherapy	1.25
4 mV linear accelerator	1.3
6 mV linear accelerator	1.8
20–24 mV betatron	6.2–7.0

* meV = million electron volts.

TABLE 3.2

Brachytherapy Sources

	Half-Life	Effective Energy (meV)*
^{226}Ra	1620 years	1.2
^{137}Cs	30 years	0.66
^{198}Au	2.7 days	0.41
^{192}Ir	74 days	0.34

* meV = million electron volts.

When utilized appropriately and meticulously, both teletherapy units and brachytherapy sources have met with a high degree of success in the permanent control of a variety of malignant diseases; there is, however, nothing inherent in any of these x-ray or gamma ray generators which will ensure success independent of the expertise of the radiation oncologist.

BIOLOGICAL BASIS OF RADIATION ONCOLOGY

The two most obvious and difficult questions that must be asked are how cells are killed by ionizing radiations and why cancer cells can be permanently eradicated without irreparable damage to the surrounding normal tissues. Some attempts can be made to answer these questions at the chemical, subcellular, and cellular levels, but it should be recognized that most progress in radiation oncology was made empirically by careful clinical monitoring and analysis of successes and failures in the treatment of patients with cancer.

Radiation Chemistry

The chemical effects of ionizing radiations are both *direct*, insofar as they involve radiative interactions with the solute, and *indirect*, as they involve interactions with the solvent. Evidence for direct effects can be seen at the macromolecular level with the irradiation of certain solids at room temperature. Subsequent heating of these solids results in emission of light proportional to the amount of radiations absorbed. This phenomenon of thermoluminescence, especially with lithium fluoride, is used as a measure of absorbed dose in clinical and experimental work. Subtle indicators of direct effects on the solute are alterations in electron spin resonance and the identification of stable damaged molecules irradiated in the solid state.

Indirect effects essentially involve the interactions with water. Highly reactive free radicals and ions are formed by the interactions between water and the electrons scattered as a result of the photon beam.The most important moieties formed are the H· and OH· radicals, positive water (H_2O+), and hydrated electrons. These transient species combine in a matter of microseconds with each other and with groups on the critical biological molecules, particularly deoxyribonucleic acid (DNA) and ribonucleic acid (RNA), and possibly nuclear enzymes.

The direct and indirect effects of radiations can be altered by temperature, water content, and especially by the presence or absence of oxygen. As will be seen, the oxygen enhancement ratio (OER), i.e., the greater effect from ionizing radiations in the presence of full oxygenation divided by the effect under anoxic or hypoxic conditions, probably has considerable significance in the irradiation of malignant tumors.

Cellular Radiation Biology

The principal cellular effect of concern is that of lethality. Sublethal effects occur and are repaired both in normal and malignant cells. However, sublethal damage and repair are very difficult to study, and the largest body of data relates to cell survival studies. This is, of course, an appropriate end point to study by the radiation oncologist since the killing of malignant cells is the sine qua non of his activities. Suffice it to say that various functions of the cell can be temporarily or permanently impaired without a lethal effect. Reparable or nonlethal chromosome breaks occur, temporary or permanent delays in mitosis can be detected, but the lethal effects are the most apparent.

The irradiated cells can undergo three types of death. With extremely high doses (in the range of 100,000 rads or more) instant, *coagulative* death occurs. At lower dose levels, but at levels well above clinical usefulness (10,000–50,000 rads) cells may undergo *interphase* death; this type of death occurs hours to days following the irradiation but without an intervening division of the cell. The most important type of death at clinical levels of irradiation is *reproductive* or *mitotic* death. Such death will not necessarily occur at the time of the first mitosis, and a cell can divide several times after irradiation, but it is no longer "clonogenic." The precise events leading to cellular death are still unknown. Eventually, the integrity of the DNA must be affected, but whether it is affected directly or by interference with critical enzyme systems is not yet clear, despite the considerable amount of work which has been and is still being carried out to elucidate the mechanisms (Kaplan, 1963).

A large body of data has developed around the cellular effects of a single exposure of ionizing radiations since the original description by Puck and Marcus (1956). There is little direct applicability of such information since there are few indications for the use of single exposures in clinical radiation oncology. However, the single exposure effects are well known and, of course, have a bearing on fractionated irradiation. Figure 3.2 shows a stylized cell survival curve. It has a shoulder region, D_q, reflecting the accumulation of sublethal damage. At doses beyond the shoulder, exponential reduction of the surviving fraction is seen with increasing dose. This curve is described by the equation $S = (1 - e^{-D/D37})^N$ where S equals the surviving fraction, N equals the number arrived at by extrapolating the straight line portion of the curve to the ordinate; D is dose and D_{37} is the increment of dose which reduces the surviving fraction to 37%. It can be seen that when $D = D_{37}$, and there is no shoulder (i.e., $N = 1$), S equals 0.37 (i.e., $S = e^{-1}$). D_{37} is also referred to as D_0, the mean lethal dose. For the sake of completeness, it should be noted that D_q equals $D_{37} \ln N$. Strictly speaking such a curve is asymptotic, and the surviving fraction never reaches zero.

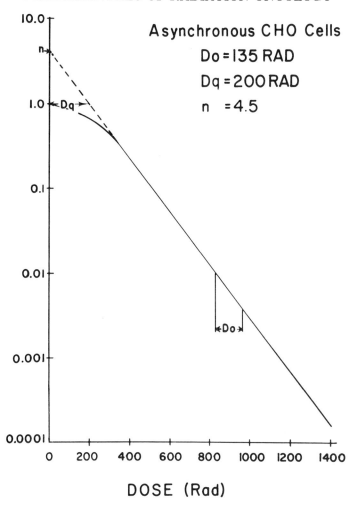

FIG. 3.2. Cell survival curve: single dose irradiation. (Courtesy L. E. Hopwood, Radiation Biology Section, Medical College of Wisconsin.)

When a second dose is given approximately 1 day after the first (Fig. 3.3) it can be seen that the shoulder has reappeared to its full extent (Elkind, 1960). (The time for complete recovery from sublethal damage is of the order of 6 hours in most cellular systems.) This figure is also stylized suggesting that there is no change in cellular radiosensitivity with successive fractions. In fact, there are changes in radiosensitivity as a result of the first dose (Whitmore and Gulyas, 1967; Kallman, 1967).

Several factors can modify the slope of the cell survival curves, i.e., modify cellular radiosensitivity. A significant endogenous factor, the

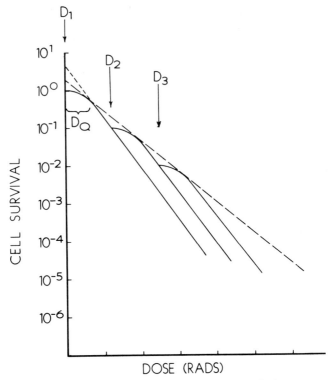

FIG. 3.3. Cell survival curve: fractionated irradiation.

position in the cell cycle, is recognized but cannot yet be put to use in clinical circumstances. In most in vivo and in vitro systems studies, mitosis (M) has proved to be the most sensitive part of the cell cycle. In practically all systems, the period of late DNA synthesis (S) has proved to be the least radiosensitive. The sensitivities of the post-mitotic-pre-synthetic phase (G_1) and of the postsynthetic-premitotic phase (G_2) vary from one cell system to another.

Another factor which is endogenous but can be altered by manipulation of the environment is the oxygen tension. As noted previously the OER is a measure of the increased radiosensitivity attending full oxygenation as compared to the anoxic state. In mammalian cells the OER ranges from 2.0 to 3.0. Attempts to utilize this knowledge clinically by employing pretreatment breathing of oxygen (Rubin et al., 1969) or treatment of the patient in hyperbaric tanks at 2–3 atmospheres of oxygen (van den Brenk, 1968; Cade and McEwen, 1967) have produced equivocal results at best. Clinical investigations of oxygen as a radiosensitizer continue in several centers.

Radiosensitizing agents such as the pyrimidine analogs and actinomycin D appear promising on the basis of cell survival studies (Tubiana and Frindel, 1965). Again, the clinical experience is much less encouraging. The combination of actinomycin D and irradiation seems to be advantageous in the treatment of pulmonary metastases (Cassady et al., 1973; Cox et al., 1972) but there is insufficient knowledge of the radiation doses required to control metastases in the absence of this drug which, itself, is cytotoxic.

The effects of fractionated irradiation, insofar as the first dose affects the second, have been noted above. Repair of sublethal damage is manifested by reappearance of the shoulder in the survival curves, and it is apparent, in vivo, that the sensitivities of the residual populations are often altered. The overall effect of multiple fractions of irradiation, as noted in Figure 3.3, is to reduce the importance of the shoulder, reduce the effective extrapolation number, N, and increase substantially the total dose which must be reached in order to achieve a given reduction in survival fraction. Interestingly the same effects occur with low dose-rate, continuous irradiation as in brachytherapy. In contrast to the clinical dose rates of 50–250 rads per minute, the irradiation from brachytherapy sources is at a rate of 25–100 rads per hour. The potential advantages of such highly protracted irradiation are the subject of both laboratory (Hall, 1972) and clinical research (Pierquin and Baillet, 1971).

Radiophysiology

The effects of ionizing radiations at the tissue level have been carefully studied for three quarters of a century. Such studies shed considerable light on clinical circumstances, but they are a long way from the mathematical expressions of modern cellular radiobiology. The first approximation of inherent radiosensitivity of cells was proposed by Bergonié and Tribondeau (1906). Their conclusion can be summarized as follows: Cells are more profoundly affected by ionizing radiations (a) the greater their mitotic activity, (b) the longer the duration of mitosis, and (c) the less well differentiated they are both morphologically and functionally. This is quite a good first expression of inherent radiosensitivity, but there are many exceptions.

Many influences can modify radiosensitivity. The largest body of information concerns variations in fractionation and volume irradiated. Although there has been little work on the effects of multiple doses in modern cellular radiobiology, years of animal and clinical investigation have given us much information about the effects of fractionated irradiation as utilized clinically.

Following the development of the concept of fractionation by Coutard, it has become apparent that, while the total dose is of great importance, its true importance is appreciated only when the (a) number of fractions in which it is administered, (b) the elapsed time over which it is given, and (c) the volume in which it is distributed are known. In short, a small total dose delivered in a few fractions over a short time can produce the same biologic effects as a larger total dose administered in a much larger number of treatments or fractions over a much longer time. A first approximation of the equivalency of such time-dose regimens has been made by Ellis (1968) and is expressed as follows:

$$\text{NSD} = \frac{D}{N^{0.24}\ T^{0.11}}$$

where NSD is nominal standard dose expressed in rets (roentgen equivalent therapy), D equals total dose in rads, N equals the number of equal fractions with which that total dose was delivered, and T equals the overall time in days required to deliver that number of fractions. A refinement and "simplification" which takes into account changes in size of the individual dose as well as interruptions during a course of irradiation has recently been presented (Orton and Ellis, 1973). It is widely recognized that a larger volume of any tissue tolerates the effects of irradiation less well than a smaller volume. However, a mathematical expression of this fact has not yet been added to the time-dose-fractionation formulas.

Table 3.3 lists in order of decreasing radiosensitivity the mature tissues of the body and is modified from Rubin and Casarett (1972). In general, embryonic or actively growing tissues are more sensitive than the corresponding mature tissue. Furthermore, it is probable that all of these tissues obey the dose-fractions-time-volume relationships noted above. A discussion in depth of the responses at various dose levels for each of the tissues listed in Table 3.3 has been carefully presented elsewhere (Lacassagne and Gricouroff, 1958; Moss et al., 1973; Rubin and Casarett, 1968;

TABLE 3.3
Relative Radiosensitivity of Mature Tissues
(Decreasing Sensitivity)

1. Bone marrow	12. Salivary gland (serous)	23. Bladder
2. Ovary	13. Heart	24. Breast
3. Lens	14. Spinal cord	25. Capillaries
4. Testis	15. Brain	26. Bone
5. Lung	16. Thyroid	27. Cartilage
6. Kidney	17. Pituitary	28. Pancreas
7. Lymph nodes	18. Larynx	29. Vagina
8. Liver	19. Oral mucosa	30. Uterus
9. Small bowel	20. Esophagus	31. Bile ducts
10. Stomach	21. Arterioles	
11. Colon	22. Skin	

Vaeth, 1972). However, a brief précis of the anticipated effects at clinical dose levels seems warranted.

Bone Marrow. Single doses of 300–500 rads profoundly affect bone marrow stem cells. Such doses will not permanently eradicate all stem cells and recovery is possible. If single exposure total body irradiation to such doses occurs, 50% of the individuals will die within 30 days (i.e., this represents the $LD_{50/30}$). Following such a dose, there is a characteristic sequence of events in the peripheral blood elements. The lymphocytes drop first and reach their nadir within a matter of several hours to a few days. The granulocytes decrease over a period of several days. The platelets decrease much more slowly and do not usually reach their minimum until the granulocytes and lymphocytes have already begun to recover, if recovery is to occur. With the long life span of the red blood cell, anemia will not begin to develop for many days or weeks. Such a sequence of events is rarely seen since total body irradiation is confined to accidental exposures or a very few clinical circumstances in which marrow elements are already abnormal (del Regato, 1974). The effects of local irradiation on peripheral blood counts will depend upon the volume of bone marrow irradiated which in turn depends upon the age of the individual. The distribution of the bone marrow in the adult has been carefully studied (Ellis, 1960; Russell et al., 1966), and serves as a rough guide to anticipate peripheral blood manifestations. Local irradiation to relatively high doses is likely to result in permanent depletion of the marrow included within the field but it does not produce significant changes in the bone marrow outside the volume irradiated (Goswitz et al., 1963). The failure of the heavily irradiated bone marrow to repopulate is probably a failure of the microcirculation of the marrow since lower doses permit repopulation in spite of a transient period of acellularity (Knospe et al., 1968).

Gonads. Doses of 500–1500 rads in 1–2 weeks profoundly affect the *ovaries.* The earliest and most marked effect is on the most mature graafian follicles, while a somewhat lesser effect is seen in the primary follicles. The interstitial gland cells seem little altered by the irradiation in the short run, but after several months diffuse atrophy occurs secondary to lack of replacement from ruptured follicles. Estrogen production slowly disappears, menstruation ceases, and an artificial menopause is effected. The doses required seem higher in young women than in those nearing the age of natural menopause. In contrast to the ovaries where the primary ovocytes are somewhat less disturbed than those undergoing maturation, in the *testis* the primary spermatogonia are the most immediately and profoundly altered by the irradiation. Since the spermatogonia are the stem cells for all of the elements of spermatogenesis, their disappearance ultimately results in disappearance of the entire germinal epithelium. The total dose of the irradiation will determine whether spermatogenesis will resume. However, complete sterility is possible without impotence. Androgen levels and secondary sexual characteristics remain unaltered.

Lens. The very earliest studies around the turn of the century suggested that the lens was relatively insensitive to ionizing radiations. In fact, quite the opposite is the case and the discrepancies arose because of the latent period for the development of changes secondary to irradiation. The change, which is seen following doses of a minimum of 200 rads to a maximum of 1000 rads depending upon the fractionation, is cataract formation. The lower the dose, the longer the latent period (Merriam and Focht, 1957). A comprehensive review of the effects of ionizing radiations on the eye has been presented by Merriam et al. (1972). If carefully sought, many asymptomatic cataracts may be detected.

Lung. At doses exceeding 2000 rads in 3 weeks, pneumonitis will frequently result from irradiation. The acute changes are often seen 2–4 weeks after the completion of high dose irradiation as in the treatment of cancer of the lung. The systemic symptoms of fever and malaise accompany local manifestations of dyspnea and nonproductive cough or one productive of thick tenacious sputum. Alveolar-capillary diffusion deficit can be demonstrated if a significant volume of the lung has been irradiated. The functional impairment is often out of proportion to radiographic findings. These changes may wax and wane, depending upon pulmonary reserve and superimposed infection, for a period of 2–3 months. The acute changes of alveolar septal thickening, hyaline membrane formation, and proliferation and shedding of alveolar septal cells, gradually resolve and are replaced by scarring which may be progressive. Contraction with loss of functional lung volume is the hallmark of the late stage.

Kidney. Radiation nephropathy has been carefully studied both in animals and in man (Maier, 1972; Mostofi, 1966). Most of the data on renal tolerance are based on the use of conventional x-irradiation of the whole kidney. The tolerance of the entire kidney to supervoltage irradiation is probably not above 3000 rads in 3–4 weeks, but subtotal supervoltage renal irradiation has been carried out with impunity to doses of 4500–5000 rads in 5–6 weeks. Acute radiation nephritis seems to begin with arteriolar necrosis; subsequent glomerular changes progress from thickening of the basement membrane to eventual hyalinization. Tubular atrophy develops later along with interstitial nephritis. These changes can lead to rapidly progressive malignant hypertension and death in weeks to months. Less severe changes are more slowly progressive. Chronic radiation nephritis may evolve as a gradual sequela of the acute process or may seemingly arise without an apparent acute phase. Gradual impairment of renal function with intermittent or persistent proteinuria and minimal elevations of blood urea nitrogen may be found in patients who are usually asymptomatic. Patients may be normotensive for years and then gradually develop mild and chronic, or occasionally severe and progressive, hypertension with attendant encephalopathy and death. Irradiation of only one kidney can result in hypertension that is relieved by removal of the irradiated kidney. The anemia which accompanies chronic radiation nephritis is probably related to decreased production of erythropoietin.

Lymph nodes. There is considerable range of radiosensitivity of the cells found in lymph nodes. Lymphoblasts and lymphocytes in the germinal centers die within the first several hours following significant irradiation of the nodes. The resulting debris is actively phagocytized and atrophy becomes apparent within a matter of a few days. This persists for varying periods of time depending upon the total dose after which the nodes become repopulated with lymphocytes and active lymphopoiesis resumes. At higher dose levels there seems to be a phase of early recovery followed by a gradual increase in the connective tissue elements. The filtering or "barrier" function of the lymph nodes can be demonstrated to be impaired in the laboratory setting but there is no clinical evidence of this with the doses usually employed. *Lymphatic vessels* seem to be quite resistant to the effects of ionizing radiations (Sherman and O'Brien, 1967); any alleged sealing off or obliteration of lymphatics as a means of containing a malignant tumor is mythical. The *spleen* seems to respond in much the same way as the lymph nodes. A large number of patients have now had prophylactic or therapeutic irradiation of the spleen for malignant lymphoid tumors and no functional deficits have resulted.

Liver. The hepatic effects of irradiation in clinical dose ranges have been difficult to derive. Irradiation of only a portion of the liver results in little functional deficit because of the considerable reserve of the organ. Irradiation of the entire liver has been uncommon except when involved with neoplastic disease, and the changes secondary to the irradiation may be difficult to separate from those related to involvement by the malignant process. Thus, the tolerance level suggested by Ingold et al. (1965) of 3000 rads in 4 weeks is open to question because of the prior hepatic involvement with Hodgkin's disease. The initial change in the liver seems to be intense hyperemia which is followed by gradual occlusion of the central vein of the hepatic lobule with secondary atrophy of the surrounding parenchymal cells (Ogata et al., 1963; Reed and Cox, 1966). Abdominal pain, hepatic enlargement, and ascites are noted a few weeks to several months following the irradiation; they may resolve with supportive care, but deaths have occurred following 2500–3000 rads in 12 fractions in 2 weeks (Wharton et al., 1973).

Small Bowel. The small intestine seems to represent the most sensitive part of the gastrointestinal tract to the effects of ionizing radiations, presumably related to the inherently high mitotic activity of the basal cells of the crypts of Lieberkühn. The acute changes are swelling of the villi with an outpouring of fluid resulting in diarrhea. The absorptive capacities for glucose and fats are impaired. Late effects include ulceration and stricture formation with partial or complete obstruction (Schier et al., 1964). They may occur with doses as low as 4500 rads in 4½ weeks (Roswit et al., 1972). The duodenum and jejunum are seemingly more sensitive at a given dose level than the ileum in rats (Baker and Mitchell, 1963), but radiation enteropathy is most frequent, clinically, in the terminal ileum. This is related to its relative fixation at the cecum and the proximity to the many pelvic neoplasms which require irradiation. Fortunately, simple bypass with anastamosis of unirradiated bowel usually corrects the complication.

Stomach. The complexity of the gastric mucosa and the differential responses of the various cellular elements make the overall response of the stomach to ionizing radiations a difficult subject. Furthermore, functional changes do not always correlate well with histologic findings. In brief, at low dose levels (1600 rads in 10 days with conventional x-rays) an asymptomatic gastritis occurs. A reduction in free hydrochloric acid is followed by a reduction in pepsin, but the zymogenic cells seem to be affected, microscopically, prior to the parietal cells. Consequently, such dose levels have been used successfully in the treatment of intractible peptic ulcer disease (Goldgraber et al., 1954). Otherwise, the gastric mucosa is not profoundly affected at doses up to 4000–5000 rads in 4–5 weeks, and the only frequent symptom is nausea. The mucosa regenerates from the neck glands and ulceration is quite uncommon. At higher dose levels, however, the risk of ulceration and, with very intense irradiation, perforation and obstruction increases precipitously. Such ulceration seems to respond poorly to conventional medical management (Roswit et al., 1972).

Large Bowel. The effects of irradiation on the large bowel are most carefully documented in the rectum and rectosigmoid. It is presumed that the entire large bowel has a similar radiosensitivity. Acutely, mucosal edema and hyperemia are associated with diarrhea, often with considerable mucus, and tenesmus without bleeding. At doses of 5000–5500 rads in 5–6 weeks, the acute reaction can be expected consistently, but late changes are minimal and rarely symptomatic. At higher dose levels, prolonged diarrhea and tenesmus, with occasional rectal ulceration, may be seen. Persistent ulceration, stricture, and perforation can be seen months or years following excessive doses. Late reactions increase precipitously with doses above 6000 rads in 6 weeks and, of course, are related to the volume irradiated (Roswit et al., 1972). Precise correlations of dose with morbidity are complicated by the frequent addition of intracavitary sources to the external irradiation; this results in very high doses to small segments of the rectum (Strockbine et al., 1970).

Salivary Glands. Rarely, following an initial dose of irradiation of 150–250 rads, the salivary glands will become markedly swollen and painful. This unusual reaction is self-limited and subsides within 24–48 hours. It is not an indication for interrupting radiation therapy. The common and predictable response of the salivary glands occurs at much higher dose levels. Transient responses are seen as low as 2000 rads in 2 weeks and are more prolonged up to 5000 rads in 5 weeks. Beyond that dose, the changes are usually permanent. A reduction in the acini of the gland occurs; the serous are more markedly affected than the mucous acini. An alteration in taste, which is at first unusual and then generally depressed, is associated with decreased amount and increased viscidity of the saliva. The aberrations of taste and the dryness may persist for as long as a year and then return to normal, but, at very high dose levels, both are permanent. Accompanying the decreased serous component of the saliva, the cleansing action on the teeth is diminished. This results in a greatly increased tendency toward development of caries at the gum, a characteristic postirradiation phenomenon first described by del Regato (1939). This is avoidable by meticulous dental prophylaxis, including topical application of fluoride.

Squamous Mucous Membrane. The lining of the oral cavity, oropharynx, hypopharynx, esophagus, nasal cavity, vagina, and cervix respond in essentially the same way although some areas seem to be slightly more susceptible than others. In general, the lining of the upper aerodigestive tract seems more sensitive to irradiation than the squamous epithelium of the female genital tract. At modest dose levels, the squamous epithelium is lost between the 11th and 14th day due to destruction of the basal, germinative cells with consequent gradual thinning and eventual disappearance of the epithelium. This is replaced by a false membrane similar to a diphtheroid membrane. Changes may at first be patchy and will eventually become confluent. With doses of the order of 6000 rads in 6 weeks, the epithelium will regenerate over a period of 2–3 weeks. At higher dose levels, prolonged denudation may occur. Such changes were classically termed "radioepithelitis" (Lacassagne and Gricouroff, 1958) and more recently have been called "mucositis." Both terms are misnomers, and use of the term "reaction" without any pathophysiologic designation is preferable.

Skin. The most carefully studied and widely recognized reaction to ionizing radiations occurs in the skin. For years it was the limiting factor in the use of radiation therapy for deep seated tumors. Fortunately this is no longer the case. Different portions of the human skin have slightly different sensitivities. Furthermore, the effects of the irradiation vary considerably with the quality (penetrability) of the radiations and the previously mentioned factors of volume, time, daily dose, and total dose. With careful observation, a transient erythema can be noted several hours following the irradiation. A more obvious, and gradually progressive erythema appears at the beginning of the 2nd week of irradiation. Around the same time, epilation begins and will usually be complete 2–3 weeks later. The pathophysiologic mechanism is similar to that of the squamous mucosa. Destruction of the basal layers of the epidermis results in a failure of replacement of the intermediate and superficial layers with gradual thinning.

The thinning and flaking of the skin, with underlying erythema and new skin formation may be all that is seen if the dose is kept to moderate levels. This condition is known as dry radioepidermitis. With larger doses, the erythema and dry reaction give way to vesicle formation with gradual coalescence and denudation around the 4th week. This moist radioepidermitis will be more intense and last longer the higher the dose; it may heal surprisingly rapidly, however, if the dose is not excessive. Islands of epidermis appear within the denuded region, and healing also occurs from the periphery. This new epidermis is thin and fragile and will remain so relative to the surrounding skin. If a moist reaction has occurred, the healed area will remain epilated. Over a period of many months, the hyperpigmented epidermis gradually fades, and eventually will appear hypochromic. Trauma with secondary infection during the moist reaction or following complete healing can lead to an ulceration which persists for months or years. Telangiectases are another hallmark of the late sequelae of intensive irradiation. The effects on the *microvasculature* of the underlying dermis are very important since the delivery of nutrients, especially oxygen, is dependent upon its integrity. The endothelial cells are moderately to markedly resistant to radiations (Reinhold, 1972). The microvascular response cannot be separated from the inflammatory response in the irradiated tissue. The scarring (fibrosis), which is a natural consequence of inflammation, may progress slowly for many years. The studies of this series of events, the magnitude of the late effects, and the relationship to the ability to control malignant tumors arising in the skin, led to the first graphic representations of biologic equivalence of different fractionation regimens (Stranqvist, 1944). Analyses emphasizing the importance of the volume irradiated have been published by von Essen (1963). The data from such studies have been the most important human component leading to the formulation of biologic isoeffectiveness of treatment regimens as in the NSD approximation of Ellis (1968).

Bone and Cartilage. Effects of irradiation on mature bone and cartilage are of little importance until the doses become quite high. The striking preferential bone absorption which occurs with low kilovoltage x-rays resulted in an appreciable frequency of osteoradionecrosis. At present, it is uncommon to see this phenomenon except following dental extractions or other types of trauma to the heavily irradiated maxilla or mandible. However, growing bone and cartilage are affected with much lower doses. The magnitude of the effect is more marked the more active the growth rate and, thus, correlates with age (Probert et al., 1973). Some degree of decreased growth and consequent stunting and/or asymmetry can be expected with the irradiation of almost any malignant condition in children less than 15 years old.

Discussions of the many other tissues and organs of less importance and lesser radiosensitivity are beyond the scope of this chapter. For such information, as well as a more exhaustive discussion of the tissues and organs mentioned above, the interested reader is referred to the classic and standard monographs.

Embryo. The embryo is very sensitive to ionizing radiations especially within the first 6 weeks. During the first 3 weeks, a single dose of the fractionated irradiation, usually given to the mother for the treatment of cancer, would be more than sufficient to kill the embryo. Irradiation during the 3rd to 6th weeks could permit continued development, but aberrations of specific organs which develop rapidly at that time could result in serious anomalies. Direct irradiation of the embryo during the treatment of a malignant process will lead to abortion during the first trimester of pregnancy. It is rare that a fetus would be irradiated after the first trimester.

Genetic Effects. As noted previously, direct irradiation of the gonads during the treatment of a malignant process will result in permanent sterility. However, scattered radiations within the body will often result in absorbed doses of a few to several hundred rads without sterility. Concern often arises as to the potential genetic effects attending a curative course of irradiation with consequent scatter to the gonads. Since the primary effect is on the genetic material, mutations can and do result. Such mutations can be assumed to be harmful. There is no demonstrable threshold dose for an increase in mutation rate so any dose of irradiation can be considered mutagenic. Well identified mutations and consequent abnormalities in the offspring have been described in lower forms, but such eventualities have not yet occurred in man. It is not widely recognized that genetic effects following the atomic bombs in Japan have not been seen. It is possible that too little time has elapsed to begin to see genetic abnormalities in the offspring of the survivors, but it is also possible that some recovery in the genetic material has occurred.

Systemic Effects of Irradiation

The effect of irradiation on immune responses is a relatively new and complex subject. When total body irradiation occurs to doses which are potentially lethal, the immune mechanisms throughout the body, both humoral and cell mediated, are depressed. This is presumably a direct result of the suppression of the stem cells of plasma cells or lymphocytes which produce immunoglobulins as well as those which participate in the cellular response. The effects of local irradiation, particularly the importance of the volume irradiated and the amount of bone marrow within that volume, are not yet defined. Furthermore, since the malignant process itself may impair both humoral and cell mediated immunity in man (Harris and Sinkovics, 1970), the contributions of the primary disease and the therapy are difficult to separate. Recent studies have rather clearly shown that irradiation of many of the common malignant conditions does not impair cellular immunity as measured by the delayed hypersensitivity reaction (Gross et al., 1973). When very large volumes are irradiated, as in patients with Hodgkin's disease, cutaneous anergy may follow temporarily (Kaplan, 1972). Patients who have anergy presumably related to the malignant process will often recover their delayed hypersensitivity response following the irradiation.

Depressions of the peripheral blood count from local irradiation are seen only when the volume irradiated is very large and encompasses a significant portion of the active bone marrow. Irradiation of small areas does not significantly influence white blood count, platelet count, or hematocrit. The assumption that local irradiation is sufficient to cause profound pancytopenia can lead to serious delay in seeking the actual causes.

Nausea and vomiting have been considered by many, patients and physicians alike, a necessary accompaniment of any sort of irradiation. This complicates the task of the radiation oncologist since nausea and vomiting may indeed accompany the irradiation as a function of the suggestibility of the patient. There is undoubtedly a considerable range of individual sensitivity to these occasional side effects of irradiation, but nausea is a likely occurrence only when the stomach or significant portions of the intestine are included within the treatment volume. The irradiation of a very large volume of tissue, even when the gastrointestinal tract is excluded, as with treatment with the "mantle" field, can also result in nausea. Nausea which is truly related to the irradiation for one of the above reasons occurs at the very start of a course of treatment. Again, serious delays in finding the causative factors can occur if one assumes that nausea and vomiting which appear well into or near the end of a course of treatment are related to the irradiation when in fact they are not.

Oncogenic Effects of Ionizing Radiations

As with most powerful agents, ionizing radiations resemble a double-edged sword. As they are capable of selectively destroying malignant cells and sparing normal tissues, they do retain the capacity to result in malignant transformation in normal tissues irradiated. Such occurrences are rare. Analyses of the prior irradiation in a patient who has developed a malignant process within a field previously treated will usually reveal either the use of low quality (poorly penetrating), caustic radiations, multiple courses of irradiation to a single area, or irradiation of an infant or child. Examples of these three influences are multicentric basal cell carcinomas developing in the skin which had dermatologic irradiation for acne, leukemia which developed in patients who received repeated courses of irradiation for ankylosing spondylitis (Court-Brown and Doll, 1957) and carcinomas of the thyroid as well as leukemia developing in children who underwent irradiation of the thymus in the neonatal period (Hemplemann et al., 1967). The survivors of the atomic bombs at Hiroshima and Nagasaki have shown a striking increase in the occurrence of several malignant processes—leukemia (Bizzozero et al., 1966), carcinoma of the thyroid (Socolow et al., 1963), carcinoma of the breast (Wanebo et al., 1968), and malignant salivary gland tumors (Belsky et al., 1972). A greater frequency of each of these neoplasms occurred as a function of higher total body dose. The atomic bomb experience probably relates more to generalized suppression of the immune processes than to specific local oncogenic influences.

Most of the conditions noted above were not associated with treatment of patients for malignant diseases and the practitioners utilizing the radiations were not primarily involved with radiation therapy and thus were unaware of the potential consequences. It is fair to say that the risk of irradiation induced or irradiation associated malignant processes with modern equipment, techniques, and confinement of radiation therapy to the treatment of malignant diseases, is a very low risk indeed, sufficiently low that it should never impede the appropriate administration of ionizing radiations for a potentially lethal condition.

Effects on Malignant Tumors

Certain generalizations can be made with regard to the effects of ionizing radiations on malignant neoplasms, both in laboratory animals and in humans. The responses of the malignant cells to ionizing radiations differ little from the responses of the normal cells. The cells tend to be most sensitive at the corresponding times of the cell cycle. With fractionated irradiation, both undergo intracellular repair of sublethal damage, repopulation as a result of the regeneration of clonogenic cells, redistribution of the cells as a function of their differing sensitivities in different phases of the cell cycle with consequent radiation-induced synchrony, and reoxygenation of hypoxic cells (Fowler, 1972). These phenomena of repair, repopulation, redistribution, and reoxygenation apply to malignant and normal tissues with the exception of the last. Normal tissues are considered to be optimally oxygenated under normal circumstances. Most malignant tumors have a proportion, perhaps one fifth of all cells, in a hypoxic state. This is more compatible for the malignant tissues since anaerobic metabolism is the norm for them. The radioprotective effect of hypoxia is assumed to be a reason for failure of local control of many malignant tumors (Suit, 1969). Fractionated irradiation is thought to destroy tumor cells close to blood vessels, which leads to closer proximity of the hypoxic cells to the vascular supply, which eliminates the hypoxia (Rubin and Casarett, 1966). Although the exact mechanisms are unknown, recovery of normal tissues from fractionated irradiation is greater than for malignant tissues—a fact which is readily demonstrable clinically. Since only normal tissue is spared, perhaps repopulation with migration into areas previously occupied by tumor is the underlying mechanism.

The other principle which is applicable to all malignant tumors is the greater the volume of the tumor, the higher the dose necessary for control. Although this has been assumed for many years, only recently has Shukovsky (1970, 1973) carefully demonstrated that squamous cell carcinomas require higher doses for control of larger tumors. This seems to be the case for most malignant tumors, particularly those which require doses very near the limits of tolerance of the normal tissues. However, this may not be true for very radiosensitive tumors such as those arising from lymphoreticular cells (Cox et al., 1974).

The sensitivities of the various malignant tumors seem to be related primarily to the radiosensitivity of the cell of origin. Although "radiosensitivity" of malignant *cells* is a meaningful term, the application of this term to malignant *gross tumors* is confusing. The confusion arises from equating radiosensitivity with the rapidity of regression of the tumor rather than with the ability to permanently sterilize the tumor. Effects on specific animal tumors are beyond the scope of this discussion and emphasis is better placed on an understanding of the radioresponsiveness of the malignant tumors in man.

CLINICAL APPLICATIONS OF RADIATION ONCOLOGY

It is important to have some definitions of the responses of various malignant cells to ionizing radiations. As just noted, *radiosensitivity* is the ability to eradicate malignant cells permanently at doses within the tolerance of the surrounding normal tissues; it has nothing to do with the rate of regression of the tumor. Radiosensitivity is a necessary, but not sufficient, condition for *radiocurability*. The latter can be achieved when sufficiently radiosensitive malignant cells are encompassed within a reasonable volume and are carried to dose levels which permanently eradicated them. The rate of regression of a malignant tumor is best termed its *radioresponsiveness*. Table 3.4 shows the interrelationships of radiosensitivity, radioresponsiveness, and radiocurability for a variety of malignant processes.

The degree of differentiation of the malignant cells can influence radioresponsiveness and profoundly influences the radiocurability. For many malignant tumors, the propensity to invade and metastasize is clearly correlated with the tumor grade; prime examples are adenocarcinomas of the breast and transitional cell carcinomas of the bladder (Bloom, 1965). A tumor which has spread beyond the irradiated volume will not be radiocurable. Therefore, the greater likelihood of invasion and metastasis will be reflected in a reduced cure rate. However, control of disease within the treated volume, in general, is not dependent upon tumor grade. An obvious exception to this is the radiocurability, or lack thereof, of malignant gliomas. The highly undifferentiated glioblastoma multiforme is much less radioresponsive and radiocurable than the more intermediate grade astrocytomas (Bouchard, 1966) (one of many exceptions to the law of Bergonié and Tribondeau). Another exception, and one where the greater radiosensitivity is associated with less differentiation, is the greater ability to achieve local control of lymphoepitheliomas of the nasopharynx as compared to the more differentiated squamous cell carcinomas (Chen and Fletcher, 1971). Although cytologic studies have suggested that prognosis following irradiation is correlated with specific histologic patterns of cancer of the cervix (Wentz and Lewis, 1965), this has not been confirmed in institutions where higher control rates have been obtained (Gunderson et al., 1974). All too frequently tumor grade and radiocurability have been related by assessing survival data following radiation therapy rather than evaluating local control. The survival data

TABLE 3.4
Radiation Interrelationships for Malignant Diseases

Disease	Radio-sensitivity	Radio-responsiveness	Radio-curability
Squamous cell carcinoma*	+++	++	+++
Adenocarcinoma*	+++	+	++
Hodgkin's disease	++++	+++	+++
Embryonal carcinoma	+++	++	++
Seminoma	++++	++++	++++
Lymphoreticular (nodular)	++++	++++	+++
Lymphoreticular (diffuse)*	++++	+++	++
Soft tissue sarcoma	++	+	++
Ewing's sarcoma	+++	++	+
Glioblastoma	±	+	±
Osteosarcoma	±	+	±
Small cell carcinoma (lung)	+++	++++	±

* Considerable difference in radiocurability depending on site of origin.

often simply reflect the greater propensity for the poorly differentiated tumor to invade and disseminate and do not reflect the ability to control the portion of disease actually irradiated. In general, as Fletcher (1973) has noted, there is probably little, if any, inherent difference in radiosensitivity for any of the epithelial tumors.

For many years, the basic determinant of total dose was the tolerance of the surrounding normal tissues, especially the skin. With the skin-sparing of the supervoltage irradiation, greater attention has been focused on the depth and distribution of dose correlated with permanent eradication of the disease. It is now apparent that tumor control probability for epithelial tumors is profoundly affected by small changes in time-dose relationships (Shukovsky, 1971, 1973), and the size of the tumor influences greatly the dose necessary to achieve a high probability of control (Fletcher, 1973).

While the time-dose relationships are of great importance for the control of epithelial tumors, the time factor seems much less significant in the treatment of very radiosensitive tumors (Hodgkin's disease, the malignant lymphoreticular tumors, seminoma, Wilms' tumor, neuroblastoma, retinoblastoma). It has been shown that the total dose seems to be a much more important determinant in the control of Hodgkin's disease (Fischer and Fischer, 1971; Johnson, et al., 1971) and nodular and diffuse malignant lymphoreticular tumors (Cox et al., 1974), while the number of fractions and the time in which the dose is delivered are of much less importance (Fig. 3.4). Since deleterious effects on normal tissues are related not just to dose, but to fractionation and time (Ellis, 1968), a much greater margin of safety attends more fractionated irradiation delivered over a longer time.

Evaluation of the effectiveness of irradiation can only be made on the basis of success or failure of *local control* of malignant disease within the irradiated volume. Although this seems obvious, effectiveness has usually been based upon survival alone. For example, Stage I squamous cell carcinoma of the cervix is controlled locally by careful radiation therapy over 95% of the time. Five-year disease-free survival rates for this disease are also of the order of 90%. By contrast, local control of disease can also be achieved in approximately 95% of patients with Stage II carcinoma of the cervix (Fletcher, 1971), but the survival rate is substantially lower. This does not reflect inability of irradiation to control the disease which it encompasses, but reflects the propensity for the more advanced cervical tumors to spread to lymph nodes and organs beyond the volume irradiated.

The only measure of failure of local control, i.e., true recurrence, is regrowth of tumor within the irradiated volume. This requires careful

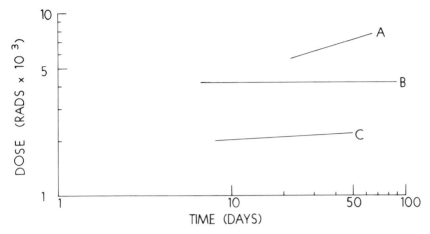

F<small>IG</small>. 3.4. Comparison of isoeffect (recurrence exclusion) *Curves*: epithelial vs. malignant lymphoreticular tumors. (*A*) Squamous cell carcinoma (Shukovsky and Fletcher, 1973). (*B*) Diffuse malignant lymphoreticular (non-Hodgkin's lymphoma) (Cox et al., 1974). (*C*) Nodular malignant lymphoreticular (non-Hodgkin's lymphoma) (Cox et al., 1974).

evaluation of the patient over months and years, but attempts to predict failure of local control by other means have been unsuccessful. The rate of regression of a tumor and, consequently, the extent of residual tumor at the completion of irradiation have been evaluated both in animals and man and have not proved to correlate with ultimate control of disease (Suit et al., 1965; Fazekas et al., 1972). Suggestions that postirradiation biopsies would help were based on the expectation that "viability" could be assessed histologically. This, too, has proved to be incorrect in that histologically intact tumor cells within the irradiated volume have been shown to have no significance (Suit and Gallager, 1964; Cox and Stoffel, 1977), unless associated with clinical evidence of regrowth.

Radiation therapy is appropriately used as the sole means of treatment in clinical circumstances where the local control rate is very high, and the likelihood of encompassing all known or suspected disease within a reasonable volume is also high. The list of examples is too long to be enumerated but includes all invasive carcinomas of the cervix (Fletcher, 1971), larynx (Stages I and II) (Bataini et al., 1971), tonsillar fossa (Shukovsky and Fletcher, 1973), anterior two-thirds of the tongue and the floor of the mouth (Pierquin et al., 1971; Fayos and Lampe, 1972), Hodgkin's disease (Stages I, II, and III) (Kaplan, 1972), and the nodular (Stages I, II, and III) and diffuse (Stages I and II) non-Hodgkin's malignant lymphoid tumors (Cox et al., 1974).

Sequential use of radiation therapy and surgery has an important place in the management of many malignant tumors. The modalities can be used to attack different portions of the disease as when radical orchiectomy is followed by irradiation to the inguinal and para-aortic lymph nodes for testicular tumors, or when irradiation is used for the primary tumor in carcinoma of the anterior tongue or floor of the mouth and radical neck dissection is used to control cervical lymph node metastases. Postoperative irradiation can also be used to reduce the risk of local or regional recurrence, e.g., following mastectomy (Fisher et al., 1970) and following a radical neck dissection (Fletcher, et al., 1973).

Preoperative irradiation has an established place in the treatment of malignant diseases where failure of local control by operation alone is significant and such failure is a major determinant of survival. Preoperative irradiation is founded upon the ability of modest doses of ionizing radiations to eradicate microscopic extensions of the disease at the margins of surgical dissection or beyond, to injure malignant cells which might be disseminated via lymphatics or the blood stream at the time of the operation, and thereby reduce regional and distant metastases. The theroretical advantages of preoperative irradiation (Nias, 1967; Powers and Palmer, 1968), have been confirmed in a variety of clinical circumstances. Local recurrences have been reduced in carcinomas of the endometrium (Moss, et al., 1973) and rectum (Allen and Fletcher, 1972), and in advanced carcinomas of the larynx and laryngopharynx (Goldman et al., 1972). Regional lymph node metastases have been reduced by preoperative irradiation of cancer of the rectum (Higgins and Dwight, 1972). Irradiated cells have been shown experimentally to have a decreased capacity to establish themselves in distant sites (Hoye and Smith, 1961; Smith and Godbee, 1968) and this has undoubtedly contributed to improved survival in patients irradiated preoperatively for carcinoma of the rectum (Roswit et al., 1973).

It may be argued that postoperative irradiation can be used as effectively as preoperative irradiation and has the advantage of permitting a more accurate pathologic staging. However, to achieve the desired effect of reducing local recurrences, a higher dose of irradiation is necessary when given postoperatively (Perez and Olson, 1970). This is likely to result in an increased complication rate in some locations, for example the pelvis (Schier et al., 1964), but the higher postoperative dose may be better tolerated in other locations (Fletcher et al., 1973). There cannot, of course, be any hope of reduced viability of cells disseminated at the time of the operation if the irradiation is given postoperatively. The importance of this reduced viability has recently been confirmed by the demonstration that patients with carcinomas of the upper respiratory and digestive tract have significantly fewer distant metastases after preoperative irradiation compared with postoperative irradiation, in spite of similar local control rates (Merino et al., 1977).

The all too frequent practice of waiting until local recurrences have appeared clinically and then using irradiation with the hope of control is quite disadvantageous. Although the reasons are poorly understood, irradiation for postoperative recurrence is relatively ineffective, while operations for postirradiation recurrences may be remarkably effective (Crews and Fletcher, 1971).

In recent years, there has been increasing interest in the combined use of cytotoxic drugs with irradiation and/or surgery. Much of the interest among radiation oncologists came from laboratory studies that suggested a variety of drugs might potentiate the effect of ionizing radiations on cells (Vermund and Gollin, 1968). Attempts to exploit the combined effects clinically have not yet met with much success. The initial enthusiasm brought about by apparent clinical effectiveness of combinations of radiation therapy and chemotherapy have subsequently given way to questioning and lack of confirmation by controlled clinical trials. For example, the remarkable improvement in ability to control retinoblastoma was long attributed to the combination of irradiation and intra-arterial triethyline melamine (TEM) (Reese, 1963). The necessity of using the drug was subsequently questioned (Tapley, 1964) and further studies failed to show any advantage of adding TEM to the irradiation (Cassady et al., 1969).

There is evidence, however, that small cell carcinoma of the lung may be controlled with lower doses when irradiated in conjunction with combination chemotherapy (Cox et al., 1978).

Current interest is less in the potentiation of irradiation and more in the early treatment of disseminated cells. For example, the treatment of Wilms' tumor in most centers involves the combination of nephrectomy for diagnosis and treatment of the primary tumor, radiation therapy for regional spread, and systemic chemotherapy from the day of operation for many months or years with the idea of "prevention" or early treatment of metastases (Farber, 1966). However, results from several centers have led to questions of the necessity of systematically using the cytotoxic agents, particularly actinomycin D (Jereb and Eklund, 1973; Maier and Aarestad, 1969; Stone and Williams, 1969). It seems apparent that metastases are not "prevented" with any consistency by the addition of actinomycin D. However, remarkable improvement in overall survival has resulted from combined treatment of pulmonary metastases from Wilms' tumor with actinomycin D and irradiation (Cassady et al., 1973).

It is essential to establish the role of combination regimens by randomized studies. Such studies have indeed confirmed the advantage of pro-phylactic irradiation of sanctuary areas, especially the central nervous system, of patients in remission from acute lymphocytic leukemia (Pinkel, 1971; Simone et al., 1972).

FUTURE DEVELOPMENTS

The progress of radiation therapy within the past 20 years and the increasing awareness of its applicability with curative intent to a wide variety of malignant diseases has been rapid. The pace of this develop-ment does not seem likely to slacken for many more years. A considerable amount of work is underway with the currently available x- and gamma-ray units to investigate different approaches to irradiation such as altered fractionation (Schlienger et al., 1968; Abramson and Cavanaugh, 1973), and alterations of the rate at which the radiations are delivered both at the very high dose (Hall, 1972) and very low dose (Pierquin and Baillet, 1971) ends of the spectrum. Radiation sensitizers that are not cytotoxic, such as oxygen and chloroquin (Kim et al., 1973), and electron affinic hypoxic cell sensitizers such as the nitrofurans and nitroimidazoles (Whit-more, 1975; Chapman and Urtasun, 1977) are being investigated in attempts to increase the ability to control marginally radiosensitive tumors. Similarly, radiation protectors, such as the thiophosphate com-pounds (Phillips et al., 1973) and heparin (Kinzie et al., 1972) will hopefully increase the tolerance of normal tissues and improve the therapeutic ratio. Hyperthermia has antitumor properties and is being studied as a radiosensitizer (Dewey et al., 1977). Satisfactory means of producing local hyperthermia and the distribution of heat within an irradiated volume require much more development and critical analysis (Conner et al., 1977).

High LET (linear energy transfer) radiations which deposit great amounts of energy per unit length in traversing biologic material are under investigation in several parts of the world. In fact, neutron radiation therapy is being evaluated in Phase II and Phase III studies at several cyclotron facilities in the United States and Europe. Irradiation with neutrons clearly has increased biologic effectiveness and a reduced OER, and therefore, should be more effective in marginally radioresponsive tumors especially where central hypoxia is felt to be a cause of decreased sensitivity. Other heavy particle accelerators are being developed which will offer possibilities of irradiation with negative pi mesons (Kaplan et al., 1973) and protons (Archambeau et al., 1974).

Combinations of cytotoxic drugs and irradiation and, in turn, their combination with operations are actively being investigated and seem fruitful in many areas. However, assumptions as to the efficacy of the combinations are not justified, nor is the use of historical controls. Many of the advances that might be attributed to adding chemotherapy to an operation or radiation therapy may, in part, be attributable to changes of the radiotherapeutic or surgical approaches themselves. In any case, the full impact of a truly multidisciplinary approach to malignant diseases has barely begun to be felt. As diseases which were long considered incurable gradually fall to the dedicated efforts of investigators in all fields of oncology, competitive approaches will give way to cooperative ones as superior results provide irresistible justification.

REFERENCES

Abramson, N., and Cavanaugh, P. J. Short-course radiation therapy in carcinoma of the lung; a second look. Radiology, 108: 685–687, 1973.

Allen, C. V., and Fletcher, W. S. A pilot study on preoperative irradiation of rectosigmoid carcinoma. A.J.R., 114: 504–508, 1972.

Archambeau, J. O., Bennett, G. W., Levine, G. S., Cowen, R., and Akanuma, A. Proton radiation therapy. Radiology, 110: 445–457, 1974.

Baker, D. G., and Mitchell, R. I. Studies of the intestine during acute radiation syndrome. Gastroenterology, 44: 291–300, 1963.

Bataini, J.-P., Ennuyer, A., and Poncet, P. Télécobaltothérapie du cancer du larynx, à propos de 289 malades traités à la Fondation Curie de 1958 à 1965. Ann. Otolaryngol. (Paris), 88: 555–568, 1971.

Belsky, J. L., Tachikawa, K., Cihak, R. W., and Yamamoto, T. Salivary gland tumors in atomic bomb survivors, Hiroshima-Nagasaki, 1957 to 1960. J.A.M.A., 219: 864–868, 1972.

Bergonié, J., and Tribondeau, L. Interprétation de quelques résultats de la radiothérapie et éssai de fixation d'une technique rationelle. C. R. Acad. Sci. (Paris) 143: 983–985, 1906.

Bizzozero, O. J., Jr., Johnson, K. G., and Ciocco, A. Radiation-related leukemia in Hiroshima and Nagasaki, 1946–1964; I. Distribution, incidence and appearance time. N. Engl. J. Med., 274: 1095–1101, 1966.

Bloom, H. J. G. The influence of tumour grade on radiotherapy results. Br. J. Radiol., 38: 227–240, 1965.

Bouchard, J. Radiation Therapy of Tumors and Diseases of the Nervous System. Lea & Febiger, Philadelphia, 1966.

Cade, I. S., and McEwen, J. B. Megavoltage radiotherapy in hyperbaric oxygen; a controlled trial. Cancer, 20: 817–821, 1967.

Cantril, S. T. The contributions of biology to radiation therapy. A.J.R. 78: 751–768, 1957.

Cassady, J. R., Sagerman, R. H., Tretter, P., and Ellsworth, R. M. Radiation therapy in retinoblastoma; an analysis of 230 cases. Radiology, 93: 405–409, 1969.

Cassady, J. R., Tefft, M., Filler, R. M., Jaffe, N., Paed, D., and Hellman, S. Considerations in the radiation therapy of Wilms' tumor. Cancer, 32: 598–608, 1973.

Chapman, J. D., and Urtasun, R. C. The application in radiation therapy of substances which modify cellular radiation response. Cancer, 40: 484–488, 1977.

Chen, K. Y., and Fletcher, G. H. Malignant tumors of the nasopharynx. Radiology, 99: 165–171, 1971.

Connor, W. G., Gerner, E. W., Miller, R. C., and Boone, M. L. M. Prospects for hyperthermia in human cancer therapy. Radiology, 123: 497–503, 1977.

Court-Brown, W. M., and Doll, R. Leukemia and aplastic anemias in ankylosing spondylitis. Medical Research Council, Report 295. Her Majesty's Stationery Office, London, 1957.

Cox, J. D., Gingerelli, F., Ream, N. W., and Maier, J. G. Total pulmonary irradiation for metastases from testicular carcinoma. Radiology, 105: 163–167, 1972.

Cox, J. D., Koehl, R. H., Turner, W. M., and King. F. M. Irradiation in the local control of malignant lymphoreticular tumors (non-Hodgkin's malignant lymphoma). Radiology, *112:* 179–185, 1974.

Cox, J. D., and Stoffel, T. J. The significance of needle biopsy after irradiation for stage C adenocarcinoma of the prostate. Cancer, *40:* 156–160, 1977.

Cox, J. D., Byhardt, R., Wilson, J. F., Eisert, D. R., Greenberg, M., and Komaki, R. Dose-time relationships in the local control of small cell carcinoma of the lung. Radiology, *128:* 205–207, 1978.

Crews, Q. E., and Fletcher, G. H. Comparative evaluation of the sequential use of irradiation and surgery in primary tumors of the oral cavity, oropharynx, larynx and hypopharynx. A.J.R., *111:* 73–77, 1971.

Dewey, W. C., Hopwood, L. E., Sapareto, S. A., and Gerweck, L. E. Cellular responses to combinations of hyperthermia and radiation. Radiology, *123:* 463–474, 1977.

Elkind, M. M. Cellular aspects of tumor therapy. Radiology, *74:* 529–541, 1960.

Ellis, F. The relationship of biological effect to dose-time-fractionation factors in radiotherapy. *In* Current Topics in Radiation Research, edited by M. Ebert and P. Howard, Vol. 4, pp. 359–399. North Holland Publishing Co., Amsterdam, 1968.

Ellis, R. E. The distribution of active bone marrow in the adult. Phys. Med. Biol., *5:* 255–258, 1960.

von Essen, C. F. A spatial model of time-dose-area relationships in radiation therapy. Radiology, *81:* 881–883, 1963.

Farber, S. Chemotherapy in the treatment of leukemia and Wilms' tumor. J.A.M.A., *198:* 826–836, 1966.

Fayos, J. V., and Lampe, I. Treatment of squamous cell carcinoma of the oral cavity. Am. J. Surg., *124:* 493–500, 1972.

Fazekas, J. T., Green, J. P., Vaeth, J. M., and Schroeder, A. F. Postirradiation induration as a prognosticator; a retrospective analysis of squamous-cell carcinomas of the oral cavity and oropharynx. Radiology, *102:* 409–412, 1972.

Fischer, J. J., and Fischer, D. B. The determination of time-dose relationships from clinical data. Br. J. Radiol., *44:* 785–792, 1971.

Fisher, B., Slack, N. H., Cavanaugh, P. J., Gardner, B., and Ravdin, R. G. Postoperative radiotherapy in the treatment of breast cancer; results of the NSABP trial. Ann. Surg., *172:* 711–732, 1970.

Fletcher, G. H. Cancer of the uterine cervix; Janeway Lecture, 1970. A.J.R., *111:* 225–242, 1971.

Fletcher, G. H. Clinical dose-response curves of human malignant epithelial tumours. Br. J. Radiol., *46:* 1–12, 1973.

Fletcher, G. H., Jesse, R. H., Jr., and Westbrook, K. C. Interaction of surgery and irradiation in head and neck cancers. *In* Textbook of Radiotherapy, edited G. H. Fletcher, pp.166–173. Lea & Febiger, Philadelphia, 1973.

Fowler, J. F. Current aspects of radiobiology as applied to radiotherapy. Clin. Radiol., *23:* 257–262, 1972.

Goldgraber, M. B., Rubin, C. E., Palmer, W. L., Dobson, R. L., and Massey, B. W. The early gastric response to irradiation, a serial biopsy study. Gastroenterology, *27:* 1–20, 1954.

Goldman, J. L., Zak, F. G., Roffman, J. D., and Birken, E. A. High dosage preoperative radiation and surgery for carcinoma of the larynx and laryngopharynx. Ann. Otol. Rhinol. Laryngol., *81:* 488–495, 1972.

Goswitz, F. A., Andrews, G. A., and Kniseley, R. M. Effects of local irradiation (Co^{60} teletherapy) on the peripheral blood and bone marrow. Blood, *21:* 605–619, 1963.

Gross, L., Manfredi, O. L., and Protos, A. A. Effect of cobalt-60 irradiation upon cell-mediated immunity. Radiology, *106:* 653–655, 1973.

Gunderson, L. L., Weems, W. S., Hebertson, R. M., and Plenk, H. P. Correlation of histopathology with clinical results following radiation therapy for carcinoma of the cervix. A.J.R., *120:* 74–87, 1974.

Hall, E. J. Radiation dose-rate; a factor of importance in radiobiology and radiotherapy. Br. J. Radiol., *45:* 81–97, 1972.

Harris, J. E., and Sinkovics, J. G. The Immunology of Malignant Disease. C. V. Mosby, St. Louis, 1970.

Hempelmann, L. H., Pifer, J. W., Burke, G. J., Terry, R., and Ames, W. R. Neoplasms in persons treated with x-rays in infancy for thymic enlargement; a report of the third follow-up survey. J. Natl. Cancer Inst., *38:* 317–341, 1967.

Higgins, G. A., and Dwight, R. W. The role of preoperative irradiation in cancer of the rectum and rectosigmoid. Surg. Clin. North Am., *52:* 847–858, 1972.

Hoye, R. C., and Smith, R. R. The effectiveness of small amounts of preoperative irradiation in preventing the growth of tumor cells disseminated at surgery. Cancer, *14:* 284–295, 1961.

Ingold, J. A., Reed, G. B., Kaplan, H. S., and Bagshaw, M. A. Radiation hepatitis. A.J.R., *93:* 200–208, 1965.

Jereb, B., and Eklund, G. Factors influencing the cure rate in nephroblastoma; a review of 335 cases. Acta Radiol. (Ther.), *12:* 84–106, 1973.

Johnson, R. E., Glover, M. K., and Marshall, S. K. Results of radiation therapy and implications for the clinical staging of Hodgkin's disease. Cancer Res., *31:* 1834–1837, 1971.

Kallman, R. F. Evidence for cyclic fluctuations in radiosensitivity and the implications. Natl. Cancer Inst. Monogr., *24:* 205–223, 1967.

Kaplan, H. S.: Biochemical basis of reproductive death in irradiated cells. A.J.R. *90:* 907–916, 1963.

Kaplan, H. S. Hodgkin's Disease, pp. 184–195. Harvard University Press, Cambridge, Mass., 1972.

Kaplan, H. S., Schwettman, H. A., Fairbank, W. M., Boyd, D., and Bagshaw, M. A. A hospital-based superconducting accelerator facility for negative pi-meson beam radiotherapy. Radiology, *108:* 159–172, 1973.

Kim, S. H., Kim, J. H., and Fried, J. Enhancement of the radiation response of cultured tumor cells by chloroquine. Cancer, *32:* 536–540, 1973.

Kinzie, J. J., Studer, R. K., Perez, B., and Potchen, E. J. Noncytokinetic radiation injury; anticoagulants as radioactive agents in experimental radiation hepatitis. Science, *175:* 1481–1483, 1972.

Knospe, W. H., Blom, J., and Crosby, W. H. Regeneration of locally irradiation bone marrow; II. Induction of regeneration in permanently aplastic medullary cavities. Blood, *31:* 400–405, 1968.

Lacassagne, A., and Gricouroff, G. Action of Radiation on Tissues; An Introduction to Radiotherapy, Ed. 2. Grune & Stratton, New York, 1958.

Maier, J. G. Effects of radiations on kidney, bladder and prostate. Front. Radiat. Ther. Oncol., *6:* 196–227, 1972.

Maier, J. G., and Aarestad, N. O. Concepts in the treatment of Wilms' tumor. Front. Radiat. Ther. Oncol., *4:* 187–194, 1969.

Merino, O. R., Lindberg, R. D., and Fletcher, G. H. An analysis of distant metastases from squamous cell carcinoma of the upper respiratory and digestive tracts. Cancer, *40:* 145–151, 1977.

Merriam, G. R., Jr., and Focht, E. F. A clinical study of radiation cataracts and the relationship to dose. A.J.R., *77:* 759–785, 1957.

Merriam, G. R., Jr., Szechter, A., and Focht, E. F. The effects of ionizing radiations on the eye. Front. Radiat. Ther. Oncol., *6:* 346–385, 1972.

Moss, W. T., Brand, W. N., and Battifora, H. Radiation Oncology: Rationale, Technique, Results, Ed. 4. C. V. Mosby, St. Louis, 1973.

Mostofi, F. K. Radiation Effects on the Kidney, Edited by F. K. Mostofi, and D. E. Smith, pp. 338–386. Williams & Wilkins, Baltimore, 1966.

Nias, A. H. W. Radiobiological aspects of pre-operative irradiation. Br. J. Radiol., 40: 166–169, 1967.

Ogata, K., Hizawa, K., Yoshida, M., Kitamuro, T., Akagi, G., Kagawa, K., and Fukada, F. Hepatic injury following irradiation; a morphologic study. Tokushima J. Exp. Med., 9: 240–251, 1963.

Orton, C. G., and Ellis, F. A simplification in the use of the NSD concept in practical radiotherapy. Br. J. Radiol., 46: 529–537, 1973.

Perez, C. A., and Olson, J. Preoperative vs. postoperative irradiation; comparison in an experimental animal tumor system. A.J.R., 108: 396–404, 1970.

Phillips, T. L., Kane, L. K., and Utley, J. F. Radioprotection of tumor and normal tissues by thiophosphate compounds. Cancer, 32: 528–535, 1973.

Pierquin, B., and Baillet, F. La téléradiothérapie continue et de faible débit: rapport préliminaire (neuf premières observations). Ann. Radiol., 14: 617–629, 1971.

Pierquin, B., Chassagne, D., Cachin, Y., Baillet, F., and Fournelle le Buis, F. Carcinomes épidermoides de la langue mobile et du plancher buccal; étude de 245 cas traités à l'Institut Gustave-Roussy. Acta Radiol. (Ther.), 9: 465–480, 1970.

Pierquin, B., Chassagne, D., and Cox, J. D. Toward consistent local control of certain malignant tumors. Radiology, 99: 661–667, 1971.

Pinkel, D. Five-year follow-up of "total therapy" of childhood lymphocytic leukemia. J.A.M.A., 216: 648–652, 1971.

Powers, W. E., and Palmer, L. A. Biologic basis of preoperative radiation treatment. A.J.R., 102: 176–192, 1968.

Probert, J. C., Parker, B. R., and Kaplan, H. S. Growth retardation in children after megavoltage irradiation of the spine. Cancer, 32: 634–639, 1973.

Puck, T. T., and Marcus, P. J. Action of x-rays on mammalian cells. J. Exp. Med., 103: 653–666, 1956.

Reed, G. B., and Cox, A. J., Jr. The human liver after radiation injury; a form of veno-occlusive disease. Am. J. Pathol., 48: 597–608, 1966.

Reese, A. B. Tumors of the Eye, Ed. 2. Harper & Row, New York, 1963.

del Regato, J. A. Dental lesions observed after roentgen therapy in cancer of the buccal cavity, pharynx and larynx. A.J.R., 42: 404–410, 1939.

del Regato, J. A. Total body irradiation in the treatment of chronic lymphogenous leukemia. A.J.R., 120: 504–520, 1974.

Regaud, C. Influence de la durée de l'irradiation sur les effets déterminés dans le testicule par le radium. C. R. Soc. Biol., 86: 787–790, 1922.

Regaud, C., Coutard, H., and Hautant, A. Contribution au traitement des cancers endolaryngés par les rayons-x. X Congr. Internat. d'Otol. pp. 19–22, 1922.

Reinhold, H. S. Radiations and the microcirculation. Front. Radiat. Ther. Oncol., 6: 44–56, 1972.

Roswit, B., Higgins, G. A., Humphrey, E. W., and Robinette, C. D. Preoperative irradiation of operable adenocarcinoma of the rectum and rectosigmoid colon. Radiology, 108: 389–395, 1973.

Roswit, B., Malsky, S. J., and Reid, C. B. Severe radiation injuries of the stomach, small intestine, colon and rectum. A.J.R., 114: 460–475, 1972.

Rubin, P., and Casarett, G. Microcirculation of tumors; II. The supervascularized state of irradiated regressing tumors. Clin. Radiol., 17: 346–355, 1966.

Rubin, P., and Casarett, G. W. Clinical Radiation Pathology. W. B. Saunders, Philadelphia, 1968.

Rubin, P., and Casarett, G. A direction for clinical radiation pathology; the tolerance dose. Front. Radiat. Ther. Oncol., 6: 1–16, 1972.

Rubin, P., Poulter, C. A., and Quick, R. S. Changing perspectives in oxygen breathing and radiation therapy. A.J.R., *105:* 665–681, 1969.

Russell, W. J., Yoshinaga, H., Antoku, S., and Mizuno, M. Active bone marrow distribution in the adult. Br. J. Radiol., *39:* 735–739, 1966.

Schier, J., Symmonds, R. E., and Dahlin, D. C. Clinicopathologic aspects of actinic enteritis. Surg. Gynecol. Obstet., *119:* 1019–1025, 1964.

Schlienger, M., Parmentier, C., Laugier, A., Schlumberger, J., Bok, B., Mathé, G., and Tubiana, M. La radiothérapie splenique dans le traitement des leucemies lymphocytaires chroniques, ses analogies avec l'irradiation extra-corporelle. Nouv. Rev. Fr. Hematol., *8:* 719–732, 1968.

Sherman, J. O., and O'Brien, P. H. Effect of ionizing irradiation on normal lymphatic vessels and lymph nodes. Cancer, *20:* 1851–1858, 1967.

Shukovsky, L. J. Dose, time, volume relationships in squamous cell carcinoma of the supraglottic larynx. A.J.R., *108:* 27–29, 1970.

Shukovsky, L. J., and Fletcher, G. H. Time-dose and tumor volume relationships in the irradiation of squamous cell carcinoma of the tonsillar fossa. Radiology, *107:* 621–626, 1973.

Simone, J., Aur, R. J. A., Hustu, H. O., and Pinkel, D. "Total therapy" studies of acute lymphocytic leukemia in children; current results and prospects for cure. Cancer, *30:* 1488–1494, 1972.

Smith, R. R., and Godbee, G. A. Alteration of tumor cell implantability by preoperative irradiation. *In* Cancer Therapy by Integrated Radiation and Operation, edited by B. F. Rush and R. H. Greenlaw, pp. 20–27. Charles C Thomas, Springfield, Ill., 1968.

Socolow, E. L., Hashizume, A., Neriishi, S., and Niitani, R. Thyroid carcinoma in man after exposure to ionizing radiation; a summary of the findings in Hiroshima and Nagasaki. N. Engl. J. Med., *268:* 406–410, 1963.

Stone, J., and Williams, I. G. The treatment of Wilms' tumour with special reference to actinomycin D. Clin. Radiol., *20:* 40–46, 1969.

Strandqvist, M. Studien über die kumulative Wirkung der Röntgenstrahlung bei Fraktionierung. Acta Radiol. (Suppl. 55), pp. 1–293, 1944.

Strockbine, M. F., Hancock, J. E., and Fletcher, G. H. Complications in 831 patients with squamous cell carcinoma of the intact uterine cervix treated with 3,000 rads or more whole pelvis irradiation. A.J.R., *108:* 293–304, 1970.

Suit, H. D. Statement of the problem pertaining to the effect of dose fractionation and total treatment time on response of tissue to x-irradiation. *In* Time and Dose Relationships in Radiation Biology as Applied to Radiotherapy, pp. vii–x. Brookhaven National Laboratory Report BNL 50203 (C-57), 1969.

Suit, H. D., and Gallager, H. S. Intact tumor cells in irradiated tissue. Arch. Pathol., *78:* 648–651, 1964.

Suit, H. D., Lindberg, R., and Fletcher, G. H. Prognostic significance of extent of tumor regression at completion of radiation therapy. Radiology, *84:* 1100–1107, 1965.

Tapley, N., duV. The treatment of bilateral retinoblastoma with radiation and chemotherapy. *In* Ocular and Adnexal Tumors, edited by M. Boniuk, pp. 158–170. C. V. Mosby, St. Louis, 1964.

Tubiana, M., and Frindel, E. Les radiosensibilisateurs et les méthodes permettant d'augmenter la radiosensibilité. Biol. Med., *54:* 493–511, 1965.

Vaeth, J. M. (ed.) Radiation effect on tolerance, normal tissue. In Frontiers in Radiation Therapy and Oncology, Vol. 6, pp. 1–526. University Park Press, Baltimore, 1972.

Van den Brenk, H. A. S. Hyperbaric oxygen in radiation therapy; an investigation of dose-effect relationships in tumor response and tissue damage. A.J.R., *102:* 8–26, 1968.

Vermund, H., and Gollin, F. F. Mechanisms of action of radiotherapy and chemotherapeutic adjuvants; a review. Cancer, *21:* 58–76, 1968.

Wanebo, C. K., Johnson, K. G., Sato, K., and Thorslund, T. W. Breast cancer after exposure to the atomic bombings of Hiroshima and Nagasaki. N. Engl. J. Med., *279:* 667–671, 1968.

Wentz, W. B., and Lewis, G. C. Correlation of histologic morphology and survival in cervical cancer following radiation therapy. Obstet. Gynecol., *26:* 228–232, 1965.

Wharton, J. T., Delclos, L. Gallager, S., and Smith, J. P. Radiation hepatitis induced by abdominal irradiation with the cobalt-60 moving strip technique. A.J.R., *117:* 73–80, 1973.

Whitmore, G. F. The potential for radiation sensitizers and possible strategy for use. Laryngoscope, *85:* 1145–1154, 1975.

Whitmore, G. F., and Gulyas, S. Studies on recovery processes in mouse L cells. Natl. Cancer Inst. Monogr., *24:* 141–156, 1967.

Chapter 4

Chemotherapeutic Principles

Therapeutic Concepts

DOUGLASS C. TORMEY, M.D., Ph.D., and JOHANNES BLOM, M.D.

The kinetic principles of animal and human tumors have been extrapolated to arrive at the clinical definitions as depicted in Figure 4.1. The ordinate of the graph is the log of the number of tumor cells present; in clinical terms this is usually expressed as a measure of the volume of the tumor mass. The abscissa is in arbitrary units of time. The curve begins with the size of a mass at the time that it is first measured clinically, approximately 10^{10}–10^{12} cells.

The percent change in tumor measurements is ideally related to the actual number of cells in the tumor. This can be approximated only if the lesions can be measured in more than one plane; however, it can be estimated from cross sectional measurements in one plane. The volume of the mass can be crudely calculated from these measurements by assuming that the lesion is an oblate spheroid. The number of cells present in the lesion is usually approximated by assuming that 1 cc of tumor mass contains 10^9 cells. Relating all known tumor volumes to cell numbers gives an estimate of the host's tumor burden. In practice tumor size is usually estimated by multiplying the largest two-dimensional measurements of the lesion. The measurements utilized would be the longest diameter of the lesion and its greatest perpendicular diameter. Percent changes from the baseline volume are then used as a measure of the effect of therapy. When a therapeutic response is achieved the minimum tumor measurements obtained are used as a new baseline for subsequent calculation, especially with relation to determining when progressive disease occurs. Accordingly, a patient who relapses during close follow-up may have fewer tumor cells present than when therapy was first initiated.

The "induction" course of therapy is designed to achieve complete

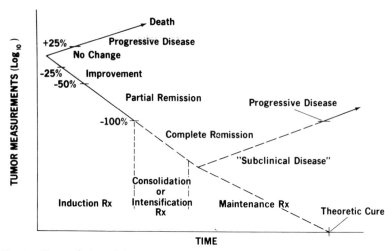

FIG. 4.1. Extrapolation of clinical definitions to tumor kinetics. See text for discussion. R_x = therapy.

clinical remission and is usually the most intensive and, potentially, the most immediately life-threatening phase of therapy. As can be seen from the graph there is considerable subclinical disease at the end of the induction phase of therapy, approximately 10^6–10^8 cells at the start of a complete remission. The patient is given "consolidation" or "intensification" courses of therapy in an attempt to further reduce the host's tumor burden. The consolidation courses may entail the same drugs used during induction, the same drugs with others added, or a completely different set of drugs. Because patients in complete remission are in better overall health, the intensification phase is usually associated with less morbidity and considerably less mortality than is the induction phase. Ideally, the consolidation phase should be continued to theoretic cure (0.01–0.001 cells) (Skipper et al., 1964); at present, this is not usually done. Instead, at a time point determined by "best available data" and/or social/medical reasons, patients are entered into a still-better-tolerated maintenance program. Many maintenance programs have intermittent reinduction or reinforcement "pulses" with the drugs used during the induction and/or consolidation phases. Many current induction and maintenance programs employ "intermittent therapy," i.e., 1 or 2 weeks of therapy followed by a 2–4-week rest. The strategy in these programs is to attempt to allow the immune response to be reactivated during the rest period to help eliminate the tumor and decrease the risk of infection (Hersh and Oppenheim, 1967; Hersh et al., 1966a, b). Such "release" of the immunologic capability of the host apparently does not occur with daily or weekly "continuous" therapy.

The above principles of therapy have been shown to be highly useful in large cooperative group studies in the acute leukemias, non-Hodgkin's lymphomas, and Hodgkin's disease. They are now being extended to certain solid tumors as we learn how to intertwine the enlarging armamentarium of effective chemotherapeutic drugs with cell kinetic and biochemical principles.

It appears that the probability of achieving a response in a given patient decreases with each subsequent relapse or with each therapeutic trial that fails. Since the survival of responders is usually better than that of nonresponders, it is generally advisable to use a maximally tolerated therapeutic approach to try to achieve a complete remission. For example, in carcinoma of the colon the median survival was shown to be 20 months in patients who responded to therapy and only 10 months in their nonresponding counterparts (Moertel and Reitemeier, 1969). Similarly, in carcinoma of the breast the responding patients experienced a 13-month median survival, whereas their nonresponding counterparts survived only 6 months (Stutz et al., 1974). The median survival in Stages III and IV ovarian carcinoma is reported to be 22 months in responders and only 8 months in nonresponders (Smith and Rutledge, 1970). In those cases in which responders survived only slightly longer than nonresponders the quality of survival is generally improved, i.e., the patient "feels" better and is able to perform better. Patients achieving complete remissions will generally survive longer than those who achieve only a partial response. For these reasons current investigations of the induction phases in diseases such as Hodgkin's disease and breast carcinoma are designed to increase the number of complete responders. At present about 60–80% of patients with Stage IV Hodgkin's disease achieve a complete response and they subsequently do better than the ones who achieve only a partial response (DeVita, 1973; Stutzman and Glidewell, 1973).

The character or quality of life in patients who are in remission is becoming increasingly important as the oncologist's armamentarium and capabilities have expanded. Patients with complete remissions are able to carry on essentially normally except for their visits to the physician. Patients with partial responses or improvements are generally able to perform as well as, and usually better than, before therapy. A drug side effect in most maintenance regimens is seldom prohibitive and is usually manifest as mild leukopenia or thrombocytopenia. The patient need not be unduly concerned about this type of side effect as it seldom interferes with his ability to carry on normally.

The concept of the 5-year cure in cancer has led many to believe that the disease is erradicated if 5 years later there is no evidence of tumor. This may be true in some situations. However, relapses after 5 years are not uncommon in a great many cancers. It should be emphasized to the patient that cancer is much like diabetes mellitus in that it will, in so far as we now know, always need to be observed closely. During each checkup the physician should also bear in mind that a patient who has been treated successfully for a first cancer appears to be at an increased risk of developing a second one.

The Cell Cycle

DOUGLASS C. TORMEY, M.D., Ph.D.

The elucidation of kinetic differences between various normal and cancer tissues is becoming increasingly important in cancer chemotherapy. The information gained from such investigations has led to new concepts in the design of effective multiple drug therapeutic programs. The interpretation and application of the burgeoning kinetic data depends upon an understanding of the cell cycle in both normal and cancer cells.

The cell cycle (Baserga, 1968; Gelfant, 1977; Mueller, 1969; Patt and Quastler, 1963; Peterson et al., 1969) can be viewed as a road-map of the past, present and future of any individual cell. A replicating cell begins its "life sequence" at the end of mitosis (M), and proceeds through the interphase ($G_1 \rightarrow S \rightarrow G_2$) to arrive at, and then complete, another mitotic event (Fig. 4.2). The time to complete this sequence of events is highly variable and is often termed the transit time. Cells at the transition point between two major phases of the cell cycle are frequently said to be at a boundary or transition zone, e.g., the G_1-S boundary or transition.

The movement of cells around the cycle is a highly ordered phenomenon which occurs in a specific temporal sequence. For example, in Figure 4.2 a cell at position B in G_1 will not arrive at position D unless it first passes through those biochemical events associated with position C. Similarly, a cell in G_1 cannot enter G_2 until it passes through the S phase. Such temporally ordered sequential requirements constitute an important

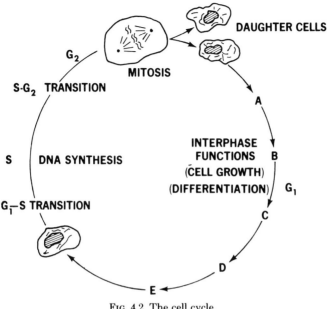

FIG. 4.2. The cell cycle.

facet in the rational design of multidrug regimens in cancer chemotherapy.

The S phase of the cell cycle is the period during which cells synthesize deoxyribonucleic acid (DNA) and double their chromosomal complement. Thus, at the end of the S phase there will be 92 chromosomes instead of the usual G_1 complement of 46. The time to complete this phase of the cell cycle may range from 6 to more than 50 hours.

After completing their chromosomal replication the cells pass through the G_2 (gap 2) phase. During this portion of the cycle the cells appear to be undergoing a sequence of biochemical events that prepare them for the ensuing mitosis. Since they have just completed the S phase the cells contain twice their normal complement of chromosomes. Although most mammalian cells tend to spend less than 6 hours in G_2, there are some which stop in G_2 and differentiate. Examples of this latter group appear to be some lymphocytes, hepatocytes, and central nervous system cells.

After completing G_2 the cells progress sequentially through the classic subdivisions of the mitotic (M) phase: prophase, metaphase, anaphase, and telophase. It is during this portion of the cell cycle that the cell undergoes nuclear and cytoplasmic division to yield two daughter cells, each with the normal complement of 46 chromosomes. Most mammalian cells appear to spend about 1 hour in the M phase of the cell cycle after which the daughter cells enter the G_1 phase.

The G_1 (gap 1) phase is the period during which most cells can be easily recognized under the microscope as being of one cell type or another, e.g., hepatocyte or granulocyte. During this period many cells express their particular differentiated function, such as insulin production and secretion by the pancreatic β cells. During the G_1 phase the major macromolecular activity of the cell is concerned with ribonucleic acid (RNA) synthesis and protein synthesis and secretion. Specific RNA and protein syntheses also occur as concomitants of the S and G_2 phases, and to a lesser degree, the M phase.

The major portion of the life span of most cells is usually spent in G_1. The time span is quite variable, however, and can range from minutes to years. Some gastrointestinal and hematopoietic cells, for example, are constantly replicating and constantly passing sequentially through the various phases of the cell cycle. However, other cells such as central nervous system neurons usually remain stationary in G_1 for their entire adult life, and muscle cells leave G_1 only if replication is called for by the death of adjacent muscle cells. Some investigators consider these stationary G_1 cells to be in a special resting phase called G_0. The G_0 state is then thought of as a pool of cells which are "out of cycle" and may, under special circumstances, be brought back into the G_1 phase of the cell cycle. From a practical chemotherapeutic standpoint it makes little difference at present to distinguish between a G_0 and a stationary G_1 state. Cells in both situations are regarded as being out of cycle in contrast to those which are clearly progressing around the cell cycle and are therefore considered to be "in cycle."

The distinction between various phases of the cell cycle as well as between cells in cycle and those out of cycle formulates a basis for the classification of chemotherapeutic agents and has important implications for the application of chemotherapy to tumor growth kinetics (see "Cell Kinetic Considerations," below.)

Cell Kinetic Considerations

DOUGLASS C. TORMEY, M.D., Ph.D.

One of the first major advances in the knowledge of the action of chemotherapeutic drugs was the observation that each dose of a drug kills a constant percentage of susceptible cells in animal and cell culture systems, i.e., drugs kill by first order kinetics (Skipper et al., 1964). A greater than 99% statistical chance of cure occurs in animal systems if all but 0.001 cells were killed (Skipper et al., 1964). Such a tumor cell kill is very difficult to achieve in advanced disease in vivo primarily because most drugs kill replicating host cells with almost the same efficiency as the tumor cells. The limitations of drug toxicity therefore provide a low therapeutic ratio for most of the effective antitumor agents. In addition the majority of drugs are most effective only against those cells which are in cycle. The number of tumor cells in a clinical mass that are in cycle, i.e., in the growth fraction, is generally less than 20%, and the number of replicating tumor cells that are in a portion of the cell cycle which is susceptible to a single dose of drug, e.g., the S phase, is still lower.

Tumor masses may be thought of as existing in four major compartments (Fig. 4.3). A constant flux of cells exists among these compartments. One compartment is composed of cells that are dying and it will receive a certain percentage of cells from each of the other compartments. It is this compartment that current chemotherapy attempts to increase.

The stationary differentiated cell compartment contains cells which theoretically have lost their capacity for further division. Such a permanently nonproliferative state is very difficult to demonstrate in nucleated cells. Some investigators doubt its existence. Others suggest cells like keratinizing epithelial cells as examples of this compartment. Although it is of little interest in designing current chemotherapeutic programs, future cancer control may entail increasing the size of this compartment.

The compartments of prime interest in designing current therapeutic programs are the proliferating and temporarily differentiated compartments. Theoretically, cells from either of these compartments could enter the permanently nonproliferative state. The temporarily differentiated compartment is composed of cells that are nonreplicating, i.e., out of cycle in a prolonged or stationary G_1 phase. Cells in this state comprise the majority of the cells in most tumors (Skipper and Perry, 1970;

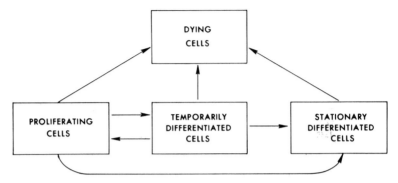

FIG. 4.3. The theoretical compartments comprising a tumor (Skinner and Perry, 1970).

Schabel, 1969). They are sensitive to being killed only by drugs that are lethal to resting cells. Drugs that require the cells to be replicating will have little effect on these nonreplicating cells. Cells in the proliferating compartment are in cycle and constitute the "growth fraction" or "proliferative pool" of the tumor. They are effectively killed by drugs active against replicating cells; the cell kill efficiency of drugs active against nonreplicating cells is even higher against cells in the proliferating cell compartment than in the nonproliferating cell compartments.

When cells from the proliferating compartment are killed there appears to be a net influx of the cells from the temporarily differentiated compartment (Schabel, 1969). This movement has the effect of increasing the percent of cells in the tumor which are in cycle. Thus, the smaller the tumor mass the greater is the percentage of the cells that are in cycle, i.e., in the growth fraction. Accordingly, as the tumor decreases in size it becomes increasingly susceptible to chemotherapeutic agents. It is for this reason that chemotherapy is most effective when used against small animal tumors. Equivalent data concerning increased effectiveness of therapy in smaller human lesions is not well documented, however, some of the adjunctive chemotherapy studies to be discussed below do lend some support to these concepts.

The growth of a tumor mass follows Gompertzian kinetics (Schabel, 1969). If the number of tumor cells are plotted on a logarithmic scale against time on a linear scale, the increase in either tumor mass or cells will initially be a straight line. After a period of time the growth will tend to fall off and may reach a near steady state in which the size of the tumor mass does not further increase. The reasons for this phenomenon are not clearly known but it is interesting that the human body follows a similar growth pattern (Skipper and Perry, 1970). It has also been observed that as the tumor mass enlarges there is an increasing percentage of cells entering the nonproliferating and dying cell compartments

(Skipper and Perry, 1970). There also appears to be a gradient in which the cells furthest from a blood vessel are in a more differentiated compartment; nearer the vessel there are more and more cells in the proliferative pool (Tannock, 1968). It is of considerable interest that the tumor cells undergoing maximum proliferation frequently appear to have cell cycle transit times approaching those of the tissue of origin.

Human tumors reach levels of clinical detection at a volume of about 1 cc, or about 10^9 cells. The percentage of tumor cells in the growth fraction of such a lesion can be anticipated to be considerably less than 40% in most instances. Below the limit of clinical detection there are a large number of cells (up to ca. 10^9) which can be thought of as constituting "subclinical disease." The growth fraction of the subclinical tumor may be quite large and, at very small cell numbers, may theoretically approach 100%.

The changes in tumor size observed during chemotherapy depend on the rate of cell destruction, the rate of cell removal, and the rate of growth of both sensitive and resistant cells. In most solid tumors the rate of dead cell removal appears to be slow. This is due in part to the poor vascularity of many tumors. It appears that as many as 99% of the tumor cells may have to be killed in order for the tumor to undergo a 50% regression in size (Skipper, 1971).

From these kinetic considerations it is not surprising to find that in animal systems, the earlier a tumor is treated, even with a single dose of drug, the longer the animal will survive (Skipper, 1971). Cures can be achieved if the animals are treated very early but seldom if they are treated late. The human corollary would be the early sustained adjunctive chemotherapy studies. A striking example is the marked increase in survival of patients with Wilms' tumor (Fernbeck and Martyn, 1966). In this disease the survival of 40% with surgery plus radiotherapy has been increased to 85–90% by adding chemotherapy in the absence of clinically demonstrable disease. Increases in survival have also been reported in gastric (Hattori et al., 1966), colon (Higgins et al., 1971), ovarian (Julian and Woodruff, 1969), and breast (Bonadonna et al., 1977) tumors treated with adjunctive chemotherapy. Current cooperative group studies are exploring this important area more fully in many human cancers.

One of the problems in extrapolating animal data to the human situation has been a lack of animal tumor systems that closely correlate with human diseases. With the new thrust in exploiting kinetic parameters such animal models are now being found and studied. At present it is possible to regularly cure many animal tumors by making use of differing drug toxicities and the above concepts concerning cell kinetics. Such systems judiciously use combinations of agents that kill cells in specific phases of the cell cycle, and other drugs that kill cells in all phases of the cycle (Skipper and Perry, 1970; Schabel, 1969). Similar approaches to the treatment of certain human tumors are under investigation but as yet the gain has not been impressive.

Classification of Chemotherapeutic Agents

DOUGLASS C. TORMEY, M.D., Ph.D., and BRUCE A. CHABNER, M.D.

The most common method of classifying cancer chemotherapeutic agents is based on either the source of the drug or its general mechanism of action (Table 4.1). The following reports are recommended for further details of chemotherapeutic agent classification: Bertino (1974), Bhuyan et al. (1972), Bruce et al. (1966), Dollinger et al. (1969), Dowling et al. (1970), Ernst and Killmann (1970), Goldberg and Friedman (1971), Harris (1970), Krakoff (1971), McIntyre et al. (1969), Pittillo et al. (1965), Schabel et al. (1965), Toby (1972), Valeriote and van Putten (1975), and van Putten (1974). Using these criteria the more common classes of agents are:

ALKYLATORS

These are highly reactive compounds characterized by alkyl side chains which form covalent bonds with nucleophilic groups. The chemical union obtained can lead to a wide variety of defects in intracellular metabolism culminating in cell death. Most of these drugs interfere with DNA function and are mutagenic. The majority of the clinically useful alkylating agents are bifunctional, i.e., they have two chemically reactive centers, and can cross-link macromolecules such as DNA; others are monofunctional or trifunctional.

ANTIMETABOLITES

These are structural analogs of normal metabolites which interfere with normal cellular metabolism either by inhibiting specific enzymatic

TABLE 4.1

Classification of Cancer Chemotherapeutic Agents by Derivation and/or Mechanism of Action[a]

Alkylating agents:	*Glutamine antimetabolites:*
BCNU (BeeCNU)[b]	Azaserine[c]
Busulfan (Myleran)	Azotomycin[c]
CCNU (CeeNu)[b]	DON[c]
Chlorambucil (Leukeran)	
Cyclophosphamide (Cytoxan)	*Antibiotics*
Dibromodulcitol[c]	Actinomycin D (Cosmegen)
Dibromomannitol[c]	Adriamycin (doxorubicin)
Hexamethylmelamine[b, c]	Azotomycin[c]
ICDT (DTIC) (dacarbazine)[b]	Bleomycin (Blenoxane)
Melphalan (Alkeran)	Daunomycin[c]
Mitomycin C (Mutamycin)	Hadacidin[c]
Nitrogen mustard (Mustargen)	Mithramycin (Mithracin)
Porfiromycin[c, d]	Mitomycin C (Mutamycin)
Thio-TEPA (TSPA)	Porfiromycin[c]
Triethylenemelamine (TEM)	Streptonigrin[c]
Uracil mustard[c]	Streptozotocin[c]
Pyrimidine antimetabolites:	*Alkaloids:*
6-Azauridine[c]	Camptothecin[c]
Cytosine arabinoside (Cytosar)	Colchicine
5-Fluorouracil (Fluorouracil)	Emetine[c]
5-FUDR[c]	Vinblastine (Velban)
	Vincristine (Oncovin)
Purine antimetabolites:	*Miscellaneous:*
Allopurinol (Zyloprim)	L-Asparaginase (Elspar)
Azathioprine (Imuran)	Hydroxyurea (Hydrea)
6-Mercaptopurine (Purinethol)	Methyl GAG[c]
6-Thioguanine (Thioguanine)	o,p'-DDD (Lysodren)
Folic acid antimetabolites:	Piposulfan[c]
Methotrexate	Procarbazine (Matulane)
Baker's Antifol[c]	

[a] The name or abbreviation under which the noninvestigational drugs are marketed is in parentheses if different from the chemical name.
[b] These agents may also have other mechanisms of action.
[c] Investigational agents.
[d] Refers to possible mechanism of action.

steps or by metabolically substituting for normal metabolites resulting in a fraudulent end product. The enzyme inhibition or fraudulent end product interferes with cellular metabolism leading to an interruption of protein, RNA, and/or DNA synthesis or function in the cell. Four major subclasses of antimetabolites are the purine, pyrimidine, folic acid, and glutamine antimetabolites. The general mechanism of action of the purine and pyrimidine antimetabolites depends on the drug used; however, as a class, they interfere with RNA and/or DNA synthesis and/or function.

The folic acid antimetabolite methotrexate competes with dihydrofolic acid to bind to the enzyme dihydrofolic acid reductase. This reaction prevents the reutilization of oxidized folates resulting in a depletion of reduced folate compounds required for synthesis of protein, RNA, and DNA. The glutamine antimetabolites compete with glutamine for the enzymes which utilize this amino acid in the biosynthesis of proteins and purines.

ANTIBIOTICS

This heterogeneous group is composed of drugs which are natural products synthesized by various bacterial and fungal species. They interfere with cellular metabolism by binding to nucleic acids (e.g., adriamycin, actinomycin), by scission of DNA (bleomycin), or by functioning as antimetabolites (azotomycin).

ALKALOIDS

These compounds are derived from plants. At least three of these, colchicine, vincristine, and vinblastine, interfere with the assembly of cytoplasmic and nuclear spindles, most notably in the mitotic apparatus.

MISCELLANEOUS

This category includes agents which do not fit any of the above classifications.

The classification of drugs by the above system does not always reflect the action of the drug in the cell cycle. Because this information is frequently considered important to the theory of designing therapeutic regimens many investigators are classifying the drugs according to how efficiently they kill cells in different phases of the cell cycle. By this classification schema there are at least two major classes of drugs (Tables 4.2 and 4.3):

1. *Cell Cycle Phase Nonspecific.* These are agents which kill cells regardless of where they are in the cell cycle—i.e., they will kill cells in S, G_2, M, G_1, or G_0. Although they are generally more effective against cells that are in cycle (the proliferating pool), they will also directly or indirectly kill cells that are out of cycle in the nonproliferating pools. Some of these agents, e.g., adriamycin, are especially lethal to cells in specific phases such as the S phase.

2. *Cell Cycle Phase Specific.* These agents will kill cells only when they are in cycle, i.e., in the proliferating pool. The important distinction from the cell cycle phase nonspecific agents is that the cell must be traversing the cell cycle in order for the drug to be effective. Most of the cell cycle phase nonspecific agents, e.g., adriamycin, are considerably more effective against cells that are in cycle than against cells that are out of cycle. The truly cell cycle phase specific agents will kill cells exposed to the drug

only in a specific phase of the cell cycle. For example, if a drug is S phase specific it will kill only those cells in the proliferative pool that are traversing the S phase of the cell cycle during their time of exposure to cytocidal levels of the agent. Cells in the G_1, G_2, and M phases would not be affected by the drug. The majority of these agents are S phase specific.

TABLE 4.2
Cell Cycle Phase Nonspecific Agents[a]

Class of Agent	Biochemical Site of Action	Drugs
Alkylators	Alkylation of DNA, RNA, and/or protein	BCNU (BeeCNU) Busulfan (Myleran) CCNU (CeeNU) Chlorambucil (Leukeran) Cyclophosphamide (Cytoxan) Dibromodulcitol[b] Dibromomannitol[b] Hexamethylmelamine[c] ICDT (DTIC) (Dacarbazine) Melphalan (Alkeran) Mitomycin C (Mutamycin) Nitrogen mustard (Mustargen) Porfiromycin[b, d] Procarbazine (Matulane)[d] Triethylenemelamine (TEM) Thio-TEPA (TSPA) Uracil mustard[b]
Antimetabolites	Pyrimidine synthesis and/or function	5-FUDR (intravenous injection)[b]
	Purine synthesis and/or function	Azathioprine (Imuran)
	Glutamine utilization	Azaserine[b] Azotomycin[b] DON[b]
Antibiotics	DNA-dependent-RNA polymerase	Actinomycin D (Cosmegen) Mithramycin (Mithracin)
	Glutamine utilization	Azotomycin[b]
	Nucleic acid synthesis and/or function	Hadacidin[b] Adriamycin (doxorubicin) Daunomycin[b]
	Alkylation	Mitomycin C (Mutamycin) Porfiromycin[b]
Miscellaneous	Asparagine degradation	L-Asparaginase (Elspar)
	Alkylation and H_2O_2 generation	Procarbazine (Matulane)
Corticosteroids	Cell membrane	Prednisone[e]

[a] The name or abbreviation under which the noninvestigational drugs are marketed is in parentheses if different from the chemical name.
[b] Investigational agents.
[c] Investigational agents which may have other mechanisms of action.
[d] Refers to possible actions.
[e] In high dose (e.g., >100 mg/sq m/day); at low doses (e.g., 20 to 50 mg/sq m/day) it may be cycle specific.

The classification of drugs by cycle specificity is relatively new and continues to generate debate. The agents listed in Tables 4.2 and 4.3 are classified on the basis of our view of the existing evidence. Some of these drugs will undoubtedly have to be reclassified in the future. Problems in classification revolve around such considerations as the differing activity of prednisone and some other drugs at different dosages, the unknown contribution of the inhibition of amino acid transport by drugs like vinblastine, and the self-limiting nature of the S phase cycle specificity of drugs like methotrexate. Additional subclassifications of drugs, based on their cell cycle specificities, have been put forward. All systems tend to focus on the biochemical mechanism of action of the agent and its implications for cellular kinetics.

TABLE 4.3
Cell Cycle Phase Specific Agents

Cycle Phase	Class of Agent	Biochemical Site of Action	Drugs
G$_1$	Corticosteroids	Cell membrane[a]	Prednisone[b]
S	Antimetabolites	Dihydrofolic acid reductase	Methotrexate
		Incorporation into DNA	6-Thioguanine (Thioguanine)
			5-FUDR (small continuous doses)[c]
		DNA polymerase inhibition and pyrimidine function	Cytosine arabinoside (Cytosar)
		Pyrimidine synthesis and/or utilization	6-Azauridine[c]
			5-Fluorouracil (Fluorouracil)
		Purine synthesis and/or function	6-Mercaptopurine (Purinethol)
	Antibiotics		Streptonigrin[a, c]
	Miscellaneous	Ribonucleotide reductase	Hydroxyurea (Hydrea)
G$_2$	Antibiotics	Protein synthesis; DNA scission	Bleomycin (Blenoxane)
M	Alkaloids	Assembly of mitotic spindle protein subunits	Colchicine
			Vinblastine (Velban)[d]
			Vincristine (Oncovin)

[a] Refers to possible actions.

[b] In low doses (e.g., 20–50 mg/sq m/day); at high doses (e.g., >100 mg/sq m/day) it may be cycle nonspecific.

[c] Investigational agents.

[d] Vinblastine has been shown to interfere with amino acid transport across the cell membrane; if this action is clinically significant, it may be cycle nonspecific. In addition, the M agents listed may have to be present during the S period to interact with the spindle protein subunits. (The name under which the noninvestigational drugs are marketed is in parentheses if it is different from the chemical name.)

Drug Dosage Guidelines

DOUGLASS C. TORMEY, M.D., Ph.D., JOHANNES BLOM, M.D., and
PATRICK R. BERGEVIN, M.D.

IMPORTANCE OF DOCUMENTING DRUG SIDE EFFECTS

The intensity of side effects varies with the drugs used (see Chapter 5) as well as the phase of therapy. Maximum toxicity usually occurs during the induction phase of therapy. The maintenance phase is generally associated with minimal toxicity, usually hematopoietic. It is of the utmost importance to closely document drug toxicity in order to avoid serious side effects from the overuse of the drug as well as to register unusual and previously undescribed side effects. Equally important is the documentation of drug toxicity when attempting to ascertain the effect of the drug or drug combination on the tumor. At the present time there are seldom more than one or two optimally effective therapeutic regimens for a given tumor, thus the host-drug interaction is crucial to decision-making in the presence of either progressive disease or relapse. This is illustrated by the four clinical situations that follow:

1. Disease Progression While Off Therapy. When this occurs in a patient who had previously responded the patient will frequently respond again to the agent(s) that initiated the previous remission. Accordingly it is usually utilized again in the trial immediately after the relapse. If, on the other hand, the patient had not responded and had not previously had an adequate trial of drug (usually 3–6 weeks) the same drug(s) is generally given again to obtain an adequate trial.

2. Disease Progression During a Period of Documented Drug Toxicity. The patient in this situation need not be further exposed to the same drug(s) since he has demonstrated refractoriness to it in the face of a biologically active dose of drug(s). A new therapeutic program should be initiated in this situation.

3. Disease Progression During a Period of Documented Lack of Drug Toxicity. When this occurs the patient may respond to increased doses of the agent(s); however, the chance of doing so is probably less than that for the patient in situation 1. If subtoxic doses have selected for the accruement of resistant cells, then experience from the infectious disease discipline would suggest that perhaps this patient should be switched to another regimen, at least temporarily, before repeating the present regimen. Theoretically, the new regimen would decrease the number of cells resistant to the first regimen thus making it more effective when it is later reinstituted. Such an approach has not been well documented. The usual practice, therefore, is to assume that selection has not occurred and increase the dose of the first agent(s) to toxicity. If this is done and disease progression continues the patient enters situation two.

4. Disease Progression in the Absence of Documentation of the Presence or Absence of Drug Side Effects. This is a most unsatisfactory situation. It is not known if the patient's tumor is refractory to the drug (situation 2) or if it is still potentially sensitive (situation 3). The physician in this setting is forced to make a judgment based on the probability of the patient's responding to another regimen. If he chooses to use the same drug(s) and the patient's tumor is refractory then it continues to increase in size, the growth fraction theoretically decreases further, and the theoretical probability of a response to another regimen also decreases. Alternatively, the physician may switch to a less desirable program and find that the patient's disease is still progressing. Theoretically, this progression may be great enough to reduce the growth fraction enough so that now the patient is unresponsive to the original agent(s) in question. Thus, this setting constitutes a most distressing therapeutic dilemma which no physician should have to face. It is important, therefore, to observe the patient closely so that his reactions to the drug(s) are definitely known.

COMMON THERAPEUTIC COMPLICATIONS

General dosage guidelines can be stated in cancer chemotherapy. Some are obvious and do not require further explanation. The most common of the dose modifying therapeutic complications are listed below.

1. Nausea and Emesis. When they occur shortly after the drug is administered nausea and vomiting can frequently be managed with antiemetics such as the phenothiazines. If nausea or emesis are severe, refractory to treatment, or are present 5–7 days after a dose of drug, the drug should be withdrawn until these symptoms abate. If it is then reintroduced it should be done so cautiously.

2. Stomatitis. A red, painful, or ulcerated oropharynx is always an indication to stop the drug until this sign of toxicity has cleared. The agent should then be reintroduced cautiously, frequently at a lower initial dose.

3. Diarrhea, Gastrointestinal Ulcerations, and/or Bleeding. These are clearly danger signals with many drugs and indicate that the agent should be withdrawn and, when reinstituted, done so at a lower dose.

4. Bone Marrow Suppression. Leukopenia and thrombocytopenia are quite common and vary in their severity. Drug-induced anemia is less common. Severe cytopenias may require transfusions of the appropriate elements. As cytopenias develop the drug(s) may be withdrawn or the dosage reduced, depending upon the tumor being treated. The "rule of halves" can usually be followed during the therapy of most tumors, especially when daily or weekly therapy is used as in the chronic leukemias, viz., each time the white blood cell or platelet count falls by 50% the drug dosage should be reduced by 50%.

5. *Central Nervous System Alterations.* Confusion, irritability, coma, ataxia, and other neurologic signs and symptoms may be seen with certain drugs and are always an indication to discontinue the agent(s).

6. *Peripheral Nervous System Changes.* Motor or sensory neuropathies are common with several agents, notably the vinca alkaloids; if severe, the dose is reduced or the drug withdrawn.

7. *Hepatorenal Injury.* The hepatic or renal toxicity of most drugs can be detected early by monitoring kidney and liver function carefully. Such toxicity is usually reversible and indicates that the agent(s) should be withdrawn at least temporarily.

8. *Pulmonary Complications.* Pulmonary fibrosis can occur during therapy with bleomycin and occasionally with alkylating agents, notably busulfan. It is always an indication to discontinue the drug. Early detection of this toxicity is extremely important and is discussed under the appropriate agents in Chapter 5. An interstitial pneumonitis is occasionally seen with methotrexate, but opinions vary as to whether or not the drug should be temporarily stopped for this complication. The role of adding steroids in the treatment of this complication is also not clear.

9. *Hyperuricemia.* This can be an early complication due to increased breakdown of host and tumor cells during chemotherapy, particularly in acute leukemias and lymphomas. It can usually be prevented by instituting allopurinol and adequate hydration 48–72 hours before beginning treatment. In other tumors these measures are not usually taken unless the uric acid level is increased at the start of therapy. Severe hyperuricemia (> 12 mg/100 ml) can cause renal insufficiency and is best treated with high doses of allopurinol (up to 1200–1600 mg daily in divided doses), urine alkalinization with oral sodium bicarbonate and diamox, and maintenance of high urine flow.

10. *Immune Suppression.* This is a common feature of chemotherapeutic drugs and may predispose the patient to an increased risk of infection. If a patient undergoing therapy becomes infected the chemotherapeutic drugs are frequently withdrawn temporarily, especially if there is an associated granulocytopenia (granulocytes < 1000/cu mm). This decision must be weighted against the risk of not continuing the chemotherapy.

11. *Hypercalcemia.* This is an unusual complication except in those diseases which have involved large segments of the bone marrow, notably breast cancer. Occasionally the initiation of therapy with chemothera-

peutic agents and/or hormones will stimulate a hypercalcemic episode within the first week of therapy. This can usually be controlled with saline diuresis and mithramycin administration but occasionally will necessitate more vigorous therapy. Most investigators would not withhold chemotherapeutic agents under this circumstance but would withhold hormone therapy. When the situation is under control the hormone would then be reinstituted at about one-third the dose and increased by 30% at weekly intervals until the therapeutic dose is reached.

12. Hyperkalemia. Hyperkalemia is an occasional complication of rapid tumor lysis in Burkitt's lymphoma and is treated medically.

13. Infection. Infection is an indirect complication of cancer chemotherapy. Predisposing factors include the immune suppression and granulocytopenia associated with chemotherapeutic agents. The development of fever with an associated granulocytopenia (< 1000/cu mm) should be considered an emergency and sepsis considered likely. After taking cultures, broad-spectrum antibiotic coverage should be initiated immediately. Many oncologists choose high dosages of Keflin and Gentamycin; and if the fever persists for 3–4 days, add carbenicillin. Obviously the therapy in this setting must be directed by positive cultures and the predominant organisms in the environment. It is not uncommon to recover no organism and have the fever persist until adequate granulocytes (> 1000/cu mm) have returned. Experience directs that withholding therapy in this situation will frequently lead to recovery of an organism in the blood too late to reverse the septic state. Cancer patients are also uniquely susceptible to rare infections, such as *Pneumocystis carinii* and toxoplasmosis. These are treated vigorously when they occur.

REFERENCES

Baserga, R. Biochemistry of the cell cycle; a review. Cell Tissue Kinet., *1:* 167, 1968.

Bertino, J. R. Folate antagonists, antineoplastic and immunosuppressive agents. *In* Handbook of Experimental Pharmacology, edited by A. C. Sartorelli, and D. G. Johns, Vol. 38. Springer-Verlag, New York, 1974.

Bhuyan, B. K., Scheidt, L. G., and Fraser, T. J. Cell cycle phase specificity of antitumor agents. Cancer Res., *32:* 398, 1972.

Bonadonna, G., Rossi, A., Valagussa, P., Banfi, A., and Veronesi, U. The CMF program for operable breast cancer with positive axillary nodes. Lancet, *1:* 2904–2915, 1977.

Bruce, W. R., Meeker, B. E., and Valeriote, F. A. Comparison of sensitivity of normal hematopoietic and transplanted lymphoma colony forming cells to chemotherapeutic agents administered in vivo. J. Natl. Cancer Inst., *37:* 233–245, 1966.

DeVita, V. T. Combined drug treatment of Hodgkin's disease: remission induction, remission duration, and survival; an appraisal. Natl. Cancer Inst. Monogr., *36:* 373–379, 1973.

Dollinger, M. R., Golbey, R. B., and Karnofsky, D. A. Cancer chemotherapy. D.M., April 1969.

Dowling, M. D., Krakoff, I. H., and Karnofsky, D. A. Mechanism of action of anticancer drugs. *In* Chemotherapy of Cancer, edited by W. H. Cole. Lea & Febiger, Philadelphia, 1970.

Ernst, P., and Killmann, S. A. Perturbation of generation cycle of human leukemic blast cells by cytostatic therapy in vivo; effect of corticosteroids. Blood, *36:* 689, 1970.

Fernbeck, D. J., and Martyn, D. T. Role of dactinomycin in the improved survival of children with Wilm's tumor. J.A.M.A., *195:* 1005, 1966.

Gelfant, S. A new concept of tissue and tumor cell proliferation. Cancer Res., *37:* 3845–3862, 1977.

Goldberg, I. H., and Friedman, P. A. Antibiotics and nucleic acid synthesis and function. In Drugs and Cell Regulation, edited by E. Mihich, p. 100. Academic Press, New York, 1971.

Harris, A. W. Differential functions expressed by cultured mouse lymphoma cells; I. Specificity and kinetics of cell response to corticosteroids. Exp. Cell Res., *60:* 341, 1970.

Hattori, T., Ito, I., Hirata, K., et al. Results of combined treatment in patients with cancer of the stomach; palliative gastrectomy, large dose mitomycin-C, and bone marrow transplantation. Gan., *57:* 441, 1966.

Hersh, E. M., and Oppenheim, J. J. Inhibition of *in vitro* lymphocyte transformation during chemotherapy in man. Cancer Res., *27:* 98, 1967.

Hersh, E. M., Carbone, P. P., and Freireich, E. J. Recovery of immune responsiveness after drug suppression in man. J. Lab. Clin. Med., *67:* 566, 1966a.

Hersh, E. M., Wong, V. G., and Freireich, E. J. Inhibition of the local inflammatory response in man by antimetabolites. Blood, *27:* 38, 1966b.

Higgins, G. A., Dwight, R. W., Smith, J. V., et al. Fluorouracil as an adjuvant to surgery in carcinoma of the colon. Arch. Surg., *102:* 339, 1971.

Julian, G. G., and Woodruff, J. D. The role of chemotherapy in the treatment of primary ovarian malignancy. Obstet. Gynecol. Surg., *24:* 1307, 1969.

Krakoff, I. H. The present status of cancer chemotherapy. Med. Clin. North Am., *55:* 683, 1971.

McIntyre, O. R., Eurenius, K., Holland, F. C., and Ebaugh, F. G. Studies on the mechanism of hydrocortisone inhibition of the RNA response. In Proceedings of the Third Annual Leukocyte Culture Conference, edited by W. Rieke, p. 307. Appleton-Century-Crofts, New York, 1969.

Moertel, C. G., and Reitemeier, R. J. Advanced Gastrointestinal Cancer—Clinical Management and Chemotherapy. Harper & Row, New York, 1969.

Mueller, G. C. Biochemical events in the animal cell cycle. Fed. Proc., *28:* 1780, 1969.

Patt, H. N., and Quastler, H. Radiation effects on cell renewal and related systems. Physiol. Rev., *43:* 357, 1963.

Peterson, D. F., Tobey, R. A., and Anderson, E. C. Synchronously dividing mammalian cells. Fed. Proc., *28:* 1771, 1969.

Pittillo, R. F., Schabel, F. M., Wilcox, W. S., and Skipper, H. E. Experimental evaluation of potential anticancer agents; XVI. Basic study of effects of certain anticancer agents on kinetic behavior of model bacterial cell populations. Cancer Chemother. Rep., *47:* 1, 1965.

Schabel, F. M., Jr. The use of tumor growth kinetics in planning "curative" chemotherapy of advanced solid tumors. Cancer Res., *29:* 2384, 1969.

Schabel, F. M., Skipper, H. E., Trader, M. W., and Wilcox, W. S. Experimental evaluation of potential anticancer agents; XIX. Sensitivity of nondividing leukemic cell populations to certain classes of drugs in vivo. Cancer Chemother. Rep., *47:* 17, 1965.

Skipper, H. E. Kinetics of mammary tumor cell growth and implications for therapy. Cancer, *28:* 1479, 1971.

Skipper, H. E., and Perry, S. Kinetics of normal and leukemia leukocyte populations and relevance to chemotherapy. Cancer Res., *30:* 1883, 1970.

Skipper, H. E., Schabel, F. M., and Wilcox, W. S. Experimental evaluation of potential anticancer agents; XIII. On the criteria and kinetics associated with "curability" of experimental leukemia. Cancer Chemother. Rep., *35:* 1, 1964.

Smith, J. P., and Rutledge, F. Chemotherapy in the treatment of cancer of the ovary. Am. J. Obstet. Gynecol., *107:* 691, 1970.

Stutz, F. H., Blom, J., and Tormey, D. C. Combination chemotherapy in disseminated carcinoma of the breast. Oncology, *29:* 139, 1974.

Stutzman, L., and Glidewell, O. Multiple chemotherapeutic agents for Hodgkin's disease. J.A.M.A., *225:* 1202, 1973.

Tannock, I. F. The relation between cell proliferation and the vascular system in a transplanted mouse mammary tumor. Br. J. Cancer, *22:* 258, 1968.

Toby, R. A. A simple, rapid technique for determination of the effects of chemotherapeutic agents on mammalian cell-cycle traverse. Cancer Res., *32:* 309, 1972.

Tubiana, M. The kinetics of tumour cell proliferation and radiotherapy. Br. J. Radiol., *44:* 325, 1971.

Valeriote, F., and van Putten, L. Proliferation-dependent cytotoxicity of anticancer agents; a review. Cancer Res., *35:* 2619–2630, 1975.

van Putten, L. M. Are cell kinetic data relevant for the design of tumor chemotherapy schedules? Cell Tissue Kinet., *7:* 493–504, 1974.

II
Chemotherapy

Chapter 5

Cancer Chemotherapeutic Agents

PATRICK R. BERGEVIN, M.D., DOUGLASS C. TORMEY, M.D., Ph.D., and
JOHANNES BLOM, M.D.

ACTINOMYCIN D, DACTINOMYCIN (COSMEGEN—MERCK)

Biochemistry. Actinomycin D is an antibiotic obtained from cultures of *Streptomyces parvulus.* It acts by combining noncovalently with deoxyguanosine residues in the helical DNA. The combination raises the energy required to separate the DNA strands. It also results in inhibition of RNA synthesis by interfering with the action of DNA-dependent RNA polymerase. At the cellular level these effects lead to mitotic abnormalities and chromosomal abnormalities (Goldberg, 1965; Reich, 1963). It is a cell cycle nonspecific antibiotic; however, cells in G_1 seem to be the most susceptible to its actions.

Pharmacology. After a single intravenous injection 85% of the drug is cleared from the blood in 2 min. Twelve to 20% is recovered in the urine and 50–90% is excreted in the bile within 24 hours.

Side Effects. Nausea and vomiting are common and may be severe. An erythematous sore mouth progressing to an ulcerative stomatitis, esophagitis and enteritis may occur with even standard dose regimens; onset of a sore mouth or one of the other gastrointestinal side effects (abdominal pain, diarrhea) is a signal to discontinue the drug, until these manifestations have cleared. It is important to remember that the severity of systemic side effects varies markedly from person to person and is only partly dependent on the dose employed. Side effects, with the exception of nausea and vomiting, usually do not become apparent until 2–4 days after the end of the usual 5–7 day course of treatment and may not be maximal until 1–2 weeks have elapsed. Leukopenia, thrombocytopenia and anemia are common, may be severe (although the anemia is usually only mild) and may occur a few days after institution of therapy. The drug is corrosive; avoid extravasation into tissues since cellulitis, phlebitis and sloughing may ensue. Erythema or other dermal changes from previous radiation may be reactivated by actinomycin D, especially when the interval between the two forms of therapy is brief. Skin eruptions at nonirradiated sites and acneiform lesions have also been reported. Alopecia may occur.

Administration. The drug is supplied in vials containing slightly more than 0.5 mg of the lyophilized powder. It should be protected from light and excessive heat and can be reconstituted by adding 1.1 ml of sterile water, which gives a drug concentration of 0.5 mg/ml. The desired dose is injected into the tubing of an intravenous infusion of 5% dextrose in water. Although the drug should be administered soon after its reconstitution, any unused portion may be kept in the refrigerator for up to 1 week without significant loss of potency.

Usual Dose. Dose is 0.010 mg/kg/day, intravenously for 7 days every 2–4 weeks, or 0.015 mg/kg/day, intravenously for 5 days every 2–4 weeks or 0.015–0.040 mg/kg/week, intravenously for 3–5 weeks.

ADRIAMYCIN (ADRIA), DOXORUBICIN HYDROCHLORIDE

Biochemistry. Adriamycin is an antibiotic isolated from cultures of a mutant *Streptomyces peucetius.* Its chemical structure is similar to that of daunomycin, differing only in the substitution of a hydrogen atom by a hydroxyl group in the acetyl radical. It binds specifically with DNA by intercalation between adjacent base pairs of the double helix. Adriamycin appears to affect cells in all phases of the cell cycle; however, those in the S phase are more sensitive than others.

Pharmacology. Adriamycin is rapidly cleared from the plasma and is widely distributed in plasma and tissue. Urinary excretion of the drug is prolonged, with only 5% of the drug excreted in the first 5 days, suggesting prolonged tissue binding. The drug is metabolized predominantly in the liver; half of the parent drug is excreted in the bile and 30% appears as conjugates. Adriamycin has been detected in malignant pleural and peritoneal effusions but does not appear in the cerebrospinal fluid in significant amounts.

Side Effects. (Middleman et al., 1971; Wang et al., 1974). Thrombocytopenia and leukopenia are mild to moderate. Anemia may occur. Marked myelosuppression has been noted in patients with liver dysfunction; thus the drug dose should be reduced by 50–75% in the presence of moderately abnormal liver function tests. Anorexia, nausea, and vomiting are commonly seen. Alopecia occurs frequently and may be severe. Stomatitis may occur; the degree of stomatitis correlates with the degree of bone marrow suppression. Myocardial damage appears to be less frequent with Adriamycin than with daunomycin; it generally occurs only when large doses are given or when the total cumulative dose of the drug has exceeded 550 mg/m^2. However, cardiac toxicity has been seen at lower total doses, especially in elderly patients. Nonspecific ST-T wave changes on the electrocardiogram (ECG) may precede severe cardiac toxicity and are generally an indication to hold the drug temporarily until the changes revert to normal. Cardiac arrhythmias and congestive heart failure are serious sequelae and may be fatal. Patients with pre-existing cardiac diseases or ECG abnormalities may be more likely to develop cardiac problems; a pretherapy ECG is desirable. If a decrease in QRS voltages greater than 30% in the standard leads in subsequent ECG occurs, the drug should probably be temporarily discontinued. The incidence of cardiotoxicity is increased when radiotherapy is administered to the heart, either previous to or concomitantly with the administration of Adriamycin, and may also be increased by the concomitant use of cyclophosphamide. In these cases the cumulative drug dose of Adriamycin should be kept less than 450 mg/m^2. An enhanced radiation reaction in normal esophagus and skin may be seen particularly when the Adriamycin is given concomitantly or shortly after radiotherapy.

Administration. The drug is supplied in vials of 10 and 50 mg as a reddish powder mixed with 50 mg of lactose and should be stored at room temperature. It is reconstituted with 5 and 25 ml, respectively, of normal saline or 5% dextrose in water and injected intravenously.

Care should be taken to avoid extravasation since the drug is an irritant and will cause cellulitis. The drug should be infused slowly over a period of several minutes. Some investigators recommend monitoring the pulse rate during the drug administration, and if tachycardia occurs to interrupt the infusion until the pulse rate returns to normal, after which the infusion is restarted at a slower rate. The unused reconstituted drug should be discarded.

Usual Dose. Dose is 60–75 mg/m^2 intravenously as a single dose every 3–5 weeks; 30 mg/m^2 intravenously daily for 3 days every 4 weeks.

ALLOPURINOL (ZYLOPRIM—BURROUGHS WELLCOME)

4-Hydroxypyrazolo-[3,4-D]pyrimidine

Biochemistry. Allopurinol is a structural analog of the natural purine base hypoxanthine. It inhibits the production of xanthine and uric acid by blocking the enzyme xanthine oxidase. It has been reported to inhibit the hepatic microsomal oxidase system, thus prolonging the half-lives of drugs like antipyrine, bishydroxycoumarin and possibly cyclophosphamide (Beardmore and Kelley, 1971; Vesel et al., 1970).

Pharmacology. Allopurinol is relatively rapidly absorbed after oral administration. It appears in the plasma in 30–60 min, with peak blood levels at 2–6 hours. It is not detectable in the intact form in the blood after 24 hours. Allopurinol is rapidly metabolized to alloxanthine, which has a plasma half-life of 23 hours. Alloxanthine appears also to be a potent inhibitor of xanthine oxidase. Both allopurinol and alloxanthine are excreted in the urine.

Side Effects. A few cases of reversible hepatic dysfunction (elevated alkaline phosphatase and SGOT) have been reported. The most common side effect is a skin rash (local or generalized), usually maculopapular, but occasionally exfoliative, urticarial or purpuric lesions are noted. All are rapidly reversible upon discontinuation of the drug. The onset of the skin rash has been reported as late as 2 years after starting the drug. The drug should be used with caution in pregnant women, since its effects on the fetus are poorly understood. Other side effects occasionally seen are: fever, nausea, diarrhea, abdominal pain, eosinophilia, arthralgias, cataracts, alopecia and peripheral neuritis. An increase in hepatic iron stores has been frequently noted in rats; for this reason, allopurinol should be used with caution in patients with hemochromatosis.

Administration. The drug is supplied in tablets of 100 mg for oral use, and vials of 500 mg (investigational) for intravenous use. The vials may be reconstituted with 10 ml of sterile water. The unused reconstituted drug is discarded.

Usual Dose. The initial dose is usually 200 mg orally 3–4 times daily, depending on the uric acid level and the amount of tumor. The maintenance dose is adjusted according to uric acid levels. The intravenous form is usually reserved for patients who are unable to take the drug orally; the dosage is the same as for the oral form.

Note. It is imperative to give one-third to one-fourth of the calculated dose of 6-mercaptopurine if allopurinol is given concurrently, since the degradation of 6-mercaptopurine depends on xanthine oxidase.

L-ASPARAGINASE (ELSPAR—MERCK SHARPE & DOHME)

Biochemistry. Partial purification of L-asparaginase has been obtained from various sources including guinea pig serum, yeast, *Escherichia coli* and *Erwinia carotovora.* These various enzymes differ with regard to physical, chemical and biologic properties. The molecular weight of L-asparaginase from guinea pig serum and from *E. coli* is approximately 130,000 and that from yeast is greater than 800,000. The preparation Elspar is from *E. coli.* Asparaginase prepared from *E. carotovora* may be used in patients who have shown an anaphylactic reaction to the *E. coli* preparation (Ohnuma et al., 1972). The enzyme causes depletion of L-asparaginase by hydrolyzing L-asparagine to L-aspartic acid and ammonia; theoretically this results in death of tumor cells lacking an endogenous synthetic capability for L-asparagine (Capizzi et al., 1970). In sensitive cells, L-asparaginase causes a rapid inhibition of protein synthesis and a delayed inhibition of DNA and RNA synthesis. Resistance to the drug is related to the cellular level of asparagine synthetase, the enzyme responsible for the endogenous synthesis of L-asparagine from L-aspartic acid. Leukemic cell populations both in vivo and in vitro appear to develop resistance rapidly to asparaginase activity. The drug appears to be cell cycle nonspecific.

Pharmacology. The half-life of L-asparaginase after intravenous injection is 8–30 hours irrespective of dose and varies depending on the commercial source of the enzyme. Measurable plasma levels are not achieved after oral administration of the enzyme, and, when given intramuscularly, the plasma level is $\frac{1}{10}$ of that achieved by intravenous injection. Twenty-four hours after an intravenous injection of 100 IU/kg blood levels of 8 to 20 IU/ml are usually found (Capizzi et al., 1970). In one study (Haskell et al., 1972), the disappearance of L-asparaginase from plasma was found to be biphasic with a rapid initial phase ($t_{1/2}$ 4–9 hours) and a prolonged second phase ($t_{1/2}$ 1.4–1.8 days). L-Asparaginase does not pass readily from the vascular to the tissue space and does not enter cells; little if any of the drug is excreted in the urine or bile. L-Asparaginase appears to cross the blood-brain barrier in only trace amounts (Ho et al., 1971).

Side Effects. Bone marrow depression is rare. Occasionally a mild anemia is noted, sometimes with a hemolytic component. The toxic manifestations of the drug are mainly due to hypersensitivity and inhibition of protein synthesis. Liver dysfunction is frequently seen and is manifested by elevated SGOT, alkaline phosphatase, bilirubin and ammonia levels and decreased albumin, fibrinogen and cholesterol. Liver biopsy invariably shows fatty metamorphosis. All of these phenomena are reversible within a few weeks when the drug is discontinued. There may be no recurrence of hepatotoxicity when the drug is restarted (Capizzi et al., 1970). Nausea and vomiting are common and may be severe. Fever after injection of the drug is occasionally noted but is transient and usually disappears with continued therapy. Hypersensitivity reactions such as urticaria, serum sickness, respiratory difficulty and anaphylactic shock are occasionally noted, perhaps on the basis of sensitivity to a contaminating endotoxin. Anaphylaxis does not usually occur after the first exposure but can occur after the second or repeated exposures to the drug. Coagulation abnormalities may be seen and include an elevated prothrombin time and partial thromboplastin time and decreased fibrinogen and plasma factors V, VII, VIII, IX, all on the basis of decreased synthesis and perhaps a limited disseminated intravascular coagulation (Gralnick and Henderson, 1971). Despite rather frequent and marked abnormalities in clotting function, severe bleeding is infrequently seen. Azotemia is frequently noted (mild elevation of BUN with normal urine sediment; rarely oliguria and renal failure), which is usually reversible when the drug is discontinued. The elevated BUN is probably in large part secondary to an elevated level of ammonia, which is metabolized into urea. Acute pancreatitis is not infrequent. Frequent serum amylase determinations should be done to pick up early evidence of pancreatitis, whereupon the drug should be permanently discontinued. Central nervous system dysfunction appears to occur mainly in adults and ranges from mild depression and drowsiness to impaired sensorium and frank coma, during which time the electroencephalogram may reveal diffuse slow wave activity. The mechanism of this dysfunction is not known but may be related to low levels of brain asparagine or to elevated ammonia levels. Hyperosmotic nonketotic hyperglycemia may be seen and is often associated with depressed serum insulin levels; it can be readily reversed by discontinuing the drug (Capizzi et al., 1970). There is no apparent effect on oral and gut mucosa or on hair follicles. The susceptibility of different patients to L-asparaginase toxicity is extremely variable with respect to dose; the toxicity may be an expression of a genetic incapability to synthesize asparagine or to adapt by increasing asparagine synthetase, rather than a strict drug dose-related phenomenon. The drug is both immunosuppressive and teratogenic in animals.

Administration. Elspar is supplied in 10-ml vials containing 10,000 IU of asparaginase as a dry powder and is stored below 8°C. It is stable at 5°C for 8 hours after reconstitution with 5 ml of sterile water or normal saline. After reconstitution, the drug is given through the side arm of an intravenous infusion. Because hypersensitivity reactions occur occasionally, a physician should remain in attendance for at least 5 min after the infusion has been completed. Resuscitative equipment, adrenalin, benadryl, and hydrocortisone should be on hand. Because of the occurrence of allergic reactions, an intradermal skin test should be performed prior to the initial administration of the drug and when it is given after an interval of a week or more has elapsed between doses. An allergic reaction even to the skin test dose may rarely occur. A negative skin test reaction does not preclude the possibility of an allergic reaction upon administration of the drug. Desensitization should be performed before administering the first dose of Elspar in a skin test positive patient and on retreatment of any patient. Instructions for skin testing and desensitization are included in the manufacturer's drug brochure and should be carefully followed.

Usual Dose. The drug is used only in the treatment of acute lymphocytic leukemia. 1000 IU/kg/day intravenously for 10 days on day 22 of an induction regimen of prednisone and vincristine, or 6000 IU/m^2 intramuscularly on days 4, 7, 10, 13, 16, 19, 22, 25 and 28 of an induction regimen of prednisone and vincristine, or 200 IU/kg/day intravenously for 28 days as the sole induction agent.

5-AZACYTIDINE

4-Amino-1-β-D-ribofuranosyl-1,3,5-triazine-2-one or
1-β-D-ribofuranosyl-5-azacytosine

Biochemistry. 5-Azacytidine is an analog of cytidine and is therefore incorporated into both RNA and DNA. It may act to disrupt protein synthesis by incorporating into mRNA, thereby interfering with the translocation process of protein synthesis (Troetel et al., 1972). It is probably an S phase specific cell cycle agent.

Pharmacology. Following an intravenous injection of the drug the plasma $t_{1/2}$ is 3.5 hours, although traces of the drug are still detectable in tissues up to 6 days after drug administration. Eighty-five percent of the drug is excreted in the urine within 48 hours. Significant levels of the drug are not attainable in the central nervous system (CNS) (Troetel et al., 1972).

Side Effects. Nausea, vomiting, and diarrhea may be severe, occurring shortly after administration of the drug; these symptoms may be ameliorated by infusing the drug intravenously over 15–30 min. Fever up to 40°C (104°F) may occur within 1–4 hours of drug administration and hypotension may also occur during or shortly after drug administration. Bone marrow suppression is usually severe and recovery may be prolonged at doses greater than 200 mg/m²/day for 5 days (Freireich, 1973). Abnormal liver function tests may be seen with treatment and even hepatic coma has been described. The drug should be used with caution in the presence of liver disease (Bellet et al., 1973b). Levi et al. (1975) described a myalgic/asthenic syndrome in 17 of 18 patients receiving 5-azacytidine by intravenous bolus or a 200 mg/m²/day times 5 schedule. On the 2nd or 3rd day of therapy the patients developed muscle tenderness, weakness, and lethargy. Some patients became confused and somnolent. This syndrome has also been reported by other investigators, although at a considerably decreased frequency. Stomatitis, phlebitis and a pruritic follicular skin rash have also been reported occasionally.

Administration. The drug is supplied in vials of 100 mg as a lyophilized powder (investigational, NSC-102816) and may be reconstituted with 19.9 ml of sterile water for immediate intravenous use. The reconstituted solution hydrolyzes at room temperature and should be used within 30 min. The reconstituted solution can be further diluted in lactated Ringer's solution and then should be used within 2–3 hours. The dry vials are stored at 4°C.

Usual Dose. For the treatment of acute myelogenous leukemia, remission rates have been seen with 100–250 mg/m² twice weekly, 150–400 mg/m²/day times 5 days and continuous infusions over 5 days.

AZATHIOPRINE (IMURAN—BURROUGHS WELLCOME)

Biochemistry. Azathioprine is an analog of the nucleic acid constituent, adenine, and the physiologic purine base, hypoxanthine. It is an imidazoyl derivative of 6-mercaptopurine, designed to be metabolized to 6-mercap-

6-(1-Methyl-4-nitro-5-imadazoyl)thiopurine

topurine. It interferes with nucleic acid synthesis by interfering with the incorporation of purines into purine nucleosides (Calabresi and Welch, 1965). The drug is probably a cell cycle nonspecific agent.

Pharmacology. In vivo the drug is cleaved to 6-mercaptopurine; its metabolism and excretion generally follow that of 6-mercaptopurine. Azathioprine is used primarily as an immunosuppressive agent.

Side Effects. The most common adverse effect is marrow depression, especially leukopenia, and, with excessive prolonged dosage, thrombocytopenia. The nadir of each is 6–10 days after the drug is discontinued. Stomatitis, progressing to oral ulcerations, may occur. Nausea and vomiting are occasionally seen but are usually mild. Diarrhea may occur.

Administration. The drug is supplied in tablets of 50 mg for oral use.

Usual Dose. Dose is 3–5 mg/kg/day, orally.

Caution. The dose of azathioprine should be reduced to one-third or one-fourth its usual dose if allopurinol is given concurrently, since the latter is a xanthine oxidase inhibitor.

BCNU, CARMUSTINE, BiCNU (BRISTOL)

$$Cl-CH_2CH_2-N-\overset{\overset{\displaystyle O}{\|}}{C}-NH-CH_2CH_2Cl$$
$$|$$
$$NO$$

1,3-Bis (2-chloroethyl)-1-nitrosourea

Biochemistry. BCNU, because of its structure, is believed to act as an alkylating agent; it has been suggested that cleavage of the nitrosated N-carboxyl carbon bond may release a highly reactive chloroethyl isocyanate group with strong potential for interaction with protein (DeVita et al., 1967). However, cross resistance in humans between BCNU and the standard alkylating agents usually is not seen. BCNU inhibits the synthesis of purine nucleotides, leading to a delayed inhibition of DNA synthesis (Wheeler and Bowdan, 1965). The drug possesses a high degree of lipid solubility, a low degree of ionization, and is thus able to cross the blood-brain barrier with ease. BCNU may be cell cycle G_2 phase specific.

Pharmacology. Plasma samples contain no detectable BCNU 15 min after an intravenous dose and extremely small amounts of the parent compound are excreted into urine, but the plasma levels of the degradation products are prolonged, and urinary excretion is moderately slow. Twenty-four hours after an intravenous dose, 38% of these products are recovered in the urine, and 63% are recovered in the first 96 hours (DeVita et al., 1967). The prolonged plasma levels of these products are probably the result of plasma protein binding plus enterohepatic recirculation. It may be that the prolonged plasma levels of the degradation products are associated with the unusual delayed bone marrow toxicity seen with the nitrosoureas. The entry of the degradation products of BCNU into the cerebrospinal fluid is prompt and closely parallels changes in the concurrent plasma levels.

Side Effects. Bone marrow depression is delayed, with the nadir of leukopenia and thrombocytopenia at about 4–5 weeks; recovery occurs in another 1–3 weeks. Nausea and vomiting occur in most patients shortly after drug administration. In some patients it is best to premedicate with an antiemetic, such as one of the phenothiazines. Venous irritation occurs frequently and is related to the concentration of drug, the alcohol solvent, and its rate of infusion. This may be very painful and is best treated by decreasing the rate of infusion; in addition, it may be necessary to give a strong analgesic such as meperidine, 50–75 mg, intramuscularly. BCNU can produce epidermal cell mutation with pigmentation changes on contact with skin; the physician should therefore be careful in handling this agent. A transient maculopapular rash occasionally occurs. Central nervous system toxicity, manifested by dizziness and ataxia, may be seen shortly after administration of the drug. Hepatic or renal toxicity is unusual (DeVita et al., 1965).

Administration. The drug is supplied in vials of 100 mg and is stored in the refrigerator. Each vial can be reconstituted for use with 3 ml of absolute ethanol (supplied with the drug) and 27 ml of sterile water. Without further dilution, it may be administered through the tubing of a running intravenous infusion of 5% dextrose in water over 5–30 min. Refrigeration of reconstituted BCNU increases the stability of the solution with only 4% decomposition at 24 hours.

Usual Dose. Dose is 200 mg/m^2 intravenously every 42 days.

BLEOMYCIN (BLENOXANE—BRISTOL)

Structure. Blenoxane is a copper-free mixture of several bleomycin species. Approximately 65% of the mixture is composed of the bleomycin A group and 35% of the B group.

Biochemistry. Bleomycin is an antibiotic isolated from *Streptomyces verticillatus.* It acts by interference with DNA synthesis (Kunimoto et al., 1967) and by causing scission of DNA strands (Suzuki et al., 1968), presumably through a preferential attack on guanine and cytosine bases. It inhibits DNA synthesis under conditions where the synthesis of RNA and protein are unimpaired. At low doses, bleomycin reversibly inhibits cell progression at the S-G_2 boundary and in the M phase.

Pharmacology. After a single intravenous injection of bleomycin, the blood level of the drug falls rapidly during the first 30 min but more slowly thereafter. About 40% of the dose is excreted in the urine within the first 24 hours. The majority of the unexcreted drug is found in the skin, lungs, peritoneum and lymph (Fujita and Kimura, 1970). This localization may depend on a lack of bleomycin-inactivating enzyme in these tissues.

Side Effects. Bone marrow depression is uncommon; usually only a mild leukopenia and thrombocytopenia occur. Pulmonary toxicity can be noted by the onset of fine rales or rhonchi, which should alert the physician to the possibility of pulmonary complications. This then progresses to fever, dyspnea, leukocytosis and nonproductive cough. Chest x-ray shows usually a bilateral lower lobe interstitial infiltrate. The process may be reversible at this point by discontinuation of the drug; treatment with high dose prednisone (100 mg/day) may hasten resolution. However, the process may progress to severe pulmonary fibrosis and death. Such grave results usually occur only in elderly patients or with total doses greater than 250 mg/m^2; however, it has been seen with total doses as low as 10–40 mg. Prior lung disease and radiotherapy to the lungs seem to predispose to the pulmonary toxicity. Pulmonary function tests seem to be of little value in predicting clinical bleomycin lung toxicity (Mosher et al., 1972), although a brisk decline in forced vital capacity (FVC) may herald the onset of pulmonary fibrosis. Some cases of pulmonary toxicity may be related to a hypersensitivity phenomenon and be more responsive to corticosteroids (Holoye et al., 1978). Dermatologic changes appear to be dose-related. An initial erythema is noted over areas of maximal pressure or abrasion (hands, feet, elbows, etc.), progressing to ulcerations of the skin. A thickened, hyperpigmented dry skin may result with dystrophic nail changes. A morbiliform rash has been reported. Alopecia is occasionally seen. Fever (occasionally as high as 41°C (106°F)) and chills may occur, usually 3–5 hours after administration of the drug and usually lasting from minutes to a few hours. Treatment with an antihistamine such as diphenylhydramine may help to resolve the fever and chills. A few patients have developed severe acute fulminant reactions following administration of bleomycin, progressing to death (Blum et al., 1973). These reported patients all had a lymphoma; after a delay of several hours following drug administration all developed profound hyperpyrexia, hypotension and sustained cardiorespiratory collapse with death. Milder acute reactions consist of hyperpyrexia, hypotension and varying degrees of respiratory distress occurring shortly after administration of bleomycin: these reactions are reversible, some spontaneously and others appearing to respond to parenteral antihistamines and steroids. Anorexia, nausea, vomiting and diarrhea may occur. Other reported side effects are: stomatitis, esophagitis, tracheitis, acute arthritis, Raynaud's phenomenon, headache and hyperesthesia of the scalp. There is no clear-cut evidence of hepatic or renal toxicity.

Administration. The drug is supplied in ampules containing 15 units of the lyophilized powder. It is stable for at least 1 year at room temperature and can be reconstituted with 2–5 ml of normal saline, 5% dextrose in water, or sterile water for injection. In solution, in 5% dextrose in water, it is stable for at least 8 hours at room temperature. The drug is given intramuscularly, intravenously or subcutaneously.

Usual Dose. Dose is 4–15 units/m^2, intravenously once or twice a week. Other dose schedules are currently under investigation.

BUSULFAN (MYLERAN—BURROUGHS WELLCOME)

$$O{-}SO_2CH_3$$
$$CH_2$$
$$(CH_2)_2$$
$$CH_2$$
$$O{-}SO_2CH_3$$

1,4-Di(methanesulfonoxy)butane

Biochemistry. Busulfan is a bifunctional alkylating agent with a mechanism of action similar to that of other alkylating agents. The drug appears to be cell cycle phase nonspecific.

Pharmacology. After intestinal absorption, over 90% of the drug is cleared from the blood within 2–3 min. Excretion is in the urine as metabolic products, chiefly methanesulfonic acid (Nadkarni et al., 1959). The primary pharmacologic effect of the drug is a depressant action on myelopoiesis.

Side Effects. Bone marrow suppression is seen mainly as leukopenia, in which the rate of fall of the white blood cell count is clearly dose-related. With continued therapy, thrombocytopenia and anemia are seen. Nausea and vomiting are uncommon and usually mild. Most menstruating women on long term busulfan therapy will develop menstrual dysfunction, usually amenorrhea. Occasionally, patients on busulfan for several years will develop a syndrome of persistent dry cough and slowly progressive dyspnea due to intra-alveolar exudation of fibrin and subsequent organization into fibrosis; this syndrome may be reversed by promptly discontinuing the drug (Kirschner and Esterly, 1971). Occasionally seen is a wasting syndrome mimicking Addison's disease, and characterized by weight loss, anorexia, hypotension, hyperpigmentation of the skin due to increased melanin, but normal adrenal function tests (Kyle et al., 1961). Following prolonged therapy with busulfan, cytologic dysplasia may be seen in various organs including cervix, lung and urinary tract (Koss et al., 1965). Other side effects reported are: glossitis, gonadal atrophy with sterility (male and female), gynecomastia, anhidrosis, alopecia and cataracts.

Administration. The drug is supplied in tablets of 2 mg, scored, for oral use.

Usual Dose. Dose is 2–8 mg/day, orally.

CCNU, LOMUSTINE (Ceenu—BRISTOL)

$$\text{cyclohexyl}-NH-\overset{\overset{\displaystyle O}{\|}}{C}-\underset{\underset{\displaystyle NO}{|}}{N}-CH_2CH_2Cl$$

1-(2-Chloroethyl)-3-cyclohexyl-1-nitrosourea

Biochemistry. CCNU is structurally related to BCNU but is more lipid-soluble, which might allow its increased passage across the blood-brain barrier. Although the active form and mechanism of action of CCNU are unknown, evidence indicates that it acts as an alkylating agent and may, as do the other nitrosoureas, inhibit key enzymatic processes leading to DNA synthesis. However, in some tumors CCNU lacks cross resistance with conventional alkylating agents and may act in a different phase of the cell cycle than alkylating agents. It has been recently found that CCNU interacts with proteins via cyclohexylcarbamylation of lysine residues (Wasserman et al., 1974). Its cell cycle specificity is not clear, but it may be cell cycle G_2 phase specific.

Pharmacology. After administration of ^{14}C-labeled CCNU (Oliverio, 1973; Sponzo et al., 1973), there is prompt absorption and a rapid rise in plasma levels of isotope with peaks at 1–4 hours, representing about 0.1% of the administered dose. About 50% of the radioactivity is excreted in the urine during the first 12 hours with nearly complete excretion by 48–72 hours. CCNU rapidly enters the cerebrospinal fluid (CSF); the CSF radioactivity:plasma radioactivity ratio is 0.3 for the chloroethyl moiety. None of the intact drug is detected at any time in the urine, plasma or CSF, which implies that the active and/or myelosuppressive form of

CCNU is not the parent compound but rather one or more of its degradation products. It is possible that the active antitumor metabolite may not be the same compound that produces the myelosuppressive effect.

Side Effects. Thrombocytopenia and leukopenia are common, with a delayed onset and a nadir at 4–6 weeks. Thrombocytopenia often appears earlier, is of shorter duration, and recovery is more rapid than from leukopenia. The hematocrit is rarely affected. Nausea and vomiting are frequently noted up to 6 hours after drug administration and are often followed by 2–3 days of anorexia. Hepatic and renal dysfunction is rarely seen in humans (Hansen et al., 1971).

Administration. CCNU is supplied in dose packs, each containing: two 100-mg caps, two 40-mg caps, and two 10-mg caps. These capsules are stable for at least 2 years when stored at room temperature in well closed containers.

Usual Dose. Dose is 130 mg/m^2 orally every 6 weeks.

CHLORAMBUCIL, CLB (LEUKERAN—BURROUGHS WELLCOME)

$$ClCH_2CH_2 \diagdown \underset{\displaystyle ClCH_2CH_2}{\overset{\displaystyle}{N}} - \langle \text{phenyl} \rangle - CH_2CH_2CH_2COOH$$

4-[*p*-[Bis(2-chloroethyl)amino]phenyl]butyric acid

Biochemistry. Chlorambucil is a bifunctional alkylating agent with a mechanism of action similar to that of other alkylating agents. It is probably a cell cycle nonspecific agent.

Pharmacology. There is incomplete information concerning the metabolism, distribution or elimination of the drug in man.

Side Effects. Bone marrow depression is seen mainly in the form of leukopenia; platelets and erythrocytes are little affected. The usual daily therapeutic doses will depress the leukocyte count (both lymphocytes and neutrophils) within 10 days; this depression can be rapidly reversed. Nausea and vomiting are mild and usually do not occur with total daily doses less than 20 mg. An occasional patient will complain of epigastric burning. Liver damage is rare and possibly a hypersensitivity reaction (Koler and Fosgren, 1958); it is an indication to stop the drug. Mutagenicity is reported (Shotten and Monie, 1964).

Administration. The drug is supplied in tablets of 2 mg for oral use.

Usual Dose. Dose is 0.1 to 0.2 mg/kg/day as a single daily oral dose.

Cis-PLATINUM

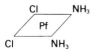

cis-Platinum (II)
diamminedichloride

Biochemistry. Cis-platinum (11) diamminedichloride is a complex formed by a central atom of platinum surrounded by an arrangement of chlorine atoms and ammonia groups in a *cis*-planar relationship. The drug interferes with DNA synthesis by causing cross linkage of DNA complementary strands. RNA and protein synthesis are inhibited to a lesser degree. The drug is cell cycle phase nonspecific.

Pharmacology. After an intravenous bolus injection of the drug, plasma levels fall in a biphasic manner with a secondary half-life of 58–73 hours. More than 90% of the drug is protein bound in its excretion phase. Twenty-seven to 45% of the drug is eliminated in the urine in the first 5 days, with platinum still detectable in tissue samples 4 months after administration of the drug (DeConti et al., 1973).

Side Effects. Bone marrow suppression is the dose-limiting factor; leukopenia is commonly seen with a mean nadir following completion of therapy of 15 days; thrombocytopenia is less common. The patient may develop a progressive anemia without evidence of hemolysis or blood loss. Nausea and vomiting are common and may be severe, especially with large doses, beginning 4–6 hours after injection and lasting 24–36 hours with variable nausea and anorexia persisting for up to a week. Nephrotoxicity is dose-dependent and did not appear following a total cumulative dose of less than 50 mg/m^2. Most commonly an elevation of the BUN was seen which was reversible upon discontinuation of the drug. Renal biopsies have shown acute tubular necrosis. The drug should be given with caution to patients with impaired renal function. Intravenous hydration along with mannitol infusion will decrease the nephrotoxicity of the drug without affecting its antitumor activity and will also allow administration of higher doses. Although the patient may not complain of hearing loss, audiologic testing has revealed frequently an impairment in the high frequency range. It is postulated that the cochlea may be the site of injury due to the drug. No mucositis or hepatotoxicity has been noted (Rossof et al., 1972). Several anaphylactic reactions to the drug have been reported, consisting of facial edema, wheezing, tachycardia and hypotension within a few minutes after drug administration and can be controlled with adrenaline, corticosteroids or antihistamines (Rozencweig et al., 1977b).

Administration. The drug is supplied in vials containing 10 mg of the drug as a white powder, investigational (NSC-119875) which may be reconstituted with 10 ml of sterile water and injected immediately intravenously. At 22°C the reconstituted solution is stable for at least 8 hours. *Usual Dose.* Dose schedules are actively under investigation.

CYCLOPHOSPHAMIDE, CTX (CYTOXAN—MEAD JOHNSON)

$$O \quad CH_2CH_2Cl$$
$$P-N-CH_2CH_2-Cl$$
$$N$$
$$H \qquad \cdot H_2O$$

2-[Bis(2-chloroethyl)amino]tetrahydro-2*H*-1,3,2,-oxazophosphorine

Biochemistry. Cyclophosphamide is an inactive cyclic phosphoramide mustard which is activated primarily by oxidation on hepatic microsomes (Brock et al., 1971). The active product alkylates cellular macromolecules. Although highly effective against cells in DNA synthesis, it kills cells in all phases of the cell cycle and is considered to be a cell cycle nonspecific bifunctional alkylating agent.

Pharmacology. The plasma half-life after intravenous administration is 6.5 hours; not more than 20% of the injected drug is excreted intact in the urine at any dose level (Bagley et al., 1973). Maximum plasma levels after oral administration are reached in 1 hour. Thirty-one to 66% of the administered dose is recovered in the stools, 17–31% as unchanged drug; the remainder is excreted in the urine mainly as metabolites (Bort et al., 1961). Allopurinol, by interfering with hepatic microsomal oxidase activation of cyclophosphamide, probably increases the half-life. Potassium iodide also prolongs the half-life of cyclophosphamide. Pretreatment with phenobarbital has been shown to enhance the metabolism of cyclophosphamide. However, prior exposure to drugs with an inducing or repressing effect on microsomal oxidase probably has little effect on the antitumor and toxic effects of cyclophosphamide (Bagley et al., 1973).

Side Effects. Nausea and vomiting are dose-related but usually mild and last less than 12 hours. Alopecia occurs in most patients given maximum regular intravenous therapy and usually occurs within a few weeks of initiation of therapy. Hair growth nearly always returns after the drug is discontinued; occasionally it begins to grow back when the dose of drug is reduced for maintenance therapy, or when the patient is placed on oral cyclophosphamide. A similar but less pronounced suppressant effect is seen with facial hair and fingernails. Leukopenia is expected, with a maximal drop 7–13 days after a large parenteral dose.

Complete restitution of counts is usual by 14–18 days. Thrombocytopenia may occur but is rarely severe. Erythrocytes are little affected. Sterile hemorrhagic cystitis is seen in 1–4% of patients. The hematuria is often preceded by a few days of urinary frequency or dysuria. The bladder mucosa is apparently injured by a cyclophosphamide metabolite which is excreted in the urine (Johnson and Meadows, 1971). Ample fluid intake on the day of and a few days after therapy may prevent it. If the cystitis does occur, the drug should be temporarily stopped and cautiously restarted after the hematuria has cleared. Fever to 38°C (101°F) may be seen shortly after a large intravenous dose. Also seen are: amenorrhea and testicular atrophy (Fairley et al., 1972), mucosal ulcerations, skin hyperpigmentation and fetal damage (Toledo et al., 1971).

Administration. The drug is supplied in vials containing 500, 200, and 100 mg of the white crystalline hydrate. The dry form decomposes at temperatures greater than 32°C (90°F). For extended stability both tablets and vials may be kept in the refrigerator. In preparing the drug for injection, add 5 ml of sterile water to a 100-mg vial, 10 ml to a 200-mg vial and 25 ml to a 500-mg vial. The drug may be used up to 3 hours after it is prepared and is given by direct intravenous injection. Too rapid injection may result in facial flushing and a feeling of faintness. The drug is also supplied in tablets of 50 mg, scored, for oral use.

Usual Dose. Dose is 1.0–1.5 g/m², intravenously, every 2–3 weeks, or 500–800 mg/m², intravenously, every 1–2 weeks, or 2–2.5 mg/kg/day, orally.

CYTOSINE ARABINOSIDE, ARA-C (CYTOSAR—UPJOHN)

1-β-D-Arabinofuranosylcytosine

Biochemistry. Cytosine arabinoside is a synthetic nucleoside pyrimidine antimetabolite which is cytotoxic to a variety of cell lines. It must gain entry to the cell and be converted to cytosine arabinoside-5'-triphosphate (ARACTP) to be active. Cytosine arabinoside decreases the conversion of uridine to deoxycytidine nucleotides and competes with deoxycytidine for deoxycytidine kinase. ARACTP inhibits DNA polymerase and thus DNA synthesis. Cytosine arabinoside will cause G_2 phase chromosomal breaks; however, at limiting doses it produces a reversible S phase block, compatible with its effect on DNA polymerase. It is primarily a cell cycle S phase specific agent.

Pharmacology. Cytosine arabinoside is distributed in total body water and is rapidly deaminated by the liver and kidneys to uracil arabinoside, which is inactive. The intravenous dose will slowly enter the cerebrospinal fluid to a slight degree. After a single intravenous injection the plasma half-life is less than 9 min, falling to unmeasurable levels within 15–60 min, with 90% of the dose excreted in 24 hours (more by the liver than the kidneys) as the deamination product. There are large variations in the half-life of cytosine arabinoside among patients receiving the same dose of drug intravenously, presumably due to variations in degradation rates related to deaminase activity. Excessive cytosine arabinoside degradation rates may be a cause of failure of drug in certain patients (Papac et al., 1965; Baguley and Falkenhaug, 1971).

Side Effects. Because of its rapid detoxification, cytosine arabinoside can be given to patients with compromised renal failure. In doses as little as 30 mg/m^2 daily, over several days, severe depression of leukocytes and platelets can occur, but there is a wide range of individual susceptibility. If large intravenous injections are given, nausea and vomiting frequently occur. In the presence of poor liver function, cytosine arabinoside should be used with extra caution, since the drug may cause worsening of hepatocellular function. If given over several days, bone marrow megaloblastosis and chromosomal disruption will inevitably occur. Because of its rapid detoxification in vivo, cytosine arabinoside is better tolerated by rapid intravenous injection than by slow infusion. Other side effects are: diarrhea, oral ulcerations, phlebitis, fever, abdominal pain, neuritis, skin rash, arthralgias, dizziness, alopecia and teratogenicity.

Administration. The drug is supplied in vials containing 100 and 500 mg of the powder. It can be reconstituted with 5 and 10 ml, respectively, of sterile water with 0.9% benzyl alcohol (packaged with each vial). After reconstitution the drug can be stored at room temperature but must be used within 48 hours and should be discarded if the solution develops a slight haze. The drug can be administered intravenously, intramuscularly, subcutaneously or intrathecally.

Usual Dose. Dose is 100 mg/m^2/day for 5–7 days as a 24-hour infusion, or 100 mg/m^2/day for approximately 10–20 days by intravenous push or as a 1-hour infusion (acute leukemia induction); 20 mg/m^2/week subcutaneously, intramuscularly or by intravenous push (solid tumors, acute leukemia maintenance); or 30 mg/m^2 intrathecally every 1–7 days (central nervous system leukemia).

DACARBAZINE (DTIC—DOME)

$$CH_3-N-N=N \quad \text{(imidazole ring with } NH_2-C=O \text{ substituent)}$$

Imidazole carboxamide dimethyl triazeno

Biochemistry. The mode of action of DTIC is not well understood. It may act (a) by inhibition of de novo purine biosynthesis, (b) as an alkylating agent by release of a mustard radical, or (c) by interacting with sulfhydryl groups (Goldsmith et al., 1972). Its cell cycle specificity is also unclear.

Pharmacology. After an intravenous injection, the plasma half-life of DTIC is about 34 min, and there is no detectable serum level of the drug at 24 hours after administration. Relatively little drug is protein bound (about 5%). DTIC is rapidly excreted by a renal tubular secretory mechanism. At 6 hours after a dose of the drug, 46% of the drug is excreted in the urine (half as DTIC and half as its metabolites). DTIC can be detected in the CSF in low concentrations (14% of serum concentration) (Loo et al., 1968b; Skibba et al., 1969).

Side Effects. Bone marrow depression is common. The nadir of leukopenia or thrombocytopenia may be delayed for as long as 5 weeks, with subsequent recovery in another 2 weeks. Nausea and vomiting may be severe, occurring within the first hour or 2 after the drug is injected, and generally decreasing in severity as the course of therapy progresses. A transient flu-like syndrome may occur, manifested by fever, chills and myalgias, beginning usually on day 2 of a course of therapy and usually ending with cessation of therapy. Occasional hepatic (elevated bilirubin and SGOT) and renal (elevated BUN) abnormalities are seen but are readily reversible. Facial flush and paresthesiae of the face may occur during or shortly after injection of the drug. Vincristine neurotoxicity may be potentiated.

Administration. The drug is supplied in vials containing 100 or 200 mg of the lyophilized powder. The 100-mg vial should be reconstituted with 9.9 ml and the 200-mg vial with 19.7 ml of sterile water; each milliliter of solution will then contain 10 mg of the drug. This solution is stable for at least 72 hours at 4°C. Any color change of the solution from its normal pale yellow color (usually to orange) indicates drug decomposition, and the solution should be discarded. The drug should be injected directly through the side arm of a running intravenous infusion.

GUIDE TO THERAPEUTIC ONCOLOGY

Usual Dose. Dose is 250 mg/m^2/day, intravenously for 5 days, repeated every 3–4 weeks.

DAUNOMYCIN (DNM), RUBIDOMYCIN, DAUNORUBICIN

Biochemistry. Daunomycin is an antibiotic isolated from *Streptomyces peucetius*. It is an anthracycline, consisting of a pigmented aglycone joined to an amino sugar by a glycosidic linkage. Daunomycin forms complexes with DNA by intercalation between base pairs and thereby inhibits both DNA replication and DNA-dependent synthesis of RNA. It also has the ability to delay the onset of mitosis in cells which have already synthesized DNA. Daunomycin appears to suppress RNA synthesis more than DNA synthesis in mammalian cells. Although the cell cycle phase specificity is not yet settled, there are suggestions that daunomycin may be a G$_2$ specific drug (Calendi et al., 1965; Whang-Peng et al., 1969).

Pharmacology. After a single intravenous injection, the blood level reaches its maximum in 15 min and the drug disappears in 12 hours. Total recovery in the urine is 85% of an injected dose in 24 hours, with the bulk appearing in the first 4–6 hours. Tissue distribution of the drug is not well understood. It probably does not enter the cerebrospinal fluid.

Side Effects. Bone marrow depression is commonly quite marked, with depression of all marrow elements. Prolonged bone marrow aplasia may occur. Myocardial damage may occur as a dose-related phenomenon; it generally occurs only when large doses are given or a total cumulative dose in excess of 550 mg/m^2. However, cardiac toxicity has been seen at total doses as low as 2 mg/kg, especially in older patients. Nonspecific ST-T wave changes on the electrocardiogram may precede severe cardiac toxicity and are an indication to temporarily stop the drug. Cardiac arrhythmias and congestive heart failure are serious sequelae and may be fatal. Patients with pre-existing cardiac disease or electrocardiographic abnormalities may be more likely to develop cardiac problems. Focal interstitial myocarditis has been noted at autopsy for acute myeloblastic leukemia in a few patients. This side effect has restricted daunomycin to remission induction regimens or to infrequent intermittent administration during maintenance. Stomatitis and hemorrhagic enterocolitis, renal tubular damage and hematuria, anorexia, nausea and vomiting, alopecia, fever, skin rash and phlebitis at the injection site are other side effects of variable frequency (Livingston et al., 1968).

Administration. The drug is supplied in vials containing 20 mg of the reddish powder (investigational, NSC-82151). It is stored frozen and is reconstituted with 10 ml of normal saline. The reconstituted drug can be stored at 4°C for up to 24 hours. It is given intravenously, and, as with Adriamycin, should be infused over at least a 5-min interval.

Usual Dose. Dose is 30–60 mg/m^2/day, intravenously, for 1–5 days, every 3–4 weeks.

o,p'-DDD (LYSODREN—CALBIO)

1,1-Dichloro-2-(o-chlorophenyl)-2-(p-chlorophenyl)ethane

Biochemistry. o,p'-DDD is a potent inhibitor of adrenocortical steroid synthesis and activity. It causes degenerative changes in the zona reticularis and fasciculata (Vilar and Tulner, 1959) and accelerates inactivation of adrenocorticoids by a peripheral tissue metabolism (Bledsoe et al., 1964); direct measurement of plasma cortisol is required to accurately estimate the effect of the drug on hormone secretion. It is used almost exclusively in the treatment of metastatic carcinomas of the adrenal cortex. The drug reduces cushingoid manifestations and may sometimes cause regression of the tumor and its metastases.

Pharmacology. Following oral administration of the drug, approximately 40% is absorbed with distribution primarily to body fat and excretion via metabolites in the bile and urine.

Side Effects. Gastrointestinal side effects are common, consisting of anorexia, nausea, vomiting and diarrhea. Neuromuscular side effects include lethargy, somnolence, vertigo, depression, muscular tremors, confusion, weakness, headaches and diplopia; all reversible with discontinuation of the drug or a reduction in dose. A skin rash may occur, which is not always dose related and may clear despite continued therapy. Renal and hepatic toxicity is rare. There is no bone marrow suppression. Lens opacity and toxic retinopathy have been reported. Hypoadrenocorticism may occur; for this reason, adrenal steroid replacement should be considered for all patients taking the drug (Hutter and Kayhoe, 1966).

Administration. The drug is supplied in tablets of 0.5 g, scored, for oral use.

Usual Dose. Begin with 2–6 g daily in divided doses and gradually increase the dose over several weeks to a maximum of 10–12 g.

DIBROMODULCITOL (DBD)

$$
\begin{array}{c}
CH_2\!-\!Br \\
H\!-\!C\!-\!OH \\
HO\!-\!C\!-\!H \\
HO\!-\!C\!-\!H \\
H\!-\!C\!-\!OH \\
CH_2\!-\!Br
\end{array}
$$

D-Galactital, 1,6-dibromo-1,6-dideoxy

Biochemistry. Dibromodulcitol is an α,ω substituted hexitol similar in structure to dibromomannitol. It may act as an alkylating agent as well as a pyrimidine antagonist. It is probably a cell cycle nonspecific agent.

Pharmacology. The drug is rapidly absorbed from the gastrointestinal tract and reaches a maximum blood level within 1 hour. Dibromodulcitol is rapidly hydrolyzed in plasma to monobromodulcitol and various epoxides, so that within 2 hours after administration less than 5% of the unchanged drug remains in the blood. The drug or its metabolites enter spinal, pleural and ascitic fluids and reach a maximum concentration in 5 hours. The drug and its metabolites are excreted by the kidney, 68–74% appearing in the urine within 48 hours (Belej et al., 1972).

Side Effects. Bone marrow suppression is the usual dose-limiting toxicity and occurs mainly as leukopenia. Nausea and vomiting are uncommon and mild. There have been no observable changes in hepatic or renal function tests in human studies (Keyes et al., 1971).

Administration. The drug is supplied in tablets of 25 mg (investigational NSC-104800) for oral use. It is stored at room temperature.

Usual Dose. Dose is 3–5 mg/kg/day, orally, or 140–210 mg/m^2 daily for 10 days, orally, repeated every 4–6 weeks.

DIBROMOMANNITOL (DBM)

$$
\begin{array}{c}
CH_2-Br \\
HO-C-H \\
HO-C-H \\
H-C-OH \\
H-C-OH \\
CH_2-Br
\end{array}
$$

1,6-Dibromo-1,6-dideoxy-D-mannitol

Biochemistry. Dibromomannitol is an α, ω substituted hexitol with alkylating ability, although it may also act as an antimetabolite (Livingston et al., 1968a, b). It is probably a cell cycle nonspecific agent.

Pharmacology. There is incomplete information concerning the pharmacology of the drug in man. In animals, following intravenous administration of the drug, 60–70% is excreted in the urine within 12 hours (Livingston et al., 1968a, b).

Side Effects. Bone marrow suppression is the usual dose-limiting toxicity and occurs mainly as leukopenia. Nausea and vomiting are uncommon and mild. There have been no observable changes in renal or hepatic function tests in human studies.

Administration. The drug is supplied in tablets (scored) of 50 and 100 mg (investigational, NSC-94100) for oral use. It is stored at room temperature.

Usual Dose. In the treatment of chronic myelogenous leukemia, 250 mg daily, PO, until the white blood cell count has been reduced to 20,000, with subsequent reduction to 250 mg, every other day for maintenance.

5-FLUOROURACIL (5-FU, FU) (FLUOROURACIL—ROCHE)

2,4-Dioxo-5-fluoropyrimidine

Biochemistry. 5-Fluorouracil is a pyrimidine antimetabolite which competes with uracil to undergo all anabolic and catabolic reactions typical for uracil, except that it will not go to thymidine. 5-Fluorouracil is converted in vivo to fluorodeoxyuridylic acid (FudRP), which inhibits thymidine synthesis by blocking the enzyme thymidylate synthetase, the rate-limiting enzyme for DNA synthesis. The presence of thymidine does not reverse growth inhibition due to 5-fluorouracil given as single daily intravenous doses (Calabresi and Parks, 1970). Some 5-fluorouracil is converted to 5-fluorouridine (FUR), which is rapidly incorporated into RNA; this compound may be responsible for some of the toxicity of 5-fluorouracil without adding to its antitumor effect (Heidelberger, 1963). One of the major forms of resistance to 5-fluorouracil is the inability of the resistant cell to synthesize FUdRP because of a decreased concentration of one of the necessary enzymes. Another mechanism of resistance is the ability to synthesize thymidylic acid by other pathways (Brockman, 1963). The drug appears to be a cell cycle phase nonspecific antimetabolite.

Pharmacology. After administration of oral 5-fluorouracil, peak plasma levels occur rapidly but are generally lower than those seen after intravenous administration of comparable doses. The drug is more extensively metabolized after oral administration, and there is more variability in absorption than with a comparable intravenous dose (Bruckner and Creasey, 1974). 5-Fluorouracil disappears rapidly from the blood after a single 15 mg/kg dose is given intravenously, with a mean plasma half-life of 10 min (Cohen et al., 1974). The average renal excretion of 5-fluorouracil is 16% of the injected dose, with much of the remaining drug expired as carbon dioxide. When 5-fluorouracil is given by prolonged continuous intravenous infusion, there is less urinary excretion, most of the drug being catabolized in the liver; its toxicity is also decreased about 2-fold compared with the equivalent dosage given by repeated single daily injections.

Side Effects. An erythematous mucocutaneous junction is frequently the first sign of toxicity, followed by a sore mouth and then an ulcerative stomatitis within a few days. Severe gastrointestinal ulcerations may occur, progressing to a bloody diarrhea. Any of these side effects is an indication that the drug should be discontinued until they have cleared. Nausea and vomiting commonly occur when the drug is given in repeated daily intravenous injections but are uncommon with weekly injections. Severe leukopenia or thrombocytopenia is uncommon with weekly doses of 15 mg/kg. Mild anemia is occasionally seen. Alopecia, usually mild and reversible, is seen in 5–20% of patients. An extensive erythematous dermatitis in exposed skin areas is occasionally noted, usually requiring temporary discontinuation of the drug until it clears. Neurotoxicity is seen occasionally in the form of a reversible cerebellar ataxia (Boileau et al., 1971); basal ganglia dysfunction has also been reported (Bergevin et al., 1975). Patients who have had a bilateral adrenalectomy may be more likely to develop toxicity from 5-fluorouracil. Tipton (1964) advised quadrupling the maintenance course of cortisone in these patients before using 5-fluorouracil.

Administration. The drug is supplied in ampules containing 500 mg in 10 ml of aqueous solution. It is administered intravenously or orally without further dilution. When used orally, some patients prefer to dilute the drug with water; the drug should not be mixed with fruit juices or other acidic solutions because of decreased solubility.

Usual Dose. Dose is 15 mg/kg/week, intravenously; or 12 mg/kg/day, intravenously, for 5 days, followed by half doses of the drug on alternate days starting with day 7 to the point of toxicity, the entire course repeated every 4–6 weeks; 30 mg/kg/day for a maximum of 5 days as a 24-hour infusion. Use of the drug as an oral preparation remains experimental.

HEXAMETHYLMELAMINE (HXM)

$$
\begin{array}{c}
CH_3 \quad\quad CH_3 \\
CH_3{-}N{\diagdown}\;N{\diagdown}\;N{-}CH_3 \\
N{\diagup}\;N \\
N{-}CH_3 \\
CH_3
\end{array}
$$

2,4,6-Tris(dimethylamino)-*S*-triazine

Biochemistry. Hexamethylmelamine structurally resembles triethylenemelamine; however, the metabolism of the two drugs appears to differ significantly. Hexamethylmelamine may function as a pyrimidine antimetabolite (Borkovec and DeMilo, 1967) and/or as an alkylating agent. It is probably a cell cycle nonspecific agent.

Pharmacology. Bryan et al. (1968) determined plasma levels and urinary metabolites of hexamethylmelamine in cancer patients after oral administration. Maximal plasma levels after a single dose of 4 mg/kg were obtained 2–3 hours later, at which time no intact drug was detectable in the plasma. Nearly 19% of a single oral dose was excreted in the urine as metabolites during the first 24 hours after administration, with an additional 12% appearing between 24 and 48 hours. After prolonged continual daily administration of the drug, 50–65% of a daily dose was recovered from the urine as metabolites.

Side Effects. Leukopenia and thrombocytopenia are usually moderate and reversible when the drug is discontinued. Nausea, vomiting and diarrhea are generally dose-limiting side effects; they may be severe and require temporary discontinuation of the drug (Bergevin et al., 1973). Antiemetics, such as the phenothiazines, are almost always required during therapy. Neurologic side effects are: (a) a delayed neuropathy manifested by paresthesia, hyporeflexia, motor weakness, and decreased position sense, vibratory sense and touch. These side effects are reported to be dose related and may not be entirely reversible (Louis, 1967). Previous vincristine neurotoxicity may be exacerbated by hexamethylmelamine. (b) Mental symptoms are depression, somnolence, dysphasia, insomnia, hallucinations and confusion. A parkinsonian-like state has been described (Wilson et al., 1970). A maculopapular skin rash and a psoriasis-like eczema have been described (Louis, 1967). Stolinsky et al. (1972b) observed abnormalities in liver function tests in a few patients. No adverse effects on kidney, lung or cardiovascular function have been noted.

Administration. The drug is supplied in capsules of 50 and 100 mg (investigational, NSC-13875) for oral use. It is stored at room temperature and is stable for at least 2 years.

Usual Dose. Dose is 4–8 mg/kg/day, orally. Other dose schedules are currently under investigation.

HYDROXYUREA (HU) (HYDREA—SQUIBB)

$$NH_2-\overset{\overset{\displaystyle O}{\|}}{C}-NH-OH$$

Biochemistry. Hydroxyurea is a highly selective inhibitor of DNA synthesis by inducing a block of deoxyribonucleotide formation from ribonucleotides (Krakoff et al., 1968). It is a cell cycle S phase specific agent.

Pharmacology. Hydroxyurea is rapidly absorbed from the gastrointestinal tract; maximum serum levels are attained within 1 hour, and there is complete urinary excretion of the drug within 24 hours. There is preferential uptake of the drug by both white and red blood cells (Rosner et al., 1971).

Side Effects. Bone marrow depression is clearly dose related. There is a marked and usually rapid fall in the white blood cell count, less so with platelets, in 24–48 hours after a dose, with subsequent recovery within 7 days. The drug is especially useful for rapid reduction of markedly elevated white blood cell counts, as in chronic myelogenous leukemia. Gastrointestinal and oral ulcerations are occasionally observed. Nausea and vomiting may occur after administration of the drug. Patients on long term maintenance treatment with hydroxyurea may develop dermatologic alterations, including partial alopecia, hyperpigmentation, dry skin and atrophy of skin and subcutaneous tissue (Kennedy, 1972).

Administration. The drug is supplied in capsules of 500 mg and is sometimes better tolerated by opening the capsules and dissolving the contents in warm tea, orange juice, etc.

Usual Dose. Dose is 80 mg/kg twice a week, orally, or 20–30 mg/kg daily, orally.

ICRF-159, RAZOXANE

(±)1,2-Di(3,5-dioxopiperazin-1-yl)propane

Biochemistry. ICRF-159 is a synthetic nonpolar derivative of the complexing agent ethylenediaminetetraacetic acid. It is active in the early mitotic phase and inhibits DNA synthesis possibly by acylation by biological nucleophils. ICRF-159 may act to prevent neovascularization of the primary tumor and so prevent metastases from occurring; perhaps a tumor angiogenesis factor is inhibited. In experimental systems it appears to protect against the cardiac toxicity of the anthracycline antibiotics. ICRF-159 may be most effective in the early mitotic (G_2/M) phases of cell growth (Bakowski, 1976).

Pharmacology. In one study, following an oral dose of 3 g/m^2, at 2 hours the peak plasma level of the drug was seen with negligible concentration at 24 hours after administration.

Side Effects. Bone marrow depression, especially leukopenia, is the dose-limiting factor. Nausea and vomiting may occur but are mild. Dermatitis and alopecia are occasionally seen. Renal or hepatic toxicity is unreported in humans (Creaven et al., 1974; Bellet et al., 1973a).

Administration. The drug is supplied in tablets of 50 and 250 mg (investigational, NSC-129943) for oral use. The drug is stored at room temperature.

Usual Dose. Dose schedules are currently under investigation.

MELPHALAN, L-PHENYLALANINE MUSTARD (L-PAM), L-SARCOLYSINE (ALKERAN—BURROUGHS WELLCOME)

p-Bis(*β*-chloroethyl)aminophenylalanine

Biochemistry. Melphalan is a bifunctional alkylating agent whose mechanism of action appears to be similar to that of other alkylating agents. It is probably cell cycle nonspecific.

Pharmacology. After a single oral dose, melphalan remains in an active form in the blood for up to 6 hours. It is taken up by body tissues, and its metabolic products are excreted in the urine.

Side Effects. Bone marrow depression is clearly dose related, affecting chiefly the white blood cells and platelets. The nadir of leukopenia or thrombocytopenia, after a single oral dose, is about 17 days, with a range of 6–41 days and a slow recovery to normal values. The dose should be decreased in the presence of renal insufficiency. Nausea and vomiting are uncommon and usually seen only after the ingestion of more than 20 mg of the drug. Oral mucosal ulceration may occur with prolonged use of large doses; it is an indication to withhold the drug until the ulceration has cleared. Amenorrhea may occur.

Administration. The drug is supplied in tablets of 2 mg, scored, for oral use. An intravenous form is currently under investigation.

Usual Dose. Dose is 0.05 mg/kg/day, orally, or 0.15 mg/kg/day, orally, for 7 days, then 0.05 mg/kg/day, after marrow depression resolves (about 3-4 weeks), or 0.25 mg/kg/day, orally, for 4 days, every 4–6 weeks, or 0.15 mg/kg/day, orally, for 7 days, every 4–6 weeks.

METHYL-CCNU (MeCCNU)

$$Cl-\overset{*}{C}H_2-\overset{*}{C}H_2-\underset{NO}{N}-\overset{O}{\overset{\|}{C}}-NH-\langle\;*\;\rangle-CH_3$$

1-(2-Chloroethyl)-3-(4-methylcyclohexyl)-1-nitrosourea

Biochemistry. Methyl-CCNU is the most lipid soluble of the nitrosoureas presently in clinical use, thus allowing its increased passage across the blood-brain barrier. Its action is not well understood, but, like BCNU and CCNU, it may function as an alkylating agent and/or as an antimetabolite. It may be cell cycle G_2 phase specific.

Pharmacology. Oliverio (1973) and Sponzo et al. (1973) have studied the disposition of methyl-CCNU radiolabeled in the chloroethyl and cyclohexyl moieties and administered at 120–290 mg/m^2 orally. Both moieties were rapidly absorbed with significant plasma levels of radioactivity appearing as early as 10 min and peak plasma levels occurring at 3-6 hours. Excretion is largely by the urinary tract. The analysis of CSF in 2 patients who received the cyclohexyl labeled moiety, at 2 and 3 hours, respectively, showed levels of 10 and 15% of concurrent plasma levels, respectively. No intact drug was found in blood, urine, CSF or ascitic samples. Methyl-CCNU is thus rapidly metabolized in vivo, and neither the active antitumor compound nor the myelosuppressive compound is likely to be the parent drug.

Side Effects. The dose-limiting toxicity of methyl-CCNU is a delayed bone marrow suppression, especially thrombocytopenia, with a nadir at 4–6 weeks. Cumulative bone marrow toxicity may be evident after several courses of the drug. Nausea and vomiting are frequent but are usually limited to the day of drug administration and are hardly ever dose limiting. Premedication with an antiemetic, such as one of the phenothiazines, may help in some patients. Hepatic and renal dysfunction are rarely seen in humans. In a few patients, mental confusion, delusions and disorientation are seen beginning within 24 hours of administration of the drug and lasting up to 2 weeks.

Administration. The drug is supplied in capsules of 10, 50 and 100 mg (investigational, NSC-9544). The drug is stored frozen in the dark until use, but storage at normal room temperature for short periods of time (30–60 days) will not affect potency of the drug. The frozen capsule is given orally on an empty stomach in a single dose.

Usual Dose. Dose is 200–225 mg/m^2, orally, every 6 weeks.

6-MERCAPTOPURINE (6-MP, MP) (PURINETHOL—BURROUGHS WELLCOME)

Biochemistry. 6-Mercaptopurine is an analog of the nucleic acid constituent adenine and the physiologic purine base hypoxanthine. 6-Mercaptopurine must first be converted to the ribonucleotide (6-MPRP) before it can exert its growth inhibitory effects. Cells that are resistant to 6-mercaptopurine have been shown in many cases to lack the enzyme inosine-guaninepyrophosphorylase necessary for this conversion. The effectiveness of 6-mercaptopurine is probably due to the multiplicity of blocks that its metabolites can produce on a nucleic acid pathway, particularly purine biosynthesis. The principle site of action of 6-mercaptopurine might be in the conversion of a hypoxanthine-containing compound to an adenine-containing compound. 6-Mercaptopurine inhibits nicotinamide-adenine dinucleotide synthesis and may by a feedback mechanism inhibit formation of a purine precursor, phosphoribosylamine. The incorporation of formate, glycine and phosphate into nucleic acid purines are inhibited by 6-mercaptopurine (Elion, 1967; Hitchings and Elion, 1972). It is a cell cycle phase nonspecific antimetabolite.

Pharmacology. After a single intravenous injection, the plasma half-life of 6-mercaptopurine is 90 min (Hamilton and Elion, 1954), whereas excretion after an oral dose takes days to weeks. 6-Mercaptopurine is rapidly metabolized in vivo to nontoxic derivatives, chiefly 6-thiouric acid, by a reaction catalyzed by xanthine oxidase. Both 6-mercaptopurine and its metabolites are excreted by the kidneys; after an intravenous dose, 20–40% of the compound appears in the urine unchanged within 6 hours (Coffey et al., 1972; Loo et al., 1968a).

Side Effects. The major side effect is leukopenia and thrombocytopenia. Stomatitis may occur; the oral ulcerations often resemble monilia infection. Nausea and vomiting may occur but are usually mild. In the presence of renal insufficiency the drug should be used cautiously and in decreased dosage. Jaundice is occasionally seen due to liver cell damage or possibly biliary stasis, and is usually accompanied by SGOT, SGPT and alkaline phosphatase elevations. If jaundice appears the drug should be discontinued; the abnormal liver function tests will then usually clear rapidly within 2 weeks. The drug may then be restarted, but if jaundice recurs again the drug should be permanently discontinued. Liver tenderness is often a useful early sign of hepatic toxicity and is a signal to discontinue the drug (Shorey, 1968). A maculopapular skin rash is seen occasionally. The drug is reported to be mutagenic (Thiersch, 1964). Gross hematuria has been reported after high dose intravenous 6-mercaptopurine (usually greater than 750 mg/m^2) due to renal damage by 6-mercaptopurine crystals (Duttera et al., 1972). Administration of the drug over several hours and maintenance of a high urine flow in the patient might serve to counteract this form of toxicity.

Administration. The drug is supplied in tablets of 50 mg, scored, for oral use and in vials of 500 mg for intravenous injection (investigational, NSC-755). Fifty milliliters of sterile water is added to each vial to reconstitute the drug; stability then lasts for up to 4 hours at room temperature.

Caution. Only one-third to one-fourth of the usual dose of oral 6-mercaptopurine should be given if allopurinol is administered concurrently, since the latter is a xanthine oxidase inhibitor (Rundles et al., 1963). Allopurinol appears to have little effect on the pharmacokinetics of large intravenous doses of 6-mercaptopurine in man (Coffey et al., 1972). With large doses, the enzyme systems responsible for 6-mercaptopurine catabolism may be approaching saturation.

METHOTREXATE (MTX), AMETHOPTERIN (LEDERLE)

4-Amino-N^{10}-methylpteroylglutamic acid

Biochemistry. Methotrexate is a folic acid analog which binds intracellularly with the enzyme dihydrofolate reductase (DHFR), thus preventing conversion of dihydrofolic acid to tetrahydrofolic acid. This interferes with the transport of single carbon fragments for purine and protein biosynthesis, as well as the methylation of the pyrimidine deoxyuridylic acid (dUMP) to thymidylic acid (TMP), which is a rate-limiting step for DNA synthesis. Methotrexate may limit its own killing ability in some cells by inhibiting not only DNA synthesis but also RNA and protein synthesis (G_1 to S transition block). Methotrexate also inhibits thymidylate synthetase, especially at high doses. Mechanisms of resistance to methotrexate include: reduction of cell permeability to the drug, increased synthesis of DHFR, and detoxification of the drug (Bertino and Johns, 1972). Methotrexate is predominantly a cell cycle S phase specific antimetabolite.

Pharmacology. Methotrexate is well absorbed when given by mouth in conventional doses (less than 30 mg/m^2), with blood levels comparable to those following intravenous administration. Following intravenous or oral administration of the drug, plasma levels fall to negligible levels within 3–7 hours; 58–90% of the drug is excreted unchanged in the urine within 24 hours and less than 10% excreted in the bile (Henderson et al., 1965). The amount of metabolites formed after intravenous administration is negligible, at 6% of the dose. In contrast, following oral administration, 35% of the absorbed dose is excreted as metabolites. Metabolism of orally administered methotrexate by bacteria in the gastrointestinal tract or during the first pass through the liver has been suggested (Wan et al., 1974). About 50% of the drug is bound to plasma albumin and is easily displaced by drugs such as sulfonamide and aspirin, with resultant increased toxicity. In addition methotrexate clearance by the kidney is inhibited by concomitant administration of other compounds utilizing the same renal tubular mechanism, e.g., salicylates. The initial excretion of methotrexate in urine represents drug which is surplus, i.e., drug in excess of the amount required to bind DHFR. There is a detectable urinary excretion rate of 1–2% of the retained dose per day for several weeks after administration of a single dose (Johns et al., 1964). Although the initial tissue distribution of methotrexate depends on specific membrane transport mechanisms, the long term tissue retention is determined by levels of DHFR, with the highest levels of this enzyme being observed in liver and kidney. In these tissues methotrexate can be detected weeks or months after administration. High dose intravenous infusions of methotrexate allow significant concentrations of the drug in the cerebrospinal fluid. When methotrexate is injected intrathecally, there is a prolonged release of the drug into the plasma, resulting in bone marrow and gastrointestinal toxicity which exceeds that of the same dose of methotrexate given orally or intravenously (Jacobs et al., 1975).

Side Effects. Nearly all side effects are dose-related, especially bone marrow depression and mucosal ulcerations. Toxicity is related more to the duration of drug contact with tissue than to the height of the blood level (Goldie, et al., 1972); the same dose, divided throughout the day or as a long constant intravenous infusion, is more toxic than when given as a single dose. Any impairment of renal function will delay excretion and maintain high blood levels for a longer period of time, thus increasing toxicity. The nadir of leukopenia after a single dose of methotrexate is about 7 days. As with any agent, a sudden onset of rapidly progressive leukopenia requires interruption of therapy. Methotrexate-induced buccal mucosal ulcerations are frequently preceded by complaints of a painful mouth, sore throat or anal pruritus. Examination may reveal an erythematous, reticulated mucosal rash; the ulcerations are typically shallow, painful, white or yellow, and red bordered. If any of these signs or symptoms are present, therapy should be interrupted until they have gone away. After severe ulcerations, the dose is generally reduced when reinstituted and slowly increased to tolerance. If the drug is not discontinued the ulcerations may progress throughout the entire gastrointestinal tract, with resultant massive mucosal bleeding and diarrhea which may be fatal. The occurrence of hepatic cirrhosis appears to be related to the dose of methotrexate administered. In one study (Tobias and Auerbach, 1973) only two patients who received more than 3.7 g total cumulative dose of methotrexate were free of any hepatic fibrosis. Dahl et al. (1971) have suggested that continuous methotrexate therapy may predispose to more severe liver damage than once a week schedules. Fatty liver infiltration is probably not a contraindication to further treatment in the absence of considerable fibrosis and portal cirrhosis. Elevations of liver function tests may occur transiently within 7–10 days after starting methotrexate and do not appear to reflect changes in liver histopathology. The routine performance of a liver biopsy every few months on patients taking methotrexate regularly is occasionally advocated in order to pick up early fibrosis before more severe and irreversible changes have occurred. Some patients develop a non-dose-related respiratory illness, characterized by acute onset of fever, cough, dyspnea, cyanosis, bilateral lung infiltrates and, occasionally, peripheral eosinophilia (Whitcomb et al., 1972). Microscopically there is diffuse alveolar damage with an interstitial mononuclear cell infiltrate. The use of other cytotoxic drugs may increase injury to the lung and produce a higher incidence of drug-related pulmonary disease (Stutz et al., 1973). Frequency of administration may be important since a large proportion of patients in one study who received daily intravenous methotrexate developed methotrexate lung (Nesbit et al., 1976). Resolution may be aided by a course of corticosteroids. The signs and symptoms usually clear even when the drug is continued, though it is usually felt that the illness is shortened by stopping the drug. It is unusual for the patient to experience a repeat episode despite reinstitution of methotrexate therapy. Uncommon side effects are: alopecia (mild, transient), perifolliculitis, transient pleural friction rub, localized peritonitis, middle ear hemorrhage, brownish skin pigmentation, urinary bladder dysfunction, loss of deep tendon reflexes, paresthesia, mental depression, menstrual dysfunction, oligospermia, and aggravation of diabetes mellitus. The drug is teratogenic. High doses of methotrexate with citrovorum factor rescue have been associated with moderate and reversible renal toxicity, associated with precipitation of methotrexate in the renal tubules and resulting tubular damage. This renal toxicity may be prevented by alkalinizing the urine and by increasing the urine volume (Frei et al., 1975). Recently, several instances of neurologic disorders following intrathecal methotrexate have been reported. A frequently noted side effect of intrathecal methotrexate has been arachnoiditis, manifested as a pain in the lower back, radiating into the lower extremities with transient weakness and sensory disturbances seen in some. A subacute form of intrathecal methotrexate toxicity may occur within a few weeks after starting treatment, characterized by motor dysfunction of the brain or spinal cord and leading to paraplegia, quadriplegia, cerebellar dysfunction, cranial nerve palsies and seizures. A necrotizing demyelinating leukoencephalopathy may occur months to years after onset of methotrexate therapy: the clinical picture is that of progressive neurologic deterioration beginning insidiously and evolving into severe dementia, dysarthria, ataxia, spasticity, seizures and coma. Many of these patients also received cranial irradiation and/or systemic methotrexate. It has been proposed that a preservative in the diluent for the drug may be to blame. However, use of a diluent not containing a preservative has not always prevented the toxicity. Elliott's B solution, an artificial cerebrospinal fluid, has been recommended for use as a diluent for methotrexate. Recent observations suggest that the neurotoxicity associated with intrathecal methotrexate may be secondary to prolonged exposure to excessive drug concentration in the central nervous system. In particular, the presence of meningeal leukemia appears to predispose to increased cerebrospinal fluid concentration and development of methotrexate neurotoxicity. Perhaps a smaller dose of intrathecal methotrexate should be administered to patients with overt meningeal leukemia.

Antidote. Citrovorum factor (Leukovorin), the N^5-formyl derivative of tetrahydrofolic acid, is frequently given to bypass the methotrexate-induced metabolic block in patients receiving intrathecal methotrexate or high dose, prolonged methotrexate infusions intravenously. Bone marrow suppression and other toxicities are thereby dramatically reduced. A progressively decreasing effect of citrovorum factor is observed when its administration is delayed from 4 to 72 hours after the administration of methotrexate is completed; little or no effect will occur after 72 hours. Citrovorum factor may be given by oral, subcutaneous, intramuscular or intravenous routes.

Administration. The drug is supplied in tablets of 2.5 mg, scored, for oral use. It is also available in vials of 5, 20 and 50 mg, which can be administered intravenously, intramuscularly or intrathecally.

Usual Dose. Dose is 12–15 mg/m^2/day, intravenously or intramuscularly, for 5 days, every 14–21 days (acute leukemia induction and consolidation), or 15–30 mg/m^2, intravenously, intramuscularly or orally, twice weekly (solid tumors, acute leukemia maintenance); 3–12 mg/m^2 intrathecally every 1–7 days with a maximum dose of 15 mg per injection (central nervous system leukemia) or as recently advocated, a maximum of 12 mg per injection (Bleyer, 1978).

The use of high doses of MTX ranging from 250 mg/m^2 to grams/m^2 with citrovorum factor rescue is investigational and in most conditions controversial and of dubious advantage over conventional doses.

Caution. Never administer methotrexate before the BUN or creatinine is known. If the BUN is between 20 and 30 mg/100 ml, or the creatinine is between 1.2 and 2.0 mg/100 ml, give only 50% of the planned dose; if the BUN is over 30 mg/100 ml, or the creatinine is over 2.0 mg/100 ml, no methotrexate should be given.

MITHRAMYCIN (MITH) (MITHRACIN—PFIZER)

Biochemistry. Mithramycin is an antibiotic derived from *Streptomyces plicatus.* It binds reversibly to guanine-rich DNA, resulting in inhibition of DNA-dependent RNA polymerase function and ultimately RNA synthesis. It probably also interacts with the complementary strand of DNA to produce a weak cross-link manifested by impaired DNA synthesis. It also appears to directly block the action of parathormone on bone calcium metabolism (Parsons et al., 1967). It appears to be a cell cycle nonspecific agent.

Pharmacology. There is insufficient data on human metabolism and excretion.

Side Effects. Thrombocytopenia is seen in approximately 50% of patients and may be a cause of bleeding. A beginning decline of the platelet count during therapy is a sign to discontinue the drug. Leukopenia is seen less frequently. A hemorrhagic disorder (Kennedy, 1970a; Monto et al., 1969), which appears to be dose related and cumulative with subsequent courses, is manifested by epistaxis and ecchymoses but also occasionally by hematemesis or melena. It is important to note that spontaneous bleeding may occur when coagulation studies are completely normal and is unexplained. Coagulation abnormalities are, however, often seen in the form of: (a) prolonged prothrombin time with decreased levels of Factors II, V, VII and X, usually on the basis of mithramycin-induced hepatic dysfunction, this is best treated with large doses of vitamin K (300 mg IV/day) and fresh frozen plasma; (b) qualitative platelet defects; (c) decreased vascular integrity, which may respond to corticosteroids; and (d) increased fibrinolytic activity. Bleeding during mithramycin treatment is an indication to stop the drug. Hypocalcemia (Parsons et al., 1967), not corrected by high dose vitamin D administration, may occur and is usually accompanied by a decreased urinary excretion of calcium. This is dose related with a rapid return of serum calcium to normal when the drug is stopped. This action is utilized in the treatment of hypercalcemia, especially in patients with malignancies. Mithramycin will correct the hypercalcemia, whether it is secondary to bone destruction from metastatic tumor or to the secretion of parathormone-like substance by the tumor. Hepatic dysfunction is manifested by an elevated SGOT, SGPT, LDH or alkaline phosphatase and is usually reversible within 2–3 weeks of discontinuation of the drug. Liver biopsies have revealed fatty metamorphosis and central lobular necrosis (Kennedy, 1970a). The presence of liver failure is a contraindication to the use of mithramycin. Renal impairment, which is usually cumulative with repeated courses, is manifested by rising BUN, hyposthenuria, proteinuria and occasionally, severe azotemia and death. Renal biopsies have revealed swelling of renal tubular epithelium and tubular necrosis (Kennedy, 1970a). Nausea and vomiting are common immediately after an intravenous injection, although some patients become conditioned to emesis with continued treatment. Anorexia, stomatitis and diarrhea may be seen. A dermatologic reaction is common. There is an initial pink flush on the face and neck with periorbital pallor progressing to a deeper blotchy plethora and coarsening of facial features. Scattered papular lesions and cutaneous excoriations are occasionally seen. When the drug is stopped, these features subside but the patient may be left with a mild hyperpigmentation. The initial facial flush has been used as an indication to stop the drug, since it often precedes by 24 hours the onset of some severe biochemical abnormalities. Other side effects are: headache, myalgias, lethargy, irritability, fever and alopecia. Aspermia has been described (Koons et al., 1966), and one patient was reported who suffered multiple arterial occlusive episodes in association with mithramycin therapy (Margileth et al., 1973).

Administration. The drug is supplied in vials of 2.5 mg and should be stored at 4°C. The drug should be reconstituted with sterile water and then used immediately. It is injected directly intravenously.

Usual Dose. Dose is 0.025–0.050 mg/kg, intravenously, daily or every other day to the point of toxicity or to a total dose of 0.250 mg/kg in each course, which is repeated generally at 2–4 week intervals. In one series (Kennedy, 1970b), the alternate day regimen resulted in less overall toxicity than the daily regimen of drug. For the treatment of hypercalcemia, a dose of 0.025 mg/kg, intravenously, suffices in most patients and can be repeated as often as every other day (Perlia et al., 1970).

MITOMYCIN (MUTAMYCIN—BRISTOL)

Biochemistry. Mitomycin is an antibiotic isolated from *Streptomyces caespitosus.* When activated it acts like a bifunctional alkylating agent with a covalent cross linking of the complementary DNA strands (Szybalski and Iyer, 1964). Its degree of cell cycle specificity is uncertain.

Pharmacology. Mitomycin disappears rapidly from the plasma after an intravenous injection, with 33% of the intact drug recovered in the urine within a few hours. Its exact metabolism in vivo is not known; there is no evidence of specific tissue localization. In vitro it is rapidly inactivated under anaerobic condition, particularly by liver homogenates (Philips et al., 1960).

Side Effects. Leukopenia and thrombocytopenia usually occur after a standard course of therapy, with a nadir at 3–5 weeks and recovery in another 2–4 weeks. Anorexia, nausea and diarrhea are occasionally noted, as well as stomatitis and enteritis. Renal toxicity may occur because of glomerular damage, manifested by elevated BUN and creatinine and proteinuria (Liu et al., 1971).

Administration. The drug is supplied in vials of 5 mg as a bluish powder and is reconstituted with 10 ml of sterile water or normal saline. The drug is injected directly intravenously. A chemical cellulitis at the injection site will occur with extravasation of the drug.

Usual Dose. Dose is 0.5 mg/kg, intravenously, every 4–6 weeks or 0.05 mg/kg/day, for 5 days. After a free interval of 2 days, the schedule is repeated for another 5 days. The entire schedule is repeated in 2–3 weeks.

NITROGEN MUSTARD (HN$_2$), MECHLORETHAMINE HCl (MUSTARGEN— MERCK SHARP & DOHME)

$$CH_3-N\begin{cases} CH_2CH_2Cl \\ \\ CH_2CH_2Cl \end{cases} \cdot HCl$$

Methylbis (β-chloroethyl)amine

Biochemistry. Nitrogen mustard is a bifunctional alkylating agent. It is a highly reactive compound capable of combining with various nucleophilic groups, such as amino and sulfhydryl groups. It directly interferes with cell replication by interstrand binding to guanine and perhaps other sites on the DNA molecule, thus preventing separation of the two strands of DNA in the double coiled helix necessary for cell replication (Pullman and Pullman, 1959). The cross-linking hypothesis explains why monofunctional alkylating agents are 50–100 times less effective antitumor drugs than bifunctional agents. Cells in late G$_1$ or early S phase are particularly sensitive to alkylating effects (Roberts et al., 1968). Resistance to the drug is related principally to decreased binding and transport of the drug into the cell and/or increased repair of the drug-induced DNA lesions. It is a cell cycle phase nonspecific agent.

Pharmacology. Ninety percent of an intravenous injection is cleared from the blood in 30–60 sec. It reacts quickly and nonspecifically with body tissues. Within 24 hours, 50% of the dose is excreted in the urine in a detoxified form (Smith et al., 1958).

Side Effects. Nausea and vomiting are common, sometimes occurring within minutes but usually noted 1–3 hours after injection of the drug, and persisting occasionally for as long as 24 hours. For this reason it is best to premedicate the patient 30–60 min before injection with an antiemetic such as a phenothiazine. Chills, fever, and diarrhea may also occur shortly after administration of the drug. Leukopenia and thrombocytopenia are common, occur within a few days, and persist for 10–21 days after a single injection. The erythrocyte count may decline during the first month after therapy but seldom significantly. Other side effects occasionally noted are: vertigo, tinnitus, convulsions, decreased hearing, alopecia and a maculopapular skin eruption. Temporary amenorrhea and impaired spermatogenesis may occur.

Administration. The drug is supplied in vials containing 10 mg of the white crystalline powder, which should be stored at room temperature. The drug may be reconstituted with 10 ml of sterile water or normal saline and should be used immediately, since it will decompose on standing. The drug should not be used if droplets of water are visible within the unreconstituted vial or if the solution appears discolored. Since the drug is a powerful vesicant, gloves should be worn when mixing and administering it. The drug should be injected over 1 min into the arm of a running intravenous infusion; avoid extravasation into surrounding tissues. If extravasation occurs, apply ice to the area. Immediate injection of m/6 sodium thiosulfate or normal saline into the area of extravasation is said to decrease swelling and reaction.

Nitrogen mustard is frequently used for the control of neoplastic effusions in the pleural cavity (Mark et al., 1964). Since there is some systemic absorption, other chemotherapy should not be given concomitantly. An attempt should be made to remove most of the fluid before injecting the nitrogen mustard. Since the alkylating effect is over within a few minutes after injection, the patient should assume several positions (prone, supine, right and left lateral) within 3–5 min of injection in order to thoroughly distribute the drug throughout the cavity before its alkylating effect is gone. A transient pleuritic pain may occur. For several days after instillation, fluid may reaccumulate as a result of pleural irritation from the drug, and one or several more taps may be needed.

Usual Dose. Dose is 0.4–0.6 mg/kg, intravenously, every 3–4 weeks, when used singly; 0.2–0.6 mg/kg for intracavitary instillation; 6 mg/m^2, intravenously, in most combination therapy regimens.

Note. Thrombosis and phlebitis may result from direct contact of the drug with the intima of the injected vein; therefore, it is not recommended to inject nitrogen mustard into the upper extremity of a patient with a superior vena cava syndrome or into an extremity with impaired venous drainage.

PIPOBROMAN, (VERCYTE—ABBOTT)

$$O$$
$$\overset{\|}{C}-CH_2CH_2Br$$

(piperazine ring with)

$$\overset{\|}{C}-CH_2CH_2Br$$
$$O$$

1,4-Bis (3-bromopropionyl)piperazine

Biochemistry. Pipobroman is a piperazine derivative with an unknown mechanism of action, although its chemical structure suggests that it is an alkylating agent. Its cell cycle specificity is unknown.

Pharmacology. Little is known regarding human metabolism and excretion of the drug.

Side Effects. Leukopenia and thrombocytopenia are usually moderate and reversible upon discontinuation of the drug. Anemia is often quite marked and is often the limiting factor in therapy; it may occur with as little as a total cumulative dose of 30 mg/kg but is generally dose related. In a few instances a hemolytic process was suggested by a rapid fall in hemoglobin and an elevated bilirubin and reticulocyte count; the process was reversible when the drug was discontinued. Occasionally noted are: nausea, vomiting, diarrhea and crampy abdominal pains. A skin rash has been reported. There is no change in renal or hepatic function in human studies (AMA, 1967).

Administration. The drug is supplied in tablets of 10 and 25 mg, scored, for oral use.

PIPOSULFAN

$$CH_3-SO_2-O-CH_2-CH_2-\overset{O}{\overset{\|}{C}}-N\underset{H_2\ H_2}{\overset{H_2\ H_2}{\diagdown}}N-\overset{O}{\overset{\|}{C}}-CH_2-CH_2-O-SO_2-CH_3$$

Piperazine, 1,4-dihydracryloyl-dimethane-sulfonate

Biochemistry. Piposulfan is a piperazine derivative with an unknown mechanism of action. It is very active against a variety of experimental tumors.

Pharmacology. Little is known regarding human metabolism and excretion of piposulfan.

Side Effects. Leukopenia and thrombocytopenia are usually moderate and reversible upon discontinuation of the drug. Nausea and vomiting after the drug is ingested may be severe. Diarrhea occurs occasionally. There is no change in renal or hepatic functions in human studies (Kenis, 1968; Nelson et al., 1967).

Administration. The drug is supplied in tablets of 10 and 25 mg (investigational, NSC-47774) for oral use.

Usual Dose. Dose is 1–4 mg/kg/day, orally. The average daily dose should not exceed 140 mg.

PROCARBAZINE (PCZ) (MATULANE—ROCHE)

$$CH_3-NH-NH-CH_2-\overset{}{\underset{}{\bigcirc}}-\overset{O}{\overset{\|}{C}}-NH-\overset{CH_3}{\underset{}{\overset{|}{CH}}}-CH_3 \quad \cdot HCl$$

N-Isopropyl-α-(2-methylhydrazino)-p-toluamide hydrochloride

Biochemistry. Procarbazine is the most active member of a group of synthetic cytotoxic compounds derived from methylhydrazine. Although its exact mechanism of action is unclear, it is an inhibitor of DNA, RNA and protein synthesis. It also inhibits transmethylation of methyl groups of methionine into transfer RNA (Kreis, 1971). It appears to be cell cycle phase nonspecific.

Pharmacology. Procarbazine is well absorbed from the gastrointestinal tract and appears in cerebrospinal fluid in peak concentrations 30–90 min after administration. The half-life of the drug is about 10 min with up to 70% excreted in the urine within 24 hours (Oliverio, 1971).

Side Effects. Bone marrow depression usually occurs 3–5 weeks after therapy is instituted. It is usually rapidly reversible with recovery in 2–3 weeks. Nausea and vomiting are common, especially at the onset of therapy, and abating usually after the first week. They can be ameliorated by starting therapy with 50 mg on day one, and increasing by 50-mg increments daily until the maximum dose is attained (Samuels et al., 1967). Procarbazine neurotoxicity may be manifest by somnolence, depression, agitation, and psychosis in up to 30% of patients, with possible synergy between the sedative effects of procarbazine and phenothiazines, barbiturates and tricyclic antidepressants. Effects of antihypertensive and sympathomimetic drugs may be potentiated in patients taking procarbazine, and foods with high tyramine content can produce hypertension in some patients, related to the fact that procarbazine is a monoamine oxidase inhibitor. Peripheral neuropathy with paresthesia and depressed deep tendon reflexes may occur. Ataxia and orthostatic hypotension occur occasionally. Neurotoxicity is most often seen with intermittent high dose intravenous procarbazine therapy (Weiss et al., 1974). Other side effects are: dermatitis, parkinsonism, azospermia, alopecia, hemorrhagic cystitis, and occasionally a flush syndrome after alcohol similar to that induced by antabuse.

Administration. The drug is supplied in capsules of 50 mg which are given orally. An intravenous form of the drug (investigational) is currently under investigation.

Usual Dose. Dose is 100–300 mg/day, orally.

QUINACRINE (ATABRINE—WINTHROP)

3-Chloro-7-methoxy-9-(1-methyl-4-diethyl aminobutylamino) acridine dihydrochloride dihydrate

Biochemistry. Quinacrine hydrochloride was first used during World War II as an antimalarial agent. It acts by uncoupling oxidative phosphorylation and inhibits a number of enzyme systems including flavin mononucleotide, red blood cell glucose-6-phosphate dehydrogenase, liver esterase and cholinesterase. It appears to be a nonspecific enzyme inhibitor that acts by binding with proteins. Quinacrine has been demonstrated to have cytotoxic action on a variety of normal and tumor cells in tissue culture. Although shown to be inactive at maximal tolerated doses against a number of animal and human neoplasms in vivo, it may be cytotoxic against free-floating tumor cells, as a peritoneal or pleural effusion. More importantly, when given intracavitary it will cause chemical inflammation of serous membranes with subsequent adhesions and fibrosis between visceral and parietal membranes, thus in many cases slowing the formation of a neoplastic effusion.

Pharmacology. The pharmacology of the drug in regard to its intracavitary administration is unknown.

Side Effects. (Dollinger et al., 1967) (intracavitary use). Local pain occurs in 50–60%, usually beginning several hours after instillation and lasting about a day. Fever as high as 40°C (104°F) occurs in nearly all patients, beginning 4–8 hours after instillation and usually lasting only a few hours but occasionally persisting for up to 10 days. It may be accompanied by leukocytosis. Intrapleural instillation may cause initial and transient dyspnea, especially in patients with reduced ventilation or with bilateral pleural effusions. Intraperitoneal instillation may cause ileus, nausea and vomiting, which all clear in a few days. Due to adhesion formation, bowel obstruction may occur. Other side effects reported have been hypotension, transient oliguria and skin hyperpigmentation. There is no hematologic depression.

Administration. The drug is supplied in vials containing 200 mg of the powder, which can be reconstituted with 10 ml of sterile water for intracavitary injection.

Usual Dose. Withdraw approximately half the pleural or peritoneal effusion before injection of quinacrine. Initially give 50–100 mg for pleural effusions and 100–200 mg for peritoneal effusions to determine patient tolerance. After instillation, have the patient assume several positions by turning to and fro, in order to distribute the drug within the cavity as much as possible. Instill the drug in only one hemithorax at a time to avoid severe dyspnea. Depending on individual tolerance, 200–400 mg is given daily for 4–5 days for pleural effusions and 400–800 mg daily for 3–5 days for ascites. Chest x-rays may be of little help in determining response because the resulting pleural fibrosis often resembles an opacified hemithorax.

STREPTONIGRIN

Biochemistry. Streptonigrin is an antibiotic obtained from cultures of *Streptomyces flocculus.* It acts by inhibiting DNA synthesis, causing extensive chromosome breakage. It may be S phase cell cycle specific.

Pharmacology. Little is known regarding human metabolism and excretion.

Side Effects. Bone marrow depression is often severe; the nadir of leukopenia and thrombocytopenia is about 23 days, with recovery in another 3-4 weeks. Nausea, vomiting and diarrhea occur frequently but can usually be controlled. Gastrointestinal ulceration occasionally occurs. The oral form of the drug produces less profound and more readily reversible bone marrow depression than does the intravenous form; however, gastrointestinal side effects are greater. Other side effects occasionally seen are: mental confusion, thrombophlebitis at the injection site, alopecia, proteinuria, azotemia, vitiligo and allergic reactions (Carter, 1968).

Administration. The drug is supplied in capsules of 0.2 mg (investigational, NSC-45383) for oral use. An intravenous form is also under investigation.

Usual Dose. Dose is 0.2 mg/day orally. Other dose schedules are under investigation.

STREPTOZOTOCIN

$$CH_2OH$$

HO OH O NO

NH—C—N—CH₃

Biochemistry. Streptozotocin is a 1-methyl, nitrosourea glucosamine antibiotic derived from *Streptomyces achromogenes.* It inhibits DNA synthesis in *E. coli*; in addition it inhibits RNA and protein synthesis but its mechanism of action is unknown (Heinemann and Howard, 1965).

Pharmacology. Following parenteral administration the drug is concentrated in the liver. It is then transported specifically into the pancreatic β cells as a result of the glucosamine moiety in the molecule, causing mitochondrial swelling, degranulation and necrosis of these cells (Brosky and Logothelopoulos, 1969); this action may account for its effectiveness in the treatment of malignant islet cell carcinoma. The serum half-life of the drug is 15 min with essentially no drug detectable by 2 hours after completion of therapy. Ten to 20% of each total dose is excreted in the urine with the N-nitroso group intact, the majority being excreted within 60 min after completion of drug administration (Schein et al., 1974).

Side Effects. Myelosuppression is unusual but has been reported in the form of leukopenia and thrombocytopenia, with a nadir of 1-2 weeks after completion of therapy. Severe nausea and vomiting usually occur within a few hours after injection of the drug. Streptozotocin has a direct toxic effect on renal tubular cells, the earliest detectable sign of which is usually hypophosphatemia or proteinuria; at this time the drug should be temporarily discontinued until the proteinuria disappears and renal function is normal. Various renal tubular defects occur usually as an early sign of toxicity and include: uricosuria, glycosuria, phosphaturia, acetonuria and renal tubular acidosis up to a full-blown Fanconi syndrome. Azotemia may occur and will occasionally proceed to oliguria or anuria; death from renal failure has been reported (Sadoff, 1970). Renal histology in these patients has demonstrated evidence of cellular degeneration and necrosis of tubular epithelium. A diuresis should be maintained during therapy to dilute the drug to the lowest possible concentration while passing through the kidney. A mild and reversible hepatotoxicity (elevated SGOT and SGPT) is frequently seen. Due to the drug's diabetogenic effect, serum insulin levels are lowered and hyperglycemia may occur, although insulin-dependent diabetes in humans is unreported. Diarrhea, stomatitis, fever, eosinophilia and hypocalcemia have occasionally been reported (Stolinsky et al., 1972a).

Administration. The drug is supplied in vials containing 2 g of the buffered powder (investigational, NSC-85998), which are stable at 4°C for at least 2 years. Reconstitution is with 18.6 ml of sterile water or normal saline, giving a concentration of 100 mg/ml of drug. The final solution is diluted with 5% dextrose in water to a volume of 200–300 ml and administered by rapid intravenous infusion. A sensation of burning at the injection site is an indication to slow the rate of infusion of the drug. Reconstituted solutions are stable for 8 hours at room temperature.

Usual Dose. Dose is 500 mg/m^2/day, intravenously, for 5 days, every 2 weeks, or 1.5 g/m^2/week, intravenously.

Caution. Patients with pre-existing renal function abnormalities should not receive the drug.

6-THIOGUANINE (6-TG) (THIOGUANINE—BURROUGHS WELLCOME)

2-Amino-6-mercaptopurine

Biochemistry. 6-Thioguanine is a purine antimetabolite which is incorporated into DNA as the deoxyribotide and into RNA as the ribotide.

Cross resistance exists between 6-thioguanine and 6-mercaptopurine. 6-Thioguanine is predominantly a cell cycle S phase specific agent (LePage and Jones, 1961).

Pharmacology. In vivo the drug is rapidly converted to 2-amino-6-methylmercaptopurine. It is excreted in the urine in part as 6-thiouric acid. Since the metabolism of the active compound does not depend on the enzyme xanthine oxidase, 6-thioguanine metabolism is not inhibited by allopurinol (Moore and LePage, 1958).

Side Effects. Bone marrow depression is in the form of leukopenia and thrombocytopenia. Use with caution and at decreased doses in patients with renal or hepatic dysfunction. Jaundice has rarely been reported and its etiology is uncertain; if it occurs the drug should be stopped. The abnormalities in liver function will usually clear in about two weeks, at which time the drug may be cautiously restarted. Gastrointestinal side effects are unusual except with large doses and consist of nausea, vomiting, stomatitis and rarely diarrhea.

Administration. The drug is supplied in tablets of 40 mg, scored, for oral use.

Usual Dose. Dose is 2.0–2.5 mg/kg/day orally in two equally divided doses.

TRIETHYLENEMELAMINE (TEM) (LEDERLE)

2,4,6-Tris(ethylenimino)-*s*-triazine

Biochemistry. Triethylenemelamine is a polyfunctional alkylating agent which is converted in vivo to a highly reactive quaternary ethyleneimonium compound. It is degraded under acid conditions and is extremely reactive with various organic materials. Its mode of action is similar to that of other alkylating agents, such as nitrogen mustard. It is cell cycle phase nonspecific.

Pharmacology. The degree of gastrointestinal absorption of triethylenemelamine is unpredictable. Absorption may be enhanced if reaction with the acid stomach pH is prevented by giving 1–2 g of sodium bicarbonate orally concurrently with the drug. Triethylenemelamine reacts quickly with tissues. Within 24 hours 50% of the dose is excreted in the urine in a detoxified form (Mandel, 1959).

Side Effects. Thrombocytopenia and leukopenia are common, with the nadir at 1–3 weeks. Nausea and vomiting are less common than with nitrogen mustard and usually occur 1–3 hours after giving the drug. Other side effects occasionally observed are: diarrhea, esophagitis, hematuria, albuminuria and azotemia, all reversible upon discontinuation of the drug. The drug may be mutagenic in man.

Administration. The drug is supplied in tablets of 5 mg, quarterscored, and should be stored in a refrigerator until use. The drug should be taken in the morning on an empty stomach, with no food ingestion for 60 min afterward. As mentioned above, sodium bicarbonate may be given concurrently for its buffering action.

Usual Dose. Dose is 2.5 mg, orally, every other day for four doses, then 2.5–5.0 mg/week.

TRIETHYLENETHIOPHOSPHORAMIDE (TSPA, TESPA)
(THIOTEPA—LEDERLE)

Tris(1-azirinidyl)phosphine oxide

Biochemistry. Thiotepa is a polyfunctional alkylating agent. Its mode of action is similar to that of other alkylating agents, such as nitrogen mustard.

Pharmacology. Following an intravenous injection most of the drug is cleared from the plasma within a few minutes, and about 90% is gone within 3 hours. It is metabolized in part to *n,n',n''*-triethylenephosphoramide (TEPA), which persists in the plasma for at least 6 hours. Within 24–48 hours most of the drug is excreted unchanged in the urine (Mellett et al., 1962).

Side Effects. The nadir of leukopenia and thrombocytopenia is about 14 days, with recovery in another 2–4 weeks. Nausea and vomiting are uncommon. Other side effects are amenorrhea, possible interference with spermatogenesis and an allergic dermatitis.

Thiotepa is occasionally used for the control of neoplastic effusions in the pleural and peritoneal cavities (Bateman et al., 1955). Since there is some systemic absorption, other chemotherapy should not be given concomitantly. An attempt should be made to remove most of the fluid before injecting the drug. The patient should assume several positions within 3–5 min of injection in order to thoroughly distribute the drug throughout the cavity before its alkylating effect is gone. Veenema (1968) has discussed the role of thiotepa in the treatment of bladder tumors by intravesical administration.

Administration. The drug is supplied in vials containing 15 mg and is stored in a refrigerator. The drug is reconstituted with 1.5–5.0 ml of sterile water; the solution is stable for 5 days when kept in the refrigerator. The reconstituted solution should be clear to slightly opaque; solutions grossly opaque or with precipitate should not be used. It is given intravenously or intramuscularly.

Usual Dose. Dose is 30–60 mg, intravenously or intramuscularly at 1–4-week intervals; 45–60 mg for intracavitary instillation.

URACIL MUSTARD (UPJOHN)

5-[Bis(2-chloroethyl)amino]uracil

Biochemistry. Uracil mustard is an orally active alkylating agent with a mechanism of action similar to that of nitrogen mustard.

Pharmacology. Gastrointestinal absorption is rapid and nearly complete. Blood levels of the drug decline rapidly; no evidence of the drug is detectable in the blood two hours after oral administration. The drug reacts quickly with tissues; less than one per cent of the administered dose is recovered unchanged in the urine (Lane, 1960).

Side Effects. Nausea and vomiting are common though not as severe as with nitrogen mustard. Diarrhea and stomatitis are occasionally seen. Mild to moderate leukopenia and thrombocytopenia may occur. Alopecia, if it occurs, is usually mild. A skin rash or hyperpigmentation may be seen. Abnormal liver function tests and jaundice have occasionally been reported.

Administration. The drug is supplied in capsules of 1 mg for oral use.

Usual Dose. Dose is 1–2 mg/day, orally.

VINBLASTINE, VINCALEUKOBLASTINE SULFATE (VLB) (VELBAN—LILLY)

Biochemistry. Vinblastine is a salt of an alkaloid extracted from the periwinkle plant *Vinca rosea.* It acts primarily by interfering reversibly with the assembly of the protein subunits of the mitotic spindle, thereby causing metaphase arrest in dividing cells (Marsden, 1972). For this reason it has been considered a cell cycle M phase specific agent; however, the interaction with the spindle proteins may occur in the S, G_2 and M phases. The drug interferes with cell membrane amino acid transport, resulting in decreased protein synthesis, and kills cells in late G_1. It has also been shown to inhibit RNA synthesis via inhibition of RNA polymerase. From this information, vinblastine may be a cell cycle phase nonspecific agent; however, its major effect appears to be in late G_1 and in the S and M phases, with lethal expression occurring principally in the M phase.

Pharmacology. After a single intravenous injection the drug is cleared from the blood within 30 min; its excretion is almost entirely by the liver into the bile.

Side Effects. Vinblastine should be given no more often than once every week, since severe leukopenia will occur with more frequent doses. The nadir of leukopenia is 5–10 days after a dose, with recovery in another 1–2 weeks. Thrombocytopenia is uncommon with conventional dose regimens unless other chemotherapy or radiation therapy has recently been administered. Thombocytosis occasionally occurs. The erythrocyte count is rarely affected. Alopecia is dose related and occurs in 5–10% of patients; it is usually partial, and occasionally hair will regrow while therapy continues. Although not as neurotoxic as vincristine, vinblastine will often cause areflexia and mild paresthesia, which do not require a change in dose; however, severe paresthesia and muscular weakness (although uncommon) do necessitate a 50% or greater reduction in dose. Extravasation during intravenous injection can cause a painful cellulitis and/or phlebitis, and tissue sloughing may occur. Other side effects appear to be dose related: oligospermia, mild nausea, constipation, stomatitis and gastrointestinal ulcerations, mental depression, convulsions and hemorrhagic cystitis. Appearance of oral or rectal mucosal ulcerations is a sign to discontinue vinblastine temporarily until the ulcers have cleared. As with vincristine there is evidence to suggest that the side effects of vinblastine may be reversed by glutamic or aspartic acid (Vaitkevicius et al., 1962).

Administration. The drug is supplied in vials containing 10 mg and is stored in the refrigerator. The drug may be reconstituted with 5-10 ml of normal saline. The reconstituted solution can be kept in the refrigerator for as long as 30 days. The drug is given by direct intravenous injection.

Usual Dose. Dose is 0.1-0.3 mg/kg/week, intravenously.

VINCRISTINE (VCR) (ONCOVIN—LILLY)

Biochemistry. Vincristine is an alkaloid extracted from the *Vinca rosea* periwinkle plant. It acts by interfering with the synthesis of spindle protein as well as with organization of preformed spindle protein, thus causing metaphase arrest (Marsden, 1972). This interference appears to occur as early as the S phase, but, unlike vinblastine, it is irreversible. It also interferes with cell membrane lipid synthesis and amino acid transport in some experimental systems; however, whether or not this leads to alterations in protein synthesis is uncertain. Vincristine also inhibits RNA polymerase and thus RNA synthesis. It is considered to be a cell cycle M phase specific agent; however, its expression of lethality in the M phase may accrue from exposure to the agent in S, G_2 or M, in which case it could be considered an S to M phase specific agent.

Pharmacology. After a single intravenous injection, the drug is cleared from the blood within 30 min; its excretion is almost entirely by the liver into the bile.

Side Effects. Mild leukopenia and thrombocytopenia may occur when the drug is given in high doses or when given over prolonged periods of time at doses of 2 mg/m^2/week. Thrombocytosis may occur. The main side effect is neurotoxicity, which is generally dose related (Sandler et al., 1969) and is manifested by: (a) constipation, due to involvement of the autonomic nervous system which may occur up to 5 days after a dose of vincristine. It is important to adequately hydrate the patient and to administer prophylactic stool softeners or laxatives. Severe constipation with paralytic ileus can mimick a surgical abdomen and necessitates cessation of therapy until it clears; (b) peripheral neuropathy: minor sensory impairments progressing to paresthesia and neuritic pain are common, and, together with loss of deep tendon reflexes, are the earliest signs of peripheral neuropathy. If paresthesiae become severe or if there is significant muscular weakness (50% objectively) and/or muscle wasting or incoordination, the subsequent doses of vincristine should be halved; if further impairment of neurologic function occurs, the drug should be discontinued until the severe neurologic dysfunction has cleared. Axonal degeneration is the primary pathologic process in vinca alkaloid neuropathy (Gottschalk et al., 1968), but the electrophysiologic observation of normal nerve conduction velocities noted in some patients would suggest localization of the neurotoxicity to the muscle spindle (Sandler et al., 1969). Hoarseness due to vocal cord paresis may occur. Cranial nerve palsies may occur (Albert et al., 1967), usually after several weeks or months of therapy and are mostly ocular, with ptosis and various ophthalmoplegias, but the pupil is spared. There may be unilateral or bilateral facial nerve palsy. The trigeminal nerve may be involved, with absent corneal reflexes and paroxysmal jaw pain. The central nervous system is relatively immune, but depression, insomnia, agitation, psychotic states, hallucinations, convulsions, cerebellar signs and coma have been described. Bladder atony with urinary retention may occur without any other neurologic signs of toxicity. Orthostatic hypotension has been reported secondary to vincristine-induced interruption of the adrenergic sympathetic nervous system with resultant low blood norepinephrine levels (Aisner et al., 1974). It has been urged that vincristine be used with extreme caution in patients with a pre-existing neuropathy (Weiden and Wright, 1972) or in patients already on a drug which is potentially neurotoxic, such as isoniazid and L-asparaginase (Hildebrand and Kenis, 1972). After stopping the drug, recovery from neurotoxic reactions usually occurs in about 6 weeks but may be delayed for as long as a year and may be incomplete. Patients with hepatic insufficiency may have increased neurotoxicity from vincristine, since the drug is cleared by the liver and excreted into the bile. If liver function tests are abnormal, the dose of vincristine should be decreased. Chiefly because of its neurologic side effects, vincristine should not be given more often than once a week. Children seem to be somewhat more resistant than adults to the neurotoxicity. Vincristine neuropathy may also be related to the physical activity of the patients (Sakamoto, 1974). Alopecia occurs in about 50% of patients on long term vincristine and is often total; regrowth usually occurs after cessation of the drug or when a lower dose is employed. Nausea, vomiting and diarrhea may occur. Oral and gastrointestinal ulcerations, skin rash and fever have been reported. Hyponatremia, felt to be associated with inappropriate secretion of antidiuretic hormone, has been noted (Nicholson and Feldman, 1972). Extravasation of the drug causes a severe and painful inflammatory reaction, usually culminating in cellulitis and phlebitis.

Administration. The drug is supplied in vials containing 1 and 5 mg and should be stored in the refrigerator. The drug may be reconstituted with 2 and 10 ml, respectively, of normal saline (as supplied with the drug). Once reconstituted it can be kept for up to 2 weeks in the refrigerator. It is given as an intravenous injection.

Usual Dose. Dose is 1.0–2.0 mg/m^2/week, intravenously. Never give more than 2.0 mg/m^2/week. Some physicians never use a total dose of more than 2.0 mg/week.

VP 16-213 (EPEG)

4′-Demethyl-epipodophyllotoxin-β-D-ethylidene glucoside

Biochemistry. VP 16-213 is a semisynthetic product derived from the root of the mayapple *Podophyllum peltatum.* It causes mitotic arrest at metaphase, producing an effect similar to that of colchicine, a spindle poison. It also acts in phases earlier in the cell cycle by inhibition of

DNA, RNA and protein synthesis (Goldsmith, 1973a). The drug is cell cycle nonspecific.

Pharmacology. Following administration of 220–290 mg/m^2 of the drug intravenously in 500 ml in 1 hour, plasma decay kinetics followed a biexponential function with a mean half-life of nearly 11.5 hours for the terminal phase. After 72 hours, 44% of the administered dose was also recovered in the urine, of which 67% was unchanged drug. Recovery in the feces ranged from less than 2% to 16% over 3 days. Levels in the cerebrospinal fluid varied from less than 1% to 10% of the plasma levels at 2–26 hours postinfusion (Creaven and Allen, 1975).

Side Effects. The predominant toxicity is myelosuppression, mainly granulocytopenia and to a lesser extent thrombocytopenia. Nausea and vomiting may occur. Other side effects mentioned are: fever, chills, alopecia, and headache. Episodes of generalized erythema and bronchospasm responding to antihistamines and cessation of the drug infusion have been reported (Rozencweig et al., 1977a). Hypotension has been described but may be avoided by infusions of the drug over 30 min.

Administration. The drug is supplied in ampules containing 100 mg of VP-16-213 dissolved in a combination of organic solvents (investigational, NSC-141540). The contents of the ampule are diluted with normal saline or 5% dextrose in water for intravenous infusion.

Usual Dose. Various dose schedules are currently under investigation. The desired dose of drug is diluted in 250 ml normal saline or 5% dextrose in water and infused intravenously over 30 min. Too rapid administration may result in hypotension. An oral preparation is currently under investigation.

VM-26 (PTG)

4'-Demethyl-epipodophyllotoxin-β-D-thenylidene glucoside

Biochemistry. VM-26 is a semisynthetic derivative of podophyllotoxin, a natural product from the mayapple plant *Podophyllum peltatum.* It causes mitotic arrest at metaphase, producing an effect similar to that of colchicine, a spindle poison. It also acts in phases earlier in the cell cycle by inhibition of DNA, RNA and protein synthesis (Goldsmith and Carter, 1973b). The drug is cell cycle nonspecific.

Pharmacology. After administration of 67 mg/m^2 of the drug intravenously plasma decay kinetics followed a triexponential function with half-life of the terminal phase ranging from 11–38 hours. After 72 hours, 44% of the administered dose was recovered in the urine of which 79% was metabolite. Recovery in the feces was zero to 10%. Levels of drug in the CSF were less than 1% of plasma levels in 3 patients at 24 hours after treatment and 27% in one patient who had had brain surgery and brain radiotherapy (Creaven and Allen, 1975).

Side Effects. The predominant toxicity is myelosuppression, mainly granulocytopenia and to a lesser extent thrombocytopenia. Nausea and vomiting may occur. Other side effects mentioned are: fever, alopecia, headache, hypotension with rapid drug administration and anaphylactic reactions (Rozencweig et al., 1977a).

Administration. The drug is supplied in vials of 50 mg dissolved in 5 ml of ethanol since the drug is water insoluble (investigational, NSC-122819). The contents of the vial are diluted with sterile water and infused slowly intravenously over 30–60 min in 5% dextrose in water or normal saline.

Usual Dose. Various dose schedules are currently under investigation.

REFERENCES

Aisner, J., Weiss, H. D., Chang, P., and Wiernik, P. H. Orthostatic hypotension during combination chemotherapy with vincristine (NSC-67574). Cancer Chemother. Rep., 58: 927–930, 1974.
Albert, D. M., Wong, V. G., and Henderson, E. S. Ocular complications of vincristine therapy. Arch. Ophthalmol., 78: 709, 1967.
AMA Council on Drugs. Pipobroman. J.A.M.A. 200: 619, 1967.
Bagley, C. M., Bostick, F. W., and DeVita, V. T. Clinical pharmacology of cyclophosphamide. Cancer Res., 33: 226–233, 1973.
Baguley, B. C., and Falkenhaug, E. M. Plasma half-life of cytosine arabinoside (NSC-63878) in patients treated for acute myeloblastic leukemia. Cancer Chemother. Rep., 55: 291–298, 1971.
Bakowski, M. T. ICRF 159, (±) 1,2-di(3,5-dioxopiperazin-1-yl) propane NSC-129943: Razoxane. Cancer Treat. Rev., 3: 95–107, 1976.
Bateman, J. C., Moulton, B., and Larsen, N. J. Control of neoplastic effusion by phosphoramide chemotherapy. Arch. Intern. Med., 95: 713–719, 1955.
Beardmore, T. D., and Kelley, W. N. Mechanism of allopurinol-mediated inhibition of pyrimidine biosynthesis. J. Lab. Clin. Med., 78: 696, 1971.
Belej, M. A., Troetel, W. M., Weiss, A. J., Stambaugh, J. E., and Manthei, R. W. The

absorption and metabolism of dibromodulcitol in patients with advanced cancer. Clin. Pharmacol. Ther., *13:* 563–572, 1972.

Bellet, R. E., Mastrangelo, M. J., Dixon, L. M., and Yarbro, J. W. Phase I study of ICRF-159 (NSC-129943) in human solid tumors. Cancer Chemother. Rep., *57:* 195–189, 1973a.

Bellet, R. E., Mastrangelo, M. J., Engstrom, P. F. et al. Hepatotoxicity of 5-azacytidine (NSC-102816) (a clinical and pathologic study). Neoplasma *20:* 303–309, 1973b.

Bergevin, P. R., Tormey, D. C., and Blom, J. Clinical evaluation of Hexamethylmelamine (NSC-13875). Cancer Chemother. Rep., *57:* 51–58, 1973.

Bergevin, P. R., Patwardhan, V. C., Weissman, J., and Lee, S. M. Neurotoxicity of 5-fluorouracil. Lancet, *1:* 410, 1975.

Bertino, J. R., and Johns, D. G. Folate antagonists. In Cancer Chemotherapy II, edited by I. Brodsky, S. B. Kahn, and J. H. Moyer, pp 9–22. Grune & Stratton, New York, 1972.

Bledsoe, T., Island, D. P., Ney, R. G., and Liddle, G. W. An effect of *o,p'*-DDD on the extra-adrenal metabolism of cortisol in man. J. Clin. Endocrinol Metab., *24:* 1301–1311, 1964.

Bleyer, W. A. The clinical pharmacology of methotrexate. A new application of an old drug. Cancer, *41:* 36–51, 1978.

Blum, R. H., Carter, S. K., and Agre, K. A clinical review of bleomycin—a new antineoplastic agent. Cancer, *31:* 903–914, 1973.

Boileau, G., Piro, A. J., Lahiri, S. R., and Hall, T. C. Cerebellar ataxia during 5-fluorouracil (NSC-19893) therapy. Cancer Chemother. Rep., *55:* 595–598, 1971.

Borkovic, A. B., and DeMilo, A. B. Insect chemosterilants; V. Derivatives of melamine. J. Med. Chem. *10:* 457–461, 1967.

Bolt, W., Ritzl, F., Toussaint, R., and Nahrmann, H. Verteilung und Ausscheidung eines cytostatisch wirkenden, mit Tritium markierten *N*-Lost—Derivates beim krebskranken Menschen. Arzneim. Forsch., *11:* 170–175, 1961.

Brock, N., Gross, R., Hohorst, H. J., Klein, H. O., and Schneider, B. Activation of cyclophosphamide in man and animals. Cancer, *27:* 1512–1529, 1971.

Brockman, R. W. Mechanisms of resistance to anticancer agents. Adv. Cancer Res., *7:* 129, 1963.

Brosky, G., and Logothelopoulos, J. Streptozotocin diabetes in the mouse and guinea pig. Diabetes, *18:* 606–611, 1969.

Bruckner, H. W., and Creasey, W. A. The administration of 5-fluorouracil by mouth. Cancer, *33:* 14–18, 1974.

Bryan, G. T., Worzalla, J. F., Gorske, A. L., and Ramirez, G. Plasma levels and urinary excretion of Hexamethylmelamine following oral administration to human subjects with cancer. Clin. Pharmacol. Ther., *9:* 777–782, 1968.

Calabresi, P., and Parks, R. E. Chemotherapy of neoplastic diseases. In The Pharmacological Basis of Therapeutics, Ed. 4, edited by L. S. Goodman and A. Gilman. Macmillan, New York, 1970.

Calabresi, P., and Welch, A. D. Cytotoxic drugs, hormones and radioactive isotopes. In The Pharmacological Basis of Therapeutics, Ed. 3, edited by L. S. Goodman and A. Gilman. Macmillan, New York, 1965.

Calendi, E., DiMarco, A., Reggiani, B., Scarpinato, B., and Valentini, L. On physiochemical interactions between Daunomycin and nucleic acids. Biochem. Biophys. Acta, *103:* 25, 1965.

Capizzi, R. L., Bertino, J. R., and Handschumacher, R. E. L-Asparaginase. Am. Rev. Med., *21:* 433–444, 1970.

Carter, S. K. Streptonigrin (NSC-45383). Chemotherapy Fact Sheet, NCI, 1968.

Coffey, J. J., White, C. A., Lesk, A. B., Rogers, W. I., and Serpick, A. A. Effect of allopurinol on the pharmacokinetics of 6-mercaptopurine (NSC-755) in cancer patients. Cancer Res., *32:* 1283–1289, 1972.

Cohen, J. L., Irvin, L. E., Marshall, G. J., Darvey, H., and Bateman, J. R. Clinical pharmacology of oral and intravenous 5-fluorouracil (NSC-19893). Cancer Chemother. Rep., *58:* 723–731, 1974.

Creaven, P. J., and Allen, L. M. EPEG, a new antineoplastic epipodophyllotoxin. Clin. Pharmacol. Ther., *18:* 221–226, 1975.

Creaven, P. J., Cohn, M. H., Hansen, H. H., Selawry, O. S., and Taylor, S. G. Phase I clinical trial of a single-dose and two weekly schedules of ICRF-159 (NSC-129943). Cancer Chemother. Rep., *58:* 393–400, 1974.

Creaven, P. J., and Allen, L. M. PTG, a new antineoplastic epipodophyllotoxin. Clin. Pharmacol. Ther., *18:* 227–233, 1975.

Dahl, M. G. C., Gregory, M. M., and Scheuer, P. J. Liver damage due to methotrexate in patients with psoriasis. Br. Med. J. *1:* 525–630, 1971.

DeConti, R. C., Toftness, B. R., Lange, R. C., et al. Clinical and pharmacological studies with *cis*-diamminedichloroplatinum (II). Cancer Res., *33:* 1310–1315, 1973.

DeVita, V. T., Carbone, P. P., Owens, A. H., et al. Clinical trials with 1,3-bis-(2-chloroethyl)-1-nitrosourea, NSC-409962. Cancer Res., *25:* 1876–1881, 1965.

DeVita, V. T., Denham, C., Davidson, J. D., et al. The physiological disposition of the carcinostatic 1,3-bis-(2-chloroethyl)-1-nitrosourea (BCNU) in man and animals. Clin. Pharmacol. Ther., *8:* 566–577, 1967.

Dollinger, M. R., Krakoff, I. H., and Karnofsky, D. A. Quinacrine (Atabrine) in the treatment of neoplastic effusions. Ann. Intern. Med., *66:* 249, 1967.

Duttera, M. J., Carolla, R. L., Gallelli, J. F., Gullion, D. S., Kleim, D. E., and Henderson, E. S. Hematuria and crystalluria after high-dose 6-mercaptopurine administration. N. Engl. J. Med., *287:* 292–294, 1972.

Elion, G. B. Biochemistry and pharmacology of purine analogues. Fed. Proc., *26:* 898, 1967.

Fairley, K. F., Barrie, J. U., and Johnson, W. Sterility and testicular atrophy related to cyclophosphamide therapy. Lancet, *1:* 568–569, 1972.

Frei, E., Jaffe, N., Tattersall, M. H. N., Pitman, S., and Parker, L. New approaches to cancer chemotherapy with methotrexate. N. Engl. J. Med., *292:* 846–851, 1975.

Freireich, E. Studies in acute leukemia (5-azacytidine). Data on file at NCI, 1973.

Fujita, H., and Kimura, K. Blood levels, tissue distribution, excretion and activation of bleomycin. Proc. Int. Congr. Chemother. Sixth Congr., *2:* 25–30, 1970.

Goldberg, I. H. Mode of action of antibiotics; II. Drugs affecting nucleic acid and protein synthesis. Am. J. Med., *39:* 722, 1965.

Goldie, J. H., Price, L. A., and Harrap, K. R. Methotrexate toxicity; correlation with duration of administration, plasma levels, dose and excretion pattern. Eur. J. Cancer, *8:* 409–414, 1972.

Goldsmith, M. A. 4'-Demethyl-epipodophyllotoxin-β-D-ethylidene glucoside (NSC-14150) VP-16-213. Clinical Brochure, NCI, 1973a.

Goldsmith, M. A., and Carter, S. K. 4'-Demethyl-epipodophyllotoxin-β-D-thenylidene glucoside (VM-26)—a brief review. Eur. J. Cancer, *9:* 477–482, 1973b.

Goldsmith, M. A., Friedman, M. A., and Carter, S. K. 5-(3,3-Dimethyl-1-triazeno) imidazole-4-carboxamide (DTIC, DIC) (NSC-45388). Clinical Brochure, NCI, August 1972.

Gottschalk, P. G., Dyck, P. J., and Kiely, J. M. Vinca alkaloid neuropathy; nerve biopsy studies in rats and man. Neurology, *18:* 875, 1968.

Gralnick, H. R., and Henderson, E. Hypofibrinogenemia and coagulation factor deficiencies with L-asparaginase treatment. Cancer, *27:* 1313–1320, 1971.

Hamilton, L., and Elion, G. B. The fate of 6-mercaptopurine in man. Ann. N.Y. Acad. Sci., *60:* 304–314, 1954.

Hansen, H. H., Selawry, O. S., Muggia, F. M., and Walker, M. D. Clinical studies with 1-(2-chloroethyl)-3-cyclohexyl-1-nitrosourea (NSC-79037). Cancer Res., *31:* 223–227, 1971.

Haskell, C. M., Canellos, G. P., Cooney, D. A., and Hardesty, C. T. Pharmacologic studies in man with crystallized L-Asparaginase (NSC-109229). Cancer Chemother. Rep., 56: 611–614, 1972.

Heidelberger, C. Biochemical mechanisms of action of fluorinated pyrimidines. Exp. Cell Res. Suppl., 9: 462, 1963.

Heinemann, B., and Howard, A. J. Effect of compounds with both antitumor and bacteriophage-inducing activities on E. coli nucleic acid synthesis. Antimicrob. Agents Chemother., 5: 488–492, 1965.

Henderson, E. S., Adamson, R. H., and Oliverio, R. T. The metabolic fate of tritiated methotrexate; II. Absorption and excretion in man. Cancer Res., 25: 1018, 1965.

Hildebrand, J., and Kenis, Y. Vincristine neurotoxicity. N. Engl. J. Med., 287: 517, 1972.

Hitchings, G. H., and Elion, G. B. Mechanisms of action of purine and pyrimidine analogues. In Cancer Chemotherapy II, edited by I. Brodsky, S. B. Kahn, and J. H. Moyer, pp 23–32. Grune & Stratton, New York, 1972.

Ho, D. H. W., Carter, J. K., Thetford, B., and Frei, E. Distribution and mechanism of clearance of L-asparaginase (NSC-109229). Cancer Chemother. Rep., 55: 539–545, 1971.

Holoye, P. Y., Luna, M. A., MacKay, B., and Bedrossian, C. W. M. Bleomycin hypersensitivity pneumonitis. Ann. Intern. Med., 88: 47–49, 1978.

Hutter, A. M., and Kayhol, D. E. Adrenal cortical carcinoma. Results of treatment with o,p'-DDD in 138 patients. Am. J. Med., 41: 581–592, 1966.

Jacobs, S. A., Bleyer, W. A., Chabner, B. A., and Johns, D. G. Altered plasma pharmacokinetics of methotrexate administered intrathecally. Lancet, 1: 465–466, 1975.

Johns, D. G., Hollingsworth, J. W., Cashmore, A. R., Plenderleith, I. H., and Bertino, J. R. Methotrexate displacement in man. J. Clin. Invest., 43: 621, 1964.

Johnson, W. W., and Meadows, D. C. Urinary bladder fibrosis and telangiectasia after cyclophosphamide therapy. N. Engl. J. Med., 284: 290–294, 1971.

Kenis, Y. Effect of piposulfan (NSC-47774) on malignant lymphomas and solid tumors. Cancer Chemother. Rep., 52: 433, 1968.

Kennedy, B. J. Hydroxyurea therapy in chronic myelogenous leukemia. Cancer, 29: 1052–1056, 1972.

Kennedy, B. J. Metabolic and toxic effects of mithramycin during tumor therapy. Am. J. Med., 49: 494–498, 1970a.

Kennedy, B. J. Mithramycin therapy in advanced testicular neoplasms. Cancer, 26: 755–760, 1970b.

Keyes, J. W., Selawry, O. S., and Hansen, H. H. Initial clinical trial of dibromodulcitol (NSC-104800) in patients with advanced cancer. Cancer Chemother. Rep., 55: 583–589, 1971.

Kirschner, R. H., and Esterly, J. R. Pulmonary lesions associated with Busulfan therapy of chronic myelogenous leukemia. Cancer, 27: 1074–1080, 1971.

Koler, R. D., and Fosgren, A. L. Hepatotoxicity due to chlorambucil. J.A.M.A., 167: 816, 1958.

Koons, J. R., Sensenbrenner, L. L., and Owens, A. H. Clinical studies of mithramycin in patients with embryonal cancer. Bull. Johns Hopkins Hosp., 118: 462, 1966.

Koss, L. G., Melamed, M. R., and Mayer, K. The effect of busulfan on human epithelia. Am. J. Clin. Pathol., 44: 385–397, 1965.

Krakoff, I. H., Brown, N. C., and Reichard, P. Inhibition of ribonucleoside diphosphate reductase by Hydroxyurea. Cancer Res., 28: 1559, 1968.

Kreis, W. Mechanisms of action of procarbazine. In Proceedings of the Chemotherapy conference on Procarbazine (Matulane, NSC-77213): Development and Application, edited by S. K. Carter, pp 35–44. U.S. Government Printing Office, Washington, D.C., 1971.

Kunimoto, T., Hori, M., and Umezawa, H. Modes of action of phleomycin, bleomycin and formycin in HeLa-53 cells in synchronized culture. J. Antibiot (A), *20:* 277–281, 1967.

Kyle, R. A., Schwartz, R. S., Olimer, H. L., and Dameshek, W. A syndrome resembling adrenal cortical insufficiency associated with long term busulfan (Myleran) therapy. Blood, *18:* 497–510, 1961.

Lane, M. A preliminary report; observations on the clinical pharmacology of 5-[bis-(2-chloroethyl)amino] macil. Cancer Chemother. Rep., 9: 31, 1960.

LePage, G. A., and Jones, M. Further studies on the mechanism of action of 6-thioguanine. Cancer Res., *21:* 1590, 1961.

Levi, J. A., Wiernik, P. H., Egan, J. J., et al. A comparative study of 5-azacytidine (AZA-C) and guanazole (GNZ) in previously treated adult acute non-lymphocytic leukemia (ANLL) (abstract). Proc. Am. Assoc. Cancer Res., *16:* 83, 1975.

Lui, K., Mittelman, A., Sproul, E. E., and Elias, E. G. Renal toxicity in man treated with mitomycin C. Cancer, *28:* 1314–1320, 1971.

Livingston, R. B., Carter, S. K., Davis, R. D., Cooney, D. A., Davignon, J. P., Rall, D., Murray, B. R., Schepartz, S. A., Venditti, J. M., Wood, H. B., and Zubrod, C. G. Dibromodulcitol, NSC-94100. Clinical Brochure, NCI, August, 1968a.

Livingston, R. B., Carter, S. K., Newman, J. W., Rall, D., Cooney, D. A., Schein, P., Davis, R. D., Wood, H. B., Engle, R., Davignon, J. P., Venditti, J. M., Schepartz, S. A., Murray, B. R., and Zubrod, C. G. Daunomycin, NSC-82151. Clinical Brochure, NCI, September 1968b.

Loo, T. L., Luce, J. K., Sullivan, M. P., and Frei, E. Clinical pharmalogic observations on 6-mercaptopurine and 6-methyl-thiopurine ribonucleoside. Clin. Pharmacol. Ther. *9:* 180–194, 1968a.

Loo, T. L., Tanner, B. B., Housholder, G. E., and Shepard, B. J. Some pharmacokinetic aspects of 5-(dimethyltriazino)-imidazole-4-carboxamide in the dog. J. Pharm. Sci., *57:* 2126–2131, 1968b.

Louis, J. The clinical pharmacology of Hexamethylmelamine; phase I study. Clin. Pharmacol. Ther., *8:* 55–64, 1967.

Mandel, H. G. The physiological disposition of some anticancer agents. Pharmacol. Rev., *11:* 743–838, 1959.

Margileth, D. A., Smith, F. E., and Lane, M. Sudden arterial occlusion associated with mithramycin therapy. Cancer, *31:* 709, 1973.

Mark, J. B. D., Goldenberg, I. S., and Montague, A. C. W. Intrapleural mechlorethamine hydrochloride therapy for malignant pleural effusion. J.A.M.A., *187:* 858, 1964.

Marsden, J. H. Mechanism of action of the Vinca alkaloids. *In* Cancer Chemotherapy II, edited by I. Brodsky, S. B. Kahn, and J. H. Moyer. Grune & Stratton, New York, 1972.

Mellett, L. B., Hodgson, P. E., and Woods, L. A. Absorption and fate of C^{14}-labeled N,N',N''-triethylenethiophosphoramide (Thio-TEPA) in humans and dogs. J. Lab. Clin. Med., *60:* 818–825, 1962.

Middleman, E., Luce, J., and Frei, E. Clinical trials with Adriamycin. Cancer, *28:* 844–850, 1971.

Monto, R. W., Talley, R. W., Caldwell, M. J., Levin, W. C., and Guest, M. M. Observations on the mechanism of hemorrhagic toxicity in mithramycin (NSC-24559) therapy. Cancer Res., *29:* 697, 1969.

Moore, E. C., and LePage, G. A. Metabolism of 6-thioguanine in normal and neoplastic tissue. Cancer Res., *18:* 1075, 1958.

Mosher, M. B., DeConti, R. C., and Bertino, J. R. Bleomycin therapy in advanced Hodgkin's disease and epidermoid cancers. Cancer, *30:* 56–60, 1972.

Nadkarni, M. V., Trams, E. G., and Smith, P. K. Preliminary studies on the distribution and fate of TEM, TEPA and Myleran in the human. Cancer Res., *19:* 713–720, 1959.

Nelson, N. A., Talley, R. W., Reed, M. L., Evens, A. M., Isaacs, B. L., Huffman, P., and Louis, J. Midwest cooperative group evaluation of piposulfan (A-20968) in cancer. Clin Pharmacol. Ther., 8: 385, 1967.

Nesbit, M., Krivit, W., Heyn, R., et al. Acute and chronic effects of methotrexate on hepatic, pulmonary and skeletal systems. Cancer, 27: 1048–1054, 1976.

Nicholson, R. G., and Feldman, W. Hyponatremia in association with vincristine therapy. Can. Med. Assoc. J., 106: 356–357, 1972.

Ohnuma, T., Holland, J. F., and Meyer, P. Erwinia carotovora asparaginase in patients with prior anaphylaxis to asparaginase from E. coli. Cancer, 30: 376–381, 1972.

Oliverio, V. T. Pharmacologic disposition of procarbazine. In Proceedings of the Chemotherapy Conference on Procarbazine (Matulane, NSC-77213), development and application, edited by S. K. Carter, pp. 19–28. U.S. Government Printing Office, Washington, D.C., 1971.

Oliverio, V. T. Toxicology and pharmacology in the nitrosoureas. Cancer Chemother. Rep., 4: 13–20, 1973.

Papac, R., Creasey, W. A., Calabresi, P., and Welch, A. D. Clinical and pharmacological studies with 1-β-D-arabinofuranosylcytosine (cytosine arabinoside). Proc. Am. Assoc. Cancer Res., 6: 50, 1965.

Parsons, C., Baum, M., and Self, M. Effect of mithramycin on calcium and hydroproline metabolism in patients with malignant disease. Br. Med. J., 1: 474–477, 1967.

Perlia, C. P., Gubisch, N. J., Wolter, J., Edelberg, D., Dederick, M. M., and Taylor, S. G. Mythramycin in treatment of hypercalcemia. Cancer, 25: 389–394, 1970.

Philips, F. S., Schwartz, H. S., and Sternberg, S. S. Pharmacology of mitomycin-C. Cancer Res., 20: 1354, 1960.

Pullman, B., and Pullman, A. The electronic structure of the purine-pyrimidine pairs of DNA. Biochim. Biophys. Acta, 36: 343, 1959.

Reich, E. Biochemistry of actinomycins. Cancer Res., 23: 1428, 1963.

Roberts, J. J., Brent, T. P., and Crathorn, A. R. The mechanism of the cytotoxic action of alkylating agents on mammalian cells. In The Interaction of Drugs and Subcellular Components in Animal Cells, edited by P. N. Campbell, pp. 5–27. Churchill, London, 1968.

Rosner, F., Rubin, H., and Parise, F. Studies on the absorption, distribution and excretion of hydroxyurea (NSC-32065). Cancer Chemother. Rep., 55: 167–173, 1971.

Rossof, A. H., Slayton, R. E., and Perlia, C. P. Preliminary clinical experience with cis-diamminedichloroplatinum (II) (NSC-119875, CACP). Cancer, 30: 1451–1456, 1972.

Rozencweig, M., VonHoff, D. D., Hanney, J. E., and Muggia, F. M. VM 26 and VP-16-213: A comparative analysis. Cancer, 40: 334–342, 1977a.

Rozencweig, M., VonHoff, D. D., Slavik, M., and Muggia, F. M. Cis-diammine-dichloro-platinum (D). A new anticancer drug. Ann. Intern. Med., 86: 803–812, 1977b.

Rundles, R. W., Wyngaarden, J. B., Hitchings, G. H., Elion, G. B., and Silberman, H. R. Effect of xanthine oxidase inhibitor on thiopurine metabolism, hyperuricemia and gout. Trans. Assoc. Am. Physicians, 76: 126–140, 1963.

Sadoff, L. The nephrotoxicity of streptozotocin. Cancer Chemother. Rep., 54: 457–459, 1970.

Sakamoto, A. Physical activity; a possible determinant of vincristine (NSC-67574) neuropathy. Cancer Chemother. Rep., 58: 413–415, 1974.

Samuels, M. L., Leary, W. V., Alexandrian, R., Howe, C. D., and Frei, E. Clinical trials with procarbazine in malignant lymphoma and other disseminated neoplasia. Cancer, 20: 1187, 1967.

Sandler, S. G., Tobin, W., and Henderson, E. S. Vincristine induced neuropathy. Neurology, 19: 367, 1969.

Schein, P. S., O'Connell, M. J., Blom, J., Hubbard, S., Magrath, I. T., Bergevin, P., Wiernik,

P. H., Ziegler, J. L., and DeVita, V. T. Clinical antitumor activity and toxicity of streptozotocin (NSC-85998). Cancer, *34:* 993–1000, 1974.

Shorey, J. et al. Hepatotoxicity of mercaptopurine. Arch. Intern. Med., *122:* 54, 1968.

Shotten, D., and Monil, I. W. Possible teratogenic effect of chlorambucil on a human fetus. J.A.M.A., *188:* 423, 1964.

Skibba, J. L., Ramirez, G., Beal, D. D., and Bryan, G. T. Preliminary clinical trial and the physiologic disposition of 4 (5)-(3,3-dimethyl-1-triazeno) imidazole-5 (4)-carboxamide in man. Cancer Res., *29:* 1944–1951, 1969.

Smith, P. K., Nadkarin, M. V., Trams, E. G., and Davison, C. Distribution and fate of alkylating agents. Ann. N.Y. Acad. Sci., *68:* 834, 1958.

Sponzo, R. W., DeVita, V. T., and Oliverio, V. T. Physiologic diposition of 1-(2-chloroethyl)-3-cyclohexyl-1-nitrosourea (CCNU) and 1-(2-chloroethyl)-3 (4-methylcyclohexyl)-1-nitrosourea (MeCCNU) in man. Cancer, *31:* 1154–1159, 1973.

Stolinsky, D. C., Sadoff, L., Braunwald, J., and Bateman, J. R. Streptozotocin in the treatment of cancer; Phase II study. Cancer, *30:* 61–67, 1972a.

Stolinsky, D. C., Bogdon, D. L., Soloman, J., and Bateman, J. R. Hexamethylmelamine (NSC-13875) alone and in combination with 5-(3,3-dimethyltriazeno)imidazole-4-carboxamide (NSC-45388) in the treatment of advanced cancer. Cancer, *30:* 654–659, 1972b.

Stutz, F. H., Tormey, D. C., and Blom, J. Nonbacterial pneumonitis with multidrug antineoplastic therapy in breast carcinoma. Can. Med. Assoc. J., *108:* 710–713, 1973.

Suzuki, M., Nagai, K., Yamaki, H., Tanaka, N., and Umezawa, H. Mechanism of action of bleomycin; studies with growing culture of bacterial and tumor cells. J. Antibiot. (A), *21:* 379–386, 1968.

Szybalski, W., and Iyer, N. N. Crosslinking of DNA by enzymatically or chemically activated mitomycins and porfiromycins, bifunctionally "alkylating" antibiotics. Fed. Proc., *23:* 946–957, 1964.

Thiersch, J. B. The effect of 6-mercaptopurine on the rat fetus and on reproduction of the rat. Ann. N.Y. Acad. Sci., *60:* 220, 1964.

Tipton, J. B. Death from 5-fluorouracil (NSC-19893) given after adrenalectomy. Cancer Chemother. Rep., *36:* 55, 1964.

Tobias, H., and Auerbach, R. Hepatotoxicity of long-term methotrexate therapy for psoriasis. Arch. Intern. Med., *132:* 391–396, 1973.

Toledo, T. M., Harper, R. C., and Moser, R. H. Fetal effects during cyclophosphamide and irradiation therapy. Ann. Intern. Med., *74:* 87–91, 1971.

Troetel, W. M., Weiss, A. J., Stambough, J. E., Laucius, J. F., and Manthei, R. W. Absorption distribution and excretion of 5-azacytidine (NSC-102816) in man. Cancer Chemother. Rep., *56:* 405–411, 1972.

Vaitkevicius, V. K., Talley, R. W., Tucker, J. L., and Brennan, M. J. Cytological and clinical observations during vincaleukoblastine therapy of disseminated cancer. Cancer, *15:* 296, 1962.

Veenma, R. J. The role of Thio-TEPA instillations in bladder cancer. J.A.M.A., *206:* 2725, 1968.

Vesil, E. S., Passamanti, G. T., and Greene, F. E. Impairment of drug metabolism in man by allopurinol and nortriptyline. N. Engl. J. Med., *283:* 1484, 1970.

Vilar, O., and Tulner, W. W. Effect of *o, p'*-DDD on histology and 17-hydroxycorticosteroid output of the dog adrenal cortex. Endocrinology, *65:* 80–86, 1959.

Wan, S. H., Huffman, D. H., Azarnoff, D. L., Stepheno, R., and Hoogstraten, B. Effect of route of administration and effusions on methotrexate pharmacokinetics. Cancer Res., *34:* 3487–3491, 1974.

Wang, J. J., Cortes, E., Sinks, L. F., and Holland, J. F. Therapeutic effect and toxicity of Adriamycin in patients with neoplastic disease. Cancer, *28:* 837–843, 1974.

Wasserman, T. H., Slavik, M., and Carter, S. K. Review of CCNU in clinical cancer therapy. Cancer Treat. Rev., *1:* 131–151, 1974.

Weiden, P. L., and Wright, S. E. Vincristine neurotoxicity. N. Engl. J. Med., *286:* 1369, 1972.

Weiss, H. D., Walker, M. D., and Wiernik, P. H. Neurotoxicity of commonly used antineoplastic agents. N. Engl. J. Med., *291:* 127–133, 1974.

Whang-Peng, J., Leventhal, B., Adamson, J., and Perry, S. The effect of daunomycin on human cells in vivo and in vitro. Cancer, *23:* 113–121, 1969.

Wheeler, G. P., and Bowdon, B. J. Some effects of 1,3-bis(2-chloroethyl)-1-nitrosourea upon the synthesis of protein and nucleic acids. Cancer Res., *25:* 1770–1778, 1965.

Whitcomb, M. E., Schwartz, M. I., and Tormey, D. C. Methotrexate pneumonitis; case report and review of the literature. Thorax, *27:* 636–639, 1972.

Wilson, W. L., Bisel, H. F., Cole, D., Rochlin, D., Ramirez, G., and Madden, R. Prolonged low-dose administration of hexamethylmelamine. Cancer, *25:* 586–590, 1970.

III
Neoplastic Diseases

Chapter 6

Acute Myelocytic Leukemia

ALEXANDER W. WASHINGTON, JR., M.D., ISMAT U. NAWABI, M.D., and
AARON A. ALTER, M.D.

Acute myelocytic leukemia (AML) is a malignant neoplasm of hematopoietic cells characterized by the presence of immature, functionally abnormal leukocytes in the bone marrow and peripheral blood. For 1977 it was estimated that 21,300 (3%) of the predicted 690,000 new cancer cases and 15,000 (4%) of the predicted 385,000 cancer deaths would be due to acute leukemia (Silverberg, 1977). Based on previous patterns, AML accounts for approximately 42% of these leukemias (Ellison, 1973). In most series, males are affected at a higher rate than females in a ratio of about 3:2 (Silverberg, 1977; Wintrobe, 1974). AML chiefly is a disease of adults and most frequently affects the middle-aged and elderly but is seen at all ages. Of 2172 patients with AML registered by the Cancer and Leukemia Group B (CALGB) from 1956 to 1970, the median age was 49 years but 17% were less than 20 years old at the time of diagnosis (Ellison, 1973).

The major manifestations of AML result from infiltration of the bone marrow by leukemic cells which leads to both quantitative decreases and qualitative abnormalities of granulocytes, platelets and red blood cells. In addition, infiltration of many other organs occurs, including the liver, spleen, lymph nodes, kidneys, intestines and skin but seldom results in significant dysfunction of these organs. With the introduction of newer chemotherapeutic agents and improvement in supportive measures, approximately 50% of patients can now be expected to achieve complete remission (Wiernik, 1976; Ohno et al., 1975; Clarkson, 1972). Less dramatic improvement in the length of survival has occurred and the majority of patients are dead 1 year from the time of diagnosis. Only about 20% survive 18 months (Wiernik, 1976).

CLINICAL MANIFESTATIONS

In AML and its variants, it is the infiltration of the bone marrow and the consequent replacement of normal bone marrow elements that is usually responsible for the findings at presentation and for the ultimate death of the patient. Progressive anemia, thrombocytopenia and functional as well as absolute leukopenia are reflected in complaints of fatigue, dyspnea, headaches, palpitations, bleeding and fever. The presenting complaint may be bleeding in the form of petechiae, ecchymoses, epistaxis or occasionally frank genitourinary, gynecologic, gastrointestinal or central nervous system bleeding (Winthrobe, 1974). In addition to the quantitative reduction of normal hematopoietic elements, there is evidence of functional abnormalities of the remaining normal appearing cells. This is particularly true of the mature granulocytes (Galbraith et al., 1970) and erythrocytes (Queisser et al., 1973) but also has been described for the platelets (Cowan and Haut, 1972).

Physical Examination

The physical examination may reveal signs of anemia such as pallor and tachycardia, and evidence of a generalized bleeding disorder. Adenopathy as well as hepatic and splenic enlargement may be present but occurs less frequently than in acute lymphocytic leukemia (ALL). Patients with monocytic and myelomonocytic leukemia may have skin infiltration and gingival hypertrophy, the latter resulting from both leukemic infiltration and secondary bacterial infection or hemorrhage. Other physical findings in patients with AML may reflect specific involvement of a particular organ by leukemic infiltration or occur as a result of infection or hemorrhage.

Laboratory Findings

The diagnosis of AML is made from peripheral blood and bone marrow examination. The total leukocyte count is usually elevated but may be normal or low (leukopenic leukemia). The peripheral smear may reveal many or only a few blasts and occasionally only granulocytopenia may be found (aleukemic leukemia). The blood count often reveals anemia, which is generally normochromic and normocytic, and thrombocytopenia. Rarely, the platelet count may be elevated but in this circumstance the platelets frequently appear morphologically abnormal. The bone marrow shows an increase in the number of myeloblasts and promyelocytes which varies from a moderate increase to total replacement of the other marrow elements. More often the marrow is pleomorphic and shows some degree of white cell maturation. Red cell precursors and megakaryocytes are seen in varying number. This marrow picture contrasts with that of ALL in which the marrow is more often completely replaced by immature cells. Leukocyte alkaline phosphatase and serum and urine muramidase values may be elevated, the latter, particularly in acute monocytic and acute myelomonocytic leukemia. Hyperuricemia and hyperuricosuria due to increased nucleoprotein turnover and mild, nonspecific abnormalities of liver function may be found. It is, however, the bone marrow with evident infiltration that is most definitive in making the diagnosis.

VARIANTS OF AML

The term acute myelocytic leukemia often includes a number of variants: acute myelocytic leukemia (AML), acute promyelocytic leukemia (APL), acute monocytic leukemia (AMOL), acute myelomonocytic leukemia (AMML) and erythroleukemia (EL). Chronic myelomonocytic leukemia (CMML) and the blastic transformation stage of chronic myelocytic leukemia will not be discussed. The reader is referred to Bennett et al. (1976) who present a system of classification and nomenclature of acute leukemia which points out some of the salient morphological differences among the variants.

From a therapeutic viewpoint, there is no significant difference in our approach to these variants, however, some complications occur more frequently with specific variants, such as disseminated intravascular coagulation (DIC) in APL or gingival and skin infiltration with leukemic cells in AMOL or AMML. The prognosis also shows differences, APL generally having a poor prognosis while patients with AMOL may have a longer survival just with supportive measures alone.

LEUKOCYTE KINETICS

The cure of AML would appear to require the killing of every leukemic cell. The failure of patients to remain in remission for prolonged periods as well as relapses which occur after many years is evidence for the survival of some leukemic cells after successful therapy. The development of chemotherapeutic agents effective in AML has resulted from the investigations into normal and pathologic leukocyte physiology and the study of malignant processes, particularly the leukemias, in experimental animals.

All human cells which divide (normal and neoplastic) undergo mitosis. A mitotic cycle is divided into four phases: the (S) phase (wherein DNA synthesis takes place) followed by the premitotic phase (G_2), the phase of mitosis (M), and the postmitotic phase (G_1). For the normal myeloblast G_1 is variable but generally lasts about 4 hours, the S phase about 12 hours, G_2 about 2 hours, and mitosis or M approximately ½ hour. The generation time is the period from one mitosis to the next.

An earlier concept was that leukemic cells proliferate more rapidly than normal cells resulting in explosive, uncontrolled multiplication. This concept is refuted by the following findings. The percentage of cells in mitosis (the mitotic index) is lower in leukemic cells than in normal ones (4–14% vs. 40–70%), the duration of mitosis in leukemic cells is often longer than in normal cells (60 min vs. 36 min), the DNA synthesis time determined by tritiated thymidine (3HT) incorporation is longer in leukemic cells (15–20 hours) than normal (12–14 hours) and the average generation time of the leukemic cells is approximately 60 hours compared to 15 hours for the normal cells (Killman, 1972).

Kinetic studies in experimental stem cell leukemia have led to a clearer understanding of AML in humans. In the early phases of stem cell leukemia the stem cell divides, resulting in 2 daughter stem cells which reenter the mitotic cycle without any differentiation. Cell death is negligible, and the stem cell population expands exponentially until population density reaches a maximum, following which the doubling time takes longer and longer until eventually a stationary phase (plateau) is reached. In contrast during normal cell proliferation in a steady state, one daughter cell is committed to differentiate and goes through a series of maturation divisions to produce cells with a limited life span and a specific function. The second daughter cell returns to the stem cell compartment and may then remain in a G_1 phase for variable periods of time or may become dormant (G_0), reentering the mitotic cycle only under specific conditions. The result is a stable stem cell compartment with a remarkably constant proportion of proliferating cells.

Leukemic cell growth in humans is neither logarithmic as are stem cell cultures of L1210 experimental leukemias, nor does it follow the pattern of normal cells, but lies somewhere in between. Human leukemic cells progressively accumulate. However, individual patients show variation in kinetic patterns. This partially explains why leukemia in some patients progresses much more rapidly than in others and why as many as 10–16% of AML patients have a course which might best be described as "smoldering" or subacute (Henderson, 1969; Knospe and Gregory, 1971). These patients have recognizable disease but there is less severe interference with normal cell function and for a period of time they can survive on supportive therapy.

On the basis of cell kinetic studies, Skipper and his colleagues have been able to separate leukemic cells into four compartments (Skipper and Perry, 1970). Compartment A consists of leukemic cells engaged in uninterrupted division with failure to undergo maturation. Agents which interfere with DNA synthesis such as methotrexate, 6-mercaptopurine (6-MP), thioguanine and cytosine arabinoside exert their prime effect on these cells. Compartment B contains nonproliferating leukemic cells which can enter compartment A. These cells are insensitive or only partially sensitive to most chemotherapeutic agents. Drugs such as methotrexate have been reported to shift cells from compartment B into compartment A and thereby render them susceptible to chemotherapeutic agents. Compartment C consists of nondividing leukemic cells which have lost the capacity to proliferate, have a finite life span, and are logistically less important from a therapeutic point of view. Finally, compartment D consists of cells which are in the process of dying. Since cells in compartment A are dividing, only they are capable of adding to the total number of leukemic cells. Expansion of leukemic cell population is a result of proliferation in compartment A in excess of loss in compartment D. Remission might be thought of as a state where loss to compartment D exceeds proliferation by compartment A. In the normal state, compartment A is equal to compartment D.

The lethal number of leukemic cells in humans is estimated to be 10^{12} or approximately 1 kg of tumor mass. Successful therapy leading to remission is felt to result in a 2–3 log reduction in numbers of cells or destruction of 99–99.9% of the cells, reducing the tumor load to 10^{10} or 10^9 cells. This corresponds to approximately 10 or 1 g of tumor tissue which is generally undetectable by clinical means. The surviving cells are nonproliferating, resistant cells which correspond to compartment B, and are not sensitive to the drugs generally used in the initial induction treatments. Alkylating agents are believed to be more effective in reducing this compartment. At the time of diagnosis, when the tumor burden is large and a large number of leukemic cells are nonproliferating, greater effect is produced by cytotoxic agents which are effective in all phases of the generation cycle such as daunorubicin, cyclophosphamide, and the nitrosoureas. Once the tumor load has been reduced, a large percentage of cells enter the mitotic cycle and acquire sensitivity to S phase active drugs such as cytosine arabinoside. This drug, when given continuously, is available as cells enter the S phase and thus achieves a much higher cell kill. Therapeutic regimens in practice require empiric modification of schedules spawned from kinetic data.

Even if drug schedules are improved and refined to produce reduction of tumor mass several logs greater than currently achieved and more effective maintenance therapeutic regimens are added to such an achievement, the likelihood of a high cure rate would remain small because even this degree of cell eradication would allow for survival of significant numbers of malignant cells capable of eventually reproducing clinical disease. Finally, the existence of cells in G_1 or G_0 which are resistant to chemotherapy and the emergence of resistant clones portend the unlikelihood of cures by these drugs alone. Thus, investigators are seeking other means for achieving control of AML such as immunotherapy which will be discussed later.

Specific Therapy

Before 1948, there was no effective therapy for any type of acute leukemia. Agents such as phosphorus, benzene, nitrogen mustard, Fowler's solution and ethyl carbamite which has effect in chronic leukemias were practically without value in acute leukemia. Ionizing radiation gave equally disappointing results. Remissions were occasionally reported following severe infection or blood transfusions but these were exceedingly rare, often short lived and poorly documented.

In 1948 remission in acute leukemia, primarily ALL, by the antimetabolite aminopterin was reported by Farber. With the addition of more drugs to the armamentarium, their testing in animal leukemia models, the use of multiple drugs and improved scheduling in drug use, remissions in ALL became more the rule than the exception and has resulted in longer survivals. Although progress has been made in the treatment of AML, it has been slower and less dramatic.

Single Agent Therapy

Early attempts at specific therapy utilized single agents to achieve remission. The first drug used with some success was a purine antagonist 6-MP, which used alone achieved complete remissions in 21/146 (15%) patients with AML (Boggs et al., 1962). A review of all the reported cases of AML treated with 6-MP as a single agent up to 1970 revealed that 28% of 521 patients showed a response with 11.5% achieving complete remission (Livingston and Carter, 1970). The duration of survival varied from 61 days to 6.5 months. Methotrexate induced complete remissions in 16% of 44 patients (Vogler et al., 1967), a figure comparable to the results of treatment with 6-MP, although the overall response rate (complete and partial remissions) was lower.

Other agents reported to have equal or less effectiveness than 6-MP included vincristine, cyclophosphamide, chlorambucil, busulfan, vinblastine, procarbazine and hydroxyurea. While hydroxyurea was felt to be of no value in inducing remissions, it was found to be useful in quickly (within 24–48 hours) reducing dangerously high peripheral white counts in patients at risk of cerebral thrombosis due to leukostasis.

Cytosine arabinoside, a pyrimidine analog, was one of the first drugs to achieve a significantly better remission rate than 6-MP in AML. Reported remission rates as high as 43% were seen (Ellison et al., 1968). An overall review of 299 reported cases showed a 21% complete remission rate (Livingston and Carter, 1970). The mechanism of action of the drug appears to be on DNA synthesis by inhibition of DNA polymerase.

A second drug which shows improved remission rate is daunorubicin, an antibiotic first isolated from cultures of *Streptomyces peucetius* in 1963. The drug combines with DNA preventing its replication and preventing synthesis of DNA-dependent RNA. In a literature review 34% of 211 cases of AML treated with daunorubicin were reported to have achieved complete remission (Bernard et al., 1972). Other clinical trials employing daunorubicin alone have achieved complete remission rates as high as 56% but with a high risk of severe bone marrow suppression which may be irreversible and cardiac toxicity. The cardiac toxicity appears to be dose related and cumulative. The drug is still investigational but is available as a Group C drug from the National Cancer Institute.

Steroids

When corticosteroids were first used, they were found to be highly effective in ALL but unimpressive as single agents in patients with AML. One of the best results was the achievement of a 15% remission rate in 39 patients (Medical Research Council, 1966). In a review of 425 cases of acute leukemia treated with cortisone and ACTH, the complete response rate was 5.5% for patients with AML. It has been suggested that steroids cause deterioration in some patients (Shanbrom and Miller, 1962). In one retrospective study of 68 patients with AML, 48 of whom had received corticosteroids (Knospe and Conrad, 1966), 8 patients had an acceleration of their disease associated with an increase in the numbers of leukemic cells in the peripheral blood and bone marrow. Seven of eight patients had received steroids alone. In contrast, of 24 patients not treated with steroids, only 2 showed evidence of an accelerated course and only 1 showed unusually rapid clinical deterioration. The conclusion was that steroids alone in the treatment of AML were not only nonbeneficial, but actually dangerous in adults. The authors additionally cautioned against using corticosteroids alone when the cell type was unclear. Thus, whether or not steroids are beneficial as part of multiple drug combinations such as POMP, VAMP, COAP, etc., is equivocal. Due to a lack of proven benefit and possibly harmful effects, steroids are excluded from many regimens presently under study.

Combination Chemotherapy

The development of combination chemotherapy resulted from several observations: (1) single agents could induce complete remissions in only a few patients as just described (2) better results had been achieved using combinations of drugs for treatment of other neoplasms such as Hodgkin's disease, and (3) experimental leukemia studies in animals showed that drug combinations produced significant prolongation of survival over that seen with the same drugs used singly. Thus in AML combinations have been studied with the aim of achieving maximal cell kill by combining drugs with dissimilar toxicities to vital organs, with different sites, mechanisms and duration of action, and have been used in combination or serially in a variety of doses to forstall drug resistance, prolong disease suppression and extend survival.

Prior experience with single agents had yielded one fact in AML treatment. In contrast to ALL, successful remission developed only after the drugs had induced a severe and prolonged marrow suppression, or, "no hypoplasia of life-threatening degree, no remission."

In the late 1950s and 1960s the experimental regimens consisted of a combination of 6-MP with prednisone, methotrexate, methylglyoxal bis-guanylhydrazone (methyl GAG), or vincristine. They were abandoned because of poor response or excessive toxicity. Better results were achieved using cytosine arabinoside or daunorubicin in various combinations. A particularly favorable combination was that of cytosine arabinoside + thioguanine which in one study produced a 53% overall response rate in 36 patients with 15 complete and 4 partial remissions (Gee et al., 1969). CALGB, using the same combination reported that 38% of 66 patients achieved complete remission (Carey et al., 1975), while a complete response rate of 56% (49 of 88 patients) was later reported (Clarkson et al., 1975).

Daunorubicin, because of its encouraging remission rate as a single agent, has also been extensively studied in combinations. Daunorubicin coupled with cytosine arabinoside has produced complete response rates varying from 22 to 61% (Bernard et al., 1972). The combination of daunorubicin, cytosine arabinoside and vincristine gave 48% complete remissions in 23 patients (Rosenthal and Moloney, 1972). Similar results have been reported using daunorubicin, cytosine arabinoside, 6-thioguanine and pyrimethamine in 33 patients (Wiernik et al., 1976). Some of the other better studied combinations and their complete remission rates include cyclophosphamide, cytosine arabinoside, and vincristine, with up to 53% complete remissions (Bernard et al., 1972); cyclophosphamide, vincristine, cytosine arabinoside and prednisone (COAP), 44% in 39 patients (Whitecar et al., 1972); 6-MP, vincristine, methotrexate and prednisone, 45% in 51 patients (Henderson, 1969); cytosine arabinoside, vincristine and prednisone, 33% in 30 patients (Grozea et al., 1975).

Hydroxyl-daunorubicin (Adriamycin), while similar in its action to daunorubicin, has given disappointing results when used alone (Cortes et al., 1972) though the combination of hydroxyl-daunorubicin, vincristine, cytosine arabinoside and prednisone may prove to be quite effective (Wiernik, 1976). Another investigational drug, 5-azacytidine is under study (Levi and Wiernik, 1975). At present, the most promising therapeutic programs include cytosine arabinoside and daunorubicin with or without additional drugs for initial induction therapy. Table 6.1 lists the better studied combinations, their administration schedules and response rates.

REMISSION MAINTENANCE

Achievement of remission, that is, the reduction of tumor load to a point where the disease is no longer detectable by physical examination, laboratory evaluation, or pathologic studies, is only the first objective in the treatment of AML. Without further treatment, the duration of remission is short. CALGB reported a median unmaintained remission duration of only 5 weeks (Ellison et al., 1968). All patients, after remission induction, should be treated in an attempt to extend the length of remission, for it is clear that the extended survival in acute leukemia is directly related to the length of time spent in remission. Continuing the inducing drugs at reduced doses or altered schedules is not necessarily effective in maintaining remission (Gee et al., 1969; Rodriguez et al., 1973). Therefore in some recent studies totally different agents are chosen for maintenance (Manaster et al., 1975), while in others newer agents are added to those used in induction (Eppinger-Helft et al., 1975). Remission durations differ from study to study but most range from 6 months (Medical Research Council, 1974) to 10 months (Whitecar et al., 1972). Although some investigators have reported median remission durations up to 25 months (Grozea et al., 1975), these are not representative of the general experience. In order to further reduce tumor load, some investigators have added a period of further intensive chemotherapy after remission is achieved and before maintenance therapy is begun as a "consolidation" of the remission. The aim of consolidation is to prolong remission duration and survival. What constitutes consolidation or maintenance, however, is often arbitrary.

SUPPORTIVE THERAPY

Bacterial Infection

The primary cause of death in AML is bacterial infection resulting chiefly from neutropenia due to infiltration by leukemic cells and chemotherapy related marrow suppression. In clinical studies of leukemia patients both in relapse and remission, a relationship was demonstrated between the presence and severity of infection and the level of circulating granulocytes (Bodey et al., 1966). A less significant relationship to the level of lymphocytes was also shown. When the circulating granulocyte count fell below 1500/cu mm, the risk of developing infection increased proportionately. With a granulocyte count of 1000/cu mm, the mortality rate was 30% and it increased to 72% in those patients whose granulocyte count fell to less than 100/cu mm. The longer the duration of granulocytopenia, the greater the risk of infection.

A cardinal rule is to attempt to eradicate all infections before aggressive chemotherapy is instituted otherwise the infection will rapidly disseminate. Surgical intervention must be used to remove or drain infected areas. This is particularly true for perirectal and perianal infections because these infections carry a poor prognosis with a greater than 50% mortality rate. Seventy-five percent of the fatal infections are due to septicemia, pneumonia accounts for another 20%, while meningitis, peri-

TABLE 6.1
Some Induction Chemotherapy Combinations Used in AML Treatment

Drugs	Dose	Schedule	Route	Percent Complete Response	Reference
Cytosine arabinoside	100 mg/m²	Daily 1-hour infusion until remission, *toxicity or failure*	IV	24/66 (36%)	Carey et al., 1975 (CALGB)
Thioguanine	2.5 mg/kg	Daily in divided doses as above	PO		
Cytosine arabinoside	3.0 mg/kg	q12h for 7–10 d	IV	28/43 (65%)	Clarkson, 1972
Thioguanine	2.5 mg/kg	q12h for 7–10 d	PO		
Cytosine arabinoside	2 mg/kg	Daily × 5 d	IV	39/72 (54%)	Crowther et al., 1973
Daunorubicin	1.5 mg/kg	Day 1	IV		
Cytosine arabinoside	100 mg/m²	Daily × 7 d continuous infusion	IV	10/16 (63%)	Yates et al., 1973
Daunorubicin	45 mg/m²	Daily × 3 d			
Cytosine arabinoside	2 mg/kg	Daily × 3 d	IV	11/20 (55%)	Rosenthal and Maloney, 1972
Daunorubicin	1 mg/kg	Daily × 3 d	IV		
Vincristine	1.5 mg/kg	Day 1	IV		
Cyclophosphamide	100 mg/m²	Daily × 5 d (q8h)	IV	32/66 (48%)	Bodey et al., 1974
Vincristine (Oncovin)	2 mg	Day 1 of each course	IV		
Cytosine arabinoside (COAP)	100 mg/m²	Daily × 5 d (q8h)	IV		
Prednisone (COAP)	25 mg	4 × d × 5 d	PO		
Cyclophosphamide	100 mg/m²	Daily × 5 d (q8h)	IV	17/39 (44%)	Whitecar et al., 1972
Vincristine (Oncovin)	2 mg	Day 1 of each course	IV		
Cytosine arabinoside	100 mg/m²	Daily × 5 d (q8h)	IV		
Prednisone (COAP)	200 mg	Daily in 4 divided doses	PO		

6-Mercaptopurine	500 mg/m²	Daily × 5 d	IV	13/40 (33%)	Rodriguez et al., 1973
Vincristine (Oncovin)	2 mg	Day 1	IV		
Methotrexate	7.5 mg/m²	Daily × 5 d	IV		
Prednisone (POMP)	200 mg	Daily × 5 d	PO		
Cytosine arabinoside	2 mg/kg	Daily × 5 d (q12h)	IV	17/31 (59%)	Glucksberg et al., 1975
Thioguanine	2 mg/kg	Daily × 5 d (q12h)	PO		
Prednisone	1 mg/kg	Daily × 5 d	PO		
Vincristine	1 mg/kg	Day 1	IV		
Daunorubicin	1.5 mg/kg	Day 1	IV		
Cytosine arabinoside	2 mg/kg	Daily × 7 d (q12h)	IV	32/46 (70%)	Glucksberg et al., 1975
Thioguanine	2 mg/kg	Daily × 7 d (q12h)	PO		
Prednisone	1 mg/kg	Daily × 7 d	PO		
Vincristine	1 mg/kg	Day 1 and 7	IV		
Daunorubicin	1.5 mg/kg	Day 1, 2 and 3	IV		

tonitis, pyelonephritis, arthritis and infections of the soft-tissues account for the remaining 5% (Valdivieso, 1976).

Gram-negative bacteria, notably *Pseudomonas* species, *Escherichia coli* and organisms of the Klebsiella-Enterobacter-Serratia group, produce most of the infections in patients with AML. *Bacteroides fragilis, Clostridium perfringens* and *Bacillus cereus* also produce septicemia or serious local infection. Of the relatively infrequent gram-positive organisms identified, *Staphylococcus aureus, Enterococcus* and *Diplococcus pneumoniae* are the most common. Tuberculosis, frequently in a disseminated form and possibly due to atypical strains, occurs 20 times more frequently in patients with leukemia (Valdivieso, 1976). Thus, it has been recommended that patients with positive tuberculin skin tests or x-ray changes suggesting previous exposure to tuberculosis should be placed on prophylactic isoniazid while on chemotherapy. Other bacterial infections seen more commonly in patients with leukemia are *Nocardia* and *Listeria monocytogenes.*

Fungal and Protozoan Infections

The predisposing factors leading to bacterial infection, including neutropenia, also apply to fungal infections. Autopsy data have established that fungal infections are more commonly present than clinically suspected. Thirteen percent of 45 febrile episodes reported in 24 patients with AML were clinically diagnosed to be due to fungal infection (Goodall and Vesti, 1975). At autopsy in these patients, a 56% incidence was found. *Candida* is the most common offender, but *Aspergillus, Phycomycetes, Cryptococcus, Coccidioides immitus* and *Histoplasma capsulatum* are also seen. *Pneumocystis carinii* is another cause of life-threatening pneumonitis. Since the diagnosis may require an invasive procedure such as transbronchial, transthoracic or open lung biopsy, treatment with pentamidine isethionate and, more recently, the relatively benign combination of trimethoprim-sulfamethoxazole is often begun on the basis of clinical suspicion.

Viral Infections

Infection with rhinovirus, adenovirus and enterovirus is no more frequent or serious in patients with AML than in the normal population. However, viruses such as varicella-zoster, *Herpesvirus hominis,* cytomegalovirus, rubeola and vaccinia can be fatal in these patients. Passive immunization with zoster-immune globulin or zoster-immune plasma is usually effective against varicella virus when given within 72 hours of exposure. There are no generally accepted antiviral agents for the treatment of herpes zoster, herpes simplex, or cytomegalic inclusion disease. Treatment is usually limited to local or symptomatic measures and antibiotics are administered for superimposed bacterial infections.

Fever in patients with AML usually means infection and it may be the only indication of a septic process. Pus formation or abscesses may be absent in neutropenic patients and other signs such as alveolar rales may not be readily detectable. At the earliest suspicion of infection in patients with leukemia, samples of sputum, urine, blood and spinal fluid, and exudates from wounds, catheter tips, etc., should be obtained for bacteriologic examination because of a high incidence of gram-negative organisms. Broad-spectrum antibiotics are then immediately administered in high doses, intravenously. Carbenicillin plus a cephalosporin (cephalothin or cefazolin) or carbenicillin plus an aminoglycoside (such as gentamycin or tobramycin) or all three are given pending culture and sensitivity results. When specific organisms are identified, therapy is adjusted accordingly.

Granulocyte Transfusions

Despite the use of appropriate antibiotics, patients with AML who have severe infection often fail to respond because of neutropenia. As a result, use of granulocyte transfusions combined with antibiotics in infected neutropenic patients is gaining greater acceptance. Granulocytes collected by continuous flow centrifugation or leukocyte filtration from normal donors have produced encouraging results. The transfusions must be given for several consecutive days. HL-A matched cells might be more effective than random donor cells. Trials are underway to study the value of prophylactic granulocyte transfusions in noninfected neutropenic patients. The extent to which these measures will affect remission rates and survival is yet to be determined.

Protected Environments

A variety of methods have been used in an attempt to prevent infection from both endogenous and exogenous flora including topical antiseptics and antibiotics, bowel decontamination with nonabsorbable antibiotics, sterile diets, laminar flow rooms and life-islands. Levine (1976) reviewed the 12 major clinical studies related to protected environments carried out over the past 10 years. While a decreased incidence of infection morbidity and mortality was found, there was no firm evidence for improved remission and survival rates. Levine concluded that the ultimate utility of protected environments and prophylactic antibiotics in acute leukemia therapy remains uncertain. In addition, the present cost of establishing and maintaining protected environments is prohibitive.

Hemorrhage

The second most frequent cause of death in patients with AML is hemorrhage, most often due to thrombocytopenia. Prior to the availability of platelet transfusion, as many as 80% of patients died from blood loss or hemorrhage into a vital structure. Hemorrhage is more likely to occur when platelet counts are lower than 20,000/cu mm. In the presence of fever and infection, hemorrhage may occur at higher platelet levels. An absolute indication for platelet transfusion is bleeding due to thrombocytopenia. In the absence of bleeding, a platelet count of 20,000/cu mm. or lower is also considered an indication. Platelet concentrates produce an increment of approximately 15–20,000 platelets/cu mm/ square meter of body-surface area for each unit of platelets transfused. However, in the presence of active bleeding or infection the expected platelet count rise may not occur. Frequently, clinical bleeding will stop following platelet transfusion even in the absence of an increment in circulating platelets. With the availability of platelet transfusions, bleeding is now responsible for only about 15% of leukemia-related deaths. Antiplatelet antibodies may develop in the recipient after repeated transfusions of platelets from random donors, leading to reduced effectiveness and to severe hypersensitivity reactions. Subsequent transfusions of HL-A matched platelets will usually produce platelet increments and control bleeding. Bleeding may also occur due to liver failure or disseminated intravascular coagulation (DIC) associated with septicemia. DIC has frequently been found to be associated with acute promyelocytic leukemia (APL) and may cause the death of the patient before chemotherapeutic agents can be effective (Gralnick and Sultan, 1975). DIC is believed to be due to the release of some intracellular procoagulant from the promyelocyte which may be worsened by treatment of the leukemia. It has been recommended that heparin be given at a dose of 50 units/kg, every 4–6 hours, IV and that depleted coagulation factors be replaced by giving fresh frozen plasma, factor VIII concentrate, platelets, etc. The value of heparin in this condition remains to be proved.

CENTRAL NERVOUS SYSTEM LEUKEMIA

The magnitude of central nervous system (CNS) leukemia in ALL became recognized only after large numbers of patients achieved remission and survived longer. More than 50% of patients given only systemic chemotherapy developed CNS relapse. CNS involvement in AML was at one time considered unusual. In the early 1960s, it was reported that only 1 of 51 cases of adult AML had meningeal infiltration (Shaw et al., 1960). In a retrospective study of 200 consecutive cases of AML at M. D. Anderson Hospital from 1954 to 1970, not one clinically recognized case of leukemic meningitis was detected, but since 1970, 7 cases have been seen in 41 patients (Dawson et al., 1973). This increased incidence was felt to reflect the increased frequency of remission (50%) and the increased median survival as well as a higher index of suspicion. A more recent study found CNS leukemia to be clinically identified in 6.5% of patients but found at autopsy in 19% (Wolk et al., 1974). Thus a disparity exists between CNS involvement and clinical recognition in AML, unlike ALL where the autopsy incidence is virtually identical to the clinical incidence (39 vs. 40.5%).

The treatment of CNS leukemia consists of intrathecal administration of cytosine arabinoside, 30 mg/m^2 or methotrexate, 12 mg/m^2, (with a recommended maximal dose of 12 mg) (Bleyer, 1978), once or twice weekly until symptoms subside and spinal fluid abnormalities disappear. No conclusive studies have been done to determine if intrathecal agents, irradiation or both would constitute appropriate prophylactic therapy in AML.

Chloroma (Granulocytic Sarcoma)

Chloroma is a localized extramedullary tumor composed of early myeloid and monocytoid precursors, primarily undifferentiated myeloblasts and monoblasts, but also containing small numbers of more mature granulocytes, eosinophiles and nucleated erythrocytes. In a series of 323 cases studied at Peter Bent Brigham Hospital in Boston, chloromas were seen in 2.5% of patients at autopsy (Muss and Moloney, 1973). These green, myeloperoxidase containing tumors are seen most commonly in the bones of the skull, especially the bones of the orbit, and in the sternum, ribs, pelvis and proximal long bones, but can be seen in any location including the nervous system. Typically, chloromas are diagnosed simultaneously with acute leukemia but they may precede clinical acute leukemia. The clinical course and survival of these patients is similar to that of patients without chloromas. The tumor may regress with successful chemotherapy of the leukemia, although rapid relapse is noted, often before marrow relapse. In cases where the location of the tumor causes compression symptoms, localized radiation therapy generally produces response.

Other Complications

The patient with AML runs the risk of additional complications of disease and treatment. Among these are splenic infarction and rupture due to vascular compromise or infiltrative enlargement. Hyperuricemia with urate nephropathy, and, rarely, gout may result from the increased production of urate from cell death and nucleic acid breakdown. This is particularly risky at the initiation of chemotherapy since increased cell death produces a large urate load over a short period of time. Allopurinol, in doses of 300–900 mg daily, prior to induction therapy, and 200–300 mg daily thereafter is effective in preventing significant hyperuricemia. Adequate hydration must be maintained. 6-MP is metabolized by xanthine oxidase and thus the use of xanthine oxidase inhibitors such as allopurinol requires reduction of 6-MP dosages by 50–75%. 6-Thioguanine does not require dosage modification.

Immunotherapy

The failure of chemotherapy to produce remissions uniformly and the difficulty in maintaining them has stimulated other approaches to the treatment of AML. Clinical trials have shown that various forms of immunotherapy could stimulate the immune system to exert an antitumor effect and eradicate a small tumor burden. Mathé, reasoning that acute leukemia in remission with its reduced leukemic cell population might be a good model to test the effect of immunotherapy, used killed allogeneic leukemic cells and bacillus Calmette-Guérin (BCG) to achieve dramatically superior remission lengths over chemotherapy alone in ALL (Mathé et al., 1969). A Barts-Marsden controlled study showed that immunotherapy using BCG plus allogeneic irradiated AML cells produced a median survival after remission of 545 days compared to 303 days with chemotherapy alone (Powles, 1976). More recent follow-up analysis of these patients has shown no significant difference in the remission duration with and without immunotherapy and the prolonged survival appears to be due to length of survival after relapse and more frequently successful reinductions. Modest prolongations of remission duration and/or survival have been reported following other immunologic manipulations such as the use of neuraminidase treated AML cells (neuraminidase increases immunogenicity), MER, a nonviable derivative of BCG and xenogeneic acute leukemia antisera. At present, all such studies must be regarded as purely experimental and the ultimate value of immunotherapy in the treatment of AML is yet to be determined.

Bone Marrow Transplantation

This approach has been studied in a limited number of centers because of the enormous technical support, manpower, and expense required. Patients treated by this modality have usually been those with an HL-A identical sibling and in whom all other measures have failed. In addition to the problem of graft rejection in allogeneic recipients and the development of graft-versus-host disease, interstitial pneumonia and leukemia recurrence after transplantation have also limited the success of this method. In 100 patients with acute leukemia given bone marrow transplants leukemic relapse occurred in 31. The 1-year survival was 25% (Thomas et al., 1977). In another study, 16 transplanted identical twin patients achieved an 88% complete hematologic remission rate with 6 patients remaining in remission 11–44 months (Fefer et al., 1974). Leukemic transformation of the transplanted marrow has been reported in a few instances. Bone marrow transplantation must be considered in a patient with HL-A matched sibling particularly after relapse from the first remission.

Controversy continues as to the optimum management of the elderly patient with AML. The question is not moot, as the number of patients with AML over 50 years of age has been generally found to be between 35 and 50% (Henderson, 1969; Wiernik and Serpick, 1970). A number of investigators have reported that elderly patients are resistant to therapy (Boggs et al., 1969; Whitecar et al., 1972; Southwest Oncology Group, 1974; Wiernik et al., 1976). Those investigators who find age of prognostic value explain the poorer results in the elderly as follows: (1) older patients tend to die of infections or hemorrhagic complications before an "adequate trial" of induction therapy, however, younger patients tend to resist these hazards and die more often of drug failure; (2) older patients frequently have complicating diseases such as diabetes, hypertension and arteriosclerosis with compromised renal and cardiac function and do not tolerate the infectious complications of acute leukemia; and (3) older patients may have minimal bone marrow reserves and are unable to tolerate extensive chemotherapy.

Some groups treat the elderly patient in a manner similar to that used in younger patients because responses do occur at all ages and the response rates appear to be improving for the elderly, especially in protocols using daunorubicin. Daunorubicin reportedly induces remission in less time, thus shortening the period of risk from bone marrow hypoplasia. In addition, once a remission is induced, prognosis is unaffected by age.

SUMMARY

AML is a malignant disease which responds poorly to current therapies. The outlook, however, has improved to the point that 50% of patients achieved complete remission and the median survival has been extended. The best combination of drugs to induce remission appears to be cytosine arabinoside + daunorubicin or + thioguanine, although other combinations may be equally effective. Improvements in supportive therapy have also reduced the mortality and morbidity and have added to the potential of specific chemotherapy. Remission maintenance is generally difficult.

While current results are achieved at an often frightening cost in morbidity and mortality, patients not treated are doomed to death. Patients who do achieve complete remission live essentially normal lives until relapse and with hope for future therapeutic improvements. Bone marrow transplantation is appearing promising and offers a chance to those who have relapsed and have an HL-A compatible sibling. Immunotherapy is under investigation.

REFERENCES

Bennett, J. M., Catovsky, D., Daniel, M., Flandrin, G., Galton, D. A. G., Gralnick, H. R., and Sultan, C. Proposals for the classification of the acute leukaemias. Br. J. Haematol., *33:* 451–458, 1976.

Bernard, J., Jacquillat, C., and Weil, M. Treatment of the acute leukemias. Semin. Hematol., *9:* 181–191, 1972.

Bleyer, W. A. The clinical pharmacology of methotrexate; new applications of an old drug. Cancer, *41:* 36–51, 1978.

Bodey, G. P., Buckley, M., Sathe, Y. S., and Freireich, E. J. Quantitative relationships between circulating leukocytes and infection in patients with acute leukemia. Ann. Intern. Med., *64:* 328–340, 1966.

Bodey, G. P., Coltman, C. A., Freireich, E. J., Bonnet, J. D., Gehan, E. A., Haut, A. B., Hewlett, J. S., McCredie, K. B., Saiki, J. H., and Wilson, H. E. Chemotherapy of acute leukemia. Arch. Intern. Med., *133:* 260–266, 1974.

Boggs, D. R., Wintrobe, M. M., and Cartwright, G. E. The acute leukemias; an analysis of 322 cases and review of the literature. Medicine, *41:* 163–225, 1962.

Boggs, D. R., Wintrobe, M. M., and Cartwright, G. E. To treat or not to treat acute granulocytic leukemia. (II). Arch. Intern. Med., *123:* 568–570, 1969.

Carey, R. W., Ribas-Mundo, M., Ellison, R. R., Glidewell, D., Lee, S. T., Cuttner, J., Levy, R. N., Silver, R., Blom, J., Havrani, F., Spurr, C. L., Harley, J. B., Kyle, R., Moon, J. H., Eagan, R. T., and Holland, J. F. Comparative study of cytosine arabinoside therapy alone and combined with thioguanine, mercaptopurine or daunorubicin in acute myelocytic leukemia. Cancer, *36:* 1560–1566, 1975.

Clarkson, B. D. Acute myelocytic leukemia in adults. Cancer, *30:* 1572–1582, 1972.

Clarkson, B. D., Dowling, M. D., Gee, T. S., Cunningham, I. B., and Burchenal, J. H. Treatment of acute leukemia in adults. Cancer, *36:* 775–795, 1975.

Cortes, E. P., Ellison, R. R., and Yates, J. W. Adriamycin (NSC-123127) in the treatment of acute myelocytic leukemia. Cancer Chemother. Rep., *56:* 237–243, 1972.

Cowan, D., and Haut, M. Platelet function in acute leukemia. J. Lab. Clin. Med., *79:* 893–905, 1972.

Crowther, D., Powles, R. L., Bateman, C. J. T., Beard, M. E. J., Gauci, C. L., Wrigley, P. F. M., Malpas, J. S., Fairley, G. H., and Scott, R. B. Management of adult acute myelogenous leukaemia. Br. Med. J., *1:* 131–137, 1973.

Dawson, D. M., Rosenthal, D. S., and Moloney, W. C. Neurologic complications of acute leukemia in adults; changing rate. Ann. Intern. Med., *79:* 541–544, 1973.

Ellison, R. R. Acute myelocytic leukemia. *In* Cancer Medicine, edited by J. F. Holland and E. Frei, pp. 1199–1234. Lea & Febiger, Philadelphia, 1973.

Ellison, R. R., Holland, J. F., Weil, M., Jacquillat, C., Boiron, M., Bernard, J., Sawitsky, A., Posner, F., Gussoff, B., Silver, R. T., Karanas, A., Cuttner, J., Spurr, C., Hayes, D. M., Blom, J., Leones, L. A., Havrani, F., Kyles, R., Hutchison, J. L., Forcier, R. J., and Moon, J. H. Arabinosylcytosine; useful agent in the treatment of acute leukemia in adults. Blood, *32:* 507–523, 1968.

Eppinger-Helft, M., Pavlovsky, S., Suarez, A., Muriel, F. S., Hidalgo, G., Pavlovsky, A., and Vilaseca, G. Sequential therapy for induction and maintenance of remission in acute myeloblastic leukemia. Cancer, *35:* 347–353, 1975.

Farber, S., Diamond, L. K., Mercer, R. D., Sylvester, R. F., and Wolff, J. A. Temporary remissions in acute leukemia in children produced by folic acid antagonist 4-aminopteroyl-glutamic acid (aminopterin). N. Engl. J. Med., *238:* 787–793, 1948.

Fefer, A., Einstein, A. B., Thomas, E. D., Buckner, C. D., Clift, R. A. Glucksberg, H., Neiman, P. E., and Storb, R. Bone marrow transplantation for hematologic neoplasia in 16 patients with identical twins. N. Engl. J. Med., *290:* 1389–1393, 1974.

Galbraith, P. R., Chikkappa, G., and Abu-Zahra, H. Patterns of granulocyte kinetics in acute myelogenous and myelomonocytic leukemia. Blood, *36:* 371–384, 1970.

Gee, T. S., Yu, K., and Clarkson, B. D. Treatment of adult acute leukemia with arabino-sylcytosine and thioguanine. Cancer, *23:* 1019–1032, 1969.

Glucksberg, H., Buckner, C. D., Fefer, A., De Marsh, Q., Coleman, D., Dubrow, R., Huff, J., Kjobech, C., Hill, A. A., Dittman, W., Neiman, P. E., Cheever, M. A., Einstein, Jr., A. B., and Thomas, E. D. Combination chemotherapy for acute nonlymphocytic leukemia. Cancer Chemother. Rep., *59:* 1131–1137, 1975.

Goodall, P. T., and Vosti, K. L. Fever in acute myelogenous leukemia. Arch. Intern. Med., *135:* 1197–1203, 1975.

Gralnik, H. R., and Sultan, C. Annotation; acute promyelocytic leukemia: hemorrhagic manifestation and morphologic criteria. Br. J. Haematol., *29:* 373–376, 1975.

Grozea, P. N., Bottomley, R. H., Shaw, M. T., Tv, H., Chanes, R. E., and Condit, P. T. The role of cytosine arabinoside maintenance in acute nonlymphoblastic leukemia. Cancer, *36:* 855–860, 1975.

Henderson, E. S. Treatment of acute leukemia. Semin. Hematol., *6:* 271–319, 1969.

Killman, S. Kinetics of leukaemic blast cells in man. Clin. Haematol., *1:* 94–113, 1972.

Knospe, W. H., and Gregory, S. A. Smoldering acute leukemia. Arch. Intern. Med., *127:* 910–918, 1971.

Knospe, W. H., and Conrad, M. D. The danger of corticosteroids in acute granulocytic leukemia. Med. Clin. North Am., *50:* 1653–1668, 1966.

Levi, J. A., and Wiernik, P. H. Combination therapy with 5-azacytidine (NSC-102816) and methyl-GAG (NSC 32946) in previously treated adults with acute nonlymphocytic leukemia. Cancer Chemother. Rep., *59:* 1043–1045, 1975.

Levine, A. S. Protected environments—prophylactic antibiotic programmes; clinical studies. Clin Haematol., *5:* 409–424, 1976.

Livingston, R. B., and Cater, S. K. Single Agents in Cancer Chemotherapy. IFI/Plenum, New York, 1970.

Manaster, J., Cowan, D. H., Curtis, J. E., Hasselback, R., and Bergsagel, D. E. Remission maintenance of acute nonlymphoblastic leukemia with BCNU (NSC-409962) and cyclo-phosphamide (NSC-26271). Cancer Chemother. Rep., *59:* 537–45, 1975.

Mathé, G., Amiel, J. L., Schwarzenberg, L., Schneider, M., Cattan, A., Schlumberger, J. R., Hayat, M., and deVassal. ACtive immunotherapy for acute lymphoblastic leukemia. Lancet, *1:* 697–699, 1969.

Medical Research Council Working Party on Leukemia in Adults. Treatment of acute myeloid leukemia with daunorubicin, cytosine arabinoside, mercaptopurine, L-asparagi-nase, prednisone and thioguanine: results of treatment with five multiple-drug schedules. Br. J Haematol., *27:* 373–389, 1974.

Medical Research Council Working Party on the Evaluation of Different Methods of Therapy in Leukaemia. Treatment of acute leukaemia in adults; comparison of steroid and mercaptopurine therapy, alone and in conjunction. Br. Med. J., *1:* 1383–1389, 1966.

Muss, H. B., and Moloney, W. C. Chloroma and other myeloblastic tumors. Blood, *42:* 721–728, 1973.

Ohno, R., Hirano, M., Imai, K., Koie, K., Kamiya, T., Nishiwaki, H., Ishiguro, J., Vetani, T., Sako, F., Imamura, K., and Yamada, K. Daunorubicin, cytosine arabinoside, 6-mercap-topurine riboside and prednisolone (DCMP) combination chemotherapy for acute my-elogenous leukemia in adults. Cancer, *36:* 1945–1949, 1975.

Powles, R. L. Immunologic maneuvers in the management of acute leukemia. *In* Symposium on Immunotherapy in Malignant Diseases. Med. Clin. North Am., *60:* 463–474, 1976.

Queisser, W., Graubner, A., Hoelzer, D., Quisser, V., and Heimpel, H. Some characteristics of the proliferative activity of erythroblasts in untreated and treated acute leukaemia. Acta Haematol., 49: 271–280, 1973.

Rodriguez, V., Hart, J. S., Freireich, E. J., Bodey, G. P., McCredie, K. B., Whitecar, J. P., and Coltman, C. A. POMP combination chemotherapy of adult acute leukemia. Cancer, 32: 69–75, 1973.

Rosenthal, D. S., and Moloney, W. C. The treatment of acute granulocytic leukemia in adults. N. Engl. J. Med., 286: 1176–1178, 1972.

Shanbrom, E., and Miller, S. Critical evaluation of massive steroid therapy of acute leukemia. N. Engl. J. Med., 266: 1354, 1962.

Shaw, R. K., Moore, E. W., Freireich, E. J., and Thomas, L. B. Meningeal leukemia; a syndrome resulting from increased intracranial pressure in patients with leukemia. Neurology, 10: 823–833, 1960.

Silverberg, E. Cancer statistics 1977. CA, 26: 26–41, 1977.

Skipper, H. E., and Perry, S. Kinetics of normal and leukemic leukocyte populations and relevance to chemotherapy. Cancer Res., 30: 1883–1897, 1970.

Southwest Oncology Group. Cytarabine for acute leukemia in adults; effect of schedule on therapeutic response. Arch. Intern. Med., 133: 251–259, 1974.

Thomas, E. D., Buckner, C. D., Banaji, M., Clipt, R. A., Fefer, A., Flournoy, N., Goodell, B. W., Hickman, R. D., Lerner, K. G., Neiman, P. E., Sale, G. E., Sanders, J. E., Singer, J., Stevens, M., Storb, R., and Weiden, P. L. One hundred patients with acute leukemia treated by chemotherapy, total body irradiation, and allogeneic marrow transplantation. Blood, 49: 511–533, 1977.

Valdivieso, M. Bacterial infection in haematologic diseases. Clin. Haematol., 5: 229–248, 1976.

Vogler, W. R., Huguley, C. M., Jr., and Rundles, R. W. Comparison of methotrexate with 6-mercaptopurine-prednisone in treatment of acute leukemia in adults. Cancer, 20: 1221–1226, 1967.

Whitecar, J. P., Bodey, G. P., Freireich, E. J., McCredie, K. B., and Haut, J. S. Cyclophosphamide (NSC-26271), vincristine (NSC-67574), cytosine arabinoside (NSC 63878) and prednisone (NSC-10023) (COAP) combination chemotherapy for acute leukemia in adults. Cancer Chemother. Rep., 56: 543–550, 1972.

Wiernik, P. H. Advances in the management of acute nonlymphocytic leukemia. Arch. Intern. Med., 136: 1399–1403, 1976.

Wiernik, P. H., Schimpff, S. C., Schiffer, C. A., Lichtenfeld, J. L., Aisner, J., O'Connell, M. J., and Fortner, C. Randomized clinical comparison of daunorubicin (NSC-82151) alone with combination of daunorubicin, cytosine arabinoside (NSC 63878), 6-thioguanine (NSC-752) and pyrimethamine (NSC-3061) for the treatment of acute nonlymphocytic leukemia. Caocer Treat. Rep., 60: 41–53, 1976.

Wiernik, P. H., aod Serpick, A. A. Factors affecting remission and survival in adult acute nonlymphocytic leukemia (ANNL). Medicine, 49: 505–513, 1970.

Wintrobe, M. M. Clinical Hematology, Ed. 7, pp. 1472–1499. Lea & Febiger, Philadelphia, 1974.

Wolk, R. W., Masse, S. R., Conklin, R., and Freireich, E. J. The incidence of central nervous system leukemia in adults with acute leukemia. Cancer, 33: 863–869, 1974.

Yates, J. W., Wallace, Jr., H. J., Ellison, R. R., and Holland, J. F. Cytosine arabinoside (NSC-63878) and daunorubicin therapy in acute leukemia. Cancer Chemother. Rep., 57: 485–488, 1973.

Chapter 7

Acute Lymphocytic Leukemia

FREDERICK B. RUYMANN, M.D., and JOHANNES BLOM, M.D.

GENERAL ASPECTS AND ETIOLOGY

The prognosis for children with acute lymphocytic leukemia has changed dramatically since the application of the folic acid antagonist, aminopterin, by Farber et al. (1948). Prior to this pioneering work the average survival of untreated leukemia was only 3 months (Tivey, 1954). With present treatment programs a median survival of 50% at 5 years may be expected.

Leukemia is the most common malignancy of childhood; the risk for leukemia in Caucasian children under 15 years of age in the United States has been estimated at 1 in 2880 (Miller, 1967). The peak incidence is between the ages of 2 and 4, with a nadir in the second and third decade. Subsequently there is a steady rise with increasing age. The partner of an identical twin with acute leukemia has a chance of 1 in 5, while children with Bloom's syndrome have a chance of 1 in 8, and those with Down's syndrome 1 in 95 of developing leukemia (Miller, 1967). Because of these associations prezygotic factors are felt to be important in the relative risk of developing leukemia. A consistent association of histocompatibility loci with acute lymphocytic leukemia has not been shown (Lawler et al., 1971). Increased chromosomal fragility in human fibroblasts exposed to oncogenic viruses has been implicated as an indicator of leukemia risk by Todaro et al. (1966). A family history of leukemia increases the risk for other family members (Miller, 1967). An increased incidence of abnormal dermatoglyphics has been noted in children with leukemia compared with a control group (Menser and Purvis-Smith, 1969).

Prenatal exposure to x-rays may carry an increased risk for the development of leukemia and other malignancies (MacMahon, 1962). Other factors shown to increase the risk for leukemia have been reviewed by Miller (1967) and include exposure to atomic bomb irradiation, benzene, and alkylating agents. The association of animal leukemia with viruses has stimulated interest in the viral etiology of human leukemia. The frequent occurrence of leukemia in cats has prompted a review of contacts with household animals. Bross and Gibson (1970) reported a 2-fold increased risk of leukemia in children exposed to a sick cat. At the present, however, a causal relationship between animal oncogenic viruses and human leukemia has not been demonstrated. Kessler and Lilienfeld (1969) have made an extensive review of epidemiologic factors in leukemia, including the cluster phenomena.

CLINICAL PRESENTATION AND DIAGNOSIS

Evans and Wolman (1971) described typical presenting signs and symptoms in 100 children with acute leukemia. The average child is 6 years old, either male or female with a history of pallor, fever, fatigue, and pain for the past 4 weeks. On physical examination there is moderate enlargement of the spleen, liver and lymph nodes. Laboratory studies reveal a hemoglobin of 6 g/100 ml, hematocrit of 20%, white blood cell count of 12,000/cu mm, and platelet count of 35,000/cu mm. The peripheral blood smear will show 50% blasts, and a bone marrow aspirate will have 90% blasts. The average or typical patient constitutes no great diagnostic dilemma, but the spectrum of acute leukemia is varied. Symptomatology and physical findings in adults do not differ from those in the pediatric group. Subcutaneous nodules are more frequent in younger patients and can simulate disseminated neuroblastoma, the rubella syndrome, and post-steroid panniculitis (Jaffe et al., 1971). Arthritis as a presenting symptom of malignancy has been reviewed by Schaller (1972). She reported a child with a positive latex fixation test who after 12 months of therapy for "arthritis" developed overt leukemia. Any child with the suspected diagnosis of juvenile rheumatoid arthritis should have a bone marrow aspirate to rule out occult leukemia. Pancytopenia can be present in acute leukemia as well as in bone marrow aplasia. Preleukemic states may evolve through an aplastic anemia (Melhorn et al., 1970). Although not diagnostic, 21% of 191 children presenting with acute lymphocytic leukemia had unusual roentgenographic findings (Aur et al., 1972c). These findings include prominent transverse metaphyseal lucent bands, intramedullary osteolytic mottling, and periosteal reaction, which can be similar to primary bone tumors, traumatic injury, and osteomyelitis. Meningeal leukemia with associated headache, vomiting, and weight gain can imitate a primary central nervous system (CNS) malignancy, aseptic meningitis, or Cushing's syndrome. Priapism has also been associated with CNS relapse (Vadakan and Ortega, 1972). Chloromas in the orbit, although more common in acute myelocytic or monocytic leukemia may occur and resemble histiocytosis X or metastatic neuroblastoma

(Lusher, 1964). The peripheral atypical lymphocytosis of infectious mono-
nucleosis closely mimics acute lymphocytic leukemia. Similarly, the
marrow lymphocytosis of acquired pure red cell aplasia may be mistaken
for leukemia (Miale and Bloom, 1975). Other classical mimics include
infectious lymphocytosis and pertussis. A marrow lymphocytosis of 50–
60% may occur normally under 5 years of age, which indicates the marked
lymphoid reactivity of young children. The leukemoid reaction of tuberculosis or of overwhelming infection may mimic leukemia (McMillan,
1971). Therefore, the diagnosis of acute leukemia in a child should be
made with appropriate reservations.

An adequate bone marrow aspirate properly stained with a Wright or
Giemsa stain is a prerequisite to the diagnosis of acute leukemia. A bone
marrow biopsy with touch preps should be performed if the aspirate is
insufficient. In a review of 1263 children with acute leukemia, four major
categories of leukemia were identified by Fraumeni et al. (1971), (Table
7.1). Shaw (1976) has shown that the combination of cytochemical
staining reactions with cytomorphological features reduces subjectivity
and improves the accuracy of diagnosis. Feldges et al. (1974) have
correlated prolonged complete remissions with a strongly periodic acid-
Schiff (PAS)-positive marrow. Other authors have reported PAS-positiv-
ity to be of no significant prognostic value (Humphrey et al., 1974).
Strong positivity for PAS and α-naphthylacetate esterase has been observed in 7 of 78 cases of acute lymphocytic leukemia by Shaw and
Ishmael (1975); these features may represent a subclassification of acute
lymphocytic leukemia. Analysis of leukemia cells for their content of
terminal deoxynucleotidyltransferase may be helpful in differentiating
acute lymphoblastic leukemia (ALL) from acute myelocytic leukemia
(AML) since almost 100% of patients with ALL had this enzyme and only
a few with AML (P.C. Kung et al., 1978).

Several other features may indicate greater heterogenicity of this
disease than heretofore considered. Mathé et al. (1971) have reported
longer survival of patients with microlymphoblastic leukemia. Proliferative patterns in untreated acute lymphocytic leukemia vary considerably
with regard to the duration of S phase, mitotic time, and relative numbers

TABLE 7.1
*Major Categories of Acute Leukemia in 1263 Children**

Category	Percent
Lymphocytic	43.9
Undifferentiated	24.6
Myelogenous	23.8
Monocytic	7.8

* From Fraumeni et al. (1971).

of immediately recycling cells (Wagner et al., 1972). Since the demonstration by Minowada et al. (1972) that human leukemia cell lines had surface characteristics of T lymphocytes, numerous investigators have attempted to determine whether acute leukemia of childhood is a T or a B cell disease. Many leukemic cells appear to be of the null cell type and do not express cell surface characteristics allowing identification of specific lymphoid cell subpopulations. About 20% of patients have receptors for sheep erythrocytes, a T cell marker. Sen and Borella (1975) examined the clinical features of children with lymphoblasts that formed rosettes with sheep erythrocytes and found that these were predominantly older males with a thymic mass and a high white blood cell count at diagnosis. Tsukimoto et al. (1976) have confirmed these findings and have clearly demonstrated a poorer prognosis for this group of patients. It has been known for some time that children with massive leukemic infiltration, high blast-cell count, and a mediastinal mass respond poorly to induction and maintenance therapy (Hardisty and Till, 1968). The E-rosette technique makes possible a classification based on cell membrane receptors which may have practical implications for diagnosis and treatment (Mann et al, 1974).

TREATMENT

Although great progress has been made in chemotherapy since the use of folic acid antagonists in 1948, these advances have not reached all patients, as evidenced by Ingelfinger's editorial in 1972. Progress in combination chemotherapy has been attributable largely to the thousands of patients who have been participants in co-operative group studies both in the United States and abroad. Holland (1969) has urged referral of these patients to treatment centers, so that further progress in diagnosis and management can be made.

INDUCTION

The primary goal of induction chemotherapy in childhood as well as adult acute lymphocytic leukemia is to obtain a complete remission. A complete remission is defined as a normal distribution of platelets, erythroid and myeloid marrow precursors with 5% or fewer lymphoblasts in the bone marrow aspirate. Periodic bone marrow examinations during induction chemotherapy are necessary to assess progress. A bone marrow inaspirable prior to treatment may become aspirable during therapy. The complete response rates of single agents and combination regimens are summarized in Table 7.2 adapted from Goldin et al. (1971). The mainstay of induction treatment is the combination of prednisone and vincristine. Although individual series have reported slightly higher induction rates, with three and four drug combinations, statistically most of these are not

TABLE 7.2
Effectiveness of Induction Chemotherapy in Untreated Acute Lymphocytic Leukemia of Childhood

One Drug	CR† (%)	Two Drugs	CR (%)	Three or Four Drugs	CR (%)
Prednisone	48	Prednisone + Vincristine	88	Prednisone + vincristine + daunorubicin	96
Vincristine	47	Prednisone + 6-mercapto-purine	78		
L-Asparaginase	38–75	Prednisone + daunorubicin	65	Prednisolone + vincristine + methotrexate + 6-mercaptopurine (POMP)	91
Daunorubicin	40				
6-Mercaptopurine	36	Prednisone + cyclophosphamide	59	Prednisone + vincristine + methotrexate + 6-mercaptopurine (VAMP)	88
Methotrexate	25‡	Prednisone + methotrexate	57		
Cyclophosphamide	23	Vincristine + cyclophosphamide	52		
Cytosine arabinoside	17				

* Adapted from Goldin et al. (1971).
† CR = complete remission.
‡ Intermittent therapy.

better and in some instances they carry a greater risk of toxicity (Berry et al., 1975). Ortega et al. (1977) writing for Children's Cancer Study Group have demonstrated a superior induction of 93% using the three drug combination of vincristine, prednisone, and L-asparaginase. These excellent results in 815 children with acute lymphocytic leukemia were obtained in a nonrandom study and compared to earlier data. Jones et al. (1977) writing for Cancer and Leukemia Group B (CALGB) has shown that the late use of L-asparaginase following 3 weeks of a conventional vincristine and corticosteroid induction is optimal. The median complete remission duration of the 275 patients receiving subsequent L-asparaginase was estimated at 45 months. This was significantly longer than three other treatment regimens. Patients treated with subsequent L-asparaginase had a 5-year projected complete remission rate of 50%.

Following the attainment of a complete remission, maintenance therapy is necessary to prevent relapse of the leukemia. An unmaintained remission following a single drug induction lasts 40–60 days, while a multiple drug induction with vincristine, amethopterin, 6-mercaptopurine and prednisone (VAMP) results in an unmaintained median remission duration of 150 days (Goldin et al., 1971). These data suggest a 2–4 log reduction in leukemic cells for the single drug and 8–10 log reduction for the quadruple drug program. A patient in relapse with acute lymphocytic leukemia has approximately 10^{12} neoplastic cells (DeVita et al., 1975). Frequently a more intensive maintenance regimen or consolidation phase is used prior to the routine maintenance program. One such program utilizing repetitive intensive 5-day courses of methotrexate for 8 months had a median survival in excess of 2 years (Holland, 1969). These treatment regimens result in only 50–60% complete remissions in patients 15 years and older with considerably shorter durations of remission. Although some investigators have reported higher complete remissions, the remission duration and survival were similar to those reported by others (Scavino et al., 1976; Gee et al., 1976). Trials of combinations containing cytosine arabinoside (Gingrich et al., 1978) or Adriamycin (Jacquillat et al., 1973; Lister et al., 1978) yielded somewhat higher complete remissions, but remission durations were not significantly prolonged. Simultaneous prednisone, Oncovin, methotrexate, and purinethol (POMP) followed by four additional courses over 2 months and single monthly courses for 12 months yielded a median survival of 147 weeks (Henderson and Samaha, 1969).

MAINTENANCE

Methotrexate (MTX) and 6-mercaptopurine (6-MP) are the main drugs used in maintenance chemotherapy. MTX has been particularly effective in an intermittent dosage schedule. Oral MTX at 30 mg/m^2 twice weekly was considerably more effective than small doses and as effective as the same dose given parenterally (Burgert et al., 1969). Suboptimal dosages of maintenance chemotherapy will result in shorter remissions. This has been emphasized in single drug regimens (Nagao et al., 1970) and in multiple drug maintenance regimens (Pinkel et al., 1971).

Goldin et al. (1971) have summarized 7 studies with 6-MP and found an average median remission of 23 weeks. Improvement in 6-MP maintained remissions with additional monthly pulses of prednisone and vincristine has been reported by Chevalier and Glidewell (1967) who obtained a median remission duration of 85 weeks using vincristine and prednisone periodically with a 6-MP maintenance.

With intensive chemotherapy Memorial Hospital has achieved median survivals in excess of 42 months. Following a prednisone, vincristine, and daunorubicin induction, consolidation was achieved with cytosine arabinoside, 6-thioguanine, L-asparaginase and 1,3-bis-(2-chloroethyl)-1-nitrosourea (BCNU), followed by a multidrug maintenance regimen incorporating intrathecal methotrexate and cranial irradiation (Haghbin et al., 1974). This important study, the L-2 protocol, demonstrated that consolidation need not be limited to conventional MTX and 6-MP therapy.

Meningeal Leukemia. The development of meningeal leukemia has been identified in the past 15 years as the main reason for treatment failure in acute lymphocytic leukemia. Nieri et al. (1968) noted in a review of the CNS complications of leukemia from 1882 through 1951 that only 31 patients with meningeal leukemia had been described. Improved response to combination chemotherapy and longer survival have permitted this serious complication to be observed with greater frequency. Without central nervous system prophylaxis it has been estimated that three-fourths of patients surviving 2½ years from diagnosis would be likely to develop meningeal leukemia (West et al., 1972). Common symptoms of this complication include headache, vomiting and weight gain with a voracious appetite; meningismus is uncommon (Hardisty and Norman, 1967). Cerebrospinal fluid examination will reveal an increased opening pressure with leukemic blasts on stained smear and an elevated protein. Use of the cytocentrifuge for the assessment of meningeal leukemia is mandatory since routine chamber counts have been shown to be in error 30% of the time (Evans et al., 1974). In a series of 150 children with meningeal leukemia Evans et al. (1964) were able to demonstrate a response to a single dose of intrathecal methotrexate at 0.5 mg/kg or radiotherapy at 400 rads. A course of intrathecal methotrexate as a prophylaxis against CNS leukemia was suggested by these authors. The application of 1200 rads of cranial irradiation early in the maintenance resulted in a median remission duration of 78 weeks (George et al., 1968). The superiority of intrathecal MTX in the treatment of meningeal leukemia to low dose irradiation of the cerebrospinal axis at 500 and 1000 rads was demonstrated by Sullivan et al. (1969). A major breakthrough in leukemia therapy occurred when Aur et al. (1972a) reported prevention of CNS leukemia and prolonged complete remissions in children receiving 2400 rads craniospinal irradiation. In this randomized study only 2 of 45 children receiving prophylactic craniospinal irradiation developed CNS leukemia, compared to 27 of 49 children not irradiated. For the first time the projection of a 50% long term, leukemia-free remission rate was made by Simone et al. (1972a). This projection represented an appreciable advance over the earlier 7-year leukemia-free remission rate of 17%. Hematological relapse was a major problem despite the demonstrated value of 2400 rads cranial irradiation and intrathecal methotrexate in preventing CNS leukemia (Muriel et al., 1974). The differences between intensification and maintenance regimens make comparisons with Simone's data more difficult.

Methotrexate is the primary chemotherapeutic agent used intrathecally in the prophylaxis and treatment of CNS leukemia. BCNU, because of its ability to cross the blood-brain barrier, was expected to be effective in preventing CNS leukemia. In a prospective, randomized study intravenous BCNU was inferior to intrathecal methotrexate in preventing meningeal leukemia (Sullivan et al., 1971). Although inferior to cyclophosphamide as a maintenance drug, dibromodulcitol, an alkylating agent appeared to reduce the incidence of CNS leukemia (Sitarz et al., 1975). Using intrathecal cytosine arabinoside, Wang and Pratt (1970) demonstrated improvement in 7 of 11 children with previously treated CNS leukemia. Intrathecal hydrocortisone and cytosine arabinoside in combination with intrathecal methotrexate have been highly effective in the treatment of CNS leukemia (Sullivan et al., 1975).

The administration of intrathecal methotrexate to virtually every child with ALL has prompted scrutiny of its toxicity. In 24 of 51 children who received intrathecal methotrexate Sullivan et al. (1969) have observed ulceration of oral mucosa, nausea, vomiting, fever, intensification of headache, and meningismus. Infrequent complications include seizures and paralysis of the lower extremities (Saiki et al., 1972). Neurotoxicity has also been ascribed to preservations in the diluent; the use of preservation-free diluent is usually recommended. Studies on the pharmacokinetics of intrathecal methotrexate suggest that neurotoxicity may be due to the excessively high spinal fluid concentrations of methotrexate (Bleyer et al., 1973). This has led to a recommended dose of 12 mg/m^2 with a maximum dose of 15 mg, 2 or 3 times per week. More recently the same author has recommended 6 mg for patients under the age of 1, 8 mg for 1-year-olds, 10 mg for 2-year-old patients, and a maximum of 12 mg for all patients over the age of 2 (Bleyer, 1978).

Pathologic examination of the arachnoid in 126 children with ALL demonstrated leukemic infiltrates in 70 cases (Price and Johnson, 1973). The severity of these arachnoid infiltrates was proportional to the number of CNS relapses. Occult involvement of the arachnoid in patients dying during induction was demonstrated at autopsy in about one-third of patients. This comprehensive pathologic study also suggests that intrathecal medications may not reach the deep extensions of grades 2 or 3 arachnoid leukemia. With these observations, "prophylactic" treatment of the CNS becomes a misnomer, since arachnoid infiltration may already have occurred in many instances. Jacquillat et al. (1973) reported a 33% incidence of CNS leukemia in 89 children treated prophylactically with a schedule of intrathecal methotrexate alone; the duration of the median hematologic remission was 34 months. In a more recent study of 117 children treated with craniocervical irradiation and intrathecal methotrexate only 6.8% developed CNS leukemia (Dritschilo et al., 1976).

Irradiation of the CNS has been shown to be associated with a period of transient somnolence occurring 4–8 weeks following the cessation of radiotherapy (Freeman et al., 1973). Despite a transiently abnormal EEG the somnolence resolves without apparent sequelae. A disturbance in myelin synthesis has been suggested as responsible for the somnolence syndrome. A more serious disorder of neurologic deterioration has been reported with parenchymatous degeneration of the central nervous system (Hendin et al., 1974). The severity of these findings has correlated with cranial irradiation, intrathecal methotrexate, intrathecal cytosine arabinoside, and oral pyrimethamine. Generally, the individuals most severely effected have had repeated episodes of CNS leukemia over several years. Characteristic symptoms include spasticity, ataxia, convulsions and dementia. At autopsy destruction of the white matter with vacuolization is prominent; intense fibrillary gliosis occurs peripherally. A multifactorial relationship between leukemic infiltration, intrathecal medication, irradiation, folic acid antagonists, and altered CNS dynamics is probably responsible for this tragic complication. Healthy debate on the quality of life has been evoked by these reports of neurologic sequelae (Freeman and Malpas, 1975). No abnormalities of intelligence, cytology or growth characteristics have been reported in children, surviving 2–10 years after treatment (Verzosa et al., 1974). Children receiving spinal irradiation did show some stunting of growth.

Leukemic infiltration, although most apparant in the CNS, has been reported in every organ. Of special note is the involvement of the testis, which was reported by Stoffel et al. (1975) in 8.0% of their cases. In 8 of 13 patients the testis was the first site of relapse after the initial bone marrow remission. Although associated with sterility, 1200 rads to both testis is effective in treating the leukemia and preserving Leydig cell function.

With sophistication in treatment regimens has come identification of prognostic factors. Zuelzer's (1964) observation that children with initial white blood cell counts above 20,000/cu mm had a poorer prognosis has been confirmed by numerous studies (Pierce et al., 1969; Haghbin et al., 1974; Miller et al., 1974). It is customary to intensify the induction regimen with daunorubicin and L-asparaginase for individuals with a high initial white blood cell count (Aur et al., 1971). A distinctly poorer prognosis was reported for Negro children as compared with Caucasian children; the median survival was 14 months in 46 Negro children compared to 23 months for 288 Caucasian children (Walters et al., 1972). Factors related to advanced disease and poverty, as well as variables in host-disease interaction, were suggested as responsible for those differences. Children under 2 years of age and 8 years or older have been shown to have a poorer prognosis (Pierce et al., 1969). Increased bone marrow lymphocytes, a favorable prognostic sign in neuroblastoma, has shown no correlation with prognosis in ALL of childhood (Green, 1974). The presence of radiological findings in skeletal surveys has been shown to have no correlation with prognosis (Aur et al., 1972c). Hepatosplenomegaly, a mediastinal mass, or symptomatic leukemic infiltrates appear to have a poorer prognosis. In 48 infants under the age of 2, splenomegaly was the single significant factor predicting a shorter survival (Cangir et al., 1975). Chemotherapy protocols have not consistently stratified for these variables. The utilization of cell size as a single prognostic factor has not been reproducible (Pantazopoulos and Sinks, 1974; Murphy et al., 1975). Increased steroid receptors correlate with a longer median survival (Konior et al., 1976). In acute myelogenous leukemia intact cell mediated immunity has been shown to correlate with a favorable response to chemotherapy (Hersh et al., 1971). Konior and Leventhal (1976) have recently reviewed the status of immunocompetence and prognosis in acute leukemia. Serum copper levels taken during early induction have been shown to have a positive correlation with the percentage of lymphoblasts in simultaneous bone marrow aspirates (Tessmer et al., 1972). A significantly increased number of long term survivors with acute lymphocytic leukemia have been reported to have the histocompatibility antigen, HL-A9 (Lawler et al., 1974; Cohen et al., 1974).

IMMUNOTHERAPY

The role of immunotherapy in the treatment of ALL of childhood remains undefined. In two randomized trials of immunotherapy BCG was no better than no further therapy and significantly inferior to continued methotrexate (British Medical Research Council, 1972; Heyn et al., 1973). Professor Mathé et al. (1969), following intensive cytoreductive chemotherapy, randomized patients to receive no further therapy or BCG plus allogeneic leukemia cells. Within 130 days all 10 patients receiving no further chemotherapy had relapsed while 7 of the 20 receiving specific immunotherapy remained in remission over 1000 days. These results are inferior to conventional maintenance chemotherapy where the median survival at 5 years is 51% (Simone et al., 1975). The small percentage of patients relapsing from conventional chemotherapy protocols after 3 years may be helped by continuing specific immunotherapy (Leventhal, 1975). Hope remains that a larger role for immunotherapy may be found in the treatment of acute lymphocytic leukemia of childhood.

CESSATION OF TREATMENT

The ideal time for cessation of chemotherapy in ALL has not been determined. Randomized studies have shown there is a significant advantage in continuing maintenance therapy beyond 2 and 6 months from bone marrow remission (Lonsdale et al., 1975). In a small series of 15 children in complete remission for 2¾–3⅓ years, randomization into a continued or no therapy group revealed no significant differences during 2 years of observation (Krivit et al., 1970). One hundred and thirty two children were removed from therapy after 2–3 years of complete remission (Aur et al., 1974). With a median period of 21 months off therapy 21 of the 132 patients had relapsed. Eighteen of the 21 patients relapsing did so in the first year off therapy. In response to a question by Ragab (1975), Aur (1975) provided greater details on the length of prior treatment in those patients taken off therapy. These results with attendant relapse rates are summarized in Table 7.3. Interestingly, therapy beyond 24–28 months appears to be associated with an increased relapse rate in these preliminary results. The policy in CALGB has been to treat patients for 5 years with maintenance chemotherapy and then randomize to continue chemotherapy or observations without further treatment. Questions regarding the total treatment time should be answered in the next several years. Underlying such questions are serious concerns for growth retardation, perceptual motor disorders, hepatic fibrosis and secondary malignancies as well as the incidence of relapse.

TABLE 7.3
*Duration of Therapy in Relation to Frequency of Relapse after Stopping Therapy in Acute Lymphocytic Leukemia of Childhood**

Duration of Therapy (months)	No. of Patients at Risk	No. of Patients Relapsing	Percent of Patients Relapsing
24–28	13	1	7.7
30	34	4	11.8
36	72	13	18.1
36+	13	3	23.1
Total	132	21	15.9

* Compiled from Dr. Aur's response to Dr. Ragab (Aur, 1975).

RECURRENT LEUKEMIA

The trend in present generation protocols has been to utilize as many chemotherapeutic agents as possible over the shortest period of time permitted by the patient's physical state. This approach has been highly effective and is based on the hypothesis that an early maximum leukemia cell-kill is necessary for prolonged remission or cure. The two major problems evolving from this therapy have been toxicity and the paucity of therapeutic alternatives for resistant or advanced leukemia. A standard reinduction with vincristine and prednisone is often effective in obtaining a second or third remission. This is especially true if the patient has been off all chemotherapy for several months prior to the relapse. Daunorubicin has been shown to be effective in advanced leukemia when used as a single agent. Jones et al. (1971), writing for CALGB, obtained remission rates of 43% and 38% with daunorubicin at 45 and 60 mg/m^2, respectively, administered daily for 5 days. Ragab et al. (1975) writing for the Southwest Oncology Group (SWOG) achieved a 37% complete remission rate in advanced acute lymphocytic leukemia using the hydroxymethyl analog of daunorubicin, Adriamycin. Vietti et al. (1971) in SWOG had a remission reinduction of 69% using daunorubicin in combination with vincristine and prednisone. A complete remission was obtained in 14 of 26 children relapsing with acute lymphocytic leukemia using daunorubicin, vincristine, and prednisone (Aur et al., 1972b). Life threatening myelosuppression has been consistently encountered with daunorubicin. Remissions obtained with daunorubicin alone were brief with a median of 66 days. Using L-asparaginase, vincristine, and prednisone CALGB has achieved a 73% remission rate in children with ALL following relapse (F.H. Kung et al., 1978). Neither of the two nitrosoureas, BCNU or CCNU were effective in preventing central nervous system leukemia or prolonging the remission duration over randomized controls (F.H. Kung et al., 1978).

Although cytosine arabinoside as a single inducing agent has had a response rate of only 16% (Table 7.2) impressive responses have been obtained in refractory ALL when used in combination with L-asparaginase alone (Ortega et al., 1972; Ekert et al., 1972), with L-asparaginase and cyclophosphamide (Lay et al., 1975) and with L-asparaginase and 6-thioguanine (Bryan et al., 1974). Of the 65 children reported in these four representative studies, 37, or 57%, entered a complete remission. The median remission duration varied from 28 days to 98 days. Long term second remissions beyond 3 years may be expected in 25% (Aur et al., 1972b) to 8% (Leventhal et al., 1975) of patients placed on intensive multiple drug induction and maintenance protocols. Cranial irradiation and/or intrathecal methotrexate should be incorporated to control occult or overt meningeal leukemia in children relapsing from a primary treatment protocol (Table 7.4).

TABLE 7.4
Sample Treatment Plan for Acute Lymphocytic Leukemia of Childhood

Phase (Reference)	Avg Time	Treatment	Dosage	Route	Schedule	Comments
Induction						
(Ortega et al., 1977)	28 days	Prednisone	40 mg/m²	PO	Daily	Bone marrow in relapse with 50% lymphoblasts
		Vincristine	2.0 mg/m²	IV	Weekly for 4-6 doses, day 1, 8, 15, 22, etc.	2.0 mg/dose—maximum
(Jones et al., 1977)		L-Asparaginase	6,000 IU/m² or	IM	3 times a week for 9 doses	Hyperglycemia in older children with high white counts
			1000 IU/kg/day	IV	10-day course after 3rd or 4th vincristine	Remission achieved in 87-93% of cases by day 42
Intensification (Aur et al., 1971)		6-Mercaptopurine	1.0 G/m²	IV	Daily on 3 successive days	
	7 days	Methotrexate	10 mg/m²	IV	Daily on next 3 days	
		Cyclophosphamide	600 mg/m²	IV	Once on the 7th day	
CNS-treatment (Aur et al., 1971)	5 weeks	Cranial irradiation	2,400 rads		200 rads daily 5 of 7 days to complete 2400 rads	Below 2 years of age the dose is held below 2000 rads. Field extended to upper cervical vertebrae by Dritschilo et al. (1976) May be given weekly beginning day 8 of induction
		Methotrexate	12 mg/m²	IT	Weekly for 5 doses	
Maintenance (Aur et al., 1971)	Continued	6-Mercaptopurine	50 mg/m²	PO	Daily	A high risk continuation protocol. Cyclophosphamide may be deleted for standard risk patients
	2 years or more	Methotrexate	20 mg/m²	PO	Weekly	
		Cyclophosphamide	200 mg/m²	PO	Weekly	
		Prednisone	40 mg/m²	PO	Daily for 15 days	
		Vincristine	2.0 mg/m²	IV	Weekly for 3 doses	Pulsed every 10 weeks

BONE MARROW TRANSPLANTATION

In instances where the patient has an HL-A compatible sibling and has become refractory to chemotherapy, bone marrow transplantation has been attempted. Recurrent leukemia arising in the donor marrow has been reported by Fialkow et al. (1971); this finding suggests the transmission of a leukemogenic agent to donor cells. Wide application of bone marrow transplantation as a routine therapeutic alternative in acute lymphocytic leukemia is presently not advocated by any investigator. High mortality, immunological complications, emotional problems, high cost, and need for further experience require that these investigations be limited to centers skilled in this technique. Gratifyingly, long term survival has been reported in a few patients. Thomas et al. (1977a, 1977b) recently reviewed this experience at the Fred Hutchinson Cancer Research Center in Seattle. Their results have now been sufficiently encouraging that they adopted a procedure in January 1976 for marrow transplantation for patients with AML in the first remission and for patients with ALL in their second or subsequent remission.

IMMEDIATE COMPLICATIONS

Bleeding

Severe thrombocytopenia is a common accompanient of combination chemotherapy. The predictable bleeding secondary to this planned bone marrow hypoplasia has been greatly alleviated by the institution of platelet transfusions. Alvarado et al. (1965) administered 213 units of fresh human platelet concentrates on 34 occasions to 19 patients with acute leukemia. Hemostasis was achieved in the majority of cases using a dose of 7-8 units/45 kg (100 lb) of body weight. Repeat transfusions will be necessary every 2-3 days if bleeding is to be controlled. Prophylactic platelet transfusions are recommended when the platelet count falls below 15,000/cu mm to 10,000/cu mm and to prevent CNS hemorrhage. In long term platelet transfusion support use of a single HL-A compatible donor improves effectiveness and decreases the development of platelet antibodies. Infection is associated with bleeding by increasing vascular fragility and triggering disseminated intravascular coagulation. Subsequent hypotension and shock will prove fatal unless the underlying infection is properly treated. Corrigan and Jordan (1970) have emphasized the ineffectiveness of heparin therapy in improving the mortality of bacterial sepsis with hypotension. Maintenance of an adequate intravascular blood volume and normal blood pressure is essential. A hematocrit of 35-40% can be achieved by the use of packed red cells during induction chemotherapy. Adequate erythropoiesis to maintain a normal red cell volume cannot be expected before the 3rd or 4th week from onset of therapy. Assessment of urinary output and blood pressure determinations are necessary during induction chemotherapy. If the child is too small for a conventional blood pressure measurement, a Doppler or flush reading should be recorded.

Infections

Infection is the major cause of death in leukemia and should be anticipated by those treating the malignancy. In a consecutive series of 100 patients studied during a 6-week induction at St. Jude Children's Research Hospital, Hughes and Smith (1973), encountered 51 cases of proven infection, 19 instances of fever without detectable cause, and 30 children with no evidence of infection. Seven of the 51 cases of proven infection were considered life-threatening; *Pseudomonas aeruginosa* and *Staphylococcus aureus* were the most commonly isolated pathogens. Pneumonia and urinary tract infections comprised over-half of the moderate infections. In the 35 instances of proven mild infection, 16 were attributable to respiratory tract infections, followed in decreasing order by skin abcesses and cellulitis, oral candidiasis, sinusitis, and otitis media. During the initial 2 weeks of induction, 77% of the children with infections experienced an absolute neutropenia of less than 1000 neutrophils/cu mm. The children with either fever of unknown etiology or with no infection had a 64% and 47% incidence of absolute neutropenia, respectively. Despite management of 70% of the children as outpatients, 10% of the patients acquired *Pseudomonas aeruginosa* in the rectal flora during the 6-week induction period. Any recommendation for antibiotic coverage must consider the bacterial flora isolated from the hospital in which the patient resides. At Walter Reed Army Medical Center patients with fever over 38°C (101°F) and an absolute neutropenia of less than 500/cu mm are given a complete sepsis workup, including a spinal tap, and started empirically on gentamicin, ampicillin, and nafcillin. Coverage for gram-negative bacteria and penicillinase producing *Staphlococcus aureus* is the primary concern during initial induction chemotherapy. If no organism is isolated antibiotic therapy is discontinued after 5 days. The recovery of an organism from the blood or spinal fluid requires a minimum of 10 days of therapy.

Opportunistic Infections

With increased immunosuppression and alteration of cellular immunity the patient relapsing after extended maintenance chemotherapy will have an increased number of opportunistic organisms. A shift in pathogens recovered from one institution is illustrated by the work of Frei et al. (1965); isolates of penicillinase producing staphylococci and gram-negative enteric organisms gave way to increasing fungal infections. In part this experience may be due to the increased survival of patients on

chemotherapy. The routine use of amphotericin B in the febrile, neutropenic patient with malignancy seems unwarranted. If candidiasis is suspected by the demonstration of mycelial or budding yeast forms in
tracheal aspirates or stools and the patient remains febrile with conventional antibiotics, therapy with amphotericin B or 5-fluorocytosine should
be considered. Disseminated histoplasmosis has been reported in 6 children with acute lymphocytic leukemia by Cox and Hughes (1974). In all
cases the organism was recovered from bone marrow cultures.

Pneumocystis carinii has emerged in recent years as a common cause
of pneumonia while the patient is in remission. Symptoms of hyperpnea
and persistent cough are associated with radiographic signs of a progressive interstitial pneumonia and arterial hypoxemia. Studies in an autopsy
series of 195 cases of childhood leukemia revealed an incidence of 4.6%
(Sedaghatian and Singer, 1972). Using percutaneous transthoracic needle
aspiration from infected lung and postmortem examination Hughes et al.
(1973) obtained an incidence of 6.5%. Three-quarters of the cases developed within 2 years from the date of diagnosis of the leukemia. Sulfa-
methoxazole-trimethoprim has been shown to be comparable to pentamidine in a report by Hughes et al. (1976). Additional causes of interstitial
pneumonitis with associated capillary-alveolar block include leukemic
infiltration, aspergillosis, candidiasis, cytomegalovirus infection, and congestive heart failure. The frequent occurrence of these entities alone or
in combination with P. carinii necessitates an adequate tissue diagnosis
by percutaneous transthoracic needle aspiration or open lung biopsy
before starting appropriate therapy.

Cytomegalovirus has been shown to have a definite association with
childhood leukemia (Bodey et al., 1971; Cangir and Sullivan, 1966). Since
its successful propagation in 1956, cytomegalovirus has been shown to be
a ubiquitous agent with high seropositivity in adults and children (Weller,
1971). In a longitudinal study of leukemic children, Sullivan et al. (1968)
showed that patients on chemotherapy longer than one month had
increased levels of cytomegalovirus complement fixing antibodies compared to children under treatment less than 1 month. Although symptoms
of a respiratory infection may be accompanied by seroconversion, many
infections have no outward manifestations (Armstrong et al., 1971). The
significance of cytomegalovirus infection in acute leukemia remains unclear; there is no specific therapy available at the present time.

Specialized Treatment

The use of protective environments and prophylactic, oral, nonabsorbable antibiotics has caused a significant reduction in the microbial
burden of patients undergoing chemotherapy (Bodey et al., 1971). A
longer survival was obtained, thus enabling a more adequate trial of
chemotherapy in the treated group. Levine et al. (1973) in a randomized

trial confirmed the findings of Bodey et al. (1971) with respect to incidence of severe infection in the treated group. They were unable, however, to demonstrate an increased remission rate or duration of remission in the group treated in a protected environment with prophylactic antibiotics. Another controversial, but promising, therapeutic modality has been the use of granulocyte transfusion therapy. Graw et al. (1972) demonstrated an increased survival in patients with gram-negative septicemia receiving more than three granulocyte transfusions. Similar results have been reported by Maybee et al. (1977) who have shown an increased granulocyte recovery in smaller children. A randomized study utilizing filtration-leukopheresis has shown no increased survival in patients receiving granulocyte transfusions (Alavi et al., 1974). The recently demonstrated inferiority of granulocytes collected by filtration leukopheresis has complicated interpretations of results (Klock and Bainton, 1976). Prophylactic applications of granulocyte transfusions continue under investigation at the present time.

Metabolic Complications

With the increasing effectiveness of cancer chemotherapy has come a spectrum of metabolic disorders related to the rapid destruction of malignant cells. Foremost among these entities is hyperuricemia with its possible attendant nephropathy. Allopurinol, a competitive inhibiter of xanthine oxidase, allows for an increased formation and urinary excretion of the more soluble oxypurines, xanthine and hypoxanthine. Use of allopurinol in 15 patients with leukemia and lymphoma resulted in a consistent reduction in serum uric acid (Krakoff and Meyer, 1965). Carlson and Jones (1966) have reviewed the management and prevention of uric acid nephropathy. More recently Zusman et al. (1973) have drawn attention to the increased endogenous phosphorus load resulting from lymphoblast destruction. Hyperphosphatemia, hypocalcemia, and marked hyperphosphaturia were observed within 48 hours of initial chemotherapy in 6 children with acute lymphocytic leukemia. The incidence of hypocalcemia in acute lymphocytic leukemia is 10% in a study by Jaffe et al. (1972). Although the changes in serum phosphorus and calcium may occur in the presence of a normal serum creatinine and blood urea nitrogen, renal insufficiency will aggravate the metabolic changes and increase the likelihood of seizures. Dialysis may be required with progressive renal insufficiency to control hyperphosphatemia in patients with a high leukemic burden and renal infiltration.

Surgical Problems

Surgical emergencies arising in the course of induction and remission are not uncommon. The ileocecal syndrome, the most frequent cause of an acute abdomen, is associated with inflammation, perforation and necrosis of the terminal ileum, appendix or cecum (Sherman and Woolley, 1973; Kingry et al., 1973). Early surgical intervention under aerobic and anaerobic antibiotic coverage is necessary for survival. Transfusion support with platelets and white blood cells combined with surgery has been successfully applied in perforation of the sigmoid colon with associated *Pseudomonas aeruginosa* sepsis and meningitis (Maybee et al., 1977). Subdural hematomas are a common but often unsuspected complication in acute leukemia of childhood. In an autopsy series of 177 cases, 29 were noted to have a subdural hematoma (Pitner and Johnson, 1973). All 13 of the chronic subdural hematomas occurred in children with acute lymphocytic leukemia. Any episode of systemic bleeding in association with thrombocytopenia carries the risk of a complicating subdural hematoma. Individuals failing to respond to the treatment of CNS leukemia or those presenting with cerebral symptoms and an acellular spinal fluid should be suspected of having a chronic subdural effusion (Pitner and Johnson, 1973). Diagnosis by CAT scan is easily made. Surgical therapy seems warranted by the improved survival in acute lymphocytic leukemia.

LATE COMPLICATIONS

Complications in long term survivors with acute leukemia will be under close scrutiny in coming years. An overview of these problems has been presented by Vietti and Ragab (1975). Table 9.5 illustrates the spectrum of these complications and related factors. In 24 of 26 children dying in remission, infection was the immediate cause of death (Simone et al., 1972b). The progressive increase in remission fatalities has corresponded to the increased intensity of radiotherapy and chemotherapy. Long term survival has, of course, increased as a consequence of this intensive therapy. An encouraging report from Verzosa et al. (1974) noted no impairment of intelligence or growth in children receiving chemotherapy and cranial irradiation. Soni et al. (1975) reported no psychological impairment 18 months after irradiation in a prospective study of 34 patients. Eleven patients studied retrospectively had no significant neuropsychologic impairment four years after irradiation. Recent studies of growth hormone response in patients receiving more than 2400 rads has shown no response to either arginine or insulin (Dickinson et al., 1978).

The eventual risk for secondary malignancies is anticipated to be above average. The occurrence of a hepatoma in a child with methotrexate-induced hepatic fibrosis over 5 years from the diagnosis of ALL underlines the need for long term follow-up of these children (Ruymann et al., 1977b). As in economics it has become increasingly apparent to pediatric oncologists that there is no such thing as a free lunch. A continuing price is to be paid for any treatment modality.

TABLE 7.5
Late Complications in Acute Lymphocytic Leukemia

System	Complication	Factors
Dermatological	Alopecia	Cranial irradiation and most chemotherapy, especially cyclophosphamide, Adriamycin, daunorubicin, and vincristine (usually reversible)
	Rash	Chemotherapy, graft vs. host after white cell transfusion or marrow transplantation
Cardiopulmonary	Cardiomyopathy	Adriamycin, daunorubicin, radiotherapy including the heart, other radiomimetic chemotherapy
	Pneumonitis	Methotrexate, opportunistic infections
Hematological	Myelosuppression	Chemotherapy and radiotherapy
	Recurrent leukemia	Sequestered leukemia in CNS, gonads, etc. Constitutional factors in interaction with host immunity, stem cell injury by nitrosoureas, other agents
Immunological	Immunosuppression	Chemotherapy and radiotherapy
	Secondary malignancy	Constitutional factors interacting with chemotherapy and radiotherapy
Gastrointestinal	Ulceration of mucous membrane and gastrointestinal tract	Methotrexate, 6-mercaptopurine, Adriamycin, cyclophosphamide, and other agents
	Hepatitis	Methotrexate, 6-mercaptopurine
	Hepatic fibrosis	Methotrexate
Nervous	Paresthesias, ataxia	Vincristine and intrathecal methotrexate (usually reversible)
	Convulsions, paraplegia dementia, gliosis	Multifactorial recurrent CNS leukemia, intrathecal methotrexate, cranial irradiation, oral folic acid antagonists
Skeletal	Osteoporosis	Corticosteroids and methotrexate (usually reversible)
	Growth retardation	Long term intensive chemotherapy, corticosteroids, and craniospinal axis irradiation
Urogenital	Toxic cystitis, constricted bladder, hydroureters	Cyclophosphamide
	Toxic nephropathy	Cyclophosphamide and methotrexate
	Sterility	Cyclophosphamide and craniospinal irradiation if gonads in the field

EMOTIONAL ASPECTS

Although the emphasis in this chapter has been on physical agents used in the treatment of ALL, the emotional aspects of care often preempt the choice of chemotherapeutic agent. Decision making at the psychological and emotional cross-roads has a critical effect not only on the patient and his family but on the entire treatment team (Toch, 1964). Team members should have an understanding of the changing patterns of fear in childhood and their own attitudes toward death and dying (Kubler-Ross, 1969). Optimism must remain within the bounds of probability when explaining new treatment plans. When death and dying are being discussed, honesty and openness must not become shades of bluntness. Participation of all team members in these sessions is desirable. Parent groups have been of great value in improving communication, expressing fear, and gaining insight. The value of special sessions for health professionals dealing with oncology patients may be appreciable (Artiss and Levine, 1973). Home care of the dying child has been a recent trend gaining in popularity (Ruymann et al., 1977a). Prospective analysis of the emotional and economic variables has rediscovered many advantages of this ancient practice (Martinson et al., 1978).

FUTURE PROSPECTS

In the past 30 years astounding progress has been made in extending the lives of children diagnosed with ALL (Pinkel, 1976). Major advances have come through the application of chemotherapeutic agents and radiotherapy at cancer treatment centers and through cooperative study groups. The dissemination of this information to the community is a primary goal (Holland and Glidewell, 1972). The continuation of randomized studies will be necessary for patients who have leukemias of poor prognosis. Fuller exploitation of basic research on cell cycle, drug action, and metabolic peculiarities of leukemic cells should be expected (Frei, 1972). Karon (1975) has emphasized that followup of children beyond 5 years will determine the true mortality and morbidity of ALL and its treatment.

REFERENCES

Alavi, J. B., Root, R. K., Remischovsky, J., Djerassi, I., Evans, A. E., Schreiber, A. D., Guerry, D., and Cooper, R. A. Leukocyte transfusions in acute leukemia. American Society of Hematology, Atlanta, Georgia, A317, 1974.

Alvarado, J., Djerassi, I., and Farber, S. Transfusion of fresh concentrated platelets to children with acute leukemia. J. Pediatr., *67:* 13–22, 1965.

Armstrong, D., Haghbin, M., Balakrishnan, S. L., and Murphy, M. L. Asymptomatic cytomegalovirus infection in children with leukemia. Am. J. Dis. Child., *122:* 404–407, 1971.

Artiss, K. L., and Levine, A. S. Doctor-patient relation in severe illness; A seminar for oncology fellows. N. Engl. J. Med., *288:* 1210–1214, 1973.

Aur, R. J. A. Relapses in children with ALL off treatment. N. Engl. J. Med., *292:* 431, 1975.

Aur, R. J. A., Simone, J. V., and Pratt, C. B. Successful remission induction in children with acute lymphocytic leukemia at high risk for treatment failure. Cancer, *27:* 1332-1336, 1971.

Aur, R. J. A., Simone, J. V., Hustu, H. O., and Verzosa, M. S. A comparative study of central nervous system irradiation and intensive chemotherapy early in remission of childhood acute lymphocytic leukemia. Cancer, *29:* 381-391, 1972a.

Aur, R. J. A., Verzosa, M. S., Hustu, H. O., and Simone, J. V. Response to combination therapy after relapse in childhood acute lymphocytic leukemia. Cancer, *30:* 334-337, 1972b.

Aur, R. J. A., Westbrook, H. W., and Riggs, W. Childhood acute lymphocytic leukemia. Am. J. Dis. Child., *124:* 653-654, 1972c.

Aur, R. J. A., Simone, J. V., Hustu, H. O., Verzosa, M. S., and Pinkel, D. Cessation of therapy during complete remission of childhood acute lymphocytic leukemia. N. Engl. J. Med., *291:* 1230-1234, 1974.

Berry, D. H., Pullen, J., George, S., Vietti, T. J., Sullivan, M. P., and Fernbach, D. Comparison of prednisolone, vincristine, methotrexate, and 6-mercaptopurine vs. vincristine and prednisone induction therapy in childhood acute leukemia. Cancer, *36:* 98-102, 1975.

Bleyer, W. A. The clinical pharmacology of methotrexate. New applications of an old drug. Cancer, *41:* 36-51, 1978.

Bleyer, W. A., Drake, J. C., and Chabner, B. A. Neurotoxicity and elevated cerebrospinal fluid methotrexate concentration in meningeal leukemia. N. Engl. J. Med., *289:* 770-773, 1973.

Bodey, G. P., Gehan, E. A., Freireich, E. J., and Frei, E., III. Protected environment-prophylactic antibiotic program in the chemotherapy of acute leukemia. Am. J. Med. Sci., *262:* 138-151, 1971.

British Medical Research Council Working Party on Leukaemia in Childhood. Treatment of acute lymphoblastic leukaemia; comparison of immunotherapy (BCG) intermittent methotrexate and no therapy after five month intensive cytotoxic regimen (Concord Trial). Br. Med. J., *2:* 189-194, 1971.

Bross, I. D. J., and Gibson, R. Cats and childhood leukemia. J. Med., *1:* 180-187, 1970.

Bryan, J. H., Henderson, E. S., and Leventhal, B. G. Cytosine arabinoside and 6-thioguanine in refractory acute lymphocytic leukemia. Cancer, *33:* 539-544, 1974.

Burgert, E. O., Glidewell, O., and Mills, S. D. Acute Leukemia Group B. Acute lymphocytic leukemia in children. Maintenance therapy with methotrexate administered intermittently. J.A.M.A., *207:* 923-928, 1969.

Cangir, A., and Sullivan, M. P. Occurrence of cytomegalovirus infections in childhood leukemia; report of three cases. J.A.M.A., *195:* 616-622, 1966.

Cangir, A., George, S., and Sullivan, M. Unfavorable prognosis of acute leukemia in infancy. Cancer, *36:* 1973-1978, 1975.

Carlson, D. J., and Jones, B. Uric acid nephropathy complicating acute leukemia in children; personal cases, pathogenesis, management, prevention. Clin. Pediatr., *5:* 736-742, 1966.

Chevalier, L., and Glidewell, O. Schedule of 6-meracaptopurine and effect of inducer drugs in prolongation of remission maintenance in acute leukemia. Proc. Am. Assoc. Cancer Res., *8:* 10 (A 19), 1967.

Cox, F., and Hughes, W. T. Disseminated histoplasmosis and childhood leukemia. Cancer, *33:* 1127-1133, 1974.

Cohen, E., Singal, D., Khurana, U., Gregory, S. G., Fitzpatrick, J. E., Sinks, L. F., and Henderson, E. S. Frequency of HL-A9 histocompatibility antigen in leukemic populations (abstr. 327). Am. Soc. Hematol., Atlanta, Georgia, 1974.

Corrigan, J. J., and Jordan, C. M. Heparin therapy in septicemia with disseminated

202   GUIDE TO THERAPEUTIC ONCOLOGY

intravascular coagulation. N. Engl. J. Med., *283:* 778–782, 1970.

DeVita, V. T., Young, R. C., and Canellos, G. P. Combination versus single agent chemotherapy; a review of the basis for selection of drug treatment of cancer. Cancer, *35:* 98–110, 1975.

Dickinson, W. P., Berry, D. H., Dickinson, L., Irvin, M., Schedemie, H., and Elders, M. J. Effect of cranial radiation dose on growth hormone response to arginine and insulin infusion (abstr. 600). Pediatr. Res., *12:* 463, 1978.

Dritschilo, A., Cassady, J. R., Camitta, B., Jaffe, N., Furman, L., and Traggis, D. The role of irradiation in central nervous system treatment and prophylaxis for acute lymphoblastic leukemia. Cancer, *37:* 2729–2735, 1976.

Ekert, H., Colebatch, J. H., and Mathews, R. N. Short courses of cytosine arabinoside and L-asparaginase in children with acute leukemia. Cancer, *30:* 643–647, 1972.

Evans, A. E., and Wolman, I. J. Problems in the diagnosis and management of acute leukemia in childhood. Clin. Pediatr., *10:* 571–575, 1971.

Evans, A. E., D'Angio, G. J., and Mitus, A. Central nervous system complications of children with acute leukemia; an evaluation of treatment methods. J. Pediatr., *64:* 94–96, 1964.

Evans, D. I. K., O'Rourke, C., and Jones, P. M. Cerebrospinal fluid in acute leukemia of childhood; studies with the cytocentrifuge. J. Clin. Pathol., *27:* 226–230, 1974.

Farber, S., Diamond, L. K., Mercer, R. D., Sylvester, R. F. J., and Wolff, J. A. Temporary remissions in acute leukemia in children produced by folic acid antagonist, 4-aminopteroyl-glutamic acid (aminopterin). N. Engl. J. Med. *238:* 787–793, 1948.

Feldges, A. J., Aur, R. J. A., Verzosa, M. S., and Daniels, S. Periodic acid-Schiff reaction a useful index of duration of complete remission in acute childhood lymphocytic leukemia. Acta Haematol., *52:* 8–13, 1974.

Fernbach, D. J., George, S. L., Sutow, W. W., Ragab, A. H., Lane, D. M., Haggard, M. E., and Lonsdale, D. Long-term results of reinforcement therapy in children with acute leukemia. Cancer, *36:* 1552–1559, 1975.

Fialkow, P. J., Bryant, J. I., Thomas, E. D., and Neiman, P. E. Leukaemic transformation of engrafted human marrow cells in vivo. Lancet, *1:* 251–255, 1971.

Fraumeni, T. F., Manning, M. D., and Mitus, W. J. Acute childhood leukemia; epidemiologic study by cell type of 1,263 cases at the Children's Cancer Research Foundation in Boston, 1947–65. J. Natl. Cancer Inst., *46:* 461–478, 1971.

Freeman, J., and Malpas, J. S. Long survival from acute leukaemia in childhood. Br. Med. J., *1:* 625, 1975.

Freeman, J. E., Johnston, P. G. B., and Voke, J. M. Somnolence after prophylactic cranial irradiation in children with acute lymphoblastic leukaemia. Br. Med. J., *4:* 523–525, 1973.

Frei, E. Prospectus for cancer chemotherapy. Cancer, *30:* 1656–1661, 1972.

Frei, E., Levin, R. H., Bodey, G. P., Morse, E. E., and Freireich, E. J. The nature and control of infections in patients with acute leukemia. Cancer Res., *25:* 1511–1515, 1965.

Gee, T. S., Haghbin, M., Dowing, M. D. Jr., Cunningham, I., Middleman, M. P., and Clarkson, B. D. Acute lymphoblastic leukemia in adults and children. Cancer, *37:* 1256–1264, 1976.

George, P., Hernandez, K., Hustu, O., Borella, L., Holton, C., and Pinkel, D. A study of "total therapy" of acute lymphocytic leukemia in children. J. Pediatr., *72:* 399–408, 1968.

Gingrich, R. D., Armitage, J. O., and Burns, C. P. Treatment of adult acute lymphoblastic leukemia with cytosine arabinoside, vincristine and prednisone. Cancer Treat. Rep., *62:* 1389–1391, 1978.

Goldin, A., Sandberg, J. S., Henderson, E. S., Newman, J. W., Frei, E., and Holland, J. F. The chemotherapy of human and animal acute leukemia. Cancer Chemother. Rep., *55:* 309–507, 1971.

Graw, R. G., Herzig, G., Perry, S., and Henderson, E. S. Normal granulocyte transfusion therapy; treatment of septicemia due to gram-negative bacteria. N. Engl. J. Med., *287:* 367–371, 1972.

Green, A. A. The prognostic value of bone marrow lymphocytes in acute lymphocytic leukemia of childhood. Cancer, *34:* 2009-2013, 1974.

Haghbin, M., Tan, C. C., Clarkson, B. D., Mike, V., Burchenal, J. H., and Murphy, M. L. Intensive chemotherapy in children with acute lymphoblastic leukemia (L-2 protocol). Cancer, *33:* 1491-1498, 1974.

Hardisty, R. M., and Norman, P. M. Meningeal leukaemia. Arch. Dis. Child., *42:* 441-447, 1967.

Hardisty, R. M., and Till, M. M. Acute leukaemia 1959-64; factors affecting prognosis. Arch. Dis. Child., *43:* 107-115, 1968.

Hartman, J. R. Leukemia in childhood; introduction and etiology. Cancer, *35:* 996-999, 1975.

Henderson, E. S., and Samaha, R. J. Evidence that drugs in multiple combination have materially advanced the treatment of human malignancies. Cancer Res., *29:* 2272-2280, 1969.

Hendin, B., DeVivo, D. C., Torack, R., Lell, M., Ragab, A. H., and Vietti, T. J. Parenchymatous degeneration of the central nervous system in childhood leukemia. Cancer, *33:* 468-482, 1974.

Hersh, E. M., Whitecar, J. P., McCredie, K. B., Bodey, G. P., and Freireich, E. J. Chemotherapy, immunocompetence, immunosuppression, and prognosis in acute leukemia. N. Engl. J. Med., *285:* 1211-1216, 1971.

Heyn, R., Borges, W., Joo, P., Karon, M., Nesbit, M., Shore, N., Breslow, N., and Hammond, D. BCG in the treatment of acute lymphocytic leukemia (ALL). Proc. Am. Assoc. Cancer Res., *14:* 45, 1973.

Holland, J. F. Who should treat acute leukemia? J.A.M.A., *209:* 1511-1513, 1969.

Holland, J. F., and Glidewell, O. Oncologist's reply; survival expectancy in acute lymphocytic leukemia. N. Engl. J. Med., *287:* 769-777, 1972.

Hughes, W. T., and Smith, D. R. Infection during induction of remission in acute lymphocytic leukemia. Cancer, *31:* 1008-1014, 1973.

Hughes, W. T., Price, R. A., Kim, Ho-K., Coburn, T. P., Grigsby, D., and Feldman, S. *Pneumocystis carinii* pneumonitis in children with malignancies. J. Pediatr., *82:* 404-415, 1973.

Hughes, W. T., Feldman, S., and Chaudhary, S. Comparison of trimethoprim-sulfamethoxazole and pentamidine in the treatment of *Pneumocystis carinii* pneumonitis. Pediatr. Res., *10:* 399A, 1976.

Humphrey, G. B., Nesbit, M. E., and Brunning, R. D. Prognostic value of the periodic acid-Schiff (PAS) reaction in acute lymphoblastic leukemia. Am. J. Clin. Pathol., *61:* 393-397, 1974.

Ingelfinger, F. J. Information about cancer treatment. N. Engl. J. Med., *287:* 101, 1972.

Jacquillat, C., Weil, M., Gemon, M. F., Auclere, G., Loisel, J. P., Delobel, J., Flandrin, G., Schaison, G., Izrael, V., Bussel, A., Dresch, C., Weisgerber, C., Rain, D., Tanzer, J., Najean, Y., Seligmann, M., Boiron, M., and Bernard, J. Combination therapy in 130 patients with acute lymphoblastic leukemia (protocol 06 LA 66-Paris). Cancer Res., *33:* 3278-3284, 1973.

Jaffe, N., Hann, H. W. L., and Vawter, G. F. Post-steroid panniculitis in acute leukemia. N. Engl. J. Med., *284:* 366-367, 1971.

Jaffe, N., Kim, B. S., and Vawter, G. F. Hypocalcemia; a complication of childhood leukemia. Cancer, *29:* 392-398, 1972.

Jones, B., Holland, J. F., Morrison, A. R., Lee, S. L., Sinks, L. F., Cuttner, J., Rausen, A., Kung, F., Pluss, H. J., Haurani, F. I., Patterson, R. B., Blom, J., Burgert, E. O., Moon, J. H., Chevalier, L., Sawitsky, A., Albala, M. M., Forcier, R. J. Falkson, G., and Glidewell, O. Daunorubicin (NSC-82151) in the treatment of advanced childhood lymphoblastic leukemia. Cancer Res., *31:* 84-90, 1971.

Jones, B., Holland, J. F., Glidewell, O., Jacquillat, C., Weil, M., Pochedly, C., Sinks, L.,

Chevalier, L., Maurer, H. M., Koch, K., Falkson, G., Patterson, R., Seligman, B., Sartorius, J., Kung, F., Haurani, F., Stuart, M., Burgert, E. O., Ruymann, F., Sawitsky, A., Forman, E., Pluss, H., Truman, J., and Hakami, N. Optimal use of L-asparaginase (NSC-109229) in acute lymphocytic leukemia. Med. Pediatr. Oncol., *3:* 387–400, 1977.

Karon, M. The treatment of acute childhood leukemia; predictions for the future based on extrapolations from the past. Cancer, *35:* 1000–1006, 1975.

Kessler, I. I., and Lilienfeld, A. M. Perspectives in epidemiology of leukemia. Adv. Cancer Res., *12:* 225–302, 1969.

Kingry, R. L., Hobson, R. W., and Muir, R. W. Cecal necrosis and perforation with systemic chemotherapy. Am. Surgeon, *39:* 129–133, 1973.

Klock, F. C., and Bainton, D. F. Degranulation and abnormal bactericidal function and granulocytes procured by reversible adhesion to nylon wool. Blood, *48:* 149–167, 1976.

Konior, G. S., and Leventhal, B. G. Immuno-competence and prognosis in acute leukemia. Semin. Oncol., *3:* 283–288, 1976.

Konior, G. S., Lippman, M. L., Johnson, G., and Leventhal, B. G. Glucocorticoid receptors in childhood acute lymphocytic leukemia. Clin. Res., *24:* 377 (A), 1976.

Krakoff, I. H., and Meyer, R. L. Prevention of hyperuricemia in leukemia and lymphoma; use of allopurinol, a xanthine oxidase inhibitor. J.A.M.A., *193:* 1–6, 1965.

Krivit, W., Gilchrist, G., and Beatty, E. C. The need for chemotherapy after prolonged complete remission in acute leukemia of childhood. J. Pediatr. *76:* 138–141, 1970.

Kubler-Ross, E. On Death and Dying. Macmillan, New York, 1969.

Kung, F. H., Nyhan, W. L., Cuttner, J., Falkson, G., Lanzkowsky, P., DelDuca, V., Nawabi, I. U., Koch, K., Pluss, H., Freeman, A., Burgert, E. O., Leone, L. A., Ruymann, F., Patterson, R. B., Degnan, T., Hakami, N., Pajak, T. F., and Holland, J. Vincristine, prednisone and L-asparaginase in the induction of remission in children with acute lymphoblastic leukemia following relapse. Cancer, *41:* 428–434, 1978.

Kung, P. C., Long, J. C., McCaffrey, R. P., Ratliff, R. L., Harrison, T. A., and Baltimore, D. Terminal deoxynucleotidyl transferase in the diagnosis of leukemia and malignant lymphoma. Am. J. Med., *64:* 788–793, 1978.

Lawler, S. D., Klouda, P. T., Hardisty, R. M., and Till, M. M. Histocompatibility and acute lymphoblastic leukaemia. Lancet, *1:* 699, 1971.

Lawler, S. D., Klouda, P. T., Smith, P. G., Till, M. M., and Hardisty, R. M. Survival and the HL-A system in acute lymphoblastic leukaemia. Br. Med. J., *1:* 547–548, 1974.

Lay, H. N., Ekert, H., and Colebatch, J. H. Combination chemotherapy for children with acute lymphocytic leukemia who fail to respond to standard remission-induction therapy. Cancer, *36:* 1220–1222, 1975.

Leventhal, B. G. New looks in leukemia. Cancer, *35:* 1015–1021, 1975.

Leventhal, B. G., Levine, A. S., Graw, R. G., Simon, R., Freireich, E. J., and Henderson, E. S. Long-term second remissions in acute lymphatic leukemia. Cancer, *35:* 1136–1140, 1975.

Levine, A. S., Siegels, S. E., Schreiber, A. D., Hauser, J., Preisler, H., Goldstein, I. M., Seidler, F., Simon, R., Perry, S., Bennett, J. E., and Henderson, E. S. Protected environments and prophylactic antibodies; a prospective controlled study of their utility in the therapy of acute leukemia. N. Engl. J. Med. *288:* 477–483, 1973.

Lister, T. A., Whitehouse, J. M. A., Beard, M. E. J., Brearley, R. L., Wrigley, P. F. M., Oliver, R. T. D., Freeman, J. E., Woodruff, R. K., Malpas, J. S., Paxton, A. M., and Crowther, D. Combination chemotherapy for acute lymphoblastic leukaemia in adults. Br. Med. J., *1:* 199–203, 1978.

Lonsdale, D., Gehan, E. A., Fernbach, D. J., Sullivan, M. P., Lane, D. M., and Ragab, A. H. Interrupted vs. continued maintenance therapy in childhood acute leukemia. Cancer, *36:* 341–352, 1975.

Lusher, J. M. Chloroma as a presenting feature of acute leukemia. Am. J. Dis. Child., *108:* 62–66, 1964.

MacMahon, B. Prenatal x-ray exposure and childhood cancer. J. Natl. Cancer Inst., *28:* 1173–1191, 1962.

Mann, D. L., Halterman, R., and Leventhal, B. Acute leukemia-associated antigens. Cancer, *34:* 1446–1451, 1974.

Martinson, I. M., Armstrong, G. D., Geis, D. P., Anglim, M. A., Gronseth, E. C., MacInnis, H., Kersey, J. H., and Nesbit, M. E. Home care for children dying of cancer. Pediatrics, *62:* 106–113, 1978.

Maybee, D. A., Millan, A. P., and Ruymann, F. B. Granulocyte transfusion therapy in children. South. Med. J., *70:* 320–324, 1977.

Mathé, G., Amiel, J. L., Schwarzenberg, L., Schneider, M., Cattan, A., Schlumberger, J. R., Hayat, M., and DeVassal, F. Active immunotherapy for acute lymphoblastic leukaemia. Lancet, *1:* 697–699, 1969.

Mathé, G., Pouillart, P., Sterescu, M., Amiel, J. L., Schwarzenberg, L., Schneider, M., Hayat, M., DeVassal, F., Jasmin, C., and LaFleur, M. Subdivision of classical varieties of acute leukaemia; correlation with prognosis and cure expectancy. Eur. J. Clin. Biol. Res., *16:* 554–560, 1971.

McMillan, C. W. Is it leukemia? Clin. Pediatr., *10:* 589, 1971.

Melhorn, D. K., Gross, S., and Newman, A. J. Acute childhood leukemia presenting as aplastic anemia; response to corticosteroids. J. Pediatr., *77:* 647–652, 1970.

Menser, M. A., and Purvis-Smith, S. G. Dermatoglyphic defects in children with leukaemia. Lancet, *1:* 1076–1078, 1969.

Miale, T. D., and Blom, G. E. The significance of lymphocytosis in congenital hypoplastic anemia. J. Pediatr., *87:* 550–553, 1975.

Miller, D. R., Sonley, M., Karon, M., Breslow, N., and Hammond, D. Additive therapy in the maintenance of remission in acute lymphoblastic leukemia of childhood; the effect of the initial leukocyte count. Cancer, *34:* 508–517, 1974.

Miller, R. W. Persons with exceptionally high risk of leukemia. Cancer Res., *27:* 2420–2423, 1967.

Minowada, J., Ohnuma, T., and Moore, G. E. Rosette-forming human lymphoid cell lines; I. Establishment and evidence for origin of thymus-derived lymphocytes. J. Natl. Cancer Inst., *49:* 891–895, 1972.

Muriel, F. S., Pavlovsky, S., Penalver, J. A., Hidalgo, G., Bonesana, A. C., Eppinger-Helft, M., deMacchi, G. H., and Pavlovsky, A. Evaluation of induction of remission, intensification, and central nervous system prophylactic treatment in acute lymphoblastic leukemia. Cancer, *34:* 418–426, 1974.

Murphy, S. B., Borella, L., Sen, L., and Mauer, A. Lack of correlation of lymphoblast cell size with presence of T-cell markers or with outcome in childhood acute lymphoblastic leukaemia. Br. J. Haematol., *31:* 95–102, 1975.

Nagao, T., Lampkin, B. C., and Mauer, A. M. Maintenance therapy in acute childhood leukemia. J. Pediatr., *76:* 134–137, 1970.

Nieri, R. L., Burgert, E. O., and Groover, R. V. Central-nervous-system complications of leukemia; a review. Mayo Clin. Proc., *43:* 70–79, 1968.

Ortega, J. A., Finklestein, J. Z., Ertel, I., Hammond, D., and Karon, M. Effective combination treatment of advanced acute lymphocytic leukemia with Cytosine Arabinoside (NSC-63878) and L-asparaginase (NSC-109229). Cancer Chemother. Rep., *56:* 363–368, 1972.

Ortega, J. A., Nesbit, M. E., Donaldson, M. H., Hittle, R. E., Weiner, J., Karon, M., and Hammond, D. L-Asparaginase, vincristine, and prednisone for induction of first remission in acute lymphocytic leukemia. Cancer Res., *37:* 535–540, 1977.

Pantazopoulos, N., and Sinks, L. F. Morphological criteria for prognostication of acute lymphoblastic leukaemia. Br. J. Haematol., *31:* 95–102, 1974.

Pierce, M. I., Borges, W. H., Heyn, R., Wolff, J. A., and Gilbert, E. S. Epidemiological factors and survival experience in 1770 children with acute leukemia. Cancer, *23:* 1296–1304, 1969.

Pinkel, D. Treatment of acute leukemia. Pediatr. Clin. North Am., *23:* 117–130, 1976.

Pinkel, D., Hernandez, K., Borella, L., Holton, C., Aur, R., Samoy, G., and Pratt, C. Drug dosage remission duration in childhood lymphocytic leukemia. Cancer, *27:* 247–256, 1971.

Pitner, S. E., and Johnson, W. W. Chronic subdural hematoma in childhood acute leukemia. Cancer, *32:* 184–190, 1973.

Price, R. A., and Johnson, W. W. The central nervous system in childhood leukemia; I. The arachnoid. Cancer, *31:* 520–533, 1973.

Ragab, A. H. Relapses in children with ALL off treatment. N. Engl. J. Med., *292:* 431, 1975.

Ragab, A. H., Sutow, W. W., Komp, D. M., Starling, K. A., Lyon, G. M., and George, S. Adriamycin in the treatment of childhood acute leukemia; a southwest oncology group study. Cancer, *36:* 1223–1226, 1975.

Ruymann, F. B., Mease, A. D., and Mosijczuk, A. D. At home with death; antidote for anxiety. J. Pediatr., *91:* 354–355, 1977a.

Ruymann, F. B., Mosijczuk, A. D., and Sayers, R. J. Hepatoma in a child with methotrexate-induced hepatic fibrosis. J.A.M.A., *238:* 2631–2633, 1977b.

Saiki, J. H., Thompson, S., Smith, F., and Atkinson, R. Paraplegia following intrathecal chemotherapy. Cancer, *29:* 370–374, 1972.

Scavino, H. F., George, J. N., and Sears, D. A. Remission induction in adult acute lymphocytic leukemia. Cancer, *38:* 672–677, 1976.

Schaller, J. Arthritis as a presenting manifestation of malignancy in children. J. Pediatr., *81:* 793–797, 1972.

Sedaghatian, M. R., and Singer, D. B. *Pneumocystis carinii* in children with malignant disease. Cancer, *29:* 772–777, 1972.

Sen, L., and Borella, L. Clinical importance of lymphoblasts with T markers in childhood acute leukemia. N. Engl. J. Med., *292:* 828–832, 1975.

Shaw, M. T. The cytochemistry of acute leukemia; a diagnostic and prognostic evaluation. Semin. Oncol., *3:* 219–228, 1976.

Shaw, M. T., and Ishmael, D. R. Acute lymphocytic leukemia with atypical cytochemical features. Am. J. Clin. Pathol., *63:* 415–420, 1975.

Sherman, N. J., and Woolley, M. W. Ileocecal syndrome in acute childhood leukemia. Arch. Surg., *107:* 39–42, 1973.

Simone, J. V., Aur, R. J. A., Hustu, H. O., and Pinkel, D. "Total therapy" studies of acute lymphocytic leukemia in children; current results and prospects for cure. Cancer, *30:* 1488–1494, 1972a.

Simone, J. V., Holland, E., and Johnson, W. W. Fatalities during remission of childhood leukemia. Blood. *39:* 759–770, 1972b.

Simone, J. V., Aur, R. J. A., Hustu, H. O., Verzosa, M., and Pinkel, D. Combined modality therapy of acute lymphocytic leukemia. Cancer, *35:* 25–35, 1975.

Sitarz, A. L., Albo, V., Movassaghi, N., Karon, M., Hammond, D., Weiner, J., and Reed, A. Dibromodulcitol (NSC-104800) compared with cyclophosphamide (NSC-26271) as remission maintenance therapy in previously treated children with acute lymphoblastic leukemia or acute undifferentiated leukemia; possible effectiveness in reducing the incidence of central nervous system leukemia. Cancer Chemother. Rep., *59:* 989–994, 1975.

Soni, S. S., Marten, G. W., Pitner, S. E., Duenas, D. A., and Powazek, M. Effects of central nervous system irradiation on neuropsychologic functioning of children with acute lymphocytic leukemia. N. Engl. J. Med., *293:* 113–118, 1975.

Stoffel, T. J., Nesbit, M. E., and Levitt, S. H. Extramedullary involvement of the testes in childhood leukemia. Cancer, *35:* 1203–1211, 1975.

Sullivan, M. P., Hanshaw, J. B., Cangir, A., and Butler, J. J. Cytomegalovirus complement fixation antibody levels of leukemic children; results of a longitudinal study. J.A.M.A., *206:* 569–574, 1968.

Sullivan, M. P., Vietti, T. J., Fernbach, D. J., Griffith, K. M., Haddy, T. B., and Watkins, W. L. Clinical investigations in the treatment of meningeal leukemia; radiation therapy regimens vs. conventional intrathecal methotrexate. Blood, *34:* 301–319, 1969.

Sullivan, M. P., Vietti, T. J., Haggard, M. E , Donaldson, M. H., Krall, J. M., and Gehan, E. A. Remission maintenance therapy for meningeal leukemia; intrathecal methotrexate vs. intravenous bisnitrosourea. Blood, *38:* 680–688, 1971.

Sullivan, M. P., Humphrey, G. B., Vietti, T. J., Trueworthy, R., and Komp, D. Combination intrathecal (IT) therapy for meningeal leukemia; two vs. three drugs. Proc. Am. Assoc. Cancer Res., (A 340), 1975.

Tessmer, C. F., Hrgovcic, M., Thomas, F. B., Wilbur, J. R., and Mumford, D. M. Long-term serum copper studies in acute leukemia in children. Cancer, *30:* 358–365, 1972.

Thomas, E. D., Buckner, C. D., Banaji, M., Clift, R. A., Fefer, A., Flournoy, N., Goodell, B. W., Hickman, R. O., Lerner, K. G., Neiman, P. E., Sale, G. E., Sanders, J. E., Singer, J., Stevens, M., Storb, R., and Weiden, P. L. One hundred patients with acute leukemia treated by chemotherapy, total body irradiation, and allogeneic marrow transplantation. Blood, *49:* 511–533, 1977a.

Thomas, E. D., Fefer, A., Buckner, C. D., and Storb, R. Current status of bone marrow transplantation for aplastic anemia and acute leukemia. Blood, *49:* 671–681, 1977b.

Tivey, H. The natural history of untreated acute leukemia. Ann. N.Y. Acad. Sci., *60:* 322–358, 1954.

Toch, R. Management of the child with a fatal disease. Clin. Pediatr., *3:* 418–427, 1964.

Todaro, G. J., Green, H., and Swift, M. R. Human diploid fibroblasts transformed with SV-40 or hybrid Adeno-7 × SV-40. Science, *153:* 1252–1254, 1966.

Tsukimoto, I., Wong, K. Y., and Lampkin, B. C. Surface markers and prognostic factors in acute lymphoblastic leukemia. N. Engl. J. Med., *294:* 245–248, 1976.

Vadakan, V. V., and Ortega, J. Priapism in acute lymphoblastic leukemia. Cancer, *30:* 373–375, 1972.

Verzosa, M., Aur, R., Hustu, O., Simone, J., and Pinkel, D. Central nervous system (CNS) status 5 years after preventive CNS therapy for childhood acute lymphocytic leukemia (ALL). Proc. Assoc. Cancer Res., (A 389,) 1974.

Vietti, T. J., Starling, K., Wilbur, J. R., Lonsdale, D., and Lane, D. M. Vincristine, prednisone, and daunomycin in acute leukemia of childhood. Cancer, *27:* 602–607, 1971.

Vietti, T. J., and Ragab, A. H. Complications and total care of a child with acute leukemia. Cancer, *35:* 1007–1014, 1975.

Wagner, H. P., Cottier, H., and Cronkite, E. P. Variability of proliferative patterns in acute lymphoid leukemia of children. Blood, *39:* 176–186, 1972.

Walters, T. R., Bushore, M., and Simone, J. Poor prognosis in Negro children with acute lymphocytic leukemia. Cancer, *29:* 210–214, 1972.

Wang, J. J., and Pratt, C. B. Intrathecal arabinosyl cytosine in meningeal leukemia. Cancer, *25:* 531–534, 1970.

Weller, T. H. The cytomegaloviruses; ubiquitous agents with protean clinical manifestations. N. Engl. J. Med., *285:* 203–214, 267–274, 1971.

West, R. J., Graham-Pole, J., Hardisty, R. M., and Pike, M. C. Factors in pathogenesis of central nervous system leukaemia. Br. Med. J., *3:* 311–314, 1972.

Zuelzer, W. W. Implications of long-term survival in acute stem cell leukemia of childhood treated with composite cyclic therapy. Blood, *24:* 477–494, 1974.

Zusman, J., Brown, D. M., and Nesbit, M. E. Hyperphoshatemia, hyperphosphaturia and hypercalcemia and acute lymphoblastic leukemia. N. Engl. J. Med., *289:* 1335–1340, 1973.

Chapter 8

Chronic Granulocytic Leukemia

GEORGE P. CANELLOS, M.D.

A consideration of the management of chronic granulocytic leukemia (CGL) is best divided into two phases to coincide with the natural history and biologic characteristics of the disease. There are approximately 3000 to 4000 new cases in the United States per year. The medium age of the patients is 53 years.

The initial phase of CGL is characterized by the excessive proliferation and accumulation of granulocytic precursors of intermediate maturity as well as mature polymorphonuclear leukocytes. Myeloblasts are usually less than 10% of the peripheral blood or marrow cells. In addition, at least half the cases will present with an elevated platelet count. The signs and symptoms of the disease at this stage are related to the expansion by the increased granulocytic mass in the marrow and extramedullary sites such as spleen and liver. As a result of this, symptomatic splenomegaly, bone-articular pain, anemia, and hypermetabolic symptoms such as weight loss, sweats and fever, are the usual presenting symptoms. Twenty percent of the cases will present with no symptoms and with only an elevated white count.

Over 90% of the patients who present with hematologic features of CGL will have a characteristic chromosome abnormality known as the Philadelphia, or Ph[1], chromosome. It consists of deletion of some of the chromosomal material of the G22 chromosome. In studies using banding techniques Rowley in 1973 and others subsequently demonstrated that the deleted material has been translocated onto the distal end of the long arm of a number 9 chromosome. It remains throughout the natural history of the disease regardless of the extent and duration of hematologic remission. The Ph[1] chromosome is present in erythroid as well as mega-karyocytic cells but has not been found in circulating lymphocytes or skin fibroblasts. In addition to the hematologic characteristics of the disease, most patients will present with a low or undetectable level of leukocyte alkaline phosphatase which will revert to normal or even elevated levels with the induction of hematologic remission. All patients with CGL who present with granulocytic counts over 50,000/cu mm will have elevated levels of serum B_{12}. The level is proportional to the white count but will return to normal levels during hematologic remission. The increased levels of B_{12} are related to a markedly increased binding capacity of leukemic serum for the vitamin. This, in turn, is related to increased content of B_{12} transport protein, so-called transcobalamin I, which is an α-globulin-like protein derived from granulocytes.

The accelerated or blastic phase of CGL has also been called the terminal phase, since most patients die with evolution of the disease from a stage of hyperplasia of mature cellular elements to frank dedifferentiation with increased numbers of myeloblasts and promyelocytes. The hematologic features of this phase are the result of actual displacement of cells capable of maturation or a progressive attrition of the precursor cells themselves, or both. This results in progressive anemia and thrombocytopenia. These events may evolve abruptly with a rapid proliferation of blast cells in a so-called blastic crisis which resembles acute granulocytic leukemia. In the majority of cases, however, the blastic phase is heralded by a myeloproliferative acceleration of the disease with a rather slowly progressive anemia, thrombocytopenia, splenomegaly, and leukocytosis which is refractory to previously effective therapy. There may be increased numbers of basophils accompanying or preceding the accelerated phase. Approximately 40% of patients will develop myelofibrosis during the natural course of the disease.

In addition to the Ph^1 chromosome which is retained, cell lines with further chromosomal additions or deletions (aneuploidy) may be detected during the blastic phase in about half the patients.

Duplication of the Ph^1 chromosome is the most common abnormality. Rarely blastic transformation may present as an extramedullary granulocytic tumor such as a lymph node mass, osteolytic bone lesion, or skin nodule even in the absence of systemic transformation.

The diagnosis of CGL in the patient with the typical findings as described earlier is not difficult. However, this may be more difficult or nearly impossible as long as the white blood cell count is barely elevated, the leukocyte alkaline phosphatase borderline elevated and chromosome studies do not reveal any abnormalities.

The overall median survival for patients with Ph^1 chromosome positive CGL is about 40–45 months from diagnosis. To date, the goals of chemotherapy have been to control the symptoms of the chronic phase by decreasing the extent of granulocytic proliferation. Intensive antileukemic chemotherapy is reserved for the treatment of blastic transformation. Less than 10% of patients with the otherwise typical finding of CGL do not have the Ph[1] chromosome. These patients are usually over the age of 60 years. They respond less readily to the usual treatment, even in the chronic phase and have a median survival of only 18 months (Ezdinli et al., 1970).

MANAGEMENT OF THE CHRONIC PHASE OF CGL

Splenic Irradiation

Before the introduction and more widespread use of oral cytotoxic drugs for the treatment of CGL, splenic irradiation was the principal mode of therapy. Although effective in reducing spleen size and leukocyte count in some patients, the duration of remission was relatively short and often required intermittent courses of repeat treatment. With the expanded utilization of cytotoxic drugs for CGL, some comparative trials of splenic irradiation and chemotherapy, usually busulfan, have been published (Conrad, 1973; Gollerkeri and Shah, 1971). The best study was the randomized Medical Research Council (MRC) trial which demonstrated a superiority for busulfan in maintaining normal hemoglobin levels as well as overall survival. The median survival for the drug-treated group was 170 weeks as opposed to 120 weeks for the irradiated patients. Both equally reduced spleen size and white count and the incidence of blastic transformation was the same for both (MRC Working Party, 1968).

Splenic irradiation for patients refractory to prior cytotoxic chemotherapy administered for prolonged periods is usually ineffective and has an added risk of hemopoietic toxicity (Wilson and Johnson, 1971).

Chemotherapy

Most patients in the chronic phase of CGL will respond to a number of chemotherapeutic agents. However, busulfan remains the drug of choice for the treatment of this phase of the disease. There have been a number of randomized trials which have compared busulfan with splenic irradiation, chlorambucil, and or 6-mercaptopurine (Southeastern Cancer Group, 1963; Kaung et al., 1971; Rundles et al., 1959). Busulfan emerged as the most useful agent when compared to the other commonly available drugs. Dibromomannitol, a newer agent, appears to be as effective but is not widely used and still available only for investigational use (Casazza et al., 1967).

Most patients in the chronic phase of CGL do not require immediate reduction of their elevated white count. Thus large doses of oral busulfan or other parenteral cytotoxic drugs are not indicated and may be associated with serious complications such as uric acid nephropathy and marrow aplasia. Similarly there are a small number of patients who, with even small doses of busulfan, will experience prolonged pancytopenia.

With these factors as a background, the most effective means of treating CGL in the chronic phase would entail the daily oral administration of busulfan 4–6 mg with weekly determinations of the blood count (Galton, 1969). On this regimen most patients will reduce their white count to the range of 10–20,000/cu mm by the 3rd or 4th week of treatment. Accompanying this change, a depressed hemoglobin level will rise toward normal. In the same patients the hemoglobin may rise to 16 or 18 g/100 ml. Thrombocytosis (i.e., platelet count sustained in excess of 450,000/cu mm) which often accompanies the initial phase of CGL can be equally well controlled with busulfan therapy. However, in about one-third of these cases intermittent thrombocytosis will remain through the course of the disease. The subjective symptoms of the disease as well as splenomegaly will abate as the white count returns to and remains in the normal range. In addition, the elevated serum B_{12} level and increased serum content of the B_{12}-binding protein transcobalamin I will return to normal levels. The low or absent leukocyte alkaline phosphatase which characterizes the disease will often return to normal or even increased levels. As a general rule, patients with an elevated leukocyte count have an increased tendency to bleed even in the absence of abnormal clotting tests. It is worthwhile to postpone routine surgical procedures until the white count is under control.

The attainment of a "complete" hematologic remission is not essential for prolonged survival in CGL. Although it is not uncommon for the marrow morphology and myeloid/erythroid ratio to return to normal, many patients would require continued higher doses of busulfan with the risk of thrombocytopenia to attain this state. Very adequate peripheral remission can be attained with marrow morphology which can still be described as granulocytic hyperplasia. After the white blood count falls below 15,000/cu mm, busulfan should be discontinued since the initial induction course can result in prolonged control of the blood count for up to 2 years without further therapy. With periodic follow-up the physician can ascertain the extent of disease control and reinstitute therapy when the white blood count begins to rise above 20–25,000/cu mm.

Maintenance therapy involves the intermittent or continuous administration of low doses of busulfan, usually 2–4 mg, to keep the white blood count in the range of 10–15,000/cu mm. Allopurinol therapy would be necessary during the phase of remission induction, but, depending on the uric acid level, it may be discontinued in some patients in the maintenance phase.

Primary refractoriness to busulfan is very unusual and may reflect an early transition to the accelerated or blastic phase of the disease. After even prolonged periods of disease control, the onset of blastic transformation is usually heralded by progressive refractoriness to busulfan. In some cases progressive leukocytosis and splenomegaly occur without clear morphologic evidence of blastic leukemia. In these cases where the red cell and platelet counts are adequate, therapy with hydroxyurea, 0.5–2.0 g, given as a daily oral medication may control the proliferative components of the disease without marked suppression of the other elements (Kennedy, 1972). The agent is well tolerated and its effects are rapidly reversible upon discontinuation of the drug. This stands in contrast to busulfan where the hemopoietic suppression may persist for weeks. Satisfactory control of this intermediate phase of the disease may persist from 3 to 6 months on the average before frank blastic transformation supervenes.

Complications of Busulfan

Busulfan is associated with some unique side effects which are rarely severe enough to limit therapy. About one-third of all patients receiving the drug for over 2 years will have some degree of increased skin pigmentation. There are rare instances when anorexia, nausea, and weakness accompany the increased skin pigmentation so as to resemble adrenocortical insufficiency. Adrenocortical function tests are usually normal. In addition, amenorrhea is very common in patients receiving the drug continuously for at least 2 months.

Patients who receive busulfan for long periods are also liable to develop some degree of anhidrosis and dryness of the mucous membranes. When subjected to careful ophthalmoscopic examination, some patients may have a higher incidence of lenticular changes suggestive of early cataract formation (Podos and Canellos, 1969). Busulfan lung is a rare clinico-pathologic entity characterized by extensive inter- and intra-alveolar fibrosis with alveolar cell atypia and pulmonary functional impairment (Littler and Ogilvie, 1970). This potentially fatal complication may result from an unusual sensitivity of the host tissues rather than a cumulative dose effect. Some cases have benefited with corticosteroid treatment.

Splenectomy

This procedure is rarely indicated in the treatment of CGL. However, instances of profound thrombocytopenia following standard doses of busulfan which prevent adequate control of the white count may represent a possible indication for splenectomy (Canellos et al., 1972). These patients are best treated with hydroxyurea in their subsequent course since they may still develop marked thrombocytopenia with busulfan due to an inherent marked sensitivity to the drug. Removal of an enlarged spleen especially in the presence of thrombocytopenia can be dangerous and should be attempted only if the patient is still in the chronic phase of the disease (Spiers, 1973). In frank blastic transformation removal of an enlarged spleen is associated with a high mortality and should be avoided except in life-threatening situations such as splenic rupture or massive infarction.

Other Drugs

If the patient is intolerant of busulfan, a number of other agents are available. Adequate disease control can also be attained with phenylalanine mustard, cyclophosphamide or chlorambucil but these are second-line drugs. If dibromomannitol becomes more generally available then this would also represent a suitable alternative.

THERAPY OF THE BLASTIC PHASE OF CGL

This represents one of the most refractory forms of leukemia. As mentioned above, the blastic phase can be quite heterogeneous in its appearance and thus one standard drug regimen might appear suitable for one form and not for the other.

The most dangerous form of blastic crisis of CGL is the abrupt transition of the disease to acute blastic leukemia with a rapidly rising white blood count composed mainly of blasts. The risk of fatal leukostasis lesions in the cerebral vasculature is great and aggressive therapy to lower the counts must be immediately employed. In addition to hydration and allopurinol therapy, intravenous hydroxyurea (75 mg/kg) or intravenous cyclophosphamide (20 mg/kg) are effective in rapidly reducing the blood count. If there is clinical evidence of central nervous system bleeding with or without retinal hemorrhages, whole brain irradiation should also be employed.

In most cases, however, this emergency therapy is not required and the presentation and therapeutic approach is similar to acute myeloblastic leukemia (AML). The patient with blastic CGL may also have myelofibrosis which complicates his tolerance of cytotoxic therapy even further.

One of the newer but simpler approaches has been the use of vincristine and prednisone alone (Canellos et al., 1971). Vincristine is given as a weekly intravenous dose of 1.4–2.0 mg/m^2 with prednisone at 60 mg/m^2 daily times 5 in the initial course. Maintenance therapy with either daily oral hydroxyurea 0.5 g/day or twice weekly methotrexate 15–20 mg/m^2 may delay relapse. This program can result in up to 30% remissions especially if the disease is accompanied by hypodiploidy on cytogenetic evaluation at the onset of blastic crisis. In addition one group has correlated response to these drugs with the extent of "granularity" in the blast cells (Marmont and Damasio, 1973). The median survival of responders to this regimen is 8–10 months, whereas for nonresponders it is usually 2–3 months. A number of other combined drug programs have been tried in the blastic phase (Table 10.1). There does not seem to be an advantage to adding other myelotoxic drugs including thioguanine, daunorubicin, cytosine arabinoside, methotrexate, prednisone, Cytoxan, vincristine and L-asparaginase. The TRAMPCO(L) regimen, however, appears to have effected remissions in patients failing to respond to vincristine-prednisone (Spiers et al., 1974). In a prospective randomized trial comparing vincristine-prednisone with cytosine arabinoside and 6-thioguanine, there were no responders to the latter combination in those who failed vincristine-prednisone (Canellos et al., 1975). In addition there did not appear to be an advantage for those patients who had a prior splenectomy during the chronic phase of the disease. A number of morphologic and biochemical criteria have been demonstrated to predict the effectiveness of vincristine-prednisone therapy in the blastic phase of CGL. It has been shown that approximately one-third of all patients in the blastic phase will have blast cells that at least morphologically resemble lymphoblasts. When one large series was reviewed for morphologic criteria that correlate with vincristine and prednisone response as well as survival, the lymphoblastic variants emerged to be clearly the more favorable (Rosenthal et al., 1977). An explanation for lymphoblastic appearance of these Philadelphia chromosome-positive cells is lacking, but a number of other studies including the enzyme, terminal transferase, as well as serologic reactivity with an anti-acute lymphoblastic leukemia (ALL) serum suggest that these cells may have other characteristics of the lymphoid cell. The enzyme, terminal transferase, which has been previously noted to occur in a high percentage of ALL patients as well as in normal human thymus is elevated in approximately one-third of patients entering the blastic phase of CGL. In addition, a predetermination of this enzyme seems to predict for responsiveness to vincristine and prednisone (Marks and McCaffrey, 1977). Reactivity with a non-B, non-T anti-ALL antiserum seems to correlate both with terminal transferase positivity and response to vincristine and prednisone (Janossy et al., 1976). Response to vincristine and prednisone is usually of short duration averaging no more than 6 months and, despite reinduction and maintenance chemotherapy, resistance develops and the disease is usually refractory to most other regimens. It may be more useful in the future to treat these lymphoblastic variants of CGL as adult ALL including an anthracycline antibiotic in addition to vincristine and prednisone.

Transplantation of cryopreserved autologous bone marrow harvested during the chronic phase has been attempted in 2 cases after high dose cyclophosphamide and total body irradiation (Buckner et al., 1974). One patient achieved engraftment but both patients died of sepsis 48 and 83 days after transplantation. One patient had myelofibrosis which may have interfered with graft acceptance and both patients had marked

TABLE 8.1
Chemotherapy of Blastic Transformation of Chronic Granulocytic Leukemia

Regimen	No. of Patients	Complete Remission	Partial Remission	Reference
Vincristine and Prednisone	30	6	3	Canellos et al., 1971
Vincristine and Prednisone	24	9	—	Marmont and Damasio, 1973
Prednisone, Vincristine, Methotrexate, and 6-mercaptopurine	13	1	2	Foley et al., 1969
Cytosine arabinoside infusion	30	2	—	Southwest Group, 1974; Carbone et al., 1970
Cytosine arabinoside and BCNU	35	2	3	Vogler, 1971; Carbone et al., 1970
Cytosine arabinoside and BCNU	47	3	5	Hayes et al., 1974
Cytosine arabinoside, BCNU, vincristine, and prednisone	39	1	4	Hayes et al., 1974
Multiple regimens (M.D. Anderson Hospital)	39	4	6	Vallejos et al., 1974
TRAMPCO(L)(Hammersmith—London)	9	4	1	Spiers et al., 1974
Vincristine and prednisone	19	2	5	Canellos, et al., 1975
Cytosine arabinoside and 6-thioguanine	12	1	3	
	297	35	32	

lymphopenia. This technique could be theoretically useful in the treatment of the blastic phase of CGL if the entire blastic marrow could be obliterated and replaced by preserved autologous immunocompetent marrow cells.

With a large number of patients the experience with autologous marrow transplantation has been somewhat disappointing (Buckner et al., 1978). Recently, it has been demonstrated that patients with chronic myelogenous leukemia in the chronic phase can be successfully transplanted with marrow from their normal, genetically identical twin. At least within a 1–2-year follow-up, the Philadelphia chromosome appears to have been eliminated using total body irradiation, cyclophosphamide and dimethyl busulfan. The ultimate success of this latter regimen will depend on the continued absence of the Philadelphia chromosome from the marrow of these patients (Fefer et al., 1977).

Meningeal leukemia is almost never seen in the chronic phase of CGL. However, with the increase in survival as a result of good responses to chemotherapy more cases have been noted (Schwartz et al., 1975). The therapeutic benefit of intrathecal methotrexate or cytosine arabinoside with or without cranial irradiation is considerable so that meningeal leukemia in these patients should be treated aggressively.

REFERENCES

Buckner, C. D., Clift, R. A., Fefer, A., Neiman, P. E., Storb, R., and Thomas, E. D. Treatment of blastic transformation of chronic granulocytic leukemia by high dose cyclophosphamide, total body irradiation and infusion of cryopreserved autologous marrow. Exp. Hematol., 2: 138–146, 1974.

Buckner, C. D., Stewart, P., Clift, R. A., Fefer, A., Neiman, P. E., Singer, J., Storb, R., and Thomas, E. D. Treatment of blastic transformation of chronic granulocytic leukemia by chemotherapy, total body irradiation and infusion of cryopreserved autologous marrow. Exp. Hematol., 6: 96–109, 1978.

Canellos, G. P., DeVita, V. T., Whang-Peng, J., and Carbone, P. P. Hematologic and cytogenetic remission of blastic transformation in chronic granulocytic leukemia. Blood, 38: 671–679, 1971.

Canellos, G. P., Nordland, J., and Carbone, P. P. Splenectomy for thrombocytopenia in chronic granulocytic leukemia. Cancer, 29: 660–665, 1972.

Canellos, G. P., Young, R. C., Chabner, B. A., Schein, P. S., Whang-Peng, J., and DeVita, V. T. Chemotherapy of the blastic phase of chronic granulocytic leukemia; prospective comparison of vincristine/prednisone with cytosine arabinoside-6-thioguanine and the effect of prior splenectomy. Sci. Proc. Am. Soc. Clin. Oncol., 16: 252, 1975.

Carbone, P. P., Canellos, G. P., and DeVita, V. T. Therapy of the blastic phase of chronic granulocytic leukemia. In Recent Results in Cancer Research, edited by G. Mathé, pp. 142–148. Springer-Verlag, New York, 1970.

Casazza, A. R., Cahn, E. L., and Carbone, P. P. Preliminary studies with dibromomannitol (NSC-94100) in patients with chronic myelogenous leukemia. Cancer Chemother. Rep., 51: 91–96, 1967.

Conrad, F. G. Survival in chronic granulocytic leukemia; splenic irradiation vs. busulfan. Arch. Intern. Med., 131: 684–685, 1973.

Ezdinli, E., Sokal, J. E., Crosswhite, L., and Sandberg, A. A. Philadelphia-chromosome-positive and -negative chronic myelocytic leukaemia. Ann. Intern. Med., 72: 175–182, 1970.

Fefer, A., Cheever, M., Thomas, E. D., Boyd, C., Rambera, R., Glucksberg, H., Buckner, C. D., Sanders, J., and Storb, R. Disappearance of Ph¹-positive cells from marrows of 4 CML patients after chemotherapy, radiation, and marrow transplantation from an identical twin. Blood, 50: Supp. I, 314, 1977.

Foley, H. T., Bennett, J. M., and Carbone, P. P. Combination chemotherapy in accelerated phase of chronic granulocytic leukemia. Arch. Intern. Med., 123: 166–170, 1969.

Galton, D. A. Chemotherapy of chronic myelocytic leukemia. Semin. Hematol., 6: 323–343, 1969.

Gollerkeri, M. P., and Shah, G. B. Management of chronic myeloid leukemia; a five-year survey with a comparison of oral busulfan and splenic irradiation. Cancer, 27: 596–601, 1971.

Hayes, D. M., Ellison, R. R., Glidewell, O., Holland, J. F., and Silver, R. T. Chemotherapy for the terminal phase of chronic myelocytic leukemia. Cancer Chemother. Rep., 4: 233–247, 1974.

Janossy, G., Greaves, M. F., Revesz, T., Lister, T. A., Roberts, M., Durrant, J., Kirk, B., Catovsky, D., and Beard, M. E. J. Blast crisis of chronic myeloid leukaemia (CML). Br. J. Haematol., 34: 179–192, 1976.

Kaung, D. T., Close, H. P., Whittington, R. M., and Patno, M. E. Comparison of busulfan and cyclophosphamide in the treatment of chronic myelocytic leukemia. Cancer, 27: 608–612, 1971.

Kennedy, B. J. Hydroxyurea therapy in chronic myelogenous leukemia. Cancer, 29: 1052–1056, 1972.

Littler, W. A., and Ogilvie, C. Lung function in patients receiving busulfan. Br. Med. J., 4: 530–532, 1970.

Marks, S. M., and McCaffrey, R. Terminal transferase as a predictor of initial responsiveness to vincristine-prednisone in blastic chronic myelogenous leukemia. Blood, 50: 198, 1977.

Marmont, A. M., and Damasio, E. E. The treatment of terminal metamorphosis of chronic granulocytic leukaemia with corticosteroids and vincristine. Acta Haematol., 50: 1–8, 1973.

Medical Research Council Working Party. Chronic granulocytic leukaemia; comparison of radiotherapy and busulphan therapy. Br. Med. J., 1: 201, 1968.

Podos, S. M., and Canellos, G. P. Lens changes in chronic granulocytic leukaemia; possible relationship to chemotherapy. Am. J. Ophthalmol., 68: 500–504, 1969.

Rosenthal, S., Canellos, G. P., Whang-Peng, J., and Gralnick, H. R. Blast crisis of chronic granulocytic leukemia. Am. J. Med., 63: 542–547, 1977.

Rowley, J. D. Chromosomal patterns in myelocytic leukemia. N. Engl. J. Med., 289: 220–221, 1973.

Rundles, R. W., Grizzle, J., Bell, W. N., Corley, C. C., Frommeyer, W. B., Jr., Greenberg, B. G., Huguley, C. M., Jr., James, G. W., III, Jones, R., Jr., Larsen, W. E., Loeb, V., Leone, L. A., Palmer, J. G., Riser, W. H., and Wilson, S. J. Comparison of chlorambucil and myleran in chronic lymphocytic and granulocytic leukemia. Am. J. Med., 27: 424–432, 1959.

Schwartz, J. H., Canellos, G. P., Young, R. C., and DeVita, V. T. Meningeal leukemia in the blastic phase of chronic granulocytic leukemia. Am. J. Med., 59: 819–828, 1975.

Southeastern Cancer Chemotherapy Cooperative Study Group. Comparison of 6-mercaptopurine and busulfan in chronic granulocytic leukemia. Blood, 21: 89–100, 1963.

Southwest Oncology Group. Cytarabine for acute leukemia in adults; effect of schedule on therapeutic response. Arch. Intern. Med., 133: 251–259, 1974.

Spiers, A. D., Costello, C., Catovsky, D., Galton, D. A., and Goldman, J. M. Chronic granulocytic leukaemia; multiple-drug chemotherapy for acute transformation. Br. Med. J., *13:* 77–80, 1974.

Spiers, A. S. D. Surgery in management of patients with leukaemia. Br. Med. J., *3:* 528–532, 1973.

Vallejos, C. S., Trujillo, J. M., Cork, A., Bodey, G. P., McCredie, K. B., and Freireich, E. J. Blastic Crisis in chronic granulocytic leukemia; experience in 39 patients. Cancer, *34:* 1806–1812, 1974.

Vogler, W. R. Clinical trials of 1-β-D-arabinofuranocyl cytosine and 1,3-bis-(2-chloroethyl)-1-nitrosourea combination in metastatic cancer and acute leukemia. Cancer, *27:* 1081–1088, 1971.

Wilson, J. F., and Johnson, R. E. Splenic irradiation following chemotherapy in chronic myelogenous leukemia. Radiology, *101:* 657–661, 1971.

Chapter 9

Chronic Lymphocytic Leukemia

DANIEL B. KIMBALL, JR., M.D.

Chronic lymphocytic leukemia (CLL) is a lymphoproliferative disorder characterized by the accumulation of increasing numbers of well differentiated lymphocytes and represents the most common leukemia seen in the United States. It is a disease predominantly of the 5th decade and beyond (Boggs et al., 1966; Green and Dixon, 1965), although rarely, it is seen in infancy (Sardeman, 1972). Males predominate over females, cytogenetic abnormalities are rarely noted (Fitzgerald and Hamer, 1969; Woodliff and Cohen, 1972), although familial occurrence is recognized (Fraumeni et al., 1969) and there is a concordance rate of 39% (Gunz, 1973). Etiologically, neither ionizing radiation nor toxic marrow suppression have been implicated (Cronkite et al., 1972). The etiologic role of RNA viruses remains unknown.

The nature of the CLL lymphocyte has been under intense study. Most investigators have presented evidence that CLL is a B cell disease (Buxbaum, 1973; Catovsky et al., 1974; Harris and Bagai, 1972: Pincus et al., 1972; Preud'homme and Seligman, 1972; Utsinger, 1975; Wilson and Hurdle, 1973), although Winkelstein et al. (1974) have presented evidence that the majority of cells react to anti-thymocyte sera (suggesting a T cell origin) as well as having immunoglobulin markers (standard marker of B lymphocytes). McLaughlin and co-workers (1973) hypothesize that the immunoglobulin negative lymphocytes may be immature B cells unable to produce immunoglobulin and Catovsky and his co-workers (1974) suggest that the level of T cells may correlate with the stability of the disease and that increased T cell levels may represent an immune response to CLL. Although the precise immunological nature of the CLL cell is incompletely understood, patients with CLL may demonstrate immunologic dysfunction of B or T cells. About one-half the patients may demonstrate hypogammaglobulinemia at the time of diagnosis (Carbone and Canellos, 1972; DeSimone, 1974; Slungaard and Smith, 1974), some patients demonstrate impaired primary and secondary humoral (antibody) responses (Harris and Bagai, 1972) and impaired T cell function may be demonstrated in vitro (Aisenberg et al., 1973; Harris and Bagai, 1972; Schultz et al., 1974; Shaw et al., 1974; Smith et al., 1973; Utsinger, 1975; Winkelstein et al., 1974). There is also an increased incidence of second tumors in CLL (Manusow and Weinerman, 1975; Mulligan, 1970). There is little correlation between impaired T cell responses and percentage of T lymphocytes (Utsinger, 1975) and dilution with B cells does not account for the degree or pattern of impaired T cell function (Schultz et al., 1974; Utsinger, 1975). An unconfirmed report (Utsinger, 1975) suggests that there may be a circulating inhibitory factor depressing T cell function, although the CLL B cell does not appear to be the source of that factor. Since CLL may represent a syndrome and not just one disease, discordant results concerning the nature of the CLL cell can easily be understood.

In man, most circulating lymphocytes are long lived, recirculating for months to years between the blood and thoracic duct via lymph nodes and spleen, with only a small proportion of lymphocytes being rapidly dividing. In CLL, the increased lymphocytes are found in the nondividing, recirculating pool (Manaster et al., 1973; Zimmerman et al., 1968) and the disease can be thought of as an accumulative disease (Dameshek, 1967).

The patient presenting with CLL usually has no specific complaints and one-fourth of the patients diagnosed with CLL have no presenting complaints (Wintrobe et al., 1974). The usual history is one of easy fatigability, a lack of a sense of well being or generalized malaise. Some patients may present with bleeding, anemia, infection and/or mechanical complaints (Firestone and Robinson, 1972) secondary to lymphadenopathy or organomegaly. Lymphadenopathy and splenomegaly are seen in more than three-fourths of the patients. Lymphocytic infiltration may also be manifested by hepatomegaly, tonsilar enlargement, bone pain or skin lesions (more common in CLL than other leukemias). When fever is seen in CLL, it should always be presumed to be of infectious etiology.

The diagnosis of CLL requires certain minimum laboratory criteria. The absolute lymphocyte count should exceed 15,000/μl on two examinations at least 14 days apart (excluding known causes of lymphocytosis). A bone marrow specimen (biopsy preferred) should show at least 40% of the nucleated cells to be lymphocytes and be hypercellular. No more than 10% of the cells in the peripheral blood or bone marrow should be lymphoblasts. Cytochemical (Micu and Astaldi, 1973) and serum protein abnormalities (Werthamer and Amaral, 1971) have been reported to provide differential diagnostic information, but these techniques remain to be confirmed as being useful. Varying degrees of hypogammaglobulinemia may be seen in a significant (39%) number of patients (Hansen, 1973) and about one-fifth of patients demonstrate autoimmune hemolytic disease. Hansen (1973) feels that the tendency toward infection in CLL patients does not correlate well with γ-globulin levels, but instead correlates with absolute neutrophil counts. Morphologic evaluation of the lymphocyte (Peterson et al., 1974; Spiro et al., 1975; Zacharski and Linmann, 1969) has not aided differential diagnosis significantly and has given conflicting results in terms of predicting prognosis. The CLL cell is usually described as a small to medium sized lymphocyte with a narrow rim of cytoplasm, but the presence of other lymphocyte forms (other than lymphoblasts) is not clearly detrimental to prognosis. Assessment of lymph node morphology will usually allow differentiation between lymphoma and CLL.

Progress in the evaluation of CLL patients, its natural course and/or response to multiple therapies, has been hampered by the heterogeneous nature of the disease. Many investigators (Boggs et al., 1966; Dameshek, 1967; Galton, 1966; Ross et al., 1961; Zippin et al., 1973) have categorized CLL patients into groups generally characterized as "indolent" or "benign" on the one hand versus "aggressive," "active," or "malignant" on the other. Based on clinical and laboratory parameters, Rai and coworkers (1975) have proposed a staging system which provides groups of relatively homogeneous patients. In a prospective study of 125 patients, they have shown that there is a good correlation between clinical stage on one hand and survival, tumor load (consistent with the hypothesis of an accumulative disease), and symptoms on the other hand. Analysis of results of therapeutic modalities using such a staging system should allow more easy comparison between studies and for more meaningful studies.

Prognosis in CLL as a disease entity has little meaning; the median survival for all patients presenting with the disease is 4–6 years. Patients with indolent or benign disease have a median survival of 6–12 years, while patients with active disease have a median survival of 13–19 months (Rai et al., 1975). Meaningful assessment of any therapeutic modality requires at least this minimal type of stratification.

The treatment of CLL is quite controversial in two major regards. Recognizing that the disorder represents a spectrum of biologically indolent to very progressive disease, there is no general agreement as to when treatment should be initiated. Most hematologists do not recommend treatment just because the diagnosis is established or because of leukocytosis in the absence of symptoms. The presence of symptoms secondary to the disease process is a generally accepted indication for therapy. Specific clinical findings leading to symptoms include any cytopenia as a consequence of bone marrow failure and/or hypersplenism, mechanical pressure by enlarged lymph nodes or spleen, autoimmune red cell and/or platelet destruction, organ infiltration by lymphocytes and infection as a consequence of hypogammaglobulinemia and/or neutropenia. Hypogammaglobulinemia, cytopenias and skin infiltration are poorly responsive to therapy. The second controversy revolves around the fact that, once it is agreed that therapy is indicated, there is no general consensus on the best form of therapy (radiotherapy, single agent chemotherapy, combined agent therapy) or the best schedule of therapy (continuous vs. intermittent). None of these controversies is satisfactorily resolved by currently published data on prospectively randomized, staged patients. It is hoped that such studies proposed for the future will resolve these issues.

Infection is the most prominent cause of death in patients with CLL (Hansen, 1973). Miller et al. (1962) have advocated prophylactic γ-globulin and antibiotics in these patients. There is no justification for this approach, in that many of these patients remain relatively free of infection despite severe hypogammaglobulinemia. An acceptable approach is to vigorously evaluate any potential infection and treat with broad-spectrum antibiotic coverage until the etiologic agent is isolated or the patient improves. If in the face of a proven bacterial infection the response to antibiotics is not acceptable, then γ-globulin may be added to the therapeutic regimen. Miller et al. (1962) reported using 0.3 ml per pound of body weight initially, followed by 0.15 ml per pound every 2 weeks. This represents a large IM dose (particularly in the presence of thrombocytopenia) and there is also a hepatitis risk.

Two "nonsystemic" approaches can be taken to the problem of painful splenomegaly and/or hypersplenism. The surgical approach advocated by Yam and Crosby (1974) and Adler and co-workers (1975) carries an immediate mortality risk of 10–15%. Response rates approximate 80% with a greater than 1-year survival of 43–85%. Treatment with splenic irradiation as reported by Byhardt et al. (1975) has no immediate mortality but perhaps less of an overall response rate with the same 1-year survival. The patient with prior chemotherapy may be a poorer candidate for splenic irradiation. A prospective randomized study might identify those patients who are the best candidates for either of these therapeutic modalities.

A xanthine-oxidase inhibitor (allopurinol) or uricosuric agents along with adequate hydration and/or alkalinization of the urine is indicated for the control of hyperuricemia. The anemia related to bone marrow failure in CLL may be responsive to androgen therapy (Silver, 1969). Other causes of anemia naturally need to be excluded in these patients.

Radiation therapy was the main therapy of CLL until 1950 (Spiers, 1974). For reduction of spleen and/or lymph node size and relief of mechanical symptoms, localized radiation therapy has a higher therapeutic/toxic ratio than systemic chemotherapy. Systemic radiotherapy has been shown to be efficacious in CLL using the technique of total body irradiation as reported by Johnson (1970) and DelRegato (1974), or systemically administered ^{32}P as reported by Hill et al. (1964), Osgood (1964) and others (Bethell et al., 1965; Zubrod, 1968). Prospective group studies comparing ^{32}P to alkylating agents (Huguley, 1962; Sprague, 1962) suggest that ^{32}P is inferior to chlorambucil and triethylene melamine (TEM). It is not clear that the groups were comparable. Richards and co-workers (1974) and Byhardt and co-workers (1975) have shown that localized radiation to the thymus (mediastinum) and spleen can have favorable effects on the systemic disease in CLL including marrow improvement in some patients. The role of total body, thymic and splenic irradiation needs to be tested against systemic chemotherapy in a prospective randomized study involving previously untreated and treated patients.

Extracorporeal irradiation of CLL patients (Cronkite et al., 1972; Lajtha, 1972; Storb et al., 1968; Thomas et al., 1965) will uniformly lead to WBC reduction with variable improvement in other disease parameters. The response is generally transient (3–7 months) and no complete responses were seen. Cronkite et al. (1972) feel that this therapeutic modality may have its greatest role in patients with active disease that is refractory to chemotherapy.

Single chemotherapeutic agents having activity in CLL include chlorambucil (Bigley, 1963; Gardner, 1972: Kaung et al., 1964a, 1964b, 1969; Rundles et al., 1959), cyclophosphamide (Bethell et al., 1960; Gardner, 1972; Kaung et al., 1964b; Rundles et al., 1962; Solomon et al., 1963), nitrogen mustard (Burchenal et al., 1949), streptonigrin (Kaung et al., 1969), TEM (Bigley, 1963; Gardner, 1972; Rundles et al., 1959), Adriamycin (Burchenal and Carter, 1972) and prednisone (Shaw et al., 1961). Nitrogen mustard and TEM are of historical interest only because of their variable clinical responses and their side effects. Streptonigrin was compared to chlorambucil in one study (Kaung et al., 1969) and found to have equivalent activity but greater gastrointestinal toxicity. Chlorambucil is considered equivalent to or greater in activity against CLL than cyclophosphamide (Kaung et al., 1964b), but since it does not have the side effects of hemorrhagic cystitis or alopecia, it is usually considered the preferred agent. A standard beginning dose is 6.0 mg/m^2. Cyclophosphamide will give objective responses in 40–50% of the patients treated (Bethell et al., 1960; Rundles et al., 1962; Solomon et al., 1963), while chlorambucil will give objective responses in 50–75% of patients treated (Huguley, 1970; Kaung et al., 1964b, 1969; Rundles et al., 1959). Streptonigrin gave objective responses in 84% of patients treated, but its use has been reported in CLL only in this one reported study. Patients who become resistant to chlorambucil may respond to cyclophosphamide (Gardner, 1972). Complete remissions are unusual (8–10%) in the treatment of CLL (Huguley, 1970; Kaung et al., 1969; Knospe et al., 1974).

Prednisone as a single agent is active in CLL (Ezdinli et al., 1969; Freymann et al., 1960; Kyle et al., 1962; Shaw et al., 1961) with reduction of organomegaly, increased hemoglobin (particularly in the treatment of autoimmune hemolytic disease) but without control of the lymphocyte count (it often rises) and a short duration of response (4 weeks). Infection, diabetes and fluid retention were major problems.

Ineffective or minimally effective agents include L-asparaginase (Clarkson et al., 1970), actinomycin (Karnofsky, 1968), hydroxyurea (Krakoff et al., 1964) and busulfan (Rundles et al., 1959).

Knospe and co-workers (1974) have published data to support the concept of the intermittent use of chlorambucil (every 2 weeks) at an initial dose of 0.4 mg/kg/day × 1 dose every 2 weeks. Doses are increased by 0.1 mg/kg every 2 weeks until toxicity or disease control is achieved. Induction rates appear comparable to those achieved with continuous chlorambucil and survival is no worse, and, indeed, may be superior to previous experience, although direct comparison of patients is difficult. Hematologic toxicity appears less with intermittent chlorambucil therapy.

It is not surprising that with the good responses seen to steroid and chlorambucil therapy and the short duration of the steroid responses, that these two agents have been tried in combination. In two studies (Galton et al., 1961; Han et al., 1973) there is no objective evidence that the combined agents improve the initial response rate or duration of response. There was a suggestion of less anemia (Han et al., 1973) using combined therapy and there appeared to be a greater tolerance to the chlorambucil (more drug administered in the combined regimen).

A brief report (Gutterman et al., 1972) noted a high complete response rate in CLL using the combination of cyclophosphamide and cytosine arabinoside. No subsequent data have been forthcoming to allow long term evaluation.

An interesting adjunct to other modalities of therapy may well be leukapheresis. Curtis (Curtis and Freireich, 1971; Curtis et al., 1972) has reported partial remissions with decreased adenopathy and splenomegaly with stable platelet counts and no transfusion requirement. Increased phytohemagglutinin (PHA) responsiveness was also noted.

Another possible adjunct to treatment might include therapy with antilymphocyte serum. Transient reduction in lymphocyte count was achieved in several studies (Herberman et al., 1971; Laszlo et al., 1968; Tsirimbas et al., 1969) with variable improvement in other disease parameters. Significant toxicity included thrombocytopenia, severe allergic reactions and one case of fatal hepatitis.

It is difficult to make a recommendation for the current "best therapy" for CLL. If the concept of CLL as an accumulative disease is correct, then early therapy even prior to symptoms makes logical sense, but until this is proven in a controlled randomized study, therapy should probably be given only to patients who are symptomatic. Local mechanical problems can usually be controlled by local radiation therapy. If systemic chemotherapy is felt to be indicated, then intermittent chlorambucil is recommended. Steroid therapy is recommended for autoimmune destruction of red cells and/or platelets. Until a broader experience is gained with systemic radiotherapy, or thymic and/or splenic irradiations (hopefully in a controlled trial), these modalities cannot be recommended for wide usage.

REFERENCES

Adler, S., Stutzman, L., Sokal, V. E., and Mittelman, A. Splenectomy for hematologic depression in lymphocytic lymphoma and leukemia. Cancer, 35: 521–528, 1975.

Aisenberg, A. C., Bloch, K. J., Long, J. C., and Calvin, R. B. Reaction of normal human lymphocytes and chronic lymphocytic leukemia cells with an antithymocyte antiserum. Blood, 41: 417–423, 1973.

Bethell, F. H., Louis, J., Robbins, A., Donnelly, W. J., Dessel, B. H., et al. Phase II evaluation of cyclophosphamide; a study by the midwest cooperative chemotherapy group. Cancer Chemother. Rep., 8: 112–115, 1960.

Bethell, F. H., Craver, L. F., Karnofsky, D. A., Osgood, E. E., and Dameshek, W. Panels in therapy; VI. The management of chronic lymphocytic leukemia. Blood, 10: 1058–1065, 1965.

Bigley, R. H. Treatment of chronic leukemic lymphocytic leukemia with triethylene melamine (TEM) and chlorambucil (CB-1348). Cancer Chemother. Rep., 30: 27–30, 1963.

Boggs, D. R., Sofferman, S. A., Wintrobe, M. M., and Cartwright, G. E. Factors influencing the survival of patients with CLL. Am. J. Med., 40: 243–254, 1966.

Burchenal, J. H., Myers, W. P. L., Craver, L. F., and Karnofsky, D. A. The nitrogen mustards in the treatment of leukemia. Cancer, 2: 1–17, 1949.

Burchenal, J. H., and Carter, S. K. New cancer chemotherapeutic agents. Cancer, 30: 1639–1646, 1972.

Buxbaum, J. N. The biosynthesis, assembly, and secretion of immunoglobulins. Semin. Hematol., 10: 33–52, 1973.

Byhardt, R. W., Brace, K. C., and Wiernik, P. H. The role of splenic irradiation in chronic lymphocytic leukemia. Cancer, 35: 1621–1625, 1975.

Carbone, P. P., and Canellos, G. P. The chronic leukemias. In Hematology: Principles and Practice, edited by C. E. Mengel, E. Frei III, and R. Nachman, pp. 424–444. Year Book Medical Publishers, Chicago, 1972.

Catovsky, D., Miliani, E., Okos, A., and Galton, D. A. G. Clinical significance of T-cells in chronic lymphocytic leukemia. Lancet, 2: 751–752, 1974.

Clarkson, B., Krakoff, I., Burchenal, J., Karnofsky, D., Colbey, R., Dowling, M., Oettgen, H., and Lipton, A. Clinical results of treatment with E. coli L-asparaginase in adults with leukemia, lymphoma and solid tumors. Cancer, 25: 279–305, 1970.

Cronkite, E. P., Chanana, A. D., and Rai, K. R. Extracorporeal irradiation of blood in therapy of leukemia. In Cancer Chemotherapy II. Twenty-second Hahnemann Symposium, edited by I. Brodsky, S. B. Kahn, and J. H. Moyer, pp. 375–382. Grune & Stratton, New York, 1972.

Curtis, J. E., and Freireich, E. J. Leukapheresis therapy of chronic lymphocytic leukemia (CLL) (abstract). Am. Soc. Clin. Oncol. Meeting, Chicago, Ill. 1971.

Curtis, J. E., Hersh, E. M., and Freireich, E. J. Leukapheresis therapy of chronic lymphocytic leukemia. Blood, *39*: 163–175, 1972.

Dameshek, W. Chronic lymphocytic leukemia—an accumulative disease of immunologically incompetent lymphocytes. Blood, *29*: 566–584, 1967.

DelRegato, J. A. Total body irradiation in the treatment of chronic lymphogenous leukemia. A.J.R., *120*: 504–520, 1974.

DeSimone, P. A. Diagnosis and management of chronic lymphocytic leukemia. J. Ky. Med. Assoc., *72*: 325–328, 1974.

Ezdinli, E. Z., Stutzman, L., Aungst, C. W., and Firat, D. Corticosteroid therapy for lymphomas and chronic lymphocytic leukemia. Cancer, *23*: 900–909, 1969.

Firestone, F. N., and Robinson, U. J. Upper airway obstruction; a rare presentation of chronic lymphocytic leukemia. Chest, *61*: 505–507, 1972.

Fitzgerald, P. H., and Hamer, J. W. Third case of chronic lymphocytic leukemia in a carrier of the inherited Ch[1] chromosome. Br. Med. J., *3*: 752, 1969.

Fraumeni, J. F., Vogel, C. L., and DeVita, V. T. Familial chronic lymphocytic leukemia. Ann. Intern. Med., *71*: 279, 1969.

Freymann, J. G., Vander, J. B., Marler, E. A., and Meyer, D. G. Prolonged corticosteroid therapy of chronic lymphocytic leukaemia and the closely allied malignant lymphomas. Br. J. Haematol., *6*: 303–323, 1960.

Galton, D. A. G. The pathogenesis of chronic lymphocytic leukemia. Can. Med. Assoc. J., *94*: 1005–1010, 1966.

Galton, D. A. G., Wiltshaw, E., Szur, L., and Dacie, J. V. The use of chlorambucil and steroids in the treatment of chronic lymphocytic leukaemia. Br. J. Haematol., *7*: 73–98, 1961.

Gardner, F. H. Treatment of lymphoproliferative disease, *In* Cancer Chemotherapy II. Twenty-second Hahnemann Symposium, edited by I. Brodsky, S. B. Kahn, and J. H. Moyer, pp. 361–373. Grune & Stratton, New York, 1972.

Green, R. A., and Dixon, H. Expectancy for life in chronic lymphatic leukemia. Blood, *25*: 23–30, 1965.

Gunz, F. W. Chronic lymphocytic leukemia. In Cancer Medicine, edited by J. F. Holland and E. Frei, pp. 1256–1275. Lea & Febiger, Philadelphia, 1973.

Gutterman, J. U., Curtis, J. E., and Freireich, E. J. Combination chemotherapy with cytosine arabinoside (Ara-C) and cyclophosphamide (CTX) of chronic lymphocytic leukemia (CLL) (abstract). Am. Soc. Clin. Oncology Meeting, Boston, Mass., 1972.

Han, T., Ezdinli, E. Z., Shimaoka, K., and Desai, D. V. Chlorambucil vs. combined chlorambucil-corticosteroid therapy in chronic lymphocytic leukemia. Cancer, *31*: 502–508, 1973.

Hansen, M. M. Chronic lymphocytic leukemia; clinical studies based on 189 cases followed for a long time. Scand. J. Haematol., *18* (suppl.): 3–286, 1973.

Harris, J., and Bagai, R. C. Immune deficiency states associated with malignant disease in man. Med. Clin. North Am., *56*: 501–514, 1972.

Herberman, R. B., Oren, M. E., Rogentine, G. N., and Fahey, J. L. Cytolytic effects of alloantiserum in patients with lymphoproliferative disorders. Cancer, *28*: 365–371, 1971.

Hill, J. M., Loeb, E., and Speer, R. J. Colloidal zirconyl phosphate ^{32}P in the treatment of chronic leukemia and lymphomas. J.A.M.A., *187*: 106–110, 1964.

Huguley, C. M. Long-term study of chronic lymphocytic leukemia; interim report after 45 months. Cancer Chemother. Rep., *16*: 241–244, 1962.

Huguley, C. M. Survey of current therapy and of problems in chronic leukemia. *In* M. D. Anderson Hospital and Tumor Institute, 14th Clinical Conference on Cancer, pp. 337–351. Year Book Medical Publishers, Chicago, 1970.

Johnson, R. E. Total body irradiation of chronic lymphocytic leukemia; incidence and duration of remission. Cancer, *25*: 523–530, 1970.

Karnofsky, D. A. The use of actinomycin in neoplastic disease in adults. *In* Actinomycin: Nature, Formation and Activities, edited by S. A. Waksman, pp. 147–161. Interscience Publishers, New York, 1968.

Kaung, D. T., Whittington, R. M., Patno, M. E., and VA Cancer Chemotherapy Study Group. Chemotherapy of chronic lymphocytic leukemia. Ann. Intern. Med., *114:* 521–524, 1964a.

Kaung, D. T., Whittington, R. M., and Patno, M. E. Treatment of chronic lymphocytic leukemia with chlorambucil (NSC-3088) and cyclophosphamide (NSC-26271). Cancer Chemother. Rep., *39:* 41–45, 1964b.

Kaung, D. T., Whittington, R. M., Spencer, H. H., and Patno, M. E. Comparison of chlorambucil and streptonigrin (NSC-45383) in the treatment of chronic lymphocytic leukemia. Cancer, *23:* 597–600, 1969.

Knospe, W. H., Loeb, V., and Huguley, C. M. Bi-weekly chlorambucil treatment of chronic lymphocytic leukemia. Cancer, *33:* 555–562, 1974.

Krakoff, I. H., Savel, H., and Murphy, M. L. Phase II studies of hydroxyurea (NSC-32065) in adults; clinical evaluation. Cancer Chemother. Rep., *40:* 53–55, 1964.

Kyle, R. A., McFarland, C. E., and Dameshek, W. Large doses of prednisone and prednisolone in treatment of malignant lymphoproliferative disorders. Ann. Intern. Med., *57:* 717–731, 1962.

Lajtha, L. G. Extracorporeal irradiation of the blood. Mod. Trends Radiother., *2:* 98–116, 1972.

Laszlo, J., Buckley III, C. E., and Amos, D. B. Infusion of isologous immune plasma in chronic lymphocytic leukemia. Blood, *31:* 104–110, 1968.

Manaster, J., Fruhling, J., and Stryekmans, P. Kinetics of lymphocytes in chronic lymphocytic leukemia; I. Equilibrium between blood and a "readily accessible pool." Blood, *41:* 425–438, 1973.

Manusow, D., and Weinerman, B. H. 1975. Subsequent neoplasia in chronic lymphocytic leukemia. J.A.M.A., *232:* 267–269, 1975.

McLaughlin, H., Wetherly-Mein, G., Pitcher, C., and Hobbs, J. R. Non-immunoglobulin-bearing "B" lymphocytes in chronic lymphatic leukaemia? Br. J. Haematol., *24:* 7–14, 1973.

Micu, D., and Astaldi, G. Lymphocyte cyto-enzymo-chemistry in the differential diagnosis between chronic lymphocytic leukemia and lymphosarcoma. *In* Erythrocytes, Thrombocytes, Leukocytes: Recent Advances in Membrane and Metabolic Research, edited by E. Gerlach, K. Moser, E. Deutsch, and W. Wilmanns, pp. 452–455. George Thieme Publishers, Stuttgart, 1973.

Miller, D. G., Budinger, J. M., and Karnofsky, D. A. A clinical and pathological study of resistance to infection in chronic lymphatic leukemia. Cancer, *15:* 307–329, 1962.

Mulligan, R. M. Interaction of host and cancer; the potential antigenicity of cancer cells, the defense mechanisms of cancer patients, and the influence of endocrine glands and aging on cancer. Exp. Med. Surg., *28:* 1–17, 1970.

Osgood, E. E. Treatment of chronic leukemias. J. Nucl. Med., *5:* 139–153, 1964.

Peterson, L. C., Bloomfield, C. D., Sundber, R. D., and Brunning, R. D. Relationship of morphology of chronic lymphatic leukemia to survival (abstract). American Society of Hematology Meeting, Atlanta, 1974.

Pincus, S., Bianco, C., and Nussenzweig, V. Increased proportion of complement-receptor lymphocytes in the peripheral blood of patients with chronic lymphocytic leukemia. Blood, *40:* 303–310, 1972.

Preud'homme, J. L., and Seligman, M. Surface bound immunoglobulins as cell marker in human lymphoproliferative diseases. Blood, *40:* 777–794, 1972.

Rai, K. R., Sawitsky, A., Cronkite, E. P., Chanana, A. D., Levy, R. N., and Pasternack, B. S. Clinical staging of chronic lymphocytic leukemia. Blood, *46:* 219–234, 1975.

Richards, F., Spurr, C. L., Pajak, T. F., Blake, D. D., and Raben, M. Thymic irradiation; an approach to chronic lymphocytic leukemia. Am. J. Med., *57:* 862–869, 1974.

Ross, S. W., MacDonald, E. J., Davis, P., Hammarsten, J., and Levin, W. C. A method for evaluation of disease and treatment in chronic leukemia. J. Lab. Clin. Med., *58:* 559–579, 1961.

Rundles, R. W., Grizzle, J., Bell, W. N., Corley, C. C., Grommeyer, W. B., et al. Comparison of chlorambucil and Myleran in chronic lymphocytic and granulocytic leukemia. Am. J. Med., *27:* 424–432, 1959.

Rundles, R. W., Laszlo, J., Garrison, F. E., Jr., and Hobson, J. B. The antitumor spectrum of cyclophosphamide. Cancer Chemother. Rep., *16:* 407–411, 1962.

Sardeman, H. Chronic lymphocytic leukemia in an infant. Acta Paediatr. Scand., *61:* 213–216, 1972.

Schultz, E. F., Davis, S., and Rubin, A. D. The nature of circulating lymphocytes in chronic lymphocytic leukemia (CLL) (abstract). American Society of Hematology Meeting, Atlanta, 1974.

Shaw, J. M., Hagon, E. E., Vincent, P. C., and Gunz, F. W. Quantitative studies on the response of normal and leukaemic lymphocytes to phytohaemagglutinin. Aust. J. Exp. Biol. Med. Sci., *52:* 87–97, 1974.

Shaw, R. K., Boggs, D. R., Silverman, H. R., and Frei, E. A study of prednisone therapy in chronic lymphocytic leukemia. Blood, *17:* 182–195, 1961.

Silver, R. T. The treatment of chronic lymphocytic leukemia. Semin. Hematol., *6:* 344–356, 1969.

Slungaard, A., and Smith, M. J. Serum immunoglobulin levels in chronic lymphatic leukemia. Scand. J. Haematol., *12:* 112–116, 1974.

Smith, M. J., Browne, E., and Slungaard, A. The impaired responsiveness of chronic lymphatic leukemia lymphocytes to allogenic lymphocytes. Blood, *41:* 505–509, 1973.

Solomon, J., Alexander, M. J., and Steinfeld, J. L. Cyclophosphamide; a clinical study. J.A.M.A., *183:* 165–170, 1963.

Spiers, A. S. D. Management of the different forms of leukemia. *In* Leukemia, edited by F. Gunz and A. G. Baikie, Ed. 3, pp. 732–744. Grune & Stratton, New York, 1974.

Spiro, S., Galton, D. A. G., Wiltshaw, E., and Lohmann, R. C. Follicular lymphoma; a survey of 75 cases with special reference to the syndrome resembling chronic lymphocytic leukaemia. Br. J. Cancer, *31* (suppl. II): 60–72, 1975.

Sprague, C. C. Evaluation of the effectiveness of radioactive phosphorus and chlorambucil in patients with chronic lymphocytic leukemia. Cancer Chemother. Rep., *16:* 235–240, 1962.

Storb, R., Epstein, R. B., Buchner, C. D., and Thomas, E. D. Treatment of chronic lymphocytic leukemia by extracorporeal irradiation. Blood, *31:* 490–502, 1968.

Thomas, E. D., Epstein, R. B., Eschbach, J. W., Jr., Prager, D., Buckner, C. D., and Marsaglia, G. Treatment of leukemia by extracorporeal irradiation. N. Engl. J. Med., *273:* 6–12, 1965.

Tsirimbas, A. D., Pfisterer, H., Hornung, B., Thierfelder, S., Michlmayr, G., and Stich, W. Studies with heterologous antilymphocytic serum as a therapy for chronic lymphocytic leukemia. Blut, *19:* 420–423, 1969.

Utsinger, P. D. Impaired T-cell transformation in chronic lymphocytic leukemia (CLL); demonstration of a blastogenesis inhibitory factor. Blood, *46:* 883–890, 1975.

Werthamer, S., and Amaral, L. Acrylamide gel electrophoretic abnormalities in chronic lymphatic leukemia sera. Am. J. Clin. Pathol., *55:* 65–67, 1971.

Wilson, J. D., and Hurdle, A. D. F. Surface immunoglobulins on lymphocytes in chronic lymphocytic leukemia and lymphosarcoma. Br. J. Haematol., *24:* 563–569, 1973.

Winkelstein, A., Whiteside, T., and Rabin, B. S. Immunological characterization of CLL lymphocytes (abstract). American Society of Hematology Meeting, Atlanta, 1974.

Wintrobe, M. M., Lee, G. R., Boggs, D. R., Bithell, T. C., Athens, J. W., and Foerster, J. Chronic lymphocytic leukemia. *In* Clinical Hematology, pp. 1520–1534. Lea & Febiger, Philadelphia, 1974.

Woodliff, H. J., and Cohen, G. Cytogenetic studies in chronic lymphocytic leukemia; I. A study of 40 patients. Med. J. Aust., *1:* 970–974, 1972.

Yam, L. T., and Crosby, W. H. Early splenectomy in lymphoproliferative disorders. Arch. Intern. Med., *133:* 270–274, 1974.

Zacharski, L. R., and Linmann, J. W. 1969. Chronic lymphocytic leukemia versus chronic lymphosarcoma cell leukemia. Am. J. Med., *47:* 75–85, 1969.

Zimmerman, T. S., Goodwin, H. A., and Perry, S. Studies of leukocyte kinetics in chronic lymphocytic leukemia. Blood, *31:* 277–291, 1968.

Zippin, C., Cutler, S. J., Reeves, W. J., Jr., and Lum, D. Survival in chronic lymphocytic leukemia. Blood, *42:* 367–376, 1973.

Zubrod, C. G. Present and future prospects for chemotherapy of the leukemias. *In* Proceedings of the International Conference on Leukemia—Lymphoma, edited by C. J. D. Zarafornetis, pp. 477–486. Lea & Febiger, Philadelphia, 1968.

Chapter 10

Management of Multiple Myeloma

JEFFREY WEISBERG, D.O., AARON A. ALTER, M.D., and
ISMAT U. NAWABI, M.D.

Multiple myeloma is a disease resulting from an abnormal proliferation of plasma cells (B lymphocytes) usually associated with immunoglobulin abnormalities and destructive bone lesions. It is a malignant process that significantly shortens life span, and histologically has the attributes of a neoplastic process characterized by an autonomous plasma cell proliferation which is invasive and destructive. The diagnosis is made by demonstrating the abnormal plasma cell proliferation, immunoglobulin abnormalities and destructive bone changes.

Multiple myeloma is a disease of the elderly and rarely occurs in patients below the age of 40 years. Its reported incidence is 2 per 100,000 population. The pathogenesis is unknown, although at the present time an unusual response to repeated antigenic and oncogenic challenges is considered a likely etiology. Genetic influences appear to play a role in this disease because of higher than expected familial incidence (Maldonada and Kyle, 1974). An almost identical disease occurs spontaneously in animals and can be induced in mice by intraperitoneal placement of Millipore filters, injections of mineral oil, or heat-killed staphylococci (Engle and Wallis, 1969).

PLASMA CELL KINETICS AND STAGING OF MULTIPLE MYELOMA

The plasma cells in multiple myeloma usually produce a protein molecule which is measurable in the serum and in culture medium making it possible to estimate the actual number of proliferating plasma cells (Salmon, 1973). Nanogram quantities of M-components secreted by relatively small numbers of plasma cells obtained by bone marrow aspiration can be used to estimate the total body tumor load. Furthermore, applying the known metabolic turnover of the various immunoglobulins, the number of functioning plasma cells can be determined by the simple formula:

Total body tumor cell count

$$= \frac{\text{Total body M-component synthetic rate}}{\text{Cellular M-component synthetic rate}}$$

The cellular M-component synthetic rates in over 70 patients with multiple myeloma who have IgG, IgA, and IgE paraproteins have been estimated and several interesting correlations between cell number and clinical findings have been found. At the time when there is a clear M-component, 10% or more plasma cells are found in the bone marrow and there may be some degree of anemia, depression of normal serum immunoglobulins, or Bence-Jones proteinuria. At least 0.2×10^{12} plasma cells are present in the body at this time. Patients with fewer than 1×10^{12} plasma cells usually do not have weight loss or generalized lytic bone lesions but may have osteoporosis or compression fractures. Patients with more than 2×10^{12} plasma cells often have widespread osteolytic lesions and fractures, hypercalcemia and marked Bence-Jones proteinuria. The latter group has a shorter life expectancy and a less favorable response to therapy. The finding of splenomegaly correlates with a high tumor mass. Hyperviscosity syndrome occurs most often in patients with a high immunosynthetic rate.

It is important to note that the serum concentration of the M-component, its total body synthetic rate or cellular synthetic rate, individually, do not correlate with the myeloma cell number. The lower limit for recognition of M-components by electrophoretic techniques is 0.2 g/100 ml which is associated with 2×10^{10} cells or approximately 20 g of tumor.

The average tumor doubling time during the clinical phase of the disease is estimated to be about 6 months. If tumor growth were truly exponential at this rate, it would require 20 years from the time a single cell underwent malignant transformation to the time of diagnosis. Such a theory for the evolution for multiple myeloma has been proposed (Hobbs, 1975) and is supported by the findings in mouse myeloma where the growth from 2 million to 100 million tumor cells is exponential and by the observation that in man it may take up to 20 years for a solitary plasmacytoma to become disseminated. On the other hand, it has been proposed that myeloma proliferates according to a gompertzian growth curve (Salmon, 1973), that is, it initially grows at a steep exponential curve but gradually slows its rate of growth as it enlarges (Fig. 10.1). Consequently, it is estimated that the preclinical duration of the disease is much shorter. By back calculation of growth curves, a 1–2-year period from malignant transformation to diagnosis and an initial doubling time of 1–3 days is estimated. In other words myeloma has almost reached a plateau in growth during the clinical phase of the disease which has been estimated to occur at, or slightly above, the lethal cell number (5–10 ×

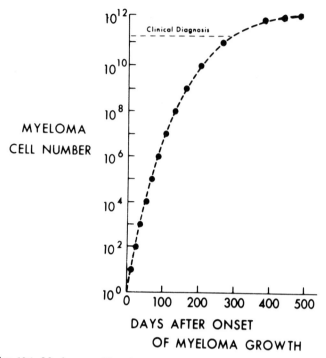

FIG. 10.1. Myeloma proliferation according to gompertzian growth curve.

10^{12}). Benign monoclonal gammopathies are believed to be similar to myeloma in their growth pattern except that the plateau occurs at a sublethal level.

The curve for tumor regression during response to treatment shows an initial rapid decrease in tumor mass and then a plateau which may persist for a period of months or years despite continuation of treatment.

A proposed system of clinical staging is shown in Table 10.1 (Durie and Salmon, 1975): in this staging system, both the stage and the subclassification correlate with response to treatment and survival. The only exception is in Stage III where the level of M-component does not appear to directly correlate with survival.

PATHOGENESIS AND CLINICAL MANIFESTATIONS

With the proliferation of an abnormal clone of plasma cells in multiple myeloma, it is postulated that there is a simultaneous decrease in the number of normal plasma cells (Salmon, 1974). The malignant cells appear not to be sensitive to an inhibitory feedback mechanism which, however, causes inhibition of the normally responding plasma cells. There is evidence to suggest that cellular products such as the immunoglobulins

TABLE 10.1
Myeloma Staging System

Stage	Criteria	Measured Myeloma Cell Mass (cells × 10^{12}/m²)
I.	*All* of the following: 1. Hemoglobin value >10 g/100 ml 2. Serum calcium value normal (≤12 mg/100 ml) 3. On roentgenogram, normal bone structure (scale 0) or solitary bone plasmacytoma only 4. Low M-component production rates a. IgG value <5 g/100 ml b. IgA value <3 g/100 ml c. Urine light chain M-component on electrophoresis <4 g/ 24 hours	<0.6 (low)
II.	Fitting neither Stage I nor Stage III	0.6–1.20 (intermediate)
III.	*One or more* of the following: 1. Hemoglobin value <8.5 g/100 ml 2. Serum calcium value >12 mg/100 ml 3. Advanced lytic bone lesions (scale 3) 4. High M-component production rates a. IgG value >7 g/100 ml b. IgA value >5 g/100 ml c. Urine light chain M-component on electrophoresis >12 g/24 hours	>1.20 (high)

Subclassification
A = Relatively normal renal function (serum creatinine value <2.0 mg/100 ml)
B = Abnormal renal function (serum creatinine value ≥2.0 mg/100 ml)
Examples
Stage IA   = low cell mass with normal renal function
Stage IIIB = high cell mass with abnormal renal function

or chalones may be the inhibiting substances (Maugh, 1972). In addition, monocytes from patients with multiple myeloma have been shown to suppress normal B lymphocytes (Broder et al., 1975). The cellular events are reflected by the increased production of a monoclonal immunoglobulin and a decrease in the levels of normal immunoglobulins.

The clinical manifestations of multiple myeloma and its pathogenesis will be discussed under two headings (Fig. 10.2): (1) those due primarily to plasma cell proliferation and (2) those related to the immunoglobulin abnormalities. This division is arbitrary and in most instances both factors and their consequent derangements play a role in the pathogenesis and clinical manifestations of multiple myeloma.

Plasma Cell Proliferation

Plasma cells and their precursors, the B lymphocytes, originate in the bone marrow and then invade the cancellous bone and other organs.

With the replacement of the normal marrow elements, anemia, leuko-penia, and thrombocytopenia can occur. Anemia, in a mild to moderate degree, is seen in the majority of cases at the time of diagnosis and progressively worsens with extension of the disease. Characteristically, the anemia is normocytic, normochromic, and unresponsive to hematin-ics. Rouleaux formation of the red cells on peripheral blood smear and a high sedimentation rate are characteristic findings. If a patient with

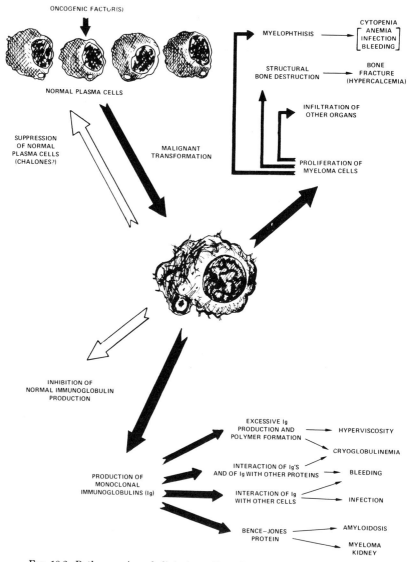

FIG. 10.2. Pathogenesis and clinical manifestations in multiple myeloma.

multiple myeloma presents with severe anemia, other causes such as blood loss, iron, vitamin B_{12}, or folate deficiency should be considered. Hemolytic anemia is rare. Renal failure and the malignant process itself may be contributory to the myelophthisic anemia by causing depression of erythropoiesis. Myelophthisis alone rarely causes severe anemia while leukopenia and thrombocytopenia are seen only in a small number of cases before the onset of therapy.

Bone Destruction. Invasion of the cortical bones by the plasma cells may be diffuse, multicentric or, rarely, solitary. The cancellous bone is invaded from within the medullary cavity and an osteoclastic activating factor (OAF) secreted by plasma cells possibly enhances destruction of bone and provides a path for tumor growth (Mundy et al., 1974). The classic bone lesion appears lytic on x-ray without any evidence of new bone formation and is not associated with an elevated serum alkaline phosphatase. This triad distinguishes the lesions from metastatic carcinoma. Osteosclerosis is rare and when accompanied by polyneuropathy, myeloid metaplasia and endocrine disturbances supposedly constitutes a different entity (Imawari et al., 1974).

Solitary plasmacytoma must be separated from the diffuse form of the disease because of its favorable outcome and potential curability by surgery or radiation. The criteria to establish the diagnosis of a solitary plasmacytoma, suggested by Snapper and Kahn (1971), are: (1) absence of plasma cell infiltration at other sites by multiple needle aspirations, (2) normal serum protein electrophoresis, and (3) absence of Bence-Jones proteins and other x-ray abnormalities. The diagnosis is confirmed unequivocally only retrospectively after years of observation.

Structural bone destruction eventually leads to bone pain, fractures and skeletal deformities, the prominent features of multiple myeloma. The pain may be fleeting from one area to another and vary in intensity from time to time and, unlike metastatic bone disease, it is less severe at night. Sharply localized pain brought on by a sudden movement is a frequent presenting symptom and usually indicates a pathologic fracture. The sites involved are predominately those with myeloid activity, i.e., the skull, vertebrae, ribs, sternum, pelvic bones, and metaphysis of long bones. X-ray studies may show osteoporosis, punched-out lesions or fractures, and frequently all three are present. In 20% of cases the x-rays may be normal. The skull lesions, the site of the classical roentgenographic findings, seldom, if ever, cause headaches.

The role of physical inactivity in aggravating bone disease requires emphasis. Over a 15-year period, not a single patient who maintained regular physical activity developed spinal cord compression (Farhangi and Osserman, 1973). Other causes which may mimic bone involvement are rheumatoid arthritis (which may antedate or accompany multiple myeloma), amyloid deposition in joints or nerve pain.

Hypercalcemia. Calcium is released as a result of bone destruction and its serum level can usually be maintained within normal limits as long as the kidneys are functioning normally. When this balance is upset by extensive and rapid bone disease or kidney impairment, the serum calcium level rises. Moreover, hypercalcemia has an anti-ADH like effect causing further dehydration, impaired renal perfusion and a further rise in serum calcium (Gordon et al., 1973).

The patient with hypercalcemia may present with constipation, weakness, polydipsia, polyuria, anorexia, nausea, vomiting and finally confusion, stupor and coma. It must be emphasized that in a comatose myeloma patient hypercalcemia and hyperviscosity, potentially reversible causes of disturbance of consciousness, should be considered in the differential diagnosis.

Uric Acid Metabolism. Increased plasma cell proliferation and destruction leads to an increased urate load which must be excreted by the kidney. The resulting hyperuricemia, aggravated by chemotherapy and radiotherapy, may result in renal failure.

Immunoglobulin Abnormalities

The Ig molecule has two identical (H) heavy and two identical (L) light polypeptide chains held together by disulfide and covalent bonds. Five varieties of heavy chains γ, α, μ, δ, and ϵ are known and are the basis on which immunoglobulins are classified as IgG, IgA, IgM, IgD, and IgE, respectively. The light chains are either of κ or λ variety. Subclasses of IgG, IgA and IgM have been defined by immunochemical techniques (Kochwa et al., 1975). In large series of patients with myelomatosis, 50–60% of the cases have IgG paraprotein, 25% IgA paraprotein and in 25% of patients, only light chains are detected in the serum or urine. Instances of IgD myeloma are rare (Jancelewicz et al., 1975) and only a few cases of IgE myeloma have been reported. Approximately 1% of cases have no paraprotein in the serum or urine. Depression of normal immunoglobulins is almost uniformly found in all patients with the disease.

Although distinctive clinical and morphologic features do not exist among these patients, those with IgG paraproteins usually show a conspicuous spike on protein electrophoresis, have a lower incidence of Bence-Jones proteinuria, renal failure and amyloidosis and have a better prognosis in spite of a higher frequency of infections (Rosen, 1975). On the other hand, IgD myeloma and patients with only light chain paraprotein have an inconspicuous paraprotein or only hypogammaglobulinemia accompanied by marked Bence-Jones proteinuria and a high incidence of renal failure and amyloidosis. In these patients the disease is rapidly progressive and early death is common. Patients with λ light chain disease have a worse prognosis than those with κ light chain disease (Shustick et al., 1976) and interestingly patients with IgG myeloma who secrete λ chains also have a worse prognosis (Cancer and Leukemia Group B, 1975).

Kidney Disease. Impaired renal function is present in the majority of patients at the time of diagnosis. A third of the patients have a serum creatinine of greater than 2 mg/100 ml. Bence-Jones proteinuria, hypercalcemia, hyperuricemia, pyelonephritis, amyloidosis and plasma cell infiltration may individually or in combination cause renal failure. The high correlation between Bence-Jones proteinuria and kidney failure is well recognized. However, in a small number of cases severe and prolonged Bence-Jones proteinuria may cause little or no renal impairment.

Recent electron microscope and immunofluorescent studies have revealed very little, if any, Bence-Jones protein in the tubular protein casts but significant amounts in the cytoplasm of the tubular epithelium thereby raising a question regarding the concept that kidney failure results from obstruction of the proximal and distal convoluted tubules (Fisher et al., 1964. Levi, et al., 1968). It is presently postulated that deposition of Bence-Jones protein in the cytoplasm of the tubular epithelial cells causes their atrophy and is primarily responsible for the renal failure. These findings may give insight into the specific tubular defects found in myeloma, such as Fanconi's syndrome, and identify the site of Bence-Jones protein catabolism and deposition of amyloid material.

Infection. The susceptibility to infection in multiple myeloma is due to a number of factors; decreased levels of normal Ig (usually less than 20% of normal); granulocytopenia, abnormal granulocyte function and possibly deranged cellular immunity. Some of these abnormalities may also occur as a consequence of therapy. The pattern of infection is similar to patients who are agammaglobulinemic, i.e., susceptibility to encapsulated pyogenic organisms such as pneumococci, staphylococci, streptococci, *Haemophilus influenzae*, etc. Recently gram-negative bacteria have been noted to occur with greater frequency (Meyers et al., 1972). Susceptibility to viral infections except herpes zoster is not increased.

Hyperviscosity Syndrome. Serum viscosity can be determined by an Oswald viscosimeter or simply by comparing the flow time of serum to water in a red pipette. A ratio of 1.4–1.8 is normal but symptoms usually do not appear until serum viscosity is above 5.0. In one large series serum viscosity was above 1.7 in 89% of cases and in 13% it was greater than 4.0 (Kyle, 1975). Hyperviscosity, although more characteristic of IgM macroglobulinemia, also occurs in patients with IgA and IgG myeloma. It may be due simply to a marked increase of immunoglobulins but more often results from abnormal amounts of immunoglobulins that tend to form polymers or due to complexes formed between the immunoglobulins and other plasma proteins or cellular components of the blood (Bloch and Maki, 1973). Of the subclasses of IgG, IgG_3 is most frequently associated with hyperviscosity syndrome. Hyperviscosity leads to sluggish blood circulation and an increase in blood volume which may result in impairment of the cerebral, retinal and renal blood flow, congestive heart failure, thrombosis and hyperglobulinemic purpura. The ocular disturbances may vary from mild to complete loss of vision. On examination of the fundi distention and tortuosity of the retinal veins, the characteristic "string of sausage appearance," retinal hemorrhages and papilledema may be present. Generalized purpura with increased bleeding from the gums, increased capillary fragility, severe uncontrollable epistaxis, oozing of blood from minor surgical wounds and tooth extraction sites may occur. Alterations in platelet function and coagulation factors may be contributory. The neurologic manifestations of hyperviscosity may vary from headache and dizziness to vertigo, nystagmus, partial or complete hearing loss, somnolence, stupor, convulsions and coma. Intractable cardiac failure has been noted which responds only to plasmapheresis. The cause and effect relationships between hyperviscosity and renal impairment is not very clear but improvement of kidney function has followed plasmapheresis.

Hemostatic Abnormalities. Hemostatic abnormalities, frequently presenting as a bleeding tendency and occasionally as thrombosis are also related to the abnormal plasma protein (Lackner, 1973). Laboratory abnormalities such as increased bleeding time, diminished platelet adhesion, diminished platelet factor III availability and poor platelet aggregation, inhibition of clotting factors I, II, V, VII, and VIII are due to interaction of immunoglobulins with platelets and clotting factors. Plasmapheresis can correct some of these abnormalities and the addition of the patient's plasma to normal platelets and clotting factors can reproduce them. At times, increased levels of factor VIII activity have also been observed. Coating of platelet membrane by immunoglobulin is thought to be responsible for the in vitro abnormality, while, in vivo, hemostatic platelet plug formation may also be inhibited by immunoglobulin coating of the connective tissue of blood vessels. Poor clot retraction may occur because of platelet abnormalities or interference with the polymerization of fibrin monomer. In addition to specific inhibitors of factors V, VII and VIII, nonspecific inhibition of thromboplastin generation, and unexplainable low levels of factors II, V, VII, VIII, and X, have been observed. Interestingly, factor X, when diminished, cannot be corrected by the infusion of large amounts of factor X. How much of a role these laboratory abnormalities play in causing clinical bleeding remains to be determined.

Cryoimmunoglobulins are serum proteins that precipitate in the cold and redissolve on warming. This is another laboratory abnormality which is frequently unaccompanied by clinical manifestations and is seen in the serum of 5% of patients. The cryoimmunoglobulins are either monoclonal or formed by complexes of IgM and IgG immunoglobulin molecules (Grey and Kohler, 1973). A very high proportion of the IgM cryoglobulins have κ light chains and IgG$_3$ is the predominant IgG component. Idiopathic cryoimmunoglobulinemia may antedate multiple myeloma by many years. The symptoms attributable to cryoimmunoglobulins may be present in various combinations and include cold urticaria, Raynaud's phenomena, dependent purpura, cutaneous vasculitis, ulcerations of the skin, thrombosis and retinal and mucocutaneous bleeding. The temperature at which the proteins precipitate is critical. Those proteins which precipitate close to the normal body temperature are associated with more frequent and more severe symptoms.

Amyloidosis. Amyloid is the eosinophilic material that stains with congo red, shows dichromism and green polarization color, and has recently been shown to be derived from amino terminal ends of light chains. Amyloidosis has been classified, on the basis of its distribution, as primary, involving mesenchymal organs (the heart, tongue, peripheral nerves, etc.) or secondary, involving the parenchymal organs (kidney, liver and spleen) (Glenner et al., 1973). Amyloidosis associated with multiple myeloma usually conforms to the primary form in distribution and chemical composition.

The increased frequency of amyloidosis with IgD myeloma may be due to the increased tendency of the light chains to form amyloid, or due to the defective proteolytic activity of the phagocytic lysozymes. The manifestations related to amyloidosis are cutaneous hemorrhages and purpura particularly in the eyelids and periorbital tissues, localized patchy thickening and alopecia of the skin, macroglossia, xerostomia, dysphagia, malabsorption syndrome, cardiac failure and cardiac arrythmias, carpal tunnel syndrome, joint stiffness, usually without pain or tenderness, and peripheral neuropathy.

Nervous System

Myeloma rarely involves the central nervous system and infiltration of the peripheral nerves is also uncommon. Compression of the spinal cord or spinal nerves by a tumor growing from the adjacent vertebrae or injury due to bone fractures and collapse is a frequent occurrence. Leukoencephalopathy, hyperviscosity, cryoglobulinemia and hypercalcemia may cause central nervous system manifestations. Complaints of fatigue, numbness, feeling of heaviness of the legs, difficulty in walking must lead to a careful neurologic examination to detect compression of the spinal cord before paralysis has occurred.

Other Malignancies

The incidence of a second malignancy in multiple myeloma varies in different reports. Snapper and Kahn (1971) noted a significantly lower than expected incidence of bronchogenic carcinoma and other malignancies, while Osserman has found a 22% incidence of a second malignancy. Others have reported that, when matched for age, the incidence of a second malignancy is not increased (Cornes et al., 1961). Recent reports suggest that there may be a higher incidence of acute leukemia in patients treated with various chemotherapeutic agents, although leukemia has occurred in those patients who have not been exposed to chemotherapy or radiotherapy (Rosner and Grunwald, 1974; Kyle, 1975).

DIAGNOSIS

The diagnosis of multiple myeloma is made by the presence of abnormally increased number of plasma cells, a monoclonal spike of immunoglobulins in the serum or urine and the presence of osteolytic lesions or osteoporosis on x-rays of the bones. In the presence of other manifestations of multiple myeloma, more than 10% plasma cells in the bone marrow may suffice to make the diagnosis. In chronic disease states, plasmacytosis of up to 20% or more may be seen and a bone marrow aspirate, unless totally infiltrated with sheets of plasma cells, is not in itself diagnostic. The different morphologic varieties of plasma cells or its immature forms are no longer considered diagnostic or helpful in differentiating the various classes of multiple myeloma, although multinucleated giant plasma cells, Mott cells, Stich cells and plasma cells with cytoplasmic or nuclear Russell bodies are seen more frequently in multiple myeloma, they can also occur in conditions associated with secondary plasmacytosis. Clusters of plasma cells surrounding the capillaries of the bone marrow are normal and should be distinguished from sheets of plasma cells. The monoclonal immunoglobulin usually exceeds 2 g/100 ml in IgG and IgA multiple myeloma, but in IgE a monoclonal spike may not be apparent and hypogammaglobulinemia may be present. In normal persons up to 50–100 mg of light chains may be secreted in the urine over a 24-hour period while greater amounts are significant and raise the possibility of myeloma. The heat test for Bence-Jones proteins has now been replaced by urine electrophoresis in many laboratories as a more sensitive and specific test. The criteria for the diagnosis of multiple myeloma proposed by Costa et al. (1973) are:

1. Cytogenic criteria
   a. Marrow morphology. Plasma cells and/or myeloma cells in excess of 10% when 1000 cells have been counted
   b. Biopsy proven plasmacytoma either in bone or soft tissues
2. a. Myeloma protein (M-component) demonstrable by electrophoresis of plasma
   b. Myeloma protein (M-component) demonstrable by electrophoresis of urine

   c. Roentgenologic evidence of osteolytic lesions. Generalized osteoporosis qualifies as a criterion if the marrow contains in excess of 30% plasma cells

   d. Myeloma cells in at least two peripheral blood smears.

The diagnosis is made in the presence of (1) 1a and 1b, or (2) 1a or 1b and either 2a, 2b, 2c, or 2d.

In addition, it is required that collagen diseases, cirrhosis, metastatic carcinoma and viral exanthemas be absent. The presence of amyloid disease does not exclude multiple myeloma. The incidence of some of the major manifestations of multiple myeloma that occur within 3 months of diagnosis as reported by Kyle et al. (1975) is: bone pain, 68%; anemia, 62%; renal insufficiency, 55%; hypercalcemia, 30%; proteinuria, 88%; Bence-Jones proteinuria, 49%; skeletal roentgenographic abnormalities, 70%; a spike on urine and serum protein electrophoresis, 75% and 76%, respectively; infections, 12%; hemostatic abnormalities, 7%; increased sedimentation rate, 90%; and increased uric acid, 61% in females and 39% in males. The lower incidence of abnormalities in these cases compared with earlier studies (Snapper and Kahn, 1971) results from reporting only those manifestations occurring within 3 months of diagnosis.

TREATMENT OF MULTIPLE MYELOMA

The most important advance in the treatment of multiple myeloma was the introduction of the alkylating agents in the early 1960s. Prior to this period, the median survival was 17 months from the onset of symptoms while life expectancy is now 3–7 times longer (Farhangi and Osserman, 1973). In addition to the use of alkylating agents, this improvement may also be attributed to the introduction of more sensitive means of diagnosis, and the availability of preventive and therapeutic measures for complications such as infection and hypercalcemia.

Surgery has virtually no role in the definitive treatment of multiple myeloma except for the very rare instance of an operable plasmacytoma. It does, however, have a role in the treatment of complications such as laminectomy for spinal cord compression. Radiotherapy is not curative but can be of considerable value in the relief of pain and neurologic complications resulting from tumor growth.

Chemotherapy is the usual treatment for the disseminated form of the disease, but is rarely, if ever, curative. All patients should be treated regardless of symptomatology because of the predictable progressive nature of the disease. However, prior to the institution of chemotherapy, time should be allowed for control of infections and localized pain, by radiotherapy, if necessary. In addition, hyperuricemia, hypercalcemia, dehydration and azotemia should be treated aggressively. The presence of these latter complications should not significantly delay the start of chemotherapy since they are secondary to the plasma cell mass.

Drugs used in the past which showed marginal benefits in the treatment of multiple myeloma are urethane and stilbamidine (Osserman, 1959; Mass, 1962). At the present time, the alkylating agents and the nitrosoureas are the most active agents. When used singly, azathioprine, streptonigrin, procarbazine, nitrogen mustard and testosterone have not been of any value. The purine and pyrimidine antagonists which are cell cycle specific agents are also of no value in the initial treatment of multiple myeloma. Thus far, newer agents such as Adriamycin, bleomycin and cytosine arabinoside have not found a well defined place in the treatment of this disease.

Salmon et al (1978) developed an in vitro tumor colony assay to measure sensitivity of myeloma cells to chemotherapeutic agents. A clear correlation between clinical response and the in vitro results are seen. This major step will mean selection of active drugs for specific cases and avoidance of the toxicity of anticancer agents to which the cells are resistant.

The alkylating agents are most effective and are usually administered with prednisone. Melphalan is most frequently used but cyclophosphamide and chlorambucil (Hammack et al., 1975) are also effective. Many regimens using melphalan have been studied. An effective protocol followed by Cancer and Leukemia Group B (CALGB) is the administration of 150 μg/kg/day for 7 days and, following recovery from leukopenia and/or thrombocytopenia, continuous oral daily maintenance of approximately one-third of the initial dose. Prednisone is concomitantly used at a dose of 0.8 mg/kg for 2 weeks and then tapered stepwise over 4–8 weeks. The 7-day melphalan loading dose will usually cause leukopenia in the range of 2000–3000/cu mm and cause the platelets to drop below 100,000/cu mm. Farhangi and Osserman (1973) believe a rest period is not advisable after the administration of the loading dose because they have observed appreciable rebound increases in the serum and urine myeloma proteins. The use of high dose intermittent intravenous melphalan does not appear to show any better response rate but may be associated with greater toxicity.

Symptomatic improvement may be noted as early as 2–3 days after instituting chemotherapy but usually requires a few weeks. Blood counts should be checked once or twice weekly for the first month and then at increasing intervals after the maintenance dose is well established (Farhangi and Osserman 1973). Controversy exists as to whether the initial dose should be reduced if leukopenia or thrombocytopenia exists prior to treatment. Other parameters to follow include hemoglobin, BUN or creatinine, serum calcium, uric acid, bone marrow examinations for cellularity and percentage of plasma cells, quantitive serum and urine immunoglobulin assays and x-rays of involved bones. Changes in pain, performance, height, weight and sense of well being are also indicators of a response.

Repeat bone x-rays during the first few months of treatment may be misinterpreted as showing progression. This finding probably represents sharper demarcation of the margins of the lesions by thickened trabeculae and does not indicate a worsened clinical state. Ten to fifteen percent of patients show recalcification of lytic lesions after 6–12 months of treatment. Continuous therapy will maintain the remission for a median of 21 months, however, disease progression eventually occurs. Indeed, therapy with melphalan and prednisone seems to be of no major value after the first year of treatment in responding patients (Alexanian et al., 1975). Prolonged periods of unmaintained remission occur primarily in patients without extensive disease at the time of diagnosis or in whom the abnormal protein disappeared from the electrophoresis strip (Alexanian et al., 1978).

The addition of prednisone to melphalan doubles the response rate and may affect survival significantly (Alexanian et al., 1969). Poor risk patients have neither increased response rate nor increased survival with the drug combination. A study by CALGB and Eastern Cooperative Oncology Group (ECOG) showed a median of 53 months of survival for the combination as compared with a median of 30 months of survival when melphalan was used alone (Costa et al., 1973). Prednisone, used alone, is not effective in the treatment of myeloma (Mass, 1962). The addition of procarbazine or testosterone to melphalan and prednisone may improve the response rate but does not seem to increase survival (Alexanian et al., 1969, 1972). Although the addition of androgens may be associated with higher hemoglobin levels, the degree of leukopenia or thrombocytopenia is unchanged.

Cyclophosphamide is as effective as melphalan in remission induction and prolongation of life. Furthermore, approximately one-third of myeloma patients resistant to melphalan show objective improvement with cyclophosphamide (Bergsagel et al., 1972). Thus, resistance to one alkylating agent does not always indicate resistance to another.

Intermittent combination induction chemotherapy has been reported to be superior to continuous treatment with alkylating agents (George et al., 1972). However, large cooperative studies by CALGB and Southwest Oncology Group (1975) have shown intermittent therapy to be less effective. In the intermittent regimen, pulse doses of melphalan and prednisone are given every 6 weeks. A schedule for this form of treatment is (Rosen, 1975):

Melphalan 0.25 mg/kg/day × 4 days orally
and
Prednisone 2 mg/kg/day × 4 days orally

This dosage is repeated every 6 weeks. A regimen recommended for continuous cyclophosphamide is:

Cyclophosphamide 200 mg orally for 5–7 days followed by maintenance therapy of 50–100 mg daily and prednisone 0.8 mg/kg daily for 2 weeks and tapered stepwise over 4–8 weeks.

An intermittent schedule for cyclophosphamide is:

Cyclophosphamide 750 mg/m^2/day orally × 4 days and prednisone 100 mg/day × 4 days orally repeated every 21 days.

Melphalan is generally preferred to cyclophosphamide. Hemorrhagic cystitis may occur in patients treated with cyclophosphamide, therefore, a vigorous urinary output is required. A current study by CALGB may determine if the combination of BCNU and prednisone is as effective as or superior to melphalan and prednisone. The combination of melphalan, BCNU and prednisone shows no clear difference in survival when compared with the combinations of melphalan and prednisone or BCNU and prednisone although the frequency of response seems to be higher when three drugs are used.

Studies are in progress using a five-drug regimen consisting of melphalan, cyclophosphamide, vincristine, BCNU and prednisone (Lee et al., 1974) and a three-drug combination of BCNU, melphalan and cyclophosphamide. Other trials comparing aklylating agents to the nitrosoureas (BCNU, CCNU, MECCNU) are also under study. The use of total bone marrow irradiation thus far has failed to be of any significant value in spite of one report of a dramatic remission.

Plasma cell kinetic studies (Salmon, 1973) have shown that a 1–2 log kill or greater in a patient who has successfully undergone treatment for multiple myeloma is associated with an increase of the growth fraction. Therefore the use of cell cycle specific agents may be of benefit at this time since a greater percentage of cells are actively proliferating. Trials with cycle active drugs during clinical remission are under study which might increase the log kill and prolong survival. Vincristine, although not an effective inducing agent in myeloma, does kill an appreciable number of tumor cells after the use of alkylating agents (Salmon, 1973). Its peak response occurs 12–24 hours after a single dose.

Different criteria are used for measuring response in this disease. CALGB defines a good response as improvement in more than half of the disease parameters which were abnormal at presentation. These parameters are the level of hemoglobin, serum protein, urine protein, number of plasma cells in the marrow, BUN, serum calcium, bone x-rays, tissue masses, Bence-Jones proteinuria, pain and performance.

The best chemotherapeutic induction regimen to date appears to be the combination of melphalan and prednisone with a 60% response rate (Wilson et al., 1971). The best maintenance regimen is continuous melphalan therapy. Most studies report no correlation of response or survival with the immunoglobulin type.

Bone Pain. The major presenting complaint is bone pain which at times is of such severity that the patient is bedridden and unable to move. It is imperative that the patient be given adequate analgesia in order to permit ambulation, thereby preventing the development of atelectasis, pneumonia, phlebitis and hypercalcemia. In order to achieve sufficient analgesia, 100–200 mg of meperidine or 15 mg of morphine sulfate may be required every 3–4 hours with careful observation for respiratory depression.

Localized severe bone pain is a frequent complaint and is, initially, very responsive to localized radiotherapy which can be given even during the course of active chemotherapy. In the absence of radiographically demonstrable bone lesions, radiotherapy should still be given to very painful bony areas if no other cause can be determined. Repeated courses may have to be given to the same bony areas.

Chemotherapy is usually unsuccessful in promoting recalcification of bones although it may decrease bone pain and prevent further destruction. Following a preliminary report by Cohen (1966) of increased bone density found in patients given fluoride with calcium supplementation, a blinded study was undertaken (Harley et al. 1972) to determine whether orally administered doses of 100 or 200 mg of sodium fluoride daily, added to chemotherapy, would result in an objective or subjective improvement in the bone complications. Chronic fluoride administration did not decrease bone pain, the need for radiotherapy for pain, the frequency of bone fractures or the loss of body height. Fluoride will improve bone density radiographically ("fluorosis") but this new bone formation is poorly mineralized and, therefore, does not improve bone strength. A recent randomized double blind study (Kyle et al., 1975) reported an increase in bone formation and bone mass in patients given a combination of fluoride and calcium in addition to melphalan and prednisone when compared with a group treated with melphalan, prednisone and placebo. No mention was made of a difference in bone pain or frequency of fractures between the two groups. The possibility of improving bone strength with a combination of fluoride, vitamin D and calcium is presently under study.

Infection. In contrast to lymphoma, fever is a very uncommon manifestation of uncomplicated multiple myeloma and its presence almost always indicates an associated infectious process. In the past, most infections were due to pyogenic organisms like *Diplococcus pneumoniae*, *Staphylococcus aureus* and *Escherichia coli*, whereas more recently opportunistic infections with gram-negative organisms, fungi and *Pneumocystis carinii* have been reported with increasing frequency. In addition to appropriate aggressive antibiotic therapy, granulocyte transfusions may be indicated in the presence of severe granulocytopenia whether due to bone marrow replacement or as a consequence of chemotherapy.

Frequently, infections occur in the presence of normal numbers of circulating granulocytes and are possibly due to qualitative granulocyte defects as well as defects in the immune system. Active infection with a specific organism does not confer immunity to that organism and patients with multiple myeloma can have repeated infections with the same strain such as *D. pneumoniae*, Type III.

In an attempt to reduce the frequency of infections, 20 ml of immune serum globulin was administered biweekly prophylactically in a double-blind study in patients treated with chemotherapy (Schilling and Finkel, 1975). There was no significant difference in the frequency or site of infection or the infecting pathogenic organisms when the study was compared with the control group. An attempt to actively immunize patients would seem to be useless at this time in the face of their demonstrated inability to adequately respond to antigenic challenges (Cohen and Rundles, 1975). The use of specific hyperimmune serum at the time of infection might be another approach. The prophylactic use of larger quantities of immune serum globulin than used in prior studies or the use of a pool of immune sera against organisms known to frequently infect these patients must be considered.

In an attempt to reduce the frequency of infections, prophylactic measures should be undertaken such as avoiding the use of indwelling urinary catheters, intravenous lines, etc. Adequate measures should be taken to ensure active bronchopulmonary drainage including sufficient thoracic pain relief in order to permit full respiratory excursions. Before chemotherapy is instituted, underlying infections should be eradicated. When a serious infection occurs, before or during chemotherapy, adequate cultures should be taken and the most likely effective antibiotics started while awaiting culture and sensitivity results. In view of the increasing incidence of gram-negative pneumonias, antibiotics should be selected initially to cover both gram-negative and gram-positive organisms even though the patient presents with lobar pneumonia.

Renal. Renal failure is a poor prognostic sign when not due to causes which are readily reversible. In an attempt to prevent renal insufficiency, patients should never be dehydrated for any reason including radiographic studies, biochemical tests and renal concentration studies. Previous reports of patients developing acute renal failure following intravenous urography were, in most instances, probably due to fluid deprivation and dehydration. In these instances, the renal failure is often readily reversible if recognized promptly and immediate steps are taken to hydrate the patient.

When a patient presents with acute renal failure, reversible etiologic factors must be searched for and treated. These include hypercalcemia, hyperuricemia, urinary tract infections, hyperviscosity and dehydration. Hemodialysis and peritoneal dialysis can be instituted while specific measures are initiated to correct these factors.

Renal failure due to amyloid deposition, plasma cell infiltration, myeloma kidney or Bence-Jones protein precipitation carry a more serious prognosis and is usually not readily responsive to treatment and generally leads to unrelenting severe uremia and death. In addition to supportive measures, specific myeloma chemotherapy should be given. During dialysis we have used 200 mg intravenous cyclophosphamide given immediately after dialysis and titrated doses against the granulocyte and platelet counts. In patients with chronic renal failure, oral chemotherapy with melphalan may be given at half the usual dose. In renal failure there is some concern that the addition of steroids might not be helpful and might even shorten the survival of the patients.

Anemia. Effective chemotherapy will reverse the anemia due to bone marrow replacement by plasma cells. In the absence of iron deficiency or megaloblastic dyserythropoiesis due to folate and vitamin B_{12} deficiency, there is no specific treatment for anemia except red blood cell transfusion. Transfusions should be used to keep the red cell mass at a level which keeps the patient comfortable. It should also be recognized that anemia may occur for the first time or may increase in severity during the period of active chemotherapy, radiotherapy, infection or uremia, and more frequent transfusions may be required.

Androgens have been used to treat anemia in patients with multiple myeloma without definite evidence of its benefit. In newly treated patients when testosterone was used in addition to melphalan and prednisone, and compared to patients receiving melphalan and steroids alone, there was no evidence that testosterone was more effective in raising hemoglobin levels. Both regimens were more effective in correcting anemia than the use of melphalan alone.

Hypercalcemia is a frequent finding in multiple myeloma and if unchecked can lead to nausea, vomiting, dehydration, renal failure, cardiac arrhythmias, coma and death. Prompt reversal of hypercalcemia may correct the renal failure. Although chemotherapy may cause a significant drop in the elevated serum calcium, it is desirable to use ancillary measures such as prompt hydration with intravenous sodium sulfate or sodium chloride solution which increase the tubular exchange for calcium. In addition, patients should be encouraged to ambulate quickly. In those instances where there is a lack of response to these measures and in the presence of a serum calcium of 12.5 mg/100 ml or higher, more active therapy is indicated. The use of oral corticosteroids such as prednisone, at a dose of 40–60 mg daily or the equivalent parenterally, in most instances will lower the serum calcium within a week. If more rapid and vigorous treatment is indicated, oral phosphate can be used at a dosage of 1.5–2.5 g per day in 3–4 divided doses which can be reduced to 0.75–1.5 g daily following a drop in the serum calcium. Blood urea nitrogen and serum calcium and phosphorus should be carefully monitored. The use of intravenous phosphate is associated with serious side effects and is used infrequently.

In very severe or resistant hypercalcemia, the cytotoxic drug mithramycin has been found to be effective at a dosage level of 15 μg per kg daily for 4 days (Stamp et al., 1975). Mithramycin is believed to exert its effect by inhibiting osteoclastic activity which is apparently independent of its antitumor activity. In a desperate situation, plasmapheresis or hemodialysis can be used to achieve temporary benefits until other therapy has become effective.

Hyperuricemia is frequently found in patients with multiple myeloma and its major serious consequence is the nephrotoxic effects of uric acid. In anticipation of chemotherapy, all patients with normal or elevated serum uric acid levels should be adequately hydrated and given allopurinol at least 3 days prior to treatment to decrease the load of uric acid presented to the kidney. Allopurinol inhibits xanthine oxidase and thereby prevents the oxidation of hypoxanthine to xanthine and the latter to uric acid. Hypoxanthine and xanthine are more soluble and are more readily cleared by the kidney. In the presence of very elevated levels of uric acid, chemotherapy should not be instituted until the uric acid has returned to normal. The initial dosage of allopurinol can range from 400–1200 mg daily. Occasionally renal shutdown may result from hyperuricemia during chemotherapy in patients not prepared by lowering the serum uric acid level. In patients whose urine shows significant numbers of uric acid crystals, alkalinization of the urine is also indicated to keep the pH above 6.0.

Neurologic. The most serious treatable neurologic complication is paraplegia which, if detected early enough, can be prevented or reversed in most instances. If paraplegia persists more than several hours, the neurologic damage may be irreversible. Frequent neurologic examinations are essential in patients who present with evidence of weakness or loss of reflexes in the lower extremities. These patients must be considered an emergency and immediate myelography and subsequent treatment must be instituted. If weakness and diminished reflexes are found, local intensive radiotherapy should be instituted to the site of the lesion. In the face of progression of the neurologic findings, emergency neurosurgery must be done. From the very outset, a neurosurgeon should be intimately involved in evaluating and following such patients. Clinically severe spinal cord and nerve root compression in the thoracic and cervical regions are much less common but a similar approach would be indicated.

Polyneuropathy is an infrequent finding which may be due to amyloidosis or be "idiopathic" as in other malignancies. It usually does not respond to any therapy. Localized neuropathy should be treated with a course of local radiotherapy even in the absence of a demonstrable lesion.

Hyperviscosity is an infrequent complication and gives rise to neurologic, bleeding and retinal manifestations as well as findings secondary to hypervolemia. These include lethargy, coma, seizures, retinopathy including venous dilation and engorgement, mucosal bleeding, congestive heart failure and renal failure. Symptoms usually do not occur until the serum viscosity approaches a value of 5.0 when compared to saline, which has a value of 1.0. Many patients are asymptomatic with serum viscosity values much above 5.0. Treatment consists of removing the paraprotein which can be done most efficiently with a blood cell separator. Plasmapheresis, using blood collection bags designed for this purpose, facilitate the removal of plasma from 2–4 liters of blood daily. These procedures permit the return of autologous red blood cells to the patient. The removal of plasma is only a temporary measure and must be accompanied by intensive chemotherapy to reduce the paraprotein load.

Hemorrhagic. The bleeding diathesis seen in multiple myeloma due to thrombocytopenia or hyperviscosity is treated with platelet transfusions or plasma removal, respectively. The other causes are not generally responsive to any treatment except, rarely, chemotherapy.

Cryoglobulinemia resulting in peripheral gangrene with occasional need for amputation has been responsive to intensive plasmapheresis. In addition, the patient's extremities should be kept warm and chemotherapy instituted.

Solitary intramedually or extramedullary plasma cell tumors (usually found in the respiratory tract) are treated by excision, if possible, and localized radiotherapy. In most instances, generalized disease appears after varying periods of time.

REFERENCES

Alexanian, R., Haut, A., Khan, A. U., McKelvey, E. M., Migliore, P. J., Stuckey Jr., W. J., and Wilson, H. E. Treatment of multiple myeloma. J.A.M.A. *208:* 1680–1685, 1969.

Alexanian, R., Bonnet, J., Gehan, E., Haut, A., Hewlett, J., Lane, M., Monto, R., and Wilson, H. Combination chemotherapy for multiple myeloma. Cancer, *30:* 382–389, 1972.

Alexanian, R., Balcerzak, S., Gehan, E., Haut, A., and Hewlett, J. Remission maintenance therapy for multiple myeloma. Arch. Intern. Med., *135:* 147–152, 1975.

Alexanian, R., Gehan, E., Haut, A., Saiki, J., and Weick, J. Unmaintained remissions in multiple myeloma. Blood, *51:* 1005–1011, 1978.

Bergsagel, D. E., Cowan, D. H., and Nasselback, R. Plasma cell myeloma; response of melphalan-resistant patients to high dose intermittent cyclophosphamide. Can. Med. Assoc. J., *107:* 851–855, 1972.

Bergsagel, D. E., Phil, D., and Pruzanski, W. Treatment of plasma cell myeloma with cytoxic agents. Arch. Intern. Med., *135:* 172–176, 1975.

Bloch, K. J., and Maki, D. G. Hyperviscosity syndromes associated with immunoglobin abnormalities. Semin. Hematol., *10:* 113–124, 1973.

Broder, S., Humphrey, R., Durm, M., Blackman, M., Meade, B., Goldman, C., Strober, W., and Waldmann, T. Impaired synthesis of polyclonal (non-protein) immunoglobulins by circulating lymphocytes from patients with multiple myeloma. N. Eng. J. Med., **293:** 887–892, 1975.

Brodsky, I., Dennis, L. H., and DeCastro, N. A., Brady, L., and Kahn, S. B. Effect of testosterone enanthate and alkylating agents on multiple myeloma. J.A.M.A., *193:* 874–878, 1965.

Cancer and Leukemia Group B. Correlation of abnormal immunoglobulin with clinical features of myeloma. Arch. Intern. Med., *135:* 46–52, 1975.

Cohen, P. Fluoride and calcium therapy for myeloma bone lesions. J.A.M.A., *198:* 583–586, 1966.

Cohen, H. J., and Rundles, R. W. Managing the complications of plasma cell myeloma. Arch. Intern. Med., *135:* 177–184, 1975.

Cornes, J. S., Jones, T. G., and Fischer, G. B. The incidence of carcinoma in patients dying from leukaemia, malignant disorders of plasma cells and malignant lymphoma. Br. J. Cancer, *15:* 200–205, 1961.

Costa, G., Engle, R. L., Jr., Schilling, A., Carbone, P., Kochwa, S., and Glidewell, O. Melphalan and prednisone; an effective combination for the treatment of multiple myeloma. Am. J. Med., *54:* 589–599, 1973.

Durie, B. G. M., and Salmon, S. E. Clinical staging system for multiple myeloma. Cancer, *36:* 842–854, 1975.

Engle, Jr., R. L., and Wallis, L. A. Immunoglobulinopathies, p. 131. Charles C Thomas, Springfield, Ill., 1969.

Farhangi, M., and Osserman, E. F. Treatment of multiple myeloma. Semin. Hematol., *10:* 149–161, 1973.

Fisher, E. R., Perez-Stable, E., and Zawadski, Z. A. Ultrastructural renal changes in multiple myeloma with comments relative to the mechanism of proteinuria. Lab. Invest., *13:* 1561–1574, 1964.

George, R. P., Poth, J. L., Gordon, D., and Schrier, S. L. Multiple myeloma—intermittent, combination chemotherapy compared to continuous therapy. Cancer, *29:* 1665–1670, 1972.

Glenner, G. G., Terry, W. D. and Isersky, C. Amyloidosis; its nature and pathogenesis. Semin. Hematol., *10:* 65–86, 1973.

Gordan, G. S., Roof, B. S., and Halden, A. Skeletal effects of cancer and their management.

In Cancer Medicine, edited by J. F. Holland and E. Frei III, p. 2018. Lea & Febiger, Philadelphia, 1973.

Grey, H. M., and Kohler, P. F. Cryoimmunoglobulins. Semin. Hematol., *10:* 87–112, 1973.

Hammack, W. J., Huguley, C. M., and Chan, Y. K. Treatment of myeloma; comparison of melphalan, chlorambucil and azathioprine. Arch. Intern. Med., *135:* 157–182, 1975.

Harley, J. B., Schilling, A., and Glidewell, O. Ineffectiveness of fluoride therapy in multiple myeloma. N. Engl. J. Med., *286:* 1283–1288, 1972.

Hobbs, J. R. Monitoring myelomatosis. Arch. Intern. Med., *135:* 125–130, 1975.

Imawari, M., Nobuharn, A., Miyuki, I., Beppu, H., Suzuki, H., and Yoshitoshi, Y. Syndrome of plasma cell dyscrasia, polyneuropathy, and endocrine disturbances. Ann. Intern. Med., *81:* 490–493, 1974.

Jancelewicz, Z., Takatsuki, K., Sugain, S., and Pruzanski, W. IgD multiple myeloma. Arch. Intern. Med., *135:* 87–93, 1975.

Kochwa, S., Makuka, E., and Frangione, B. Chemical typing of immunoglobulins and their subtypes. Arch. Intern. Med., *135:* 37–39, 1975.

Kyle, R. A. Multiple myeloma; review of 869 cases. Mayo Clinic Proc., *50:* 29–40, 1975.

Kyle, R. A., Jowsey, J., Phil, D., Kelly, P. J., and Taves, D. R. Multiple myeloma bone disease. N. Engl. J. Med., *293:* 1334–1338, 1975.

Lackner, H. Hemostatic abnormalities associated with dysproteinemias. Semin. Hematol., *10:* 125–133, 1973.

Lee, B. J., Sahakian, G., Clarkson, B. D., and Krakoff, I. H. 1974. Combination chemotherapy of multiple myeloma with Alkeran, Cytoxan, vincristine, prednisone, and BCNU. Cancer, *33:* 533–538, 1974.

Levi, D. F., William, R. C., Jr., and Lindstrom, F. D. Immunofluorescent studies of the multiple myeloma kidney with special reference to light chain disease. Am. J. Med., *44:* 922–933, 1968.

Maldonada, J. E., and Kyle, R. A. Familial myeloma. Am. J. Med., *57:* 875–884, 1974.

Mass, R. E. A comparison of the effect of prednisone and a placebo in the treatment of multiple myeloma. Cancer Chemother. Rep., *16:* 257–259,1962.

Maugh, T. H. Chalones; chemical regulation of cell division. Science, *176:* 1407–1408, 1972.

Meyers, B. R., Hirschman, S. Z., and Axelrod, J. A. Current patterns of infection in multiple myeloma. Am. J. Med., *52:* 87–92, 1972.

Mundy, G. R., Raisz, L. G., Cooper, R. A., Schechter, G. P., and Salmon, S. E. Evidence for the secretion of an osteoclast stimulating factor in myeloma. N. Engl. J. Med., *291:* 1041–1046, 1974.

Osserman, E. F. Plasma cell myeloma; II. Clinical aspects. N. Engl. J. Med., *261:* 952–960, 1959.

Rosen, B. Multiple myeloma; a clinical review. Med. Clin. North Am., *59:* 375–386, 1975.

Rosner, F., and Grunwald, H. Multiple myeloma terminating in acute leukemia. Am. J. Med., *57:* 927–939, 1974.

Salmon, S. E. Immunoglobulin synthesis and tumor kinetics of multiple myeloma. Semin. Hematol., *10:* 135–144, 1973.

Salmon, S. E. Paraneoplastic syndromes associated with monoclonal lymphocyte and plasma cell proliferation. Ann. N.Y. Acad. Sci., *230:* 228–239, 1974.

Salmon, S. E., Hamburger, A. W., Soehnlen, B., Durie, B. G. M., Alberts, D. S., and Moon, T. E. Quantitation of differential sensitivity of human tumor cells in anticancer drugs. N. Engl. J. Med., *298:* 1321–1327, 1978.

Shustik, C., Bergsagel, D. E., and Pruzanski, W. κ and λ light chain disease; survival rates and clinical manifestations. Blood, *48:* 41–51, 1976.

Schilling, A., and Finkel, H. E. Ancillary measures in treatment of myeloma. Arch. Intern. Med., *135:* 193–196, 1975.

Snapper, I., and Kahn, A. 1971. Myelomatosis, p. 308. University Park Press, Baltimore, 1971.

Southwest Oncology Group Study. Remission maintenance therapy for multiple myeloma. Arch. Intern. Med., *135:* 147–152, 1975.

Stamp, T. C. B., Child, J. A., and Walker, P. G. Treatment of osteolytic myelomatosis with mithramycin. Lancet, *1:* 719–722, 1975.

Wilson, H. E., Bonnet, J. D., and Gehan, E. A. Combination chemotherapy of multiple myeloma. *In* Proceedings of the American Society of Hematology, San Francisco, p. 45, 1971.

Chapter 11

Waldenström's Macroglobulinemia

DANIEL B. KIMBALL, JR., M.D.

Primary macroglobulinemia is a malignant lymphoproliferative disorder, characterized by lymphoid hyperplasia, including lymphocytic infiltration of the bone marrow and the presence of a monoclonal paraprotein of the IgM class in the plasma. Clinically, the syndrome has features related both to the malignant lymphomas and multiple myeloma (Osserman, 1971). Waldenström (1944) originally described three patients with anemia, increased erythrocyte sedimentation rate, lowered fibrinogen levels, and an increased level of serum globulin. Subsequent attempts at determining the antigenic specificity of these γ M antibodies have been generally unrewarding (Krause, 1970).

The clinical presentation of primary macroglobulinemia is quite variable, but is often characterized by mucosal bleeding, variable degrees of hepatosplenomegaly and lymphadenopathy, mental alterations, decreased visual acuity, anemia of a multifactorial etiology and features of the hyperviscosity syndrome (Wintrobe et al., 1974). Patients tend to be over 50 years of age, with two-thirds of the patients in most series being over 60 years of age. The symptoms and signs of the hyperviscosity syndrome may be quite nonspecific, including anorexia, easy fatigability, and extreme weakness. Specifically, with regard to the central nervous system, in addition to the mental changes and altered visual acuity already noted, headaches, vertigo, nystagmus, deafness, postural hypotention, dizziness, stupor, and generalized seizures have all been described. Cardiopulmonary manifestations include congestive heart failure. Cold sensitivity and Raynaud's phenomena are occasionally seen in this disorder secondary to cryoproperties of the IgM protein. In contrast to the situation in multiple myeloma, bone pain is not a prominent symptom, and skeletal lesions have only been rarely reported in this disorder (Bergsagel, 1977; Leb et al., 1977).

Anemia is present in at least 80–90% of patients. It is usually described as normocytic-normochromic, and, as noted above, is felt to be multifactorial in etiology, including inadequate red blood cell production with a component of decreased red cell survival, with some iron deficiency related to the bleeding syndrome. When Coombs' positive hemolytic disease occurs, it should be suspected that one is dealing with primary cold agglutinin disease (Isbister et al., 1978); we have observed such a case with Dutcher bodies in the bone marrow. The white blood cell count is usually normal, however neutropenia is occasionally found when there is marked infiltration of the bone marrow. Rouleaux or agglutination may be prominent on the peripheral smear. The sedimentation rate is usually markedly increased. Thrombocytopenia is usually mild, but again may be marked due to extensive infiltration of the marrow and/or hypersplenism. Typically the bone marrow in primary macroglobulinemia reveals an increase in lymphocytes, often described as being plasmacytoid in appearance, with often additionally an increase in mast cells.

A common hematologic manifestation is bleeding, which is usually mucosal in origin, although purpura is not uncommon. Bleeding may contribute significantly to the presentation or clinical course of these patients, and various explanations in the laboratory have been given for this clinical phenomenon. The abnormal immunoglobulin has been described as having antifactor VIII activity, antithrombin activity, and it has been suggested that inhibition of platelet function and thromboplastin may also occur (Lackner, 1973; Castaldi and Penny, 1970).

On protein electrophoresis, a sharp peak or dense band migrating in the β- or γ-globulin region is usually noted, and the Sia water test is ordinarily positive. It must be realized that this test is nonspecific, and has been associated with positive reactions in which γ-G globulins have been elevated and probably have formed complexes. Analysis of the elevated protein spike by immunoelectrophoresis should specifically identify it as an IgM protein, although exceptions do occur (Tursz et al., 1977). Gamma-M monoclonal spikes represent 4–10% of all monoclonal spikes (Alexanian, 1972; Ritzmann et al., 1970; Axelsson et al., 1966; Ameis et al., 1976). An increase in the serum viscosity is a common finding (36%) in patients with primary macroglobulinemia, and it is the level of the circulating IgM that correlates best with the presence and degree of symptomatology of the hyperviscosity syndrome (MacKenzie and Babcock, 1975; Bloch and Maki, 1973; Mannik, 1974; Franklin and Buxbaum, 1977; MacKenzie and Lee, 1977). Approximately 20–40% of these proteins have cryoproperties and correlate with the presence of Raynaud's phenomenon (Hermans, 1969). Bence-Jones proteinuria is said to be less common in macroglobulinemia than in multiple myeloma (Bergsagel, 1977), but this may depend on how carefully one seeks such findings (Krajny and Pruzanski, 1976).

Other interesting clinical manifestations are also found in this syndrome, among which are neurologic manifestations usually attributed to the hyperviscosity syndrome. A polyneuropathy has been described which has been attributed to amyloidosis, but a recent report (Iwashita et al., 1974) noted a sensorimotor polyneuropathy without amyloid deposition, but associated with the deposition of a hyalin-like substance related to IgM. These authors observed improvement in the polyneuropathy following appropriate treatment of the disorder. In addition, a malabsorption-like syndrome has been described (Bedine et al., 1973), and pleuropulmonary manifestations may include mass lesions in the lung, reticulonodular infiltrates and pleural effusions (Winterbauer et al., 1974). Renal manifestations of this disorder have been uncommon (MacKenzie and Fudenberg, 1972; Wells and Fudenberg, 1974), although recently an interesting patient was reported who had manifestations of a nephrotic syndrome with deposition of immunoglobulins G and M, as well as complement, on the kidney basement membrane (Martelo et al., 1975). The nephrotic syndrome improved following treatment of the primary macroglobulinemia. A questionable case with spontaneous splenic rupture has also been reported (Karakousis and Elias, 1974).

The disease may run a variable course, anywhere from 2 to 10 years, but in general the duration of survival is approximately 3–5 years (Cohen et al.,1966; MacKenzie and Fudenberg, 1972; Carter et al., 1977). It has been suggested that the patients who survive longest may have a benign monoclonal gammopathy of the IgM type. As noted earlier, the manifestations are generally those of a paraproteinemia and lymphoma. Therapy in general is aimed in two directions, first, against the manifestations of the hyperviscosity syndrome which basically relates to various methods of acutely and chronically reducing the paraprotein, and secondly, directed against the presumably abnormal lymphocyte, which is proliferating. As in chronic lymphocytic leukemia, it is felt that asymptomatic patients who have stable, nonaggressive disease require no therapy (Waldenström, 1965), although these are probably less common in primary macroglobulinemia than in chronic lymphocytic leukemia. The presence of symptomatic hyperviscosity requires vigorous therapeutic intervention (Perry and Hoagland, 1976) which usually includes plasmapheresis and the administration of an alkylating agent, dual therapy which is designed to remove increased amounts of immunoglobulin M in the circulation and reduce its production. Such a program might include an induction regimen, which includes the removal of two units of plasma per day for 5–7 days, and if there is symptomatic improvement at that time, a maintenance program of weekly plasmapheresis. Rapid, objective improvement of hyperviscosity retinopathy with increased retinal blood flow can be noted following plasmapheresis (Grindle et al., 1976). If, despite such a plasmapheresis program, there is not symptomatic improvement, the addition of chlorambucil, 2 mg per day, should be considered (Fudenberg, 1972). Chronic plasmapheresis is well tolerated (Lawson et al., 1968; Sakalova et al., 1973; Solomon and Fahey, 1963; Buskard et al., 1977), and, if necessary, because of the symptomatology and amount of protein present, the rapid removal of a larger volume of plasma may be accomplished utilizing a cell separator (Powles et al., 1971; Pitterman et al., 1975). Fudenberg has had excellent success in maintaining his patients on plasmapheresis alone, while other investigators have combined plasmapheresis with either single or combination agent chemotherapy. Effective chemotherapeutic agents have included chlorambucil, cyclophosphamide, phenylalanine mustard, Adriamycin, bleomycin, vincristine and prednisone. Prednisone as a single agent does not appear to be very effective, although it has reported efficacy in the treatment of hemolytic anemia and resulted in one case in improvement of the hyperviscosity syndrome secondary to cryo-gel properties of the IgM (Pitney et al., 1958; Hoogstraten, 1973; O'Reilly and MacKenzie, 1967). Most chemotherapeutic treatment experience seems to have been with chlorambucil and cyclophosphamide. Continuous cyclophosphamide (Bouroncle et al., 1964), continuous chlorambucil (Clatanoff and Meyer, 1963; Cohen et al., 1966; Fudenberg, 1972; McCallister et al., 1967) and continuous phenylalanine mustard (MacKenzie and Fudenberg, 1972) have all been successful at inducing remissions in primary macroglobulinemia. Response rates of 40–50% are expected, with durations of response averaging 2–3 years. A combination program of chlorambucil and prednisone, given on an intermittent basis for 14 days at 6–8 week intervals, combined with plasmapheresis, has recently been advocated (Ruiz and Alexanian, 1974). Because of the clinical similarity of this disorder to lymphoproliferative diseases, a patient failing to respond to a single agent may respond to a combination such as cyclophosphamide, vincristine and prednisone given on an intermittent basis, as is commonly used in the non-Hodgkin's lymphomas. Inconclusive data has been reported for a multiple alkylating agent regimen (Arlin et al., 1977). Local irradiation to the spleen has been used successfully to induce a remission in one case that had previously failed on chlorambucil (Wanebo and Clarkson, 1965), but the experience with irradiation therapy in this disorder is very limited. Again, its relationship to the other lymphoproliferative disorders suggests that, if there were a local mechanical problem due to lymphadenopathy and/or splenomegaly that was unresponsive to plasmapheresis and/or chemotherapy, a trial of local radiation would be worthwhile. Following the failure of a single alkylating agent to maintain a remission, there is probably no particular advantage in resorting to the use of another single alkylating agent administered on a continuous basis, although high dose intermittent use might be a reasonable alternative. The role of penicillamine therapy has been evaluated incompletely.

REFERENCES

Ameis, A., Ko, H. S., and Pruzanski, W. M components—a review of 1242 cases. Can. Med. Assoc. J., *114:* 889–895, 1976.

Alexanian, R. Multiple myeloma and related disorders. *In* Hematology: Principles and Practice, edited by C. E. Mengel, E. Frei III, and R. Nachman, pp. 538–539. Year Book Medical Publishers, Chicago, 1972.

Arlin, A., Lee, B. J., and Clarkson, B. Combination chemotherapy (M-2 protocol) of Waldenström's macroglobulinemia with melphalan, cyclophosphamide, vincristine and BCNU. Proc. Am. Soc. Clin. Oncol., *18:* 337, 1977.

Axelsson, U., Bachmann, R., and Hällen, J. Frequency of pathological proteins (M-components) in 6,995 sera from an adult population. Acta Med. Scand., *179:* 235–247, 1966.

Bedine, M. S., Yardley, J. H., Elliott, H. L., Banwell, J. G., and Hendrix, T. R. Intestinal involvement in Waldenström's macroglobulinemia. Gastroenterology, *65:* 308–315, 1973.

Bergsagel, D. E. Macroglobulinemia. *In* Hematology, edited by W. J. Williams, E. Beutler, A. J. Erslev, and R. W. Rundles, Ed. 2, pp. 1126–1131. McGraw-Hill, New York, 1977.

Bouroncle, B. A., Datta, P., and Frajola, W. J. Waldenström's macroglobulinemia; report of three patients treated with cyclophosphamide. J.A.M.A., *189:* 729–732, 1964.

Bloch, K. L., and Maki, D. G. Hyperviscosity syndromes associated with immunoglobulin abnormalities. Semin. Hematol., *10:* 113–124, 1973.

Buskard, N. A., Galton, D. A. G., Goldman, S. M., Kohner, E. M., Grindle, D. F. J., Newman, D. L., Twinn, K. W., and Lowenthal, R. M. Plasma exchange in the long-term management of Waldenström's macroglobulinemia. Can. Med. Assoc., J., *117:* 135–137, 1977.

Castaldi, O. A., and Penny, R. A macroglobulin with inhibitory activity against coagulation factor VIII. Blood, *35:* 370–376, 1970.

Carter, P., Koval, J. J., and Hobbs, J. R. The relation of clinical and laboratory findings to the survival of patients with macroglobulinemia. Clin. Exp. Immunol., *28:* 241–249, 1977.

Clatanoff, D. V., and Meyer, O. O. Response to chlorambucil in macroglobulinemia. J.A.M.A., *183:* 40–44, 1963.

Cohen, R. J., Bohannon, R. A., and Wallerstein, R. O. Waldenström's macroglobulinemia; a study of 10 cases. J.A.M.A., *41:* 274–284, 1966.

Dutcher, T. F., and Fahey, J. L. The histopathology of the macroglobulinemia of Waldenström. J. Natl. Cancer Inst., *22:* 887–918, 1959.

Franklin, E. C., and Buxbaum, J. Immunoglobulin structure, synthesis, secretion, and relation to neoplasms of B cells. Clin. Haematol., *6:* 503–532, 1977.

Fudenberg, H. H. Waldenström's macroglobulinemia. *In* Cancer Chemotherapy II. Twenty-second Hahnemann Symposium, edited by I. Brodsky, S. B. Kahn, and J. H. Moyer. Grune & Stratton, New York, 1972.

Grindle, D. F. J., Buskard, N. A., and Newman, D. L. Hyperviscosity retinopathy; a scientific approach to therapy. Trans. Ophthal. Soc. U.K., *96:* 216–219, 1976.

Hermans, P. E. Immunoglobulin abnormalities in man. Arch. Environ. Health, *19:* 838–848, 1969.

Hoogstraten, B. Steroid therapy of multiple myeloma and macroglobulinemia. Med. Clin. North Am., *57:* 1321–1330, 1973.

Isbister, J. P., Cooper, D. A., Blake, H. M., Biggs, J. C., Dixon, R. A., and Penny, R. Lymphoproliferative disease with IgM lamda monoclonal protein and autoimmune hemolytic anemia; a report of four cases and a review of the literature. Am. J. Med., *64:* 434–440, 1978.

Iwashita, H., Artyrakis, A., Lowitzsch, K., and Spaar, F. W. Polyneuropathy in Waldenström's macroglobulinemia. Neurol. Sci., *21:* 341–354, 1974.

Karakousis, C. P., and Elias, E. G. Spontaneous (pathologic) rupture of spleen in malignancies. Surgery, *78:* 674–677, 1974.

Krause, R. M. The search for antibodies with molecular uniformity. Adv. Immunol., *12:* 1–56, 1970.

Krajny, M., and Pruzanski, W. Waldenström's macroglobulinemia; review of 45 cases. Can. Med. Assoc. J., *114:* 899–905, 1976.

Lackner, H. Hemostatic abnormalities associated with dysproteinemias. Semin. Hematol., *10:* 125–133, 1973.

Lawson, N. S., Nosanchuk, J. S., Oberman, H. A., and Meyers, M. C. Therapeutic plasmapheresis in treatment of patients with Waldenström's macroglobulinemia. Transfusion, *8:* 174–178, 1968.

Leb, L., Grimes, E. T., Balogh, K., and Merritt, J. A. Monoclonal macroglobulinemia with osteolytic lesions; a case report and review of the literature. Cancer, *39:* 227–231, 1977.

MacKenzie, M. R., and Babcock, J. Studies of the hyperviscosity syndrome. II. Macroglobulinemia. J. Lab. Clin. Med., *85:* 227–234, 1975.

MacKenzie, M. R., and Fudenberg, H. H. Macroglobulinemia; an analysis of forty patients. Blood, *39:* 874–879, 1972.

MacKenzie, M. R., and Fudenberg, H. H. Macroglobulinemia; an analysis of forty patients. Blood, *39:* 874–879, 1972.

MacKenzie, M. R., and Lee, T. K. Blood viscosity in Waldenström macroglobulinemia. Blood, *49:* 507–510, 1977.

Mannik, M. Blood viscosity in Waldenström's macroglobulinemia. Blood, *44:* 87–98, 1974.

Martelo, O. J., Schultz, D. R., Pardo, V., and Perez-Stable, E. Immunologically mediated renal disease in Waldenström's macroglobulinemia. Am. J. Med., *58:* 567–575, 1975.

McCallister, B., Bayrd, E., Harrison, E., and McGuckin, W. Primary macroglobulinemia; review with a report on thirty-one cases and notes on the value of continuous chlorambucil therapy. Am. J. Med., *43:* 394–434, 1967.

Osserman, E. R. Multiple myeloma and related plasma cell dyscrasias. *In* Immunological Diseases, edited by M. Santer, Ed. 2, pp. 534–536. Little, Brown, Boston, 1971.

Perry, M. C., and Hoagland, H. C. The hyperviscosity syndrome. J.A.M.A., *236:* 392–393, 1976.

Pitney, W. R., O'Sullivan, W. J., and Owen, J. A. Effect of prednisolone and anaemia associated with macroglobulinaemia. Br. Med. J., *2:* 1508–1510, 1958.

Pittermann, E., Hocker, P., Lechner, K., and Stacher, A. Plasmapheresis with the continuous flow blood cell separator in the treatment of macroglobulinaemia, multiple myeloma, haemophilia and hyperlipidaemia. *In* Leucocytes: Separation, Collection and Transfusion, edited by J. M. Goldman and R. M. Lowenthal, pp. 561–567. Academic Press, New York, 1975.

Powles, R., Smith, C., Kohn, J., and Fairley, G. H. Method of removing abnormal protein rapidly from patients with malignant paraproteinaemias. Br. Med. J., *3:* 664–667, 1971.

Pronk, E. A. S., Klein, F., Elkerbout, F., Radema, H., and Cleton, F. J. Therapy of macroglobulinaemia. Acta Med. Scand., *186:* 273–281, 1969.

Ritzmann, S. E., Daniels, J. C., and Levin, W. C. Paralymphomatous disease; the syndrome of macroglobulinemia. *In* Leukemia-Lymphoma, University of Texas M. D. Anderson Hospital and Tumor Institute, pp. 169–222. Year Book Medical Publishers, Chicago, 1970.

Ruiz, V. G., and Alexanian, R. Multiple myeloma and macroglobulinemia; advances in treatment. Postgrad. Med., *55:* 179–185, 1974.

Sakalova, A., Gazova, S., Hrubisko, M., and Galikova, J. Clinical utilization of plasmapheresis and cyclophosphamide in the treatment of malignant lymphoproliferative processes. Neoplasm, *20:* 335–339, 1973.

Solomon, A., and Fahey, J. L. Plasmapheresis therapy in macroglobulinemia. Ann. Intern. Med., *58:* 789–800, 1963.

Tursz, T., Brouet, J. C., Flandrin, G., Danon, F., Clauvel, J. P., and Seligmann, M. Clinical and pathologic features of Waldenströms macroglobulinemia in seven patients with serum monoclonal IgG or IgA. Am. J. Med., *63:* 499–502, 1977.

Waldenström, J. Incipient myelomatosis or "essential" hyperglobulinaemia with fibrinogen-openia—a new syndrome? Acta Med. Scand., *117:* 216–247, 1944.

Waldenström, J. Macroglobulinemia. Adv. Metab. Disord., *2:* 115–158, 1965.

Wanebo, H. J., and Clarkson, B. D. Essential macroglobulinemia; report of a case including immunofluorescent and electron microscopic studies. Ann. Intern. Med., *62:* 1025–1045, 1965.

Wells, J. V., and Fudenberg, H. H. Paraproteinemias. DM, February: 1–45, 1974.

Winterbauer, R. H., Riggins, R. C. K., and Bauermeister, D. E. Pleuropulmonary manifestations of Waldenström's macroglobulinemia. Chest, *66:* 368–375, 1974.

Wintrobe, M. M., Lee, C. R., Boggs, D. R., Bithell, T. C., Athens, J. W., Foerster, J. (eds.): Macroglobulinemia, heavy chain diseases, and other lymphocyte and plasma cell dyscrasias. *In* Clinical Hematology, Ed. 7, pp. 1624–1630. Lea & Febiger, Philadelphia, 1974.

Chapter 12

Hodgkin's Disease

JOHANNES BLOM, M.D.

In 1832 Thomas Hodgkin described seven patients with a fatal illness in the *Medico-Chirurgical Transactions* under the title of "On some morbid appearances of the absorbent glands and spleen." A similar illness was probably described as early as 1661 by Malpighi; on subsequent histopathologic and clinical review probably only three patients had what is now considered Hodgkin's disease. Although other names have been used and are in use in other countries, the name of Hodgkin is attached to this disease in most English-speaking countries. Dorothy Reed and Carl Sternberg have given the clearest description of the characteristic binucleated giant cell associated with this disease. Although various organisms have been considered as etiologic agents, its true nature, whether infectious in the classical sense or neoplastic, remains obscure. Several investigators have been able to demonstrate a higher than normal incidence among a group of high school students and inhabitants of several geographic areas with a stable population. These were direct patient-to-patient contacts or patient-healthy intermediary-patient contacts, (Vianna et al., 1971, 1972; Heath, 1972). Prior to these epidemiologic studies, incidental cases of Hodgkin's disease among a few close contacts have been reported. More recently, Schimpff et al. (1975) have described leukemia and lymphoma patients who were interlinked by prior social contact and who were all located in stable rural areas. These and other studies favor Hodgkin's disease to be an environmental and possibly an infectious disease (Vianna, 1974; Vianna et al., 1974). Grufferman et al. (1977) detected 5 sibling pairs under the age of 45 in an incidence survey of Hodgkin's disease in Greater Boston during 1959–1973, which means a 7-fold excess. Combining literature series with their own they found that siblings of the same sex as the patient have a risk of Hodgkin's disease double that of siblings of the opposite sex and ascribe this excess of the disease in siblings to either interpersonal transmission of an etiologic agent by prolonged or intimate contact or to common source exposures. McMahon (1966) has indicated an age-specific bimodal incidence curve with a peak around age 25 and a second one around age 70. The same has been reported in other countries with the exception of Japan and the southern United States where the first peak is absent. There is a slightly higher incidence in males and in whites. The incidence in males below the age of 10 is about 4 times that in females.

PATHOLOGY

The great variations in histologic appearance may make one doubt that Hodgkin's disease is a single entity.

Jackson and Parker introduced their histopathologic classification in 1944 which divided Hodgkin's disease in paragranuloma, granuloma and sarcoma (Table 12.1). Patients with paragranuloma had the best and those with sarcoma the worst prognosis; however, since about 90% of all patients belonged in the granuloma category, this classification was of minimal benefit with regard to prognosis. Lukes et al. (1966a) and Lukes and Butler (1966) have proposed a classification with six histologic types that has a better correlation with prognosis. This was based on the evaluation of 377 U.S. Army cases from World War II registered at the Armed Forces Institute of Pathology. A simplified four-category histologic classification was accepted at the International Symposium on Hodgkin's Disease, held at Rye, New York, in 1965 (Lukes et al., 1966b). This is now the most widely used histopathologic classification and is outlined in Table 12.1.

Although the Reed-Sternberg cell has to be present to make a definite diagnosis of Hodgkin's disease, this cell can also be found in a number of other conditions, malignant as well as benign (Strum et al., 1970; McKenna and Brunning, 1975). Therefore, the Reed-Sternberg cell is diagnostic only if it is found in the proper histologic setting. The Reed-Sternberg cells are rarely so numerous that they fill the entire lymph node. The normal architecture of the lymph node may be obliterated by other cells such as lymphocytes of various sizes, histiocytes or "reticulum cells" often resembling Reed-Sternberg cells but with only a single nucleus, plasma cells, eosinophils and fibroblasts plus varying amounts of

TABLE 12.1
Histologic Classification

Rye	Jackson-Parker
Lymphocytic predominance	Granuloma
Nodular sclerosis	
Mixed cellularity	} Paragranuloma
Lymphocytic depletion	Sarcoma

fibrosis and necrosis. Reed-Sternberg cells are very large, many times the size of surrounding cells with abundant pale blue often vacuolated cytoplasm and huge multiple or bilobed nuclei. The nucleoli are large and intensely stained, often surrounded by a clear zone, the nucleoplasm is vacuolated and the nuclear membrane coarse and prominent. In the nodular sclerosing type of Hodgkin's disease, the Reed-Sternberg cell is often extremely large with the cytoplasm somewhat retracted, giving the appearance of the cell lying in a clear space or lacuna. Anagnostou et al. (1977) recently demonstrated the presence of lipid in the cytoplasm of these lacunar cells and suggest, based on their studies, that these may represent transformed lymphocytes and precursors to Reed-Sternberg cells. The nuclear chromatin is delicate and the nucleoli are smaller than in the classical Reed-Sternberg cell. The other typical feature is the presence of bands of collagen, varying from thin strands to almost complete obliteration of the lymph node. In the lymphocytic predominance type the Reed-Sternberg cells are often sparse and may be difficult to detect. The predominant stroma cell is the lymphocyte or occasionally normal-appearing histiocytes. The stroma in the mixed cellularity type is very cellular and pleomorphic with neutrophilic and eosinophilic granulocytes, lymphocytes, plasma cells, histiocytes and fibroblasts. Reed-Sternberg cells may be numerous.

The lymphocytic depletion type is characterized by a marked depletion of lymphocytes and other stromal cells and the presence of coarse, irregular fibrosis that lacks the birefringence of collagen bands present in nodular sclerosis. In areas of extreme fibrosis, the Reed-Sternberg cells may be sparse, but may be numerous in other areas. Progression from lymphocytic predominance to mixed cellularity to lymphocytic depletion in the final stage of the disease with peripheral lymphopenia occurs fairly regularly. Although patients with nodular sclerosis disease generally remain in this category the amount of collagen and the cellularity may change (Strum and Rappaport, 1971).

Lymphocytopenia in advanced Hodgkin's disease has been recognized for some time (Aisenberg, 1965). Schick et al. (1973) studied lymphocyte kinetics with tritiated thymidine autoradiographic analysis in 4 patients with lymphocytopenia and demonstrated an accelerated turnover of lymphocytes and increased lymphocytopoiesis rather than a decreased production. Bobrove et al. (1975) studied peripheral blood T and B lymphocytes in 42 untreated Hodgkin's patients and correlated the findings with the response to phytohemagglutinin (PHA) stimulation and delayed hypersensitivity skin testing. In general, antibody responses—B cell functions—are preserved until the disease is far advanced. Cell mediated immunity—a T cell function—can be disturbed even in early stages of untreated disease. Marked lymphocytopenia (counts less than

1000/cu mm) was found in 21% of the patients in this study, particularly in Stage IIIB and IVB patients, and were a combined T and B cell reduction. Cytotoxicity assay and E rosette assay yielded similar values for the proportions of T lymphocytes in the peripheral blood of normal controls, but the E rosette assay yielded considerably lower values than the cytotoxicity assay in the Hodgkin's patients. This may indicate altered surface activity of some T lymphocytes. Decreased E rosette formation correlated with decreased PHA stimulation. Only 32% and 58% of all the patients had a positive reaction to dinitrochlorobenzene (DNCB) and intradermal antigens, respectively. There was no correlation with PHA response or E rosette formation. This indicates the complexity of the altered cellular immune reactions in Hodgkin's disease and may explain some of the variations in reported abnormalities.

Rappaport and Strum (1970) and Strum et al. (1971a, 1971b) have indicated the high incidence of extranodal spread when vascular invasion could be detected in the biopsy material. Similar findings were reported by Naeim et al. (1974). However, Lamoureux et al. (1973) did not find vascular invasion in a group of 12 patients who developed extranodal disease after their primary treatment. Kirschner et al. (1974) found no evidence of extranodal spread in 4 of 91 patients with vascular invasion in the lymph node. However, 7 of 44 patients who had vascular invasion of the spleen had hepatic and bone marrow metastases, early relapse and shortened survival.

CLINICAL MANIFESTATIONS

Hodgkin's disease patients may present with an enlarged lymph node, which may have fluctuated in size over several months or which may have appeared "overnight"; most frequently this node is located in the left cervical area. A persistent, dry, irritating cough may prompt the physician to order a roentgenogram of the chest which may demonstrate a mediastinal-paratracheal mass. Fever, sometimes cyclic as described by Pel and Ebstein, night sweats, weight loss, and occasionally pruritus may cause the patient to seek medical attention. A variety of other symptoms may occur related to involvement of different sites and organs. Pain, in areas of Hodgkin's involvement, may occur in about 5% of patients minutes after the ingestion of small amounts of all types of alcoholic beverages. This discomfort is severe enough that invariably it will cause the patient to stop drinking. This phenomenon disappears when the patient is in a remission, but may recur as the first symptom of a relapse. Atkinson et al. (1976) found alcohol pain in 7% of their Hodgkin's patients, particularly in women, and in patients with nodular sclerosis and mediastinal involvement. They often found this together with other systemic symptoms and are of the opinion that if specifically asked for this complaint will be found more frequently. Essentially all organs may become involved, often causing specific symptoms and physical findings. Occasionally the patient may present with involvement of a single extranodal site. A mediastinal mass may be discovered on a routine chest roentgenogram.

DIAGNOSTIC EVALUATION

An obviously enlarged lymph node or a suspicious node should be biopsied promptly. The surgeon should be urged to select a large lymph node, by preference a deeper seated one, as small superficial nodes in a large cluster will often reveal a diagnosis of reactive hyperplasia in which case prompt rebiopsy is indicated. Partial resection of a node should also be avoided as this may greatly distort the architecture of the specimens. Prompt fixation, after bisection in case of a large specimen, will facilitate good processing. Whenever a diagnosis of Hodgkin's disease is made, a thorough and extensive evaluation to determine the extent of the disease is indicated before a treatment plan can be made.

A thorough history with particular inquiry with regard to fever, night sweats and weight loss, which connote a less favorable prognosis, is mandatory.

A physical examination with particular emphasis on all lymph node bearing areas, nasopharynx, liver and spleen can be most helpful in determining the extent and prognosis of the disease. Multiple small nodes often indicate extensive disease, mesenteric nodes included, while a limited number of large nodes connote a better prognosis; involvement of multiple nodal regions above the diaphragm with mediastinal involvement has a better prognosis than without mediastinal involvement (Peters, 1971). High cervical presentation (submental, submaxillary or jugular node involvement) may have subsequent spread to supraclavicular or occasionally axillary nodes, but mediastinal involvement was never found in 101 patients with such presentation (Teillet et al., 1971). An occasional patient may have a more or less generalized ichthyosiform eruption of the skin which will clear when the patient responds to therapy. A careful neurologic examination is indicated to detect signs indicating spinal cord compression. Occasionally peripheral neuropathy is present without Hodgkin's disease involvement of the nervous system. This will subside when the patient enters remission.

Roentgenologic examinations should include posteroanterior and lateral films of the chest with whole lung tomography, particularly if there is mediastinal-paratracheal involvement, unless there is obvious involvement of other organs, indicating advanced disease. Castellino et al. (1976) found routine full lung tomograms to have extremely low yield of pertinent additional information in patients with unequivocally normal stereographic posteroanterior (PA) and lateral chest films. Bipedal lymphangiography is indicated when there is no obvious extralymphatic disease. In a prospective study (Castellino, 1974), 149 lymphangiograms obtained in 176 unselected patients with Hodgkin's disease were evaluable with histologic correlation. There was 100% accuracy in 87 lymphograms interpreted as normal and in 11 interpreted as benign. Of 51 lymphograms interpreted as representing tumor, only in 39 patients were the histologic findings confirmative with a 76% accuracy. The overall accuracy in this group of patients was 92%. Although lymphangiography in patients with severe pulmonary dysfunction may be hazardous, LaMonte and Lacher (1973) have reported that with reduced doses (8–14 ml) of ethiodized oil satisfactory lymphograms can be obtained without oil embolization and deterioration of pulmonary function. A skeletal survey with a bone scan should be done to detect asymptomatic bone lesions. Liver and spleen scan may be helpful to detect abnormalities of both organs. Liver scan abnormalities, with or without liver function abnormalities, may require percutaneous liver biopsy or peritoneoscopy with liver biopsy under direct vision. Excretory urograms with across-the-table lateral films should be performed by preference after the lymphangiogram to determine renal size and function and the course of the ureters. However, ureteral deviation requires rather marked lymph node enlargement and this study is, therefore, rather insensitive to demonstrate abdominal lymph nodes. The inferior vena cavogram was found to be useful in defining abnormalities in the area above the confluence of lymph ducts forming the cisterna chyli which represents the blind area of lymphangiography (Abrams et al., 1968). The yield of cavography and urography was minimal with clearly negative lymphangiograms. Gallium-67 (^{67}Ga) citrate localizes in Hodgkin's disease and other malignant lymphoreticular neoplasms, but also in inflammatory tissue and some normal organs. Total body gallium scanning has, therefore, limited value in demonstrating disease below the diaphragm, but has been found to be highly accurate in demonstrating disease above the diaphragm, particularly unsuspected sites of extranodal involvement (Hoffer et al., 1973). However, most cases of pulmonary involvement are also evident on roentgenograms (Peckham, 1973). Computerized axial tomography (CAT) scanning is the most recent addition to the diagnostic armamentarium and is particularly useful for the assessment of involvement of mesenteric lymph nodes, high retroperitoneal nodes and extranodal sites in the abdomen (Jones et al., 1978). Ultrasonography can also be helpful in the detection and follow-up of abdominal masses, although it cannot differentiate between lymphoma and reactive process. Lymphangiography remains indicated for the detection of smaller node masses (Filly et al., 1976). Routine laboratory tests include a complete blood count with platelet count, sedimentation rate, urinalysis, alkaline phosphatase, with fractionation in case of abnormal values and uncertain etiology, blood urea nitrogen and serum uric acid. The sedimentation rate is one of the cheapest and most reliable indicators of activity of disease, but must be interpreted in the light of other findings and should never be taken as a single indication for treatment. The greatest value is in its use during follow-up. However, it should be kept in mind that it may remain elevated for a year or longer after extensive radiation therapy (Tubiana, 1971). Bone marrow needle biopsy plus an aspiration or a surgical biopsy should be performed, particularly in more advanced stages of the disease or if there is any indication of possible bone involvement. Nineteen of 174 patients were found to have positive bone marrow biopsies at the National Cancer Institute (Myers et al., 1974). In all cases marrow fibrosis was present. The relationship between immune parameters such as skin test reactivity, lymphocyte response to mitogen stimulation and prognosis is presently not clear (Case et al., 1976).

After this extensive evaluation a clinical assessment of the extent of the disease can be made. Several investigators have proposed classifications of Hodgkin's disease that have prognostic significance. The classification adopted at the Rye Conference in 1965 (Table 12.2) is probably the most widely used (Rosenberg, 1966). Subsequently several investigators have pointed out that localized extranodal involvement does not have the same ominous prognosis as generalized organ involvement and have proposed new classifications. These were synthesized to a new classification at the Ann Arbor Conference held in 1971 (Table 12.3) (Carbone et al., 1971). This classification is also applicable to non-Hodgkin's lymphomas. Pruritus, a complaint often voiced by Hodgkin's patients, was found not to connote a poor prognosis contrary to night sweats, unexplained temperatures over 38°C and unexplained weight loss greater than 10% of body weight in the 6 months prior to diagnosis which symptoms relegate patients to the B category. Also new were the concepts

TABLE 12.2

Rye Clinical Classification

Stage I:	Disease limited to one anatomic region or to two contiguous anatomic regions on the same side of the diaphragm
Stage II:	Disease in more than two anatomic regions or in two noncontiguous anatomic regions on the same side of the diaphragm
Stage III:	Disease on both sides of the diaphragm, but not extending beyond the involvement of lymph nodes, spleen and/or Waldeyer's ring
Stage IV:	Involvement of the bone marrow, lung parenchyma, pleura, liver, bone, skin, kidneys, gastrointestinal tract or any tissue or organ in addition to lymph nodes, spleen, or Waldeyer's ring
	A: Absence of symptoms, mentioned under B
	B: Presence of unexplained fever, night sweats, pruritus

TABLE 12.3
Ann Arbor Classification

Stage I -	*I*	One single lymph node region
	-I$_E$	One single extralymphatic organ or site
Stage II -	*II*	Two or more lymph node regions on the same side of the diaphragm
	-II$_E$	One extralymphatic organ or site plus
		One or more lymph node regions on the same side of the diaphragm
		The numbers of node regions involved may be indicated by a subscript (e.g., II$_3$)
Stage III -	*III*	Lymph node regions on both sides of the diaphragm
	-III$_E$	Lymph node involvement plus involvement of extralymphatic organ or site
	-III$_S$	Lymph node involvement plus involvement of the spleen
	-III$_{SE}$	Combination of III$_S$ and III$_E$
Stage IV -		Disseminated involvement of one or more extralymphatic organs or tissues with or without associated lymph node involvement

of clinical staging (CS) and pathological staging (PS). Clinical staging is determined by history, physical examination, laboratory data, roentgenological studies, isotopic scans and initial biopsy results. Pathological staging takes into account the results of a laparotomy with para-aortic and mesenteric node biopsies, liver biopsies and splenectomy and other biopsy data. It should be emphasized that staging classifications apply only to the patient at the time of disease presentation and prior to definitive therapy. The purposes of a classification according to Peters (1971) are: (a) for the planning of treatment, (b) to determine the prognosis and probable effect of the treatment on survival, (c) to compare results between centers, (d) to allow comprehensive studies of the patterns of presentation and the subsequent course of the disease, (e) to establish a standard characterization of the presentation of the disease to compare past, present and future experience. At the same Ann Arbor Conference an outline of required evaluation procedures was brought forth (Rosenberg et al., 1971) which are essentially the same as outlined earlier in this chapter. The value of exploratory laparotomy with splenectomy and liver biopsy was first indicated by Glatstein et al. (1969, 1970) and has been confirmed by numerous other authors. The main benefit of the laparotomy is to know the status of the spleen. Although markedly enlarged spleens are usually involved, moderately enlarged spleens are involved in about 50% of the cases. Clinically normal spleens are involved in about 25% of the cases. When the spleen is sectioned in 0.5-cm slices, involvement in almost all cases can be detected grossly so that splenic involvement rarely remains undetected by the pathologist. When the spleen is normal the liver has been found to be involved on only a rare occasion. Any nodes that are suspicious on the lymphangiogram should be attempted to be biopsied. In addition, mesenteric and celiac nodes should be looked for, particularly in lymphocytic predominance and mixed cellularity disease, that is not limited to one single region or that involves one or both supraclavicular regions (Peters, 1971). Kaplan et al. (1973) in a review of staging laparotomy in 285 consecutive, unselected, previously untreated patients with Hodgkin's disease were able to recognize the following groups of patients in whom laparotomy was contraindicated or findings were always negative: (1) Stage IV disease, (2) advanced age (usually over 65) or life-threatening medical disability, (3) lymphocytic predominance histology with negative lymphangiograms, (4) mediastinal adenopathy (alone or in association with other intrathoracic disease) without cervical or axillary adenopathy, and possibly (5) Stage I disease confined to one axilla. Complications of the procedure were minimal. For those investigators who prefer to perform peritoneoscopy to detect liver involvement, their yield of success is close to that obtained with laparotomy. If the chosen modality of treatment is radiation, the spleen will have to be included in the treatment area because of the unreliability of the clinical assessment of this organ.

It cannot be too strongly urged that therapy should not be initiated prior to a biopsy-proven diagnosis and extensive evaluation to adequately determine the stage of the disease. Occasionally, such as in patients with massive mediastinal and/or hilar adenopathy (Kaplan and Rosenberg, 1975; Piro et al., 1976) or in pregnant women (Thomas and Peckham, 1976), local therapy is indicated before the full staging evaluation can be completed. Localized primary extranodal involvement is extremely rare and amounts to less than 1% of all cases, but may have an excellent prognosis (Wood and Coltman, 1973).

THERAPY

Surgery, although at one time of benefit to patients with very limited disease, is now relegated to diagnostic procedures and occasionally laminectomy with decompression of the spinal cord. Patients with advanced Hodgkin's disease, with or without splenomegaly or demonstrable hypersplenism, who tolerate treatment poorly, are frequently benefited considerably by splenectomy with improved tolerance to therapy (Cooper et al., 1974). Patients who underwent splenectomy as part of a staging laparotomy will frequently have elevated levels of white blood cells and platelets in the peripheral blood. Several investigators have indicated less frequent interruptions of intensive courses of radiation therapy with less depression of blood counts with quicker recovery in splenectomized patients (Salzman and Kaplan, 1971; DiBella et al., 1973; Royster et al., 1974).

The principles of radiation therapy in Hodgkin's disease have been outlined by Gilbert in 1939 and were applied by Peters, Easson and others when kilovoltage equipment became available; but it was not until megavoltage equipment such as the Van de Graaff generator, the cobalt-60 teletherapy unit, the betatron and the linear accelerators came in use that extensive field radiation could be used with minimal side effects. This technique circumvents the use of multiple small treatment fields which bears the risk of overlapping or of gaps between fields.

Gilbert advocated irradiation with sufficient dose to prevent recurrences in clinically involved areas. Kaplan (1966) and others prior to him found recurrence rates of 5% or less after doses of 4000 rads delivered in 4 weeks. Johnson et al. (1969) administered this dose over a 4–7-week period and utilized the total nodal irradiation or extended field technique. Gilbert's second principle was to include adequate margins of apparent normal tissue to prevent relapse in lymph nodes in the immediate area. Peters and Middlemiss (1958) introduced the principle of prophylactic irradiation, extending the treatment fields to include clinically normal appearing adjacent lymph node areas. The extended field technique was also used by Kaplan (1962), who subsequently (Kaplan, 1965) advocated the use of the "mantle" field which covers the cervical, supra- and infraclavicular, axillary, hilar and mediastinal lymph nodes to the diaphragm and the "inverted Y" field with an extension to the left at the upper end to cover the spleen or splenic pedicle, celiac, para-aortic, iliac, inguinal and femoral nodes.

The use of high dose, large field radiation therapy is potentially hazardous and requires great technical skill. The fields have to be shaped carefully to include all the lymph node bearing areas with shielding of vital structures as much as possible. In premenopausal women, surgical oophoropexy with fixation of the ovaries in the midline preserves ovarian function in approximately 50% of these women, one of whom delivered a normal infant according to one report (Ray et al., 1970). In another report (Baker et al., 1972) 4 of 8 patients who underwent transposition of the ovaries to the midline resumed menstruation, one after 2 years of amenorrhea. One gave birth to a normal child more than 6 years after irradiation. LeFloch et al. (1976) summarized the experience at Stanford over a 10-year period: two-thirds of women retained ovarian function, 9 women became pregnant, 6 patients gave birth to 8 normal babies, 2 patients had therapeutic abortions and one a spontaneous abortion. In men prolonged and possibly permanent aspermia may occur (Speiser et al., 1973; Asbjørnsen et al., 1976a, 1976b).

Side effects that may be encountered are soreness and dryness of the mouth, dysphagia, occasionally complicated by monilial mucositis which responds readily to intensive and frequent application of mycostatic agents. Nausea, vomiting and occasionally diarrhea usually do not occur until the abdomen becomes exposed and can be alleviated with appropriate medications. Leukopenia and thrombocytopenia usually reach the nadir toward the end of the course of treatment, but occasionally may arise early necessitating interruption of therapy. As mentioned earlier splenectomy may increase the hematologic tolerance somewhat. Because the supra- and infraclavicular areas have to be included in the field of irradiation, the apices of both lungs are invariably exposed, leading to radiation pneumonitis and fibrosis of that area and other exposed areas such as mediastinal, paratracheal and pericardial areas. This may occasionally give rise to a dry, hacking, nonproductive cough with, in the acute stage, fever and moderate dyspnea on exertion (Case Records, 1971). These symptoms will gradually subside over a period of months. In severe cases treatment with corticosteroids may be indicated. Radiation pericarditis may develop gradually, remain asymptomatic and become manifested only on serial post-treatment roentgenograms of the chest. In severely, protractedly symptomatic patients pericardiectomy may be indicated. Acute onset of pericarditis during the course of treatment has been reported by several investigators; continuation of the radiation therapy is indicated as pericardial involvement with Hodgkin's disease may be the underlying etiology. Pericardial effusion may also be evidence of recurrent disease (Johnson et al., 1969). The combination of possible postradiation constrictive pericarditis plus active Hodgkin's disease was the subject of a clinicopathological exercise (Case Records, 1974). Castellino et al. (1974) observed 7 patients with radiation pneumonitis and/or radiation induced heart disease that became manifest shortly after the rapid withdrawal of corticosteroids after completion of the first or fourth cycle of MOPP (see Table 12.4) therapy. Reinstitution of high dose corticosteroids with slowly tapering of the dose over several months has been an effective form of therapy.

Hypothyroidism may develop in 5–10% of patients. The symptoms may be vague such as fatigue, lethargy and weight gain with sparse physical findings, and therefore this should be looked for because it can be treated readily (Prager et al., 1972).

Lhermitte syndrome, originally described by this French neurologist in multiple sclerosis, may develop several months after radiation to the spinal cord area and will gradually subside in 3–6 months without any residual neurologic manifestations. Patients complain of numbness and tingling and sensations of electric shocks in upper and lower extremities and sometimes in the lower back aggravated and sometimes precipitated by flexion of the head and neck. This syndrome should not be confused with symptoms secondary to a transverse myelitis which fortunately is a rare occurrence. Gradually progressing sensory changes followed by motor changes usually do not begin until 12–15 months after completion of the radiation therapy and may progress to complete paraplegia. It may be the result of an overlap of two fields over the spinal cord (Kaplan, 1972). Others (Locksmith and Powers, 1968; Maier et al., 1969) do not find this and suggest that vascular damage may be the underlying cause of parenchymal cell damage. Carmel and Kaplan (1976) found the following complications in Hodgkin's patients who received mantle irradiation: symptomatic pulmonary reactions 20%, pericarditis 13%, Lhermitte's sign 15%, and thyroid dysfunction 13%.

In 1962, the Stanford investigators (Kaplan and Rosenberg, 1966) were the first to initiate a randomized study in Stage I and II Hodgkin's disease to evaluate extended field (EF) and involved field (IF) radiation therapy in Stage I and II disease. In 1973, the same authors gave an update of their clinical experience from 1962 to 1972. Survival and freedom from relapse were not significantly different in the Stage IA and IIA group. However, for the symptomatic patients (Stages IB and IIB) both survival and relapse free period were significantly shorter in the IF treated group. An unexpected high incidence of relapse in para-aortic nodes was found in patients, treated with either modality, who had initially disease confined to cervical, supraclavicular, axillary and other supramediastinal lymph node regions. All these patients received radiation only to the mediastinal nodes as the next chain at risk. However, it became clear that cervical-supraclavicular disease can spread to areas below the diaphragm without mediastinal involvement and that EF under those circumstances should include para-aortic nodes. Therefore, in 1967 the protocol was changed with the treatment regimens being IF and total nodal radiation (TN). In September 1968, routine staging laparotomy was introduced. For Stage IA and IIA the 5-year survival figures were about 90% and essentially the same in the IF and TN group (28 and 36 patients in each group, respectively). However, the difference in relapse free period was highly significant, 80% of the TN group and 35% of the IF group at 4 years. Because of the high incidence of relapse in both the IF and EF groups of symptomatic patients, beginning in 1968 all these patients either received TN or TN plus six cycles of MOPP (see under "Chemotherapy") after a 6–8-week rest period. Results of these and subsequent studies were updated in 1975 (Rosenberg and Kaplan) and in 1977 (Glatstein). Because of apparent aggravation or initial appearance of radiation pneumonitis and/or pericarditis associated with abrupt corticosteroid withdrawal, which they reported earlier (Castellino et al., 1974), these investigators discontinued the use of prednisone in the combination chemotherapy for patients who had received mediastinal irradiation. Disease-free period and survival of the 19 Stage IB and IIB patients treated with TN were not significantly different from those of the 18 patients of the same stages treated with TN plus 6 cycles of MOPP. The 5-year survival was over 90% and the 5-year disease-free period over 85%. In several other categories of disease, survival was the same, but the disease-free survival tended to be better in the combination treatment. However, the number of patients in each category was rather small and the observation period mostly only about 3 years. With both modalities of treatment there has been a remarkable improvement in overall 5-year survival of all Stage I, II and III Hodgkin's disease patients in comparison with earlier less radical treatment and is now approaching 90% in this group of patients who were subjected to aggressive staging procedures. Goodman et al. (1976) have demonstrated that, for pathologic Stage IA and IIA with disease above the diaphragm mantle and para-aortic irradiation is sufficient treatment.

An important question is whether patients who have had a relapse and subsequently obtained another remission will ultimately have the same survival as the patients who remained in a long term remission or possibly were cured. As mentioned earlier a true recurrence in a previously irradiated area can be reduced to less than 5% with dose levels of 4000 rads delivered in 4 weeks. Spittle et al. (1973) have analyzed the 114 relapses that have occurred in 426 patients after radiation therapy with curative intent at Stanford University Hospital from 1961 until 1971. Forty-eight percent of all relapses occurred within the 1st year, 82% by the end of the 2nd year, 90% by the end of the 3rd year and all had their first relapse by the end of 5 years. Relapse rates varied from 12% in the lymphocytic predominance group to 47% in the lymphocytic depletion group. The worst prognosis was for patients with B symptoms who had their relapse within the first 12 months after completion of the radiation therapy with transdiaphragmatic or extranodal extension. Rubin et al. (1974) reported similar findings. Hopefully survival of these relapsed patients may improve with the better results obtained with combination chemotherapy. Some further trials of radiation therapy and chemother-apy combined will be discussed later.

CHEMOTHERAPY

Modern chemotherapy began during World War II with the develop-ment of nitrogen mustard. Clinical application was initiated in Hodgkin's disease and lymphomas (Jacobson et al., 1946). Adrenocorticosteroid hormones came in use at about the same time. Karnofsky summarized the experience with chemotherapy in 1968. Hall summarized new useful chemotherapeutic agents in Hodgkin's disease in 1966. These included among others the vinca alkaloids and the methylhydrazine derivative— procarbazine. Of more recent development are Adriamycin, bleomycin and the nitrosourea compounds, such as BCNU, CCNU and MeCCNU which is presently still investigational. Another investigational agent with limited usefulness is streptozotocin. For further information concerning individual drugs, please see the section on drugs (Chapter 5).

Single Agent Chemotherapy. The three most widely used alkylating agents are nitrogen mustard, cyclophosphamide and chlorambucil. The usual dose of nitrogen mustard is 0.4 mg/kg, which may be repeated after approximately 4 weeks when hematologic toxicity has cleared. However, prolonged use usually causes severe leukopenia and thrombocytopenia which in addition to the marked nausea and vomiting which occur for about 24 hours after the administration make this an unsuitable drug for maintenance therapy. Without maintenance therapy responses last an average of only 11 weeks, but Scott (1963) demonstrated a prolongation to an average of 35 weeks with daily chlorambucil in a dose of 0.2 mg/kg, initiated after satisfactory response to the nitrogen mustard.

Cyclophosphamide can also be used for induction and maintenance therapy in daily oral doses of 2.0–2.5 mg/kg, but is more effective in intermittent intravenous doses of 30–40 mg/kg given every 3–4 weeks. The gastrointestinal side effects are less than those of nitrogen mustard, but hemorrhagic cystitis may be an unpleasant and sometimes serious complication. Adequate hydration prior to the administration may avert this problem. Although leukopenia can be severe with the nadir around the 8th to the 12th day, thrombocytopenia is usually not of clinical significance. Responses may be 60–70% but are rarely complete. The vinca alkaloids, vinblastine and vincristine, came in use in the late 1950s. Because of its marked neurotoxicity and development of early refractoriness vincristine is not as suitable an agent as vinblastine for induction and maintenance therapy of Hodgkin's disease. Weekly doses of 0.1–0.2 mg/kg of the latter drug are tolerated quite well and can be prolonged to once every other week for maintenance once a remission has been obtained. Members of the Acute Leukemia Group B (Carbone and Spurr, 1968) conducted a randomized study in which 57 previously untreated Hodgkin's patients were treated with vinblastine. Fifteen obtained a complete and an additional 27 a partial remission or a total response rate of 75%. Fifty-four patients received cyclophosphamide, 10 obtained a complete remission and 19 a partial or a total response rate of 47%. However, survival was not significantly different for these two treatment regimens.

N-Methylhydrazine or procarbazine was first reported to be active in Hodgkin's disease by Martz et al. (1963) and Mathé et al. (1963). Brunner and Young (1965) reported on 51 patients. Twenty of 25 patients with Hodgkin's disease had an adequate trial with oral drug which was begun with a dose of 50–100 mg daily and then gradually increased to 200–1000 mg daily. Maintenance dosage was 100 mg every 2–3 days. It is significant that 18 of 20 adequately treated patients had received prior chemotherapy and 12 of these were resistant to vinca alkaloids and alkylating agents. Ten of these 18 patients had a clinically useful response, with 4 still in remission from 5 to 9 months. In 1974 Spivack reviewed the status of procarbazine 5 years after it was approved for noninvestigational clinical use in 1969. Its most frequent application is in combination chemotherapy.

Lessner (1968) described dramatic and rapid responses with 1,3-bis-(2-chloroethyl)-1-nitrosourea (BCNU) in 17 of 31 patients with advanced Hodgkin's disease who were resistant to standard chemotherapeutic agents. The median duration was over 120 days.

Young et al. (1971) treated 45 patients with advanced previously treated Hodgkin's disease and obtained 19 partial remissions for 16.5 weeks and 2 complete remissions for 72 and 208 weeks, respectively. There does not appear to be a cross resistance with alkylating agents. Rege and Owens (1974) described another 16 of 33 responses. Toxicity is mostly nausea and vomiting and bone marrow depression.

Although the experience with CCNU and methyl-CCNU is much less, similar responses have been described with these drugs by DeConti et al. (1973) and Young et al. (1973b). Carter (1973) gave an overview of the status of the nitrosoureas. They are also valuable agents in combination chemotherapy regimens (Bakemeier and DeVita, 1974).

Yagoda et al. (1972) reported a large series of patients treated with bleomycin. Patients with advanced Hodgkin's disease had the most impressive and prolonged responses, 32 of 64 adequately treated patients had a complete response, which lasted longer than 1 month in 20 patients. The initial dose was 0.25 mg/kg daily intravenously which was decreased to 1 mg daily intravenously or subcutaneously when there was evidence of clinical response, which was usually in 3–5 days. Blum et al. (1973) published a clinical review of bleomycin and found it to be active in all types of lymphomas. Eighty-six patients were treated in the United States, 5 had a complete and 24 a partial remission or a response rate of 43% with a median duration of 3.1 months. European investigators reported 2 complete and 14 partial remissions in 54 evaluable patients or a response rate of 30%. The usual dosages were 15–30 mg twice weekly, intravenously.

Blum and Carter (1974) reviewed the experience with Adriamycin. Twenty-three of 64 Hodgkin's patients had a response which is inferior by retrospective comparison to most other active agents; however, most of these patients had advanced disease and had failed standard therapy, including combination chemotherapy. These responses do suggest a low level of cross resistance between Adriamycin and other agents. It may by very active when used in combinations earlier in the disease. Experience in non-Hodgkin's lymphoma indicates this to be the case (McKelvey et al., 1974).

Streptozotocin, a naturally occurring nitrosourea, was found to have limited hematologic toxicity (Schein et al., 1974). Sixteen patients with advanced Hodgkin's disease, who were refractory to conventional chemotherapy or who had severe myelosuppression, prohibiting further chemotherapy received 500 mg/m^2 of the drug for 5 consecutive days. One patient achieved a complete and 6 a partial remission. The durations of response varied from 1.5 to 3.0 months. Because of its bone marrow-sparing effect it may be a valuable drug in combination regimens. Combination chemotherapy was empirically used by Lacher and Durant (1965) with good success. Sixteen evaluable patients with Stage II or III widespread Hodgkin's disease were treated with vinblastine 0.1 mg/kg weekly intravenously with chlorambucil 4 mg daily by mouth added to this in the 2nd week. Doses were gradually increased to produce a total white blood cell count of approximately 3000/cu mm. Six patients had a complete response, 7 a partial response and 3 no response. Durations of response were 13, 20 and 23 months and in 3 patients 21 months.

In order to obtain a cure with chemotherapeutic agents a large cell kill that will leave only minimal residual disease is necessary. As mentioned in the chapter on cell kinetics, a proportion rather than a fixed number of tumor cells are killed by a given dose of a chemotherapeutic agent. Chemotherapeutic agents that are presently in use have only minimal selectivity for kill of tumor cells in comparison with normal cells. Only combinations of drugs that have independent toxicities with an enhanced antitumor effect hold some promise for irradication of malignant diseases. Because of successes in animal studies and in acute leukemia (Frei, 1965; Freireich et al., 1964), trials with combination chemotherapy were initiated at the National Cancer Institute in 1963 (Moxley et al., 1967). Fourteen patients with disease stages varying from IA to IIIB received cyclophosphamide, vincristine, methotrexate and prednisone; 9 of these received additional radiation therapy. Eighty-six percent complete remissions were obtained with 9 patients remaining disease-free for as long as 40 months. With the known marginal activity of methotrexate in this disease and as more information became available about the methylhydrazine derivative, procarbazine, another study was initiated in 1964 with vincristine, nitrogen mustard, procarbazine and prednisone (MOPP) which would become probably the most widely used combination chemotherapy regimen (DeVita et al., 1970). The treatment schedule is outlined in Table 12.4. Usually the cycle of 2 weeks of treatment and 2 weeks of no treatment is repeated 6 times. In this study no further treatment was given after 6 cycles. Toxicities were moderate and as can be expected, i.e. neurotoxicity from vincristine and nausea, vomiting and myelosuppression from procarbazine and nitrogen mustard. Prednisone rarely leads to complications because of the short period of administration. The response rate was superior to that of any previous treatment regimen: 35 of 43 or 81% of patients with predominantly Stage IIIB and IVB disease achieved

TABLE 12.4

MOPP Combination Chemotherapy

Drugs (mg/m²)	Days				
	1	8	14	15–28	29
Mustargen (HN₂) (IV)	6.0	6.0		No therapy	Next
Oncovin (VCR) (IV)	1.4	1.4			cycle
Procarbazine (PO)[a]	100.0	→			
Prednisone (PO)[a, b]	40.0	→			

[a] Daily for 14 days.
[b] Cycles 1 and 4 only.

TABLE 12.5

MVPP Combination Chemotherapy

Drugs (mg/m²)	Days				
	1	8	14	15–28	29
Mustargen (HN₂) (IV)	6.0	6.0		No therapy	Next
Vinblastine (IV)	6.0	6.0	6.0		cycle
Procarbazine (PO)[a]	100.0	→			
Prednisone (PO)[a, b]	40.0	→			

[a] Daily for 14 days.
[b] Each cycle. Total dose.

a complete remission. The median duration of the complete remission from the end of 6 cycles of MOPP was 36 months, with the relapse rate being greatest in the first 18 months. None of the patients who have remained in complete remission in excess of 42 months have relapsed. Of the 35 complete responders, 41% have remained in complete remission for up to 6 years (DeVita, 1973). Similar results have been reported by individual investigators and cooperative study groups. These data were summarized by Goldsmith and Carter (1974). Patients who have received prior chemotherapy or a combination of radiation therapy plus chemotherapy have usually less favorable results, while those who received prior radiation therapy only do not respond differently from those who had no prior therapy. Other four- and five-drug combinations have had similar results. McElwain et al. (1973) from the Royal Marsden and St. Bartholomew's Hospitals in London reported on nitrogen mustard, vinblastine, procarbazine and prednisone (MVPP). The regimen is summarized in Table 12.5. The Acute Leukemia Group B studied two four-drug regimens (MOPP; BCNU-OPP) versus two three-drug regimens (BCNU + vincristine + prednisone; procarbazine + vincristine + prednisone). The complete plus partial response rate for the two four-drug regimens was 88% and 91%, and for the two three-drug regimens 71% and 69%, respectively (Nissen et al., 1973). A report from the British National Lymphoma Investigation (1975) indicated the significance of the prednisone in the MOPP regimen: 80% complete remissions in 49 patients treated with MOPP and 44% of 41 patients treated with MOP. In these regimens the procarbazine was given for 10 days and the dose of prednisone was 25 mg/m^2 given for 14 days with each cycle of treatment. Three deaths related to bone marrow depression were all in the MOPP group, suggesting that prednisone did not reduce bone marrow toxicity. Bonadonna et al. (1975) reported preliminary results of a randomized study in advanced Hodgkin's disease with MOPP versus ABVD (see Table 12.6). Nineteen of 25 (76%) evaluable patients treated with MOPP had a complete remission and three a partial remission. Fifteen of 20 (75%) patients treated with ABVD had a complete remission and 3 a partial remission. Nixon and Aisenberg (1974) reported that in their group of 52 patients treated with MOPP all patients with Stage IIIA and IVA disease remained in complete remission while 50% of those with Stage IIIB and IVB relapsed. While there is little difference of opinion concerning initial treatment of widespread Hodgkin's disease, there is considerable disagreement about further therapy once a remission has been obtained. Many investigators use 6 months of intensive therapy as an arbitrary number and then continue with less intensive maintenance therapy. Investigators at the National Cancer Institute (NCI) administer 6 cycles of therapy, but continue if no complete remission has been obtained and give an additional 2 cycles once a complete remission has been obtained, recognizing variations in the biologic characteristics of different patients. So far histopathologic differences do not seem to have a demonstrable influence on the results of treatment (DeVita, 1973). These same investigators (Young et al., 1973a) randomized 57 patients who were in complete remission after MOPP treatment to one of three regimens: no further therapy, intermittent therapy with MOPP or intermittent therapy with BCNU. The relapse figures were 24, 25 and 13%, respectively, and not significantly different. Complications and infections were more frequent in the maintenance treatment groups. The survival was not significantly different, the projected 5-year survival for the entire group being 86%. In 1976, DeVita et al. gave a 10-year progress report on 194

TABLE 12.6
ABVD Combination Chemotherapy

Drugs (mg/m^2)	Days				
	1	2–5	14	15–28	29
Adriamycin (IV)	25.0		25.0	No therapy	Next
Bleomycin (IV)	10.0		10.0		cycle
Vinblastine (IV)	6.0		6.0		
DTIC (IV)[a]	150.0	→			

[a] Daily for 5 days.

patients with advanced Hodgkin's disease who were treated with MOPP from 1964 to 1976. Because of differences in methodologies of treatment and evaluations, the results of these studies may be difficult to compare with those of other investigators. However, results between various studies by members of the same cooperative study group should vary little. The ALGB found that maintenance therapy prolonged the duration of remission in one study in comparison with a study that had similar induction treatment, but no maintenance (Nissen et al., 1973). In a report by the Southwest Oncology Group (Frei et al., 1973) 187 patients with Stage III and IV disease had a complete remission rate of 66% with MOPP therapy. After 6 months of MOPP induction therapy patients in complete remission were randomly allocated either to continued MOPP treatment every 2 months for a total of 18 months or to no further treatment. Seventy-five percent of the former and 46% of the latter group of patients were in complete remission 3 years after the onset of the study. In both groups survival was 80% at 4 years. The authors contribute this lack of difference in survival largely to effective secondary treatment in patients who relapsed after 6 months of MOPP therapy. With the prolonged survival of Hodgkin's patients, the disease-free period is a better parameter of effective therapy than survival. Although patients on maintenance therapy have a slightly increased risk of complications, particularly infections, patients who relapse early without maintenance are also at greater risk of complications and have a usually less favorable performance status, at least during the early period of reinduction. Presently it seems that maintenance therapy is beneficial, unless induction therapy is continued beyond 6 months if aggressive re-evaluation reveals residual disease. This restaging should include liver and bone marrow biopsy if they were abnormal prior to onset of treatment and biopsy of residual, accessible lymph nodes. Frei et al. (1973) also indicated a correlation with the site(s) of the initial recurrence(s). Relapse may result from persisting tumor cells rather than from reinduction of the disease. Radiation therapy to sites of major pretreatment involvement is, therefore, a rational approach. The Southwest Oncology Group is presently involved in such a study.

As mentioned earlier, because of the high incidence of relapse of symptomatic patients with radiation therapy alone, studies with radiation therapy and chemotherapy were initiated in the hope of eradicating extranodal disease that is very likely to be present, although not demonstrable in patients with Stage IB, IIB and IIIB disease. Preliminary results of treatment of Stage IIB, IIIB, III$_s$ and IV patients with mechlorethamine, Adriamycin, bleomycin, vincristine and prednisone, followed by radiation therapy by Italian investigators were favorable (DeLena et al., 1973). Van der Werf-Messing (1973) reported on the results of a trial of the European Organization for Research on Treatment of Cancer in which, between 1964 and 1971, 296 patients with Stage I and II, A and B Hodgkin's disease were randomized to two treatment modalities. All patients received 4000 rads in 4 weeks to involved areas and 3500 rads in 4 weeks to prophylactic areas on the same side of the diaphragm. Six weeks after completion of the radiation therapy, all patients were reassessed and all those who had no evidence of disease were randomly assigned to no further therapy or to chemotherapy consisting of weekly vinblastine intravenously for 2 years. None of these patients had a staging laparotomy. Five-year survival of all patients was 75% with no significant difference between the two groups yet. Disease-free survival was significantly better with the additional chemotherapy during the first 2 years. After cessation of the vinblastine the difference became less, indicating that this simple one drug chemotherapy did suppress disease in nonirradiated areas. Patients with mixed cellularity histology had a 50% 5-year survival when treated with radiation therapy alone and 75% when treated with the combination. Many of the relapses were in the nonirradiated subdiaphragmatic area, confirming Kaplan's observations which were mentioned earlier. Kaplan (1973) has pointed out the risk of not being able to administer the full dose of radiation therapy after intensive chemotherapy and prefers to administer the chemotherapy after the radiation therapy. Prosnitz et al. (1976) utilized a 6-week treatment program, as outlined in Table 12.7, followed by a 2-week rest period. After three such cycles, all areas that were involved prior to the institution of the chemotherapy, with the exception of the bone marrow, received 1500–2500 rads. After completion of the radiation therapy, another two cycles of chemotherapy were administered. The authors indicate that 4000 rads will sterilize masses of Hodgkin's disease containing 10^{11}–10^{12} cells. Even intensive chemotherapy may leave subclinical conglomerates of 10^4–10^5 cells which can readily be irradicated by 1500–2500 rads. Approximately 1500 rads are also readily tolerated by the liver and the lungs. Forty-four patients had no prior therapy, 36 had prior therapy, 34 of these had prior radiation only; this did not alter the outcome of the treatment. Sixty patients entered complete remission, only 5 of these relapsed and one developed acute leukemia. In DeVita's (1970) study, 35 of 43 previously untreated patients had a complete remission with MOPP. Twenty of these patients relapsed with a median time to relapse of 11 months.

O'Connell et al. (1975) of the Baltimore Cancer Research Center initiated a study in January 1970 in which predominantly Stage I–IIIA patients were randomized between radiation therapy only and radiation therapy followed by chemotherapy. This was based on a preliminary study at the same institution which suggested that radiation therapy

TABLE 12.7
Prosnitz Combination Chemotherapy

Drugs			1	8	15	22	29	36	43	57
							Days			
Nitrogen mustard,	0.4	mg/kg	(IV)	→						No therapy	Next cycle
Vincristine,	1.4	mg/m²	(IV)	→	→	→				
Vinblastine,	6	mg/m²	(IV)				→	→	→	
Procarbazine,	100	mg/d	(PO)							
Prednisone,	40	mg/m²	(PO)							

followed by chemotherapy was better than radiation therapy alone or chemotherapy followed by radiation therapy in Stage I and II Hodgkin's patients (Brace et al., 1973). In O'Connell's study, the radiation therapy only group received radiation to the mantle field only or, in case of mediastinal involvement, to the para-aortic nodes in addition. Stage III patients received radiation to all involved infradiaphragmatic areas plus adjacent areas. The combined modality group received radiation therapy to the mantle field only, regardless of stage of disease, plus involved areas only for disease below the diaphragm. After a 4–8-week rest period these patients were to receive 6 courses of MOPP therapy. Procarbazine was given for 10 days instead of 14 days. The toxicity was mainly hematologic and in general moderate and well tolerated. Occasional marked myelo-suppression was usually brief. No severe infections were encountered. Of 72 evaluable patients, 41 received radiation therapy only and 31 the combined treatment. Thirteen of the 41 patients relapsed from 2 to 21 months after completion of the radiation therapy. Three of 31 patients relapsed at 10, 21 and 23 months after completion of the chemotherapy. This is statistically significant. However, the differences in survival were not statistically significant. In this, as well as in several of the previously mentioned studies, it is mainly because the observation periods are still rather short and intensive chemotherapy after the first relapse is quite effective. A 32+ to 84+ months follow-up (Wiernik and Robinson, 1978) revealed that no Stage I patient relapsed. Five-year disease-free survivals for Stage I and II with radiation was 70%, with radiation + chemotherapy 95%; Stage IIIA 60% and 100%, respectively. The combination treatment was considered better for Stages II–IIIA especially if "E" disease was present (Levi and Wiernik, 1977a). Wiernik and Lichtenfeld (1975) up-dated Brace's study and found that, although combination treatment prolonged the disease-free survival, total survival was superior with radiation therapy alone because those patients who relapsed had excellent response to further radiation plus chemotherapy. Desser et al. (1977) found the addition of combination chemotherapy to total nodal irradia-tion improving the survival only in a group of Stage III patients with involvement of para-aortic, iliac or mesenteric nodes, who had a less favorable prognosis than a group of patients with abdominal disease limited to the spleen, and/or splenic, celiac or portal nodes. Theoretically, the spleen becomes involved via the splenic artery. Subsequently, the disease spreads via the existing lymph channels. Levi and Wiernik (1977b) found a similar prognosis of Stage IIIA patients with splenic involvement only and Stage IIA patients after total nodal irradiation. Patients with spleen plus node involvement had a greater relapse and poorer prognosis after total nodal irradiation alone and benefited most from post-radiation chemotherapy. Hellman (1974) reported an increase in extranodal spread in patients who had Hodgkin's disease in the spleen. Weller et al. (1976) reviewed 701 consecutive patients treated with curative intent at Stanford University Radiation Therapy Department. Of these 243 patients re- lapsed. Eighty-seven percent of these relapses occurred within 3 years of initial treatment. Relapse-free survival after second treatment which included MOPP is better than in the pre-MOPP era, although the actuarial survival at 5 years is not better. This finding also holds true for patients who relapsed only in lymph nodes. The best hope for cure of Hodgkin's disease still depends on the adequacy of the initial treatment.

Several reviews concerning pediatric Hodgkin's disease (Filler et al., 1975; Norris et al., 1975; Parker et al., 1976; Donaldson et al., 1976; Botnick et al., 1977) have indicated the need for extensive staging procedures, including laparotomy with splenectomy when indicated, and the use of localized moderate doses of radiation combined with multidrug chemotherapy to avoid altered bone growth with subsequent disfigure- ment. Randomized studies are presently ongoing in several cooperative groups.

The direct benefits of intensive radiation therapy and/or chemotherapy are now clearly evident. The immediate toxic effects are predictable and usually manageable in experienced hands. Long term effects have been studied by Arseneau et al., (1972). No long term impairment of the bone marrow function or immunocompetence were observed. Eight of 10 patients were found to be sterile. Asbjørnsen et al. (1976b) reported 7 of 8 cases of aspermia after completion of at least 6 months of chemotherapy. Sherins and DeVita (1973) evaluated reproductive function in 16 men 6 months to 7 years after they had been treated with cyclophosphamide- containing drug combinations. Libido and potency were normal, 10 men were azoospermic, 2 had minimal spermatogenesis and only 4 had normal spermatogenesis on testicular biopsy. Twelve of 26 patients had a return of spermatogenesis within 15 to 49 months after stopping cyclophospha- mide treatment (Buchanan et al., 1975).

In 425 patients treated with a variety of therapies, 12 were found to have second malignancies; this is a 3.5-fold increase over that calculated for the normal population (DeVita et al., 1973). Subsequent reports from the NCI group (Canellos et al., 1975; Canellos, 1975) have raised this total number to 18 of a total patient population of 452. Four cases of leukemia and 4 cases of solid tumors were diagnosed in 65 patients who received both radiation and intensive chemotherapy. This is an 18.6-fold increase over the expected in this group. Although these figures are impressive it should be kept in mind that the benefits of these intensive treatments in such a grave malignancy as Hodgkin's disease far outweigh the increased, but still small, risk of developing another malignancy.

Great progress has been made in the past 15 years in the diagnosis, evaluation and treatment of patients with Hodgkin's disease. Long term control and cures are obtained with radiation therapy, multiple drug chemotherapy and combinations of the two. No ideal mode of therapy can be recommended yet, but numerous studies in progress seem to indicate a trend toward best results with radiation therapy to involved areas and multiple drug chemotherapy. Careful analysis of patients treated over the past years may indicate subgroups with differing prognoses—the significance of splenic involvement was discussed earlier. Johnson et al. (1977) reviewing 58 patients with clinical Stage I-III nodular sclerosing disease found only 4 extranodal extensions. Only 1 of 12 Stage IIB patients died suggesting that "B" symptoms in the nodular sclerosing category have considerably less prognostic significance than in the other histologic categories. On the other hand, Fuller et al. (1977) had 4 pulmonary extensions in 4 of 31 patients with Stage IIA nodular sclerosing disease and in 4 of 12 Stage IIB patients.

REFERENCES

Abrams H. L., Takahashi, M., and Adams, D. F. Usefulness and accuracy of lymphangiography in lymphoma. Cancer Chemother. Rep., 52: 157-170, 1968.

Aisenberg, A. C. Lymphocytopenia in Hodgkin's disease. Blood, 25: 1037-1042, 1965.

Anagnostou, D., Parker, J. W., Taylor, C. R., Tindle, B. H., and Lukes, R. J. Lacunar cells of nodular sclerosing Hodgkin's disease. An ultrastructural and immunohistologic study. Cancer, 39: 1032-1043, 1977.

Arseneau, J. C., Sponzo, R. W., Levin, D. L., Schnipper, L. A., Bonner, H., Young, R. C. Canellos, G. P., Johnson, R. E., and DeVita, V. T. Nonlymphomatous malignant tumors complicating Hodgkin's disease; possible association with intensive therapy. N. Engl. J. Med., 287: 1119-1122, 1972.

Asbjørnsen, G., Molne, K., Klepp, O., and Aakvaag, A. Testicular functions after combination chemotherapy for Hodgkin's disease. Scan. J. Haematol., 16: 66-69, 1976a.

Asbjørnsen, G., Molne, K., Klepp, O., and Aakvaag, A. Testicular functions after radiotherapy to inverted "Y" field for malignant lymphoma. Scand. J. Haematol., 17: 96-100, 1976b.

Atkinson, K., Austin, D. E., McElwain, T. J., and Peckham, M. J. Alcohol pain in Hodgkin's disease. Cancer, 37: 895-899, 1976.

Bakemeier, R. F., and DeVita, V. T., Jr. Combination chemotherapy and immunotherapy of Hodgkin's disease; preliminary report. Proc. Am. Soc. Clin. Oncol., 15: 183, 1974.

Baker, J. W., Peckam, M. J., Morgan, R. L., and Smithers, D. W. Preservation of ovarian function in patients requiring radiotherapy for para-aortic and pelvic Hodgkin's disease. Lancet, 1: 1307-1308, 1972.

Blum, R. H., and Carter, S. K. Adriamycin; a new anticancer drug with significant clinical activity. Ann. Intern. Med., 80: 249-259, 1974.

Blum, R. H., Carter, S. K., and Agre, K. A clinical review of bleomycin—a new antineoplastic agent. Cancer, 31: 903-914, 1973.

Bobrove, A. M., Fuks, Z., Strober, S., and Kaplan, H. S. Quantitation of T and B lymphocytes and cellular immune functions in Hodgkin's disease. Cancer, 36: 169-179, 1975.

Bonadonna, G., Zucali, R., Monfardini, S., DeLena, M., and Uslenghi, C. Combination chemotherapy of Hodgkin's disease with Adriamycin, bleomycin, vinblastine and imidazole carboxamide versus MOPP. Cancer, 36: 252-259, 1975.

284   GUIDE TO THERAPEUTIC ONCOLOGY

Botnick, L. E., Goodman, R., Jaffe, N., Filler, R., and Cassady, J. R. Stages I and II Hodgkin's disease in children; results of staging and treatment. Cancer, *39:* 599–603, 1977.

Brace, K., Serpick, A. A., and Block, J. B. Combination radiotherapy and chemotherapy in the treatment of early Hodgkin's disease. Oncology, *27:* 484–492, 1973.

British National Lymphoma Investigation Report. Value of prednisone in combination chemotherapy of Stage IV Hodgkin's disease. Br. Med. J., *3:* 413–414, 1975.

Brunner, K. W., and Young, C. W. A methylhydrazine derivative in Hodgkin's disease and other malignant neoplasms. Ann. Intern. Med., *63:* 69–82, 1965.

Buchanan, J. O., Fairley, K. F., and Barrie, J. U. Return of spermatogenesis after stopping cyclophosphamide therapy. Lancet, *3:* 156–157, 1975.

Canellos, G. P. Second malignancies complicating Hodgkin's disease in remission. Lancet, *1:* 1294, 1975.

Canellos, G. P., DeVita, V. T., Arseneau, J. C., Whang-Peng, J., and Johnson, R. F. Second malignancies complicating Hodgkin's disease in remission. Lancet, *1:* 947–949, 1975.

Carbone, P. P., and Spurr, C. Management of patients with malignant lymphoma; a comparative study with cyclophosphamide and vinca alkaloids. Cancer Res., *28:* 811–822, 1968.

Carbone, P. P., Kaplan, H. S., Mushoff, K., Smithers, D., and Tubiana, M. Report of the committee on Hodgkin's disease staging classifications. Cancer Res., *31:* 1860–1861, 1971.

Carmel, J. R., and Kaplan, H. S. Mantle irradiation in Hodgkin's disease; an analysis of technique, tumor eradication and complications. Cancer, *37:* 2813–2825, 1976.

Carter, S. K. An overview of the status of the nitrosoureas in other tumors. Cancer Chemother. Rep., *4:* 35–46, 1973.

Case, D. C., Jr., Hansen, J. A., Corrales, E., Young, C. W., Dupont, B., Pinsky, C. M., and Good, R. A. Comparison of multiple in vivo and in vitro parameters in untreated patients with Hodgkin's disease. Cancer, *38:* 1807–1815, 1976.

Case records of the Massachusetts General Hospital. Case 11-1971. N. Engl. J. Med., *284:* 603–610, 1971.

Case records of the Massachusetts General Hospital. Case 49-1974. N. Engl. J. Med., *291:* 1297–1303, 1974.

Castellino, R. A. Lymphographic-histologic correlation in patients with Hodgkin's disease and non-Hodgkin's lymphoma undergoing staging laparotomy. Lymphology, *7:* 153–157, 1974.

Castellino, R. A., Glatstein, E., Turbow, M. M., Rosenberg, S., and Kaplan, H. S. Latent radiation injury of lungs or heart activated by steroid withdrawal. Ann. Intern. Med., *80:* 593–599, 1974.

Castellino, R. A., Filly, R., and Blank, N. Routine full-lung tomography in the initial staging and treatment planning of patients with Hodgkin's disease and non-Hodgkin's lymphoma. Cancer, *38:* 1130–1136, 1976.

Cooper, I. A., Ironside, P. N. J., Madigan, J. P., Morris, P. J., and Ewing, M. R. The role of splenectomy in the management of advanced Hodgkin's disease. Cancer, *34:* 408–417, 1974.

DeConti, R. C., Hubbard, S. P., Pinch, P., and Bertino, J. R. Treatment of advanced neoplastic disease with 1-(2-chloroethyl)-3-cyclohexyl-l-nitrosourea (CCNU; NSC-790377). Cancer Chemother. Rep., *57:* 201–207, 1973.

DeLena, M., Monfardini, S., Beretta, G., Fissati-Bellani, F., and Bonadonna, G. Clinical trials with intensive chemotherapy and radiotherapy in Hodgkin's disease. Natl. Cancer Inst. Monogr., *36:* 403–420, 1973.

Desser, R. K., Golomb, H. M., Ultmann, J. E., Ferguson, D. J., Moran, E. M., Griem, M. L., Vardiman, J., Miller, B., Oetzel, N., Sweet, D., Lester, E. P., Kinzie, J. J., and Blough, R. Prognostic classification of Hodgkin's disease in pathologic stage III, based on anatomic considerations. Blood, *49:* 883–893, 1977.

DeVita, V. T., Jr. Combined drug treatment of Hodgkin's disease, remission induction, remission duration and survival; an appraisal. Natl. Cancer Inst. Monogr., *36:* 373–379, 1973.

DeVita, V. T., Jr., Serpick, A. A., and Carbone, P. P. Combination chemotherapy in the treatment of advanced Hodgkin's disease. Ann. Intern. Med., *73:* 881–895, 1970.

DeVita, V. T., Arseneau, J. C., Shermin, R. J., Canellos, G. P., and Young, R. C. Intensive chemotherapy for Hodgkin's disease; long term complications. Natl. Cancer Inst. Monogr., *36:* 447–454, 1973.

DeVita, V., Canellos, G., Hubbard, S., Chabner, B., and Young R. Chemotherapy of Hodgkin's disease with MOPP, a 10-year progress report. Proc. Am. Soc. Clin. Oncol., *17:* 269, 1976.

DiBella, N.J., Blom, J., and Slawson, R. G. Splenectomy and hematologic tolerance to irradiation in Hodgkin's disease. Radiology, *107:* 195–200, 1973.

Donaldson, S. S., Glatstein, E., Rosenberg, S. A., and Kaplan, H. S. Pediatric Hodgkin's disease; II. Results of therapy. Cancer, *37:* 2436–2447, 1976.

Filler, F. M., Jaffe, N., Cassady, J. R., Traggis, D. G., and Vawter, G. F. Experience with clinical and operative staging of Hodgkin's disease in children. J. Pediatr. Surg., *10:* 321–328, 1975.

Filly, R. A., Marglin, S., and Castellini, R. A. The ultrasonographic spectrum of abdominal and pelvic Hodgkin's disease and non-Hodgkin's lymphoma. Cancer, *38:* 2143–2148, 1976.

Frei, E., III, for Leukemia Group B. The effectiveness of combinations of antileukemia agents in inducing and maintaining remission in children with acute leukemia. Blood, *26:* 642–656, 1965.

Frei, E., III, Luce, J. K., Gamble, J. F., Coltman, C. A., Jr., Constanzi, J. J., Talley, R. W., Monto, R. W., Wilson, H. E., Hewlett, J. S., Delaney, F. C., and Gehan, E. A. Combination chemotherapy in advanced Hodgkin's disease; induction and maintenance of remission. Ann. Intern. Med., *79:* 376–382, 1973.

Freireich, E. J., Karon, M., and Frei, E., III. Quadruple combination therapy (VAMP) for acute lymphocytic leukemia of childhood. Proc. Am. Assoc. Cancer Res., *5:* 20, 1964.

Fuller, L. M., Madoc-Jones, H., Gamble, J. F., Butler, J. J., Sullivan, M. P., Fernandez, C.-H., and Gehan, E. A. New assessment of the prognostic significance of histopathology in Hodgkin's disease for laparotomy—negative stage I and stage II patients. Cancer, *39:* 2174–2182, 1977.

Gilbert, R. Radiotherapy in Hodgkin's disease (malignant granulomatosis); anatomic and clinical foundations, governing principles, results. A.J.R., *41:* 198–241, 1939.

Glatstein, E. Radiotherapy in Hodgkin's disease; past achievement and future progress. Cancer, *39:* 837–842, 1977.

Glatstein, E., Guernsey, J. M., Rosenberg, S. A., and Kaplan, H. S. The value of laparotomy and splenectomy in the staging of Hodgkin's disease. Cancer, *24:* 709–718, 1969.

Glatstein, E., Trueblood, H. W., Enright, L. P., Rosenberg, S. A., and Kaplan, H. S. Surgical staging of abdominal involvement in unselected patients with Hodgkin's disease. Radiology, *97:* 425–432, 1970.

Goldsmith, M. A., and Carter, S. K. Combination chemotherapy of advanced Hodgkin's disease; a review. Cancer, *33:* 1–8, 1974.

Goodman, R. L., Piro, A. J., and Hellman, S. Can pelvic irradiation be omitted in patients with pathologic stages IA and IIA Hodgkin's disease? Cancer *37:* 2834–2839, 1976.

Grufferrman, S., Cole, P., Smith, P. G., and Lukes, R. J. Hodgkin's disease in siblings. N. Engl. J. Med., *269:* 248–250, 1977.

Hall, T. C. New chemotherapeutic agents in Hodgkin's disease. Cancer Res., *26:* 1297–1302, 1966.

Heath, C. W. The epidemiology of Hodgkin's disease (editorial). Ann. Intern. Med., *77:* 313–314, 1972.

Heublein, A. C. Preliminary report on continuous irradiation of entire body. Radiology, *18:* 1051–1060, 1932.

Hoffer, P. B., Turner, D., Gottschalk, A., Harper, P. V., and Ultmann, J.E. Whole-body radiogallium scanning for staging of Hodgkin's disease and other lymphomas. Natl. Cancer Inst. Monogr., *36:* 277–285, 1973.

Jackson, H., Jr., and Parker, F. Jr. Hodgkin's disease; II. Pathology. N. Engl. J. Med., *231:* 35–44, 1944.

Jacobson, L. O., Spurr, C. L., Guzman-Barron, E. S., Smith, T., Lushbaugh, C., and Dick, G. F. Nitrogen mustard therapy; studies on the effect of methyl-bis-(β-chloroethyl)amine hydrochloride on neoplastic disorders and allied disorders of the hemopoietic system. J.A.M.A., *132:* 263–271, 1946.

Johnson, R. E., Kagan, A. R., Hafermann, M. D., and Keyes, J. W. Patient tolerance to extended irradiation in Hodgkin's disease. Ann. Intern. Med., *70:* 1–6, 1969.

Johnson, R. E., Zimbler, H., Berard, C. W., Herdt, J., and Brereton, H. D. Radiotherapy results for nodular sclerosing Hodgkin's disease after clinical staging. Cancer, *39:* 1439–1444, 1977.

Jones, S. E., Tobias, D. A., and Waldman, R. S. Computed tomographic scanning in patients with lymphoma. Cancer, *41:* 480–486, 1978.

Kaplan, H. S. The radical radiotherapy of regionally localized Hodgkin's disease. Radiology, *78:* 553–561, 1962.

Kaplan, H. S. Radiotherapeutic management of the malignant lymphomas. Med. Rec. Ann., *58:* 43–46, 1965.

Kaplan, H. S. Evidence for a tumoricidal dose level in the radiotherapy of Hodgkin's disease. Cancer Res., *26:* 1221–1224, 1966.

Kaplan, H. S. Hodgkin's disease, p. 334. Harvard University Press, Cambridge, Mass., 1972.

Kaplan, H. S. Summary of informal discussions on current status of clinical trials. Natl. Cancer Inst. Monogr., *36:* 421–422, 1973.

Kaplan, H. S., and Rosenberg, S. A. Extended-field radical radiotherapy in advanced Hodgkin's disease; short term results of two (2) randomized clinical trials. Cancer Res., *26:* 1268–1276, 1966.

Kaplan, H. S., and Rosenberg, S. A. Current status of clinical trials; Stanford experience, 1962–72. Natl Cancer Inst. Monogr., *36:* 363–371, 1973.

Kaplan, H. S., and Rosenberg, S. A. The management of Hodgkin's disease. Cancer, *36:* 796–803, 1975.

Kaplan, H. S., Dorfman, R. F., Nelsen, T. S., and Rosenberg, S. A. Staging laparotomy and splenectomy in Hodgkin's disease; analysis of indications and patterns of involvement in 285 consecutive, unselected patients. Natl. Cancer Inst. Monogr., *36:* 291–301, 1973.

Karnofsky, D. A. Chemotherapy of the lymphomas. In Proceedings of the International Conference on Leukemia-Lymphoma, edited by C. J. D. Zaratonetis, pp. 409–422. Lea & Febiger, Philadelphia, 1968.

Kirschner, R. H., Abt, A. B., O'Connell, M. J., Sklansky, B. D., Greene, W. H., and Wiernik, P. H. Vascular invasion and hematogenous dissemination of Hodgkin's disease. Cancer, *34:* 1159–1162, 1974.

Lacher, M. J., and Durant, J. R. Combined vinblastine and chlorambucil therapy of Hodgkin's disease. Ann. Intern. Med., *72:* 468–476, 1965.

LaMonte, C. S., and Lacher, M. J. Lymphangiography in patients with pulmonary dysfunction. Arch. Intern. Med., *132:* 365–367, 1973.

Lamoureux, K. B., Jaffe, E. S., Berard, C. W., and Johnson, R. E. Lack of identifiable vascular invasion in patients with extranodal dissemination of Hodgkin's disease. Cancer, *31:* 824–825, 1973.

LeFloch, O., Donaldson, S. S., and Kaplan, H. S. Pregnancy following oophoropexy and total nodal irradiation in women with Hodgkin's disease. Cancer, *38:* 2263–2268, 1976.

Lessner, H. E. BCNU (1,3-bis(β-chloroethyl)-1-nitrosourea); effects on advanced Hodgkin's disease and other neoplasia. Cancer, 22: 451–456, 1968.

Levi, J. A., and Wiernik, P. H. Limited extranodal Hodgkin's disease; unfavorable prognosis and therapeutic implications. Am. J. Med., 63: 365–372, 1977a.

Levi, J. A., and Wiernik, P. H. The therapeutic implications of splenic involvement in stage IIIA Hodgkin's disease. Cancer, 39: 2158–2165, 1977b.

Locksmith, J. P., and Powers, W. E. Permanent radiation myelopathy. A.J.R., 102: 916–926, 1968.

Lukes, R. J., and Butler, J. J. The pathology and nomenclature of Hodgkin's disease. Cancer Res., 26: 1063–1081, 1966.

Lukes, R. J., Butler, J. J., and Hicks, E. D. Natural history of Hodgkin's disease as related to its pathologic picture. Cancer, 19: 317–344, 1966a.

Lukes, R. J., Craver, L. F., Hall, T. C., Rappaport, H., and Ruben, P. Report of the nomenclature committee. Cancer Res., 26: 1311, 1966b.

MacMahon, B. Epidemiology of Hodgkin's disease. Cancer Res., 26: 1189–1200, 1966.

Maier, J. G., Perry, R. H., Saylor, W., and Sulak, M. H. Radiation myelitis of the dorsolumbar spinal cord. Radiology, 93: 153–160, 1969.

Martz, G., D'Alessandri, A., Keil, J. H., and Bollag, W. Preliminary clinical results with a new antitumor agent RO4-6467 (NSC-77213). Cancer Chemother. Rep., 33: 5–14, 1963.

Mathé, G., Schweisguth, V., Schneider, M., Amiel, J. L., Berumen, L., Brule, G., Cattan, A., and Schwarzenberg, L. Methylhydrazine in the treatment of Hodgkin's disease and various forms of haematosarcoma and leukaemia. Lancet, 2: 1077–1080, 1963.

McElwain, T. J., Wrigley, P. F. M., Hunter, A., Crowther, D., Malpas, J. S. Peckham, M. J., Smithers, D. W., and Fairley, G. H. Combination chemotherapy in advanced and recurrent Hodgkin's disease. Natl. Cancer Inst. Monogr., 36: 395–402, 1973.

McKelvey, E. M., Gottlieb, J. A., Coltman, C. A., and Wilson, H. E. Treatment of non-Hodgkin's lymphoma with hydroxyl daunomycin (Adriamycin) combination chemotherapy. Proc. Am. Soc. Clin. Oncol., 15: 184, 1974.

McKenna, R. W., and Brunning, R. D. Reed-Sternberg-like cells in nodular lymphoma involving the bone marrow. Am J. Clin. Pathol., 63: 779–785, 1975.

Medinger, F. G., and Craver, L. F. Total body irradiation. A. J. R., 48: 651–671, 1942.

Moxley, J. H., III, DeVita, V. T., Brace, K., and Frei, E., III. Intensive combination chemotherapy and X irradiation in Hodgkin's disease. Cancer Res., 27: 1258–1263, 1967.

Myers, C. E., Chabner, B. A., DeVita, V. T., and Gralnick, H. R. Bone marrow involvement in Hodgkin's disease; pathology and response to MOPP chemotherapy. Blood, 44: 197–204, 1974.

Naeim, F., Waisman, J., and Coulson, W. F. Hodgkin's disease; the significance of vascular invasion. Cancer, 34: 655–662, 1974.

Nissen, N. I., Stutzman, L., Holland, J. F., and Glidewell, O. J. Chemotherapy of Hodgkin's disease in studies by Acute Leukemia Group B. Arch. Intern. Med., 131: 396–401, 1973.

Nixon, D. W., and Aisenberg, A. C. Combination chemotherapy of Hodgkin's disease. Cancer, 33: 1499–1504, 1974.

Norris, D. G., Burgert, E. O., Jr., Cooper, H. A., and Harrison, E. G. Hodgkin's disease in childhood. Cancer, 36: 2109–2120, 1975.

O'Connell, M. J., Wiernik, P. H., Brace, K. C., Byhardt, R. W., and Greene, W. H. A combined modality approach to the treatment of Hodgkin's disease. Cancer, 35: 1055–1065, 1975.

Parker, B. R., Castellino, R. A., and Kaplan, H. S. Pediatric Hodgkin's disease; I. Radiographic evaluation. Cancer, 37: 2430–2435, 1976.

Peckham, M. J. Invited discussion; value of radiogallium scanning in Hodgkin's disease. Natl. Cancer Inst. Monogr., 36: 287–288, 1973.

Peters, M. V. The need for a new clinical classification in Hodgkin's disease; keynote address. Cancer Res., 31: 1713–1722, 1971.

Peters, M. V., and Middlemiss, K. C. H. A study of Hodgkin's disease treated by irradiation. A.J.R., *79:* 114–121, 1958.

Piro, A. J., Weiss, D. R., and Hellman, S. Mediastinal Hodgkin's disease; a possible danger for intubation anesthesia. Intubation danger in Hodgkin's disease. Int. J. Radiat. Oncol. Biol. Phys., *1:* 415–419, 1976.

Prager, D., Sembrot, J. T., and Southard, M. Cobalt-60 therapy of Hodgkin's disease and the subsequent development of hypothyroidism. Cancer, *29:* 458–460, 1972.

Prosnitz, L. R., Farber, L. R., Fischer, J. J., and Bertino, J. R. Long term remissions with combined modality therapy for advanced Hodgkin's disease. Cancer, *37:* 2826–2833, 1976.

Rappaport, H., and Strum, S. B. Vascular invasion in Hodgkin's disease; its incidence and relationship to the spread of the disease. Cancer, *25:* 1304–1313, 1970.

Ray, G. R., Trueblood, H. W., Enright, L. P. Kaplan, H. S. and Nelson, T. S. Oophoropexy; a means of preserving ovarian function following pelvic megavoltage radiotherapy for Hodgkin's disease. Radiology, *96:* 175–180, 1970.

Rege, V. B., and Owens, A. J., Jr. BCNU (NSC-409962) in the treatment of advanced Hodgkin's disease, lymphosarcoma and reticulum cell sarcoma. Cancer Chemother. Rep., *58:* 383–392, 1974.

Rosenberg, S. A. Report of the committee on the staging of Hodgkin's disease. Cancer Res., *26:* 1310, 1966.

Rosenberg, S. A., and Kaplan, H. S. The management of stages I, II and III Hodgkin's disease with combined radiotherapy and chemotherapy. Cancer, *35:* 55–63, 1975.

Rosenberg, S. A., Boiron, M., DeVita, V. T., Jr., Johnson, R. E., Lee, B. T., Ultmann, J. E., and Viamonte, M., Jr. Report of the committee on Hodgkin's disease staging procedures. Cancer Res., *31:* 1862–1863, 1971.

Royster, R. L., Jr., Wassum, J. A., and King, E. R. An evaluation of the effects of splenectomy in Hodgkin's disease in patients undergoing extended field or total lymph node irradiation. A.J.R., *120:* 521–530, 1974.

Rubin, P., Keys, H., Mayer, E., and Antemann, R. Nodal recurrence following radical radiation therapy in Hodgkin's disease. A.J.R., *120:* 536–548, 1974.

Salzman, J. R., and Kaplan, H. S. Effect of prior splenectomy on hematologic tolerance during total lymphoid radiotherapy of patients with Hodgkin's disease. Cancer, *27:* 471–478, 1971.

Schein, P. S., O'Connell, M. J., Blom, J., Hubbard, S., Magrath, I. T., Bergevin, P., Wiernik, P. H., Ziegler, J. L., and DeVita, V. T. Clinical antitumor activity and toxicity of streptozotocin (NSC-85998). Cancer, *34:* 993–1000, 1974.

Schick, P., Trepel, F., Theml, H., Benedek, S., Trumpp, P., Kaboth, W., Begemann, H., and Fliedner, T. M. Kinetics of lymphocytes in Hodgkin's disease. Blut, *28:* 223–235, 1973.

Schimpf, J. C., Schimpf, C. R., Brager, D. M., and Wiernik, P. H. Leukaemia and lymphoma patients interlinked by prior social contact. Lancet, *1:* 124–129, 1975.

Scott, J. L. The effect of nitrogen mustard and maintenance chlorambucil in the treatment of advanced Hodgkin's disease. Cancer Chemother. Rep., *27:* 27–32, 1963.

Sherins, R. J., and DeVita, V. T. Effect of drug treatment for lymphoma in male reproductive capacity; studies of men in remission after therapy. Ann Intern. Med., *79:* 216–220, 1973.

Shipley, W. U., Piro, A. J., and Hellman, S. Radiation therapy of Hodgkin's disease; significance of splenic involvement. Cancer, *34:* 223–229, 1974.

Speiser, B., Rubin, P., and Casarett, G. Aspermia following lower truncal irradiation in Hodgkin's disease. Cancer, *32:* 692–698, 1973.

Spittle, M. F., Harmer, C. L., Cassady, J. R., and Kaplan, H. S. Analysis of primary relapse after radiotherapy in Hodgkin's disease. Natl. Cancer Inst. Monogr., *36:* 497–508, 1973.

Spivack, S. D. Procarbazine. Ann. Intern. Med., *81:* 795–800, 1974.

Strum, S. B., and Rappaport, H. Interrelations of the histologic types of Hodgkin's disease. Arch. Pathol., *91:* 127–134, 1971.

Strum, S. B., Park, J. K., and Rappaport, H. Observation of cells resembling Sternberg-

Reed cells in conditions other than Hodgkin's disease. Cancer, *26:* 176–190, 1970.

Strum, S. B., Allen, L. W., and Rappaport, H. Vascular invasion in Hodgkin's disease; its relationship to involvement of the spleen and extranodal sites. Cancer, *28:* 1329–1334, 1971a.

Strum, S. B., Hutchinson, G. B., Park, J. K., and Rappaport, H. Further significance of vascular invasion in Hodgkin's disease. Cancer, *27:* 1–6, 1971b.

Teillet, F., Boiron, M., and Bernard, J. A reappraisal of clinical and biological signs in staging of Hodgkin's disease. Cancer Res., *31:* 1723–1729, 1971.

Thomas, P. R. M., and Peckham, M. J. The investigation and management of Hodgkin's disease in the pregnant patient. Cancer, *38:* 1443–1451, 1976.

Tubiana, M. Summary of informal discussion on staging procedures in Hodgkin's disease. Cancer Res., *31:* 1751–1754, 1971.

VanderWerf-Messing, B. Morbus Hodgkin's disease, stage I and II; trial of the European Organization for Research on Treatment of Cancer. Natl. Cancer Inst. Monogr., *36:* 381–386, 1973.

Vianna, N. J. Is Hodgkin's disease infectious? Cancer Res., *34:* 1149–1155, 1974.

Vianna, N. J., Davies, J. N. P., Polan, A. K., and Wolfgang, P. Familial Hodgkin's disease; an environmental and genetic disorder. Lancet, *2:* 854–857, 1974.

Vianna, N. J., Greenwald, P., Brady, J., Polan, A. K., Dwork, A., Mauro, J., and Davis, J. N. P. Hodgkin's disease; cases with features of a community outbreak. Ann. Intern. Med., *77:* 169–180, 1972.

Vianna, N. J., Greenwald, P., and Davis, J. N. P. Extended epidemic of Hodgkin's disease in high-school students. Lancet, *1:* 1209–1211, 1971.

Wiernik, P. H., and Lichtenfeld, J. L. Combined modality therapy for localized Hodgkin's disease; a seven-year update of an early study. Oncology, *32:* 208–213, 1975.

Wiernik, P. H., and Robinson, I. Radiotherapy (R) vs radiotherapy + MOPP (R+C) for Hodgkin's disease (HD) confined to lymphnodes. Proc. Am. Soc. Clin. Oncol., *19:* 369, 1978.

Weller, S. A., Glatstein, E., Kaplan, H. S., and Rosenberg, S. A. Initial relapses in previously treated Hodgkin's disease; I. Results of second treatment. Cancer, *37:* 2840–2846, 1976.

Wood, N. L., and Coltman, C. A. Localized primary extranodal Hodgkin's disease. Ann. Intern. Med., *78:* 113–118, 1973.

Yagoda, A., Mukherji, B., Young, C., Etcubanas, E., Lamonte, C., Smith, J. R., Tan, C. T. C., and Krakoff, I. H. Bleomycin, an antitumor antibiotic; clinical experience in 274 patients. Ann. Intern. Med., *77:* 861–870, 1972.

Young, R. C., DeVita, V. T., Jr., Serpick, A. A., and Canellos, G. P. Treatment of advanced Hodgkin's disease with (1,3-bis-(2-chloroethyl)-1-nitrosourea) BCNU. N. Engl. J. Med., *285:* 475–478, 1971.

Young, R. C., Canellos, G. P., Chabner, B. A., Schein, P. S., and DeVita, V. T. Maintenance chemotherapy for advanced Hodgkin's disease in remission. Lancet, *1:* 1339–1343, 1973a.

Young, R. C., Walker, M. D., Canellos, G. P., Schein, P. S., Chabner, B. A., and DeVita, V. T. Initial clinical trials with methyl-CCNU 1-(2-chloroethyl)-3-(4-methyl cyclohexyl)-1-nitrosourea (MeCCNU). Cancer, *31:* 1164–1169, 1973b.

Chapter 13

Malignant Lymphomas Other than Hodgkin's Disease

JOHANNES BLOM, M.D.

Malignant lymphoma comprises a group of disorders of lymphoproliferative character arising from lymph nodes and lymphoid elements in other tissues. In 1845, Virchow described lymphosarcoma, distinguishing this from leukemia which is characterized by involvement of the bone marrow with or without spilling of these abnormal cells into the peripheral blood. Histologic criteria for the diagnosis of lymphosarcoma was published by Kundrat in 1893, and those for reticulum cell sarcoma by Roulet in 1930. Brill et al. in 1925 and Symmers in 1938 described giant follicle hyperplasia of lymph nodes and spleen, an entity subsequently labeled with the eponym Brill-Symmers disease until more recent classifications by Rappaport et al. (1956) and Rappaport (1966).

The etiology is uncertain, although, based on experimental studies in animals, radiation exposure studies and development of lymphomas in immunologically depressed patients, viruses, radiation exposure, defects in immunologic surveillance and carcinogenesis by immunosuppressive drugs have been implicated (Peckham, 1974). The incidence of malignant lymphoma is about 6 per 100,000, occurring particularly in the 50–60-year-old age group.

PATHOLOGY

Lymphoreticular neoplasms arise from lymphocytes or histiocytes or more immature precursor cells. These cells are found particularly in bone marrow, lymph nodes, spleen, liver, thymus and in the submucosa of the gastrointestinal tract and bronchial tree, and in smaller foci in almost all tissues. Although lymphomas may present in one single area, commonly the disease is widespread at the time of diagnosis. Brill et al. (1925) and Symmers (1938) described lymphadenopathy and splenomegaly which microscopically were characterized by giant hyperplasia of the lymphoid follicles. Initially they were considered to be benign disorders, but subsequent reports have indicated their malignancy. Rappaport et al. (1956) found a marked diversity of cell types among the 253 cases of follicular lymphoma they reviewed. They used the term nodular rather than follicular. One category was Hodgkin's disease which Lukes et al. (1966) termed nodular lymphocytic and histiocytic Hodgkin's disease. Rappaport's (1966) classification (Table 13.1), with minor variations, is presently most widely used and is outlined in Table 13.2. Recent information on lymphocyte markers and thymus-derived and bone marrow-derived lymphocytes, T and B cell systems, respectively, has lead to newer, functional approaches in the classification of lymphomas (Lukes and Collins, 1974a, 1975). B cells are concentrated in the follicular centers of lymph nodes and the spleen, are prominent in the lamina propria of the gastrointestinal tract and are interspersed among other bone marrow cells. T cells are particularly located in the paracortical areas of lymph nodes and perivascular region of the spleen and in small foci in the gastrointestinal tract (Lukes and Collins, 1974b). Jaffe et al. (1974), Levine and Dorfman (1975) and Leech et al. (1975) have indicated a follicular center cell of the B cell type to be the predominant cell type in the nodular lymphomas. Micro-

TABLE 13.1
Rappaport Classification

Malignant Lymphoma, Cell Type	Nodular	Diffuse	Old Terminology
Lymphocytic well differentiated	No	Yes	
Lymphocytic poorly differentiated	Yes	Yes	Lymphosarcoma
Mixed lymphocytic-histiocytic	Yes	Yes	Reticulum cell sarcoma
Histiocytic	Yes	Yes	Reticulum cell sarcoma
Undifferentiated	No	Yes	
Undifferentiated, Burkitt's lymphoma	No	Yes	

TABLE 13.2
Modified Rappaport Classification[a]

Malignant Lymphoma, Cell Type	Nodular	Diffuse
Lymphocytic well differentiated	No	Yes (F)
Lymphocytic poorly differentiated	Yes (F)	Yes (U)
Mixed	Yes (F)	Yes (U)
Histiocytic	Yes (U)	Yes (U)
Undifferentiated	No	Yes (U)
Undifferentiated, Burkitt's type	No	Yes
Lymphoblastic		Yes
Immunoblastic		Yes
Mycosis fungoides		Yes

[a] F = favorable histology; U = unfavorable histology.

scopically these germinal center cells have distinct features such as nuclear blebs and nuclear indentations. Most of the so-called histiocytic lymphomas consist of transformed lymphocytes. True histiocytic lymphomas consisting of dendritic reticulum cells are rare and may comprise less than 5% of all lymphomas (Editorial, 1974).

Differentiation between reactive follicular hyperplasia and nodular (follicular) lymphoma may be difficult, but the major criteria for malignancy are the following: (a) effacement of the normal nodal architecture, (b) uniform nodularity with little variation in size and shape, (c) indistinct peripheral margins of the follicles, (d) compression of reticulin fibers and small blood vessels in the stroma surrounding the follicles, (e) absence of the macrophages, (f) a paucity of mitotic figures, and (g) cellular monotony; usually only one or two distinct cell types can be recognized. They are usually of the poorly differentiated, lymphocytic type, or of the larger "histiocytic" type which several investigators now believe to be activated lymphocytes rather than true reticulum cells. Immunological studies suggest that lymphomas of the T and B cell systems develop from either a block or a "switch on" (derepression) in lymphocyte transformation rather than from alterations in cellular differentiation. Differences in cell forms are expressions of differences in metabolic state of lymphocytes rather than variations in histologic differentiation on which the older classifications were based.

Hodgkin's disease, mycosis fungoides and Sézary's syndrome have been mentioned as possible T cell lymphomas. Chronic lymphocytic leukemia, Waldenström's macroglobulinemia, Burkitt's lymphoma, nodular and diffuse lymphocytic and histiocytic lymphoma would all belong to the B cell system. This functional classification based on different stages of lymphocyte transformation gives better insight into the growth characteristics of these lymphocyte disorders and will hopefully lead to better and more differentiated forms of therapy.

Lukes and Tindle (1975) and others subsequently have described immunoblastic lymphadenopathy in patients who present with fever, sweats and weight loss and who are found to have hepatosplenomegaly, polyclonal hyperglobulinemia, and often Coombs positive hemolytic anemia. This condition may develop as a hypersensitivity reaction after exposure to certain drugs, such as penicillin (Schultz and Yunis, 1975). Immunoblastic sarcoma has been described in patients with immunological abnormalities such as those that develop while on immunosuppressive drugs, in patients with α-chain disease and macroglobulinemia of Waldenström and in patients with pre-existing immunoproliferative processes such as Sjögren's syndrome and angioimmunoblastic lymphadenopathy.

Dorfman (1977) reviewed all the new classifications of the non-Hodgkin's lymphomas at a lymphoma conference in San Francisco. Bloomfield et al. (1977) at the same conference found the best survival prediction to be based on a combination of the Rappaport histologic classification and surface marker studies. Subsequent roundtable discussions (Berard, 1977) raised many questions and indicated inadequacies of the various classifications, but for the present time the Rappaport classification with some additions as outlined remains the most practical and clinically the most useful.

The criteria for nodular lymphoma may vary somewhat at different institutions, but Warnke et al. (1977) have indicated that in the poorly differentiated lymphocytic and mixed histiocytic-lymphocytic categories any degree of nodularity imparts a more favorable prognosis than diffuse lymphoma. An exception is histiocytic lymphoma in which diffuse areas in otherwise nodular disease behaves more like diffuse than nodular disease.

CLINICAL MANIFESTATIONS

Rosenberg et al. reviewed 1269 cases of lymphoma from Memorial Hospital in 1961, and Mukherji et al. (1974) 76 cases with lymphosarcoma (LSA) and 112 cases with reticulum cell sarcoma (RCS) from the same hospital. These reviews antedate the Rappaport classification. About 50% of patients with LSA presented with adenopathy, but only about 30% of patients with RCS presented in this manner and had more frequently an extranodal site of presentation, with or without nodal involvement. Retroperitoneal involvement was the same for both disorders and amounted to approximately 70% as found with lymphangiography and/or laparotomy. Presentation with a mediastinal mass is not as common as in Hodgkin's disease. Epitrochlear nodes, which are rarely involved in Hodgkin's disease, are frequently abnormal in other lymphomas, particularly in those of the nodular variety. Bone marrow infiltration with normal lymphocytes does not seem to influence survival, however, invasion with immature cells usually indicates a worse prognosis. Symptoms such as fever, night sweats, and weight loss were present in approximately 10% of patients with LSA and 18.5% of patients with RCS. Usually these patients had widely disseminated disease. The systemic symptoms did not seem to influence the poor prognosis of this group of patients. Jones et al. (1973a) found symptoms in 17% of patients with nodular and in 24% with diffuse disease, predominantly Stage III and IV, among 405 cases they analyzed. Presence of symptoms did not adversely affect survival. Patchefsky et al. (1974) reported higher incidences: 26% in the nodular and 30% in the diffuse lymphomas, also mostly in patients with Stage III and IV disease. Six-year survival rates in nodular lymphomas were 16% for patients with symptoms and 47% for those without. In diffuse lymphomas the figures were 2% and 24%. These were all significant differences. Peters et al. (1975) found elevated levels of erythrocyte sedimentation rate (ESR) to be associated with systemic symptoms rather than with greater extent of the disease. In a large group of patients treated with radiation therapy, all patients with an ESR (Westergren method) less than 35 mm per hour, survived 1 year. When the ESR was 35–69 mm per hour the survival rate dropped to 56% at the end of the first year. Involvement of a single extranodal site bears as good a prognosis as single nodal involvement. This has also been demonstrated by other investigators (Cox et al., 1972). Diffuse involvement of several extranodal-intraabdominal areas bears as poor a prognosis as disseminated disease. Generalized nodal involvement had a relatively good prognosis. In LSA the median survival was 35 months and in RCS 23 months in patients with nodal disease. Eventually all organs may become involved. Lymph node involvement in certain areas may lead to symptoms of obstruction and neurologic manifestations. Reticulum cell sarcoma of the bone is a separate entity and will be discussed under malignancies of the bone.

DIAGNOSTIC EVALUATION

As has been discussed under Hodgkin's disease, an obviously enlarged node or a mass should be biopsied promptly in order to establish a diagnosis. Not infrequently patients will mention that a node or nodes have been present for many months or even longer, with considerable fluctuation in size. This should not be a deterrent to biopsy, as this is a history perfectly compatible with particularly a nodular lymphoma.

Symptoms like fever, night sweats and weight loss are not as common and do not seem to worsen the prognosis as much as in Hodgkin's disease. Careful questioning concerning abdominal discomfort, back ache, and gastrointestinal symptoms may establish a presumptive diagnosis of gastrointestinal or retroperitoneal involvement.

A thorough physical examination is as necessary as in Hodgkin's disease. Epitrochlear and popliteal nodes are more commonly involved than in Hodgkin's disease. Nasopharyngeal masses can often be detected early in the disease, before they are large enough to cause nasal speech or other symptoms. A careful neurologic examination is indicated to detect signs of spinal and/or peripheral nerve involvement. Lymphomatous intracranial involvement is more common than in Hodgkin's disease and is particularly prevalent in patients with leukemic transformation, retroperitoneal involvement (Law et al., 1975), or Burkitt's lymphoma.

Roentgenologic examinations should include posteroanterior and lateral films of the chest with whole lung tomography, particularly if there is mediastinal-paratracheal involvement. Lung parenchymal involvement with otherwise limited disease would be a definite contraindication to radiation therapy. Indications for lymphangiography, excretory urogram, liver and spleen scan, bone scan and bone survey are similar to those in Hodgkin's disease.

In a prospective study lymphangiography was performed in 93 patients with previously untreated non-Hodgkin's lymphoma (Castellino et al., 1974). Sixty-nine patients underwent staging laparotomy; radiologic-pathologic correlation was possible in 63 cases. Of 30 lymphangiograms interpreted as normal, only in 1 case was microscopic evidence of lymphoma found. Two cases interpreted as benign were confirmed, so there was 97% accuracy of the negative lymphangiograms. Of 31 abnormal lymphangiograms, 27 were histologically proven to contain lymphoma and the remaining 4 had striking benign reactive changes. The accuracy of the positive examinations was 87% and the overall lymphangiographic accuracy was 92%. In the study by Abrams et al. (1968), the accuracy of the negative studies was 70% and of the positive studies 91% with an overall accuracy of 80%. This lower accuracy is partially the result of misinterpretation of earlier lymphangiograms. Total body scanning utilizing ^{67}Ga-citrate can be helpful, although the rate of positive scans in individual sites was 53% in lymphomas compared with 65% in Hodgkin's disease (Greenlaw et al., 1974). The positive scans ranged from 36% in poorly differentiated lymphocytic lymphoma to 70% in histiocytic lymphoma. Positive scans were confirmed histologically or clinically in almost 90%. Demonstration of disease, otherwise undetected, accounted for only about 10% and is more commonly located above the diaphragm than below. Similar findings have been reported by others (Levi et al., 1975; Horn et al., 1976). As mentioned in the chapter on Hodgkin's disease, computerized axial tomography (CAT) scanning is the most recent addition to the diagnostic armamentarium and is particularly useful for the evaluation of the upper abdomen, where the lymphangiogram is usually not helpful, and for mesenteric nodes which are frequently involved in non-Hodgkin's lymphoma contrary to Hodgkin's disease (Jones et al., 1978).

Routine laboratory tests include a complete blood count with platelet count, sedimentation rate, urinalysis, alkaline phosphatase with fractionation in case of abnormal values and uncertain etiology, blood urea nitrogen or serum creatinine, and serum uric acid. At least a single, but by preference a bilateral, iliac crest bone marrow needle biopsy plus an aspiration or a surgical biopsy should be performed. Bone marrow involvement in clinical Stage I and II disease is very rare. Ninety-four percent of patients with bone marrow involvement had at least Stage III disease (Jones et al., 1973a). Vinciguerra and Silver (1973) found bone marrow involvement in 63% of 75 patients with lymphosarcoma. These were not subdivided into nodular or diffuse disease. Contrary to other investigators, they found higher incidences in a small number of patients with Stage I and II disease: 4 of 9 and 9 of 12, respectively. Patients with lymphocytic lymphoma have a higher incidence of marrow involvement than those with histiocytic or mixed lymphoma, and those with nodular disease higher than those with diffuse (Dick et al., 1974). The significance of an increased number of normal lymphocytes is uncertain. Also the significance of the early finding of bone marrow involvement is still uncertain, as patients with nodular lymphomas and bone marrow involvement have considerably longer survival than those with diffuse lymphomas and marrow involvement. Sexauer et al. (1975), in a retrospective review of 76 cases of both nodular and diffuse lymphocytic lymphomas, found a much shorter survival of patients with B symptoms than of patients without symptoms (A) regardless of bone marrow involvement. Severe leukopenia and/or thrombocytopenia at the time of diagnosis were found in only 3% of 550 non-Hodgkin's lymphoma patients (Koziner et al., 1975). Five patients with well differentiated lymphoma did well. The median survival of 12 patients with diffuse poorly differentiated lymphoma was only 4 months. Although with bone marrow involvement the bone scan with technicium-99^m is usually positive, Schechter et al. (1976) found it a helpful procedure in the detection of bone involvement even when clinically not suspected. The usefulness of ultrasonography was discussed in the chapter on Hodgkin's disease. After this extensive evaluation a clinical assessment of the extent of the disease can be made, as described under Hodgkin's disease. The Ann Arbor classification is the one most widely used also in non-Hodgkin's lymphomas. The significance of the "B symptoms" is not as clear as in Hodgkin's disease and in most series are not taken into account.

Although reports on staging laparotomy for Hodgkin's disease are more numerous, several reports concerning this procedure in large groups of patients with non-Hodgkin's lymphomas have recently been published. This topic was discussed extensively at a symposium on non-Hodgkin's lymphomas, held in London in October 1973 and published in the *British Journal of Cancer, 31:* Supplement II, 1975. Moran et al. (1975) performed a staging laparotomy in 57 lymphoma patients. Thirty-one of these patients had a lymphangiogram. One hundred and four sites were analyzed on the lymphangiograms. In 83% of these a correct interpretation of abnormality was made. Normal lymphangiograms were accurately interpreted in 67% of the sites. The sensitivity of the lymphangiograms in detecting lymphoma was only 49%. Positive interpretation of the gallium scan was correct in 82% and negative interpretation in 59%. The sensitivity of the gallium scan to detect lymphoma was only 31%. The accuracy of the clinical evaluation of the liver and spleen status is similar to that in Hodgkin's disease, however, splenomegaly was highly predictive of liver involvement (Chabner et al., 1975). Liver involvement with a normal spleen is a rare occurrence. Liver and spleen were more frequently involved in lymphocytic lymphomas than in histiocytic lymphomas. With para-aortic node involvement celiac and mesenteric nodes were involved in, respectively, 100% and 86% of the cases with poorly differentiated lymphocytic lymphoma and in 66% and 50% of the cases with histiocytic lymphoma. Lymphocytic lymphomas have a greater tendency toward contiguous spread than histiocytic lymphomas. The mediastinum is less frequently involved than in Hodgkin's disease. Similar findings have been reported by others (Rosenberg et al., 1975; Bonadonna et al., 1975; Goffinet et al., 1977). Johnson et al. (1975) reviewed the results of the prospective staging of 100 consecutive patients. Only 2 were found to be Stage I (one nodular lymphocytic poorly differentiated and one diffuse histiocytic) and 11 Stage II (one diffuse lymphocytic poorly differentiated, three diffuse histiocytic, two nodular mixed, two extranodal diffuse lymphocytic and three extranodal histiocytic). The authors stress that only rarely intensive radiation therapy with fields as used in Hodgkin's disease is indicated because of the widespread nodal and extranodal involvement at time of diagnosis in most patients.

Laparotomy after percutaneous liver biopsy and after peritoneoscopy reveals liver involvement in a small percentage of patients with Hodgkin's disease and histiocytic lymphomas, but revealed liver involvement in 7 of 17 patients with lymphocytic lymphomas (Chabner et al., 1975).

It is clear that staging laparotomy in lymphomas, contrary to Hodgkin's disease, is necessary only in a limited number of patients because evaluation of liver and bone marrow frequently reveals Stage IV disease. Moreover, the age and the general medical condition of the patient who might benefit from laparotomy are often contraindications. Most Stage III patients with a positive lymphangiogram have extensive intra-abdominal or organ involvement so that a laparotomy is rarely required.

THERAPY

Indications for surgical treatment and splenectomy are similar to those discussed under Hodgkin's disease. Extranodal involvement of the gastrointestinal tract, particularly a single lesion of the stomach without regional node involvement, may best be treated with radical excision. Reportedly the 5-year survival is approximately 65% (Naqvi et al. 1969; Loehr et al., 1969; Burgess et al., 1971). Postoperative radiation therapy in these cases with limited disease is of dubious value. More advanced disease of the stomach and other areas of the gastrointestinal tract that is resectable, with postoperative radiation therapy, has a 5-year survival of approximately 40%. Survival of unresectable disease is approximately 6 months with only an occasional patient surviving for several years.

Spontaneous regressions of these lymphomas have been reported (Tietjen and McAllister, 1974). These lesions should be differentiated from pseudolymphoma (Smith and Helwig, 1958; Jacobs, 1963).

The principles of high dose-large field radiation therapy have also been discussed under Hodgkin's disease. The indications for radiation therapy in the lymphomas are far less certain than in Hodgkin's disease. As discussed earlier, thorough evaluation will often reveal extranodal involvement which precludes radiation therapy as the sole form of treatment. However, the approximately 15% of patients who present with Stage I disease may be curable with radiation therapy and have a 4-year disease-free survival of over 80% (Peters et al., 1975). The results with Stage II disease are very similar to those with Stage III disease—approximately 50% 4-year survival. This probably indicates that most patients with Stage II disease have in reality more advanced disease. Similar results have been reported by others (Hellman et al., 1977; Bush et al., 1977; Bitran et al., 1977). Since Stage I and IIB patients may also have a greater chance of having more extensive disease, these patients might better be treated with chemotherapy. The value of radiation to areas of bulky disease, in addition to chemotherapy in patients with Stage III and IV disease is presently under investigation; although local control may be improved overall survival does not seem to be benefited.

Results of radiation therapy in patients who present with extranodal disease, without regional lymph node involvement, is very similar to those of Stage IA nodal disease and very favorable. Involvement of regional nodes decreases the 4-year survival to approximately 50%. Doses employed usually are in the range of 3000 rads delivered in approximately 20 fractions, although smaller doses can be used in nodular lymphomas with small discrete nodes.

Results in other studies are mostly reported for lymphosarcoma and reticulum cell sarcoma, however with the Rappaport classification patients with favorable and unfavorable histologies can be identified. Rosenberg and Kaplan (1975) reported on preliminary results of controlled clinical trials in 127 patients divided in 7 experimental groups. These groups were based on pathological stages and histological subgroups as defined by Rappaport. They also made a retrospective analysis of 405 patients treated at Stanford between 1960 and 1971 (Jones et al., 1973a). The fact that these investigators found Stage II patients prognostically similar to Stage I patients, as opposed to Peters et al.'s findings, may be the result of aggressive staging procedures. Although the number of patients in each treatment category is limited, several interesting observations were made. As mentioned previously extensive evaluation reduces the number of patients with Stage I, II and III disease. Stage I and II disease, both favorable and unfavorable histology, can be well controlled with radiation therapy. So far addition of chemotherapy has not improved the results. Patients with advanced disease and favorable histology can be well controlled with single agent chemotherapy, combination chemotherapy or combination chemotherapy plus radiation therapy. The results in Stage IV disease with unfavorable histology are poor with both multiple drug chemotherapy and chemotherapy plus radiation therapy. The employed chemotherapy and more recent results of some of these studies will be discussed further under the chemotherapy section.

Because of early spread after local radiation therapy and relapses after chemotherapy, particularly when fewer effective drugs were available, Johnson and his group at the National Cancer Institute (NCI) reactivated the interest in total body irradiation (TBI). The principles of TBI were described as early as 1907 (Dessauer), 12 years after the discovery of x-rays. Reports on clinical results followed in 1923 (Chaoul and Lange), 1927 (Teschendorf), 1932 (Heublein) and 1942 (Medinger and Craver). In 1975 Johnson reported his results in 57 patients with lymphocytic lymphomas. Thirty-one of these received TBI, 18 "comprehensive" lymph node irradiation (CNI) and 8 a combination of the two. All patients had Stage III or IV disease. Complete remission rate was 100% in 18 patients treated with CNI and 68% in 31 patients treated with TBI. The author ascribes this to the better risk patients in the CNI group. The survival rates for patients with poorly differentiated nodular disease are similar to those described in Rosenberg and Kaplan's study, referred to earlier. Patients with diffuse histology did better in the Johnson study, however histiocytic lymphomas were excluded from that study, while they were included in the Rosenberg-Kaplan study. TBI is well tolerated and toxicity compares favorably with that of chemotherapy. Similar results were observed by Chaffey et al. (1977) in 78 patients. Brace et al. (1974) reported 7 responses of short duration in 9 patients. Contrary to the experience of the previous authors they found the delivery of subsequent chemotherapy seriously compromised. Quasim (1975) observed 12 complete remissions in 14 previously treated patients with Stage IV lymphosarcoma. The remissions lasted from 1 to 17 months after one course of therapy. They found TBI effective therapy in a number of patients who were resistant to conventional forms of therapy.

CHEMOTHERAPY

Effective chemotherapy for both Hodgkin's disease and lymphomas was first described by Jacobson et al. in 1946. Most of the agents that are effective in Hodgkin's disease also have activity in lymphomas, although some of them to a lesser degree than in Hodgkin's disease. Asparaginase, which has no role in Hodgkin's disease, has some activity in lymphomas.

Single Agent Chemotherapy

The three most widely used alkylating agents are nitrogen mustard, cyclophosphamide and chlorambucil. The usual dose of nitrogen mustard is 0.4 mg/kg which may be repeated after approximately 4 weeks when hematologic toxicity has cleared. However, prolonged use usually causes severe leukopenia and thrombocytopenia which in addition to the marked nausea and vomiting which occur for about 24 hours after the administration make this an unsuitable drug for maintenance therapy.

Cyclophosphamide can be used for induction and maintenance therapy in daily oral doses of 2.0 to 2.5 mg/kg or 15 mg/kg intravenously once weekly, but is more effective in intermittent intravenous doses of 30–40 mg/kg given every 3–4 weeks (Mendelson et al., 1970). These authors reported a complete response rate of 38% with a mean duration of 20.4 months. The gastrointestinal side effects are less than those of nitrogen mustard, but hemorrhagic cystitis may be an unpleasant and sometimes serious complication. Adequate hydration prior to the administration may help avert this problem. Although leukopenia can be severe with the nadir around the 8th to the 12th day, thrombocytopenia is usually not of clinical significance.

Carbone (1972) reviewed the response to various single agents, which is summarized in Table 13.3. Complete responses were usually only 10% or less and short lived, less than 30 weeks, even with maintenance. Jones et al. (1972) in a retrospective analysis of 110 patients with non-Hodgkin's lymphoma, who received primary or secondary treatment with either daily cyclophosphamide or chlorambucil, found the proportion of complete responders significantly higher and the duration of response longer in patients with nodular disease compared to those with diffuse lymphoma. In a prospective study Rosenberg and Kaplan (1975) found daily chlorambucil as effective as combination chemotherapy with or without

TABLE 13.3
Relative Sensitivity of the Lymphomas to Chemotherapy

	Hodgkin's Disease		Lymphocytic Lymphoma		Histiocytic Lymphoma	
	%	no.	%	no.	%	no.
Nitrogen mustard	63	432	49	154	18	17
Cyclophosphamide	54	452	65	276	56	219
Vinblastine	65	380	27	84 (L.-H.)		
Vincristine	60	92	53	93	61	72
Procarbazine	69	347	40.5	42	36	33
Prednisone	54	40	74	47		

[a] Adapted from Livingston and Carter (1970) by Carbone (1972).

radiation therapy in Stage IV nodular lymphoma. It is imperative, therefore, that Rappaport's classification is utilized when results of various studies are compared. Portlock and Rosenberg (1978) recently reported that careful observation without initial therapy is an appropriate option in the management of patients with relatively asymptomatic advanced non-Hodgkin's lymphomas with favorable histologies. Median time to treatment was 31 months, varying from 9 months for nodular mixed lymphocytic-histiocytic to 8+ years for well differentiated diffuse lymphoma.

From the same institutions (Portlock et al., 1976) it was reported that in a prospective randomized trial in patients with Stage IV favorable histology 4-year survival was as good with single agent therapy as with combinations of chemotherapeutic agents or chemotherapy plus radiation therapy. However it should be kept in mind that 4 years of observation is still rather short for this type of lymphoma.

N-Methylhydrazine or procarbazine has been used predominantly in Hodgkin's disease. Spivack (1974) reported a 36% overall response rate in a small group of patients with reticulum cell sarcoma and a 40% response rate in lymphosarcoma. Although predominantly used in combination with other drugs for the treatment of Hodgkin's disease, the same combinations have activity also in non-Hodgkin's lymphomas.

The experience with the nitrosoureas is also considerably less in the non-Hodgkin's lymphomas than in Hodgkin's disease with lesser response rates in a very limited number of patients. Carter (1973) in an overview reported a 50% response rate in 149 patients with Hodgkin's disease and a 28% response rate in 107 patients with other lymphomas. Tranum et al. (1975) in a Southwest Oncology Group study had only 10 patients with lymphoma, one of whom responded.

Blum and Carter's (1974) review of Adriamycin revealed 19 of 34 responses in previously treated advanced reticulum cell sarcoma and 12 of 35 in lymphosarcoma. These promising results led to the combination of Adriamycin with other drugs analogous to the MOPP regimen for the treatment of Hodgkin's disease.

Streptozotocin caused 2 of 5 partial remissions in poorly differentiated nodular lymphoma and 1 complete remission in 6 patients with diffuse disease; none of 3 patients with diffuse histiocytic lymphoma responded (Schein et al., 1974).

Few responses of short duration were described by Yagoda et al. (1972) and by Blum et al. (1973) with bleomycin. Better results were reported by Rudders (1972) who observed greater than 50% regression in 18 of 33 patients. Because of its bone marrow sparing effect it has been incorporated in several combination regimens.

Combination Chemotherapy

Because of the efficacy of alkylating agents, vincristine and cortico-steroids as single agents and because of improved efficacy of vincristine plus corticosteroids in acute lymphocytic leukemia of childhood, Hoog-straten et al. (1969) compared weekly intravenous cyclophosphamide 15 mg/kg with a combination of the same dose of cyclophosphamide plus vincristine 0.025 mg/kg weekly and prednisone 1 mg/kg daily and a low dose combination consisting of cyclophosphamide 10 mg/kg weekly, vincristine 0.017 mg/kg weekly and prednisone 0.67 mg/kg daily. Com-plete plus partial responses were 43% in lymphosarcoma and 45% in reticulum cell sarcoma with cyclophosphamide alone. With the high dose combination the results were 100% and 85%; with the low dose combina-tion results in lymphosarcoma were essentially the same—90%, but in reticulum cell sarcoma significantly less—54%. The median remission duration was about 100 days and essentially the same for unmaintained remissions as for maintenance with twice weekly methotrexate.

Similar results with somewhat higher complete response rates were reported by Luce et al. (1971) with cyclophosphamide 800 mg/m^2 and vincristine 2 mg/m^2 on day 1 and prednisone 60 mg/m^2 daily for 5 days (COP) repeated every 14 days. Maintained complete remissions lasted more than twice as long as unmaintained remissions in lymphosarcoma and were not significantly different in reticulum cell sarcoma. Survival of previously untreated patients was significantly better with this regimen than with single agent regimens. Twelve-month survival for previously untreated patients with lymphocytic lymphoma who were in complete remission (CR) was as high as 90%.

Schein et al. (1974) reported on 80 patients staged according to Ann Arbor criteria with Rappaport's histologic classification. Treatment con-sisted of either cyclophosphamide 400 mg/m^2 daily intravenously for 5 days, vincristine 1.4 mg/m^2 intravenously on day 1 plus prednisone 100 mg/m^2 daily orally for 5 days (CVP, Table 13.4), MOPP or CMOPP (Table 13.5) in which cyclophosphamide 650 mg/m^2 on days 1 and 8 was substituted for nitrogen mustard. Four patients with diffuse well differ-

TABLE 13.4
CVP Combination Chemotherapy

Drugs (mg/m^2)	Days						
	1	2	3	4	5	6–21	22
Cyclophosphamide (PO or IV)	400	400	400	400	400	No ther-apy	Next cycle
Vincristine (IV)	1.4						
Prednisone (PO)	100	100	100	100	100		

TABLE 13.5
C-MOPP Combination Chemotherapy

Drugs (mg/m²)	Days			
	1	8	15–28	29
Cyclophosphamide (IV)	650	650	No therapy	Next cycle
Vincristine (IV)	1.4	1.4		
Procarbazine (PO)[a]	100	→		
Prednisone (PO)[a]	40	→		

[a] Daily for 14 days.

TABLE 13.6
BACOP Combination Chemotherapy

Drugs (mg/m²)	Days					
	1	8	15	22	28	29
Bleomycin (IV)			5	5		Next cycle
Adriamycin (IV)	25	25				
Cyclophosphamide (IV)	650	650				
Vincristine (IV)	1.4	1.4				
Prednisone[a]			60	→		

[a] Daily for 14 days.

entiated lymphoma survived for prolonged periods of time regardless whether they obtained a complete or a partial remission, contrary to other histologic categories where patients with complete remissions survive longer than those with partial remission. Patients with nodular disease do better than those with diffuse disease and lymphocytic better than histiocytic. Twenty-seven patients with the latter histology were reported separately (DeVita et al., 1975). In general patients with histiocytic lymphoma tend to respond dramatically, but also tend to relapse rapidly, often before the next course of treatment can be started. However, the patients who do obtain a sustained complete remission will remain in remission for prolonged periods of time and may be cured since no relapses have occurred in ten patients 24 months after the end of treatment. Subsequent reports from the same group (Anderson et al., 1977) and others have confirmed this prolonged survival in patients with Stage III and IV histiocytic lymphoma. Careful restaging is absolutely necessary to confirm the clinical impression of a CR as much as possible (Herman and Jones, 1977).

Because of the propensity to rapid relapse in between cycles and the less than 50% complete remission rate in these lymphomas, Schein et al. (1976) designed the BACOP regimen (Table 13.6) which yielded 12 of 25 complete remissions.

Skarin et al. (1977) with a slightly different BACOP regimen observed 66% complete remissions in 44 patients with diffuse disease.

TABLE 13.7
CAT Combination Chemotherapy

Drugs	Days						
	1	2	3	4	5	6–21	22
Adriamycin (mg/m², IV)	60					No therapy	Next cycle
Cytosine arabinoside (mg/kg, IV)		3.0	3.0	3.0	3.0		
6-Thioguanine (mg/kg, PO)		2.5	2.5	2.5	2.5		

The same NCI group (Canellos et al., 1975) reported on a randomized clinical trial comparing intensive CVP treatment with total body radiation therapy in Stage III and IV lymphocytic lymphoma. Fifteen of 27 or 55% of patients treated with CVP had a CR and 24 or 81% a CR + PR. Overall survival was not significantly different between the two treatment modalities. Patients with nodular lymphoma responded more frequently than those with diffuse and had a significantly longer survival. The combination of total body radiation and multiple drug chemotherapy was not any better than each modality alone in a randomized trial (Brereton et al., 1978). Lenhard et al. (1976) found 43% complete remissions with COP, but only 17% with CO; this latter regimen also had shorter remission durations and decreased survival. This indicates the importance of prednisone in combination regimens.

Portlock and Rosenberg (1976) reported on their experience with CVP at Stanford Medical Center. The addition of bleomycin to the regimen in 17 patients did not improve the results. Overall response rate was 78.5% with 33.9% complete remission. Best results were seen in the nodular lymphomas with 96.6% responses, 43.3% of which were complete. In general, survival of patients with complete remissions is better than those with a partial response, however for nodular lymphomas there is no significant difference, probably because the main difference between CR and PR is the persistence of bone marrow infiltration after all evidence of peripheral disease has gone. These same authors (Portlock and Rosenberg, 1977) observed 44.4% complete remissions in previously untreated patients with nodular and diffuse histiocytic and mixed lymphomas utilizing the CAT regimen (Table 13.7). Responses in previously treated patients were few and the duration of complete responses were disappointingly short, contrary to the experience with other regimens.

McKelvey et al. (1976) reported on a randomized study by the Southwest Oncology Group between cyclophosphamide, Adriamycin, vincristine plus prednisone (CHOP, Table 13.8), and Adriamycin, vincristine and prednisone (HOP, Table 13.9). Complete remission rates were 71% and 60% and CR + PR 92% and 88%. Patients with nodular disease had somewhat higher rates of CR with both regimens. Subsequently the same author (McKelvey, 1978) reported higher complete remissions with CHOP in nodular and diffuse lymphocytic lymphomas and with HOP in nodular and diffuse histiocytic lymphomas, including longer duration of remission and survival.

The addition of bleomycin to the CHOP regimen (Rodriguez et al., 1977) does not seem to be of particular benefit.

Garrett et al. (1977) at Memorial Cancer Center have utilized 1000–1200 mg/m^2 of cyclophosphamide followed by cyclophosphamide, vincristine, prednisone and daunorubicin with radiation therapy to massively

TABLE 13.8
CHOP Combination Chemotherapy

Drugs	Days		
	1	5	
Cyclophosphamide (mg/m², IV)	750		Repeat every 2–3 weeks
Adriamycin (mg/m², IV)	50		
Vincristine(mg/m², IV)[a]	1.4		
Prednisone (PO)[b]	100	→	

[a] Maximum, 2 mg.
[b] Daily for 5 days.

TABLE 13.9
HOP Combination Chemotherapy

Drugs	Days		
	1	5	
Adriamycin (mg/m², IV)	80		Repeat every 2–3 weeks
Vincristine (mg/m², IV)[a]	1.4		
Prednisone (PO)[b]	100	→	

[a] Maximum, 2 mg.
[b] Daily for 5 days.

involved areas. Prophylactic intrathecal methotrexate or cytosine arabinoside is given to all patients under 40 and to all patients with bone marrow involvement. L-Asparaginase and BCNU are added later, followed by a maintenance of multiple courses of various drugs. Results in diffuse lymphocytic lymphomas are similar to and in histiocytic lymphomas worse than in other reported series with a greater amount of toxicity.

Berd et al. (1975) treated 15 evaluable reticulum cell sarcoma patients with a regimen outlined in Table 13.10. Nine had a CR and 6 a partial remission (PR). It is interesting that upon reclassification according to Rappaport's criteria, 8 patients had diffuse and 2 had nodular histiocytic lymphoma; the remaining 6 had lymphocytic lymphoma. Of the 8 patients with diffuse histiocytic lymphoma 6 attained a CR and 1 a PR. One of the CR patients had a short survival; the remaining ones are in continued remission greater than 39 months.

MOPP, although used predominantly in Hodgkin's disease, reportedly has activity in lymphocytic and histiocytic lymphomas (Lowenbraun et al., 1970). Anderson et al. (1977) reviewed the experience with CVP (Table 13.4), C-MOPP (Table 13.5) and BACOP (Table 13.6) at the NCI, confirming their previous observations.

With the better regimens and longer survivals in diffuse histiocytic lymphomas central nervous system (CNS) involvement is becoming a more frequent complication. Prophylactic radiation therapy to the brain and/or chemotherapy intrathecally seems to be of benefit with considerable reduction of CNS involvement (Sweet et al., 1978; Bunn and DeVita, 1978), contrary to the experience in children as will be discussed later.

Various other combination chemotherapy regimens have been described, many have only limited number of patients and lack the previously mentioned detailed histologic analysis. Taking these histologic groups and the clinical stages into account requires large numbers of patients to perform randomized studies, as was pointed out by Rosenberg and Kaplan (1975), however these studies are clearly indicated.

Contrary to Hodgkin's disease, non-Hodgkin's lymphomas in children are quite different from those in adults. They are almost exclusively of the diffuse variety. Immunological studies have been quite helpful in providing some differentiation.

Diffuse undifferentiated non-Burkitt type or lymphoblastic lymphoma predominantly affects boys over 6 years old. There is usually mediastinal and thymic involvement as well as early development of the CNS and bone marrow involvement with high peripheral blast counts. This is a disease of the T lymphocytes that demonstrate marked convolutions of the nucleus. It is far less responsive to chemotherapy than "B" or "null" cell lymphomas.

The "null" cell lymphoblastic lymphomas have none of the "T" or "B" cell characteristics. They are found equally in boys and girls, mostly under the age of six. The patients are usually anemic with low white blood cell counts and early bone marrow involvement. They respond promptly to chemotherapy and tend to have prolonged complete remissions. "B" lymphocytic lymphoma is usually of the poorly differentiated nodular variety, is quite rare, usually localized and curable with local radiation therapy. Histiocytic lymphoma in children is similar to the adult form and is treated, stage for stage, in a similar fashion (Kaplan et al., 1974; Murphy et al., 1975; Pinkel et al., 1975, 1977). Wollner et al. (1976) have reported median survivals of 25+ months with sequential multi-drug-radiation therapy (LSA$_2$L$_2$ protocol, Memorial Cancer Center) compared with 6.5 months for a group treated earlier, less intensively. Patients with Stage I and II can be properly treated with local radiation therapy, with less than 10% risk of developing a first relapse in the CNS, contrary to Stage III and IV patients. CNS prophylaxis with both radiation therapy and/or chemotherapy has not been as beneficial as in acute lymphocytic leukemia and are of no benefit in Burkitt's lymphoma (Ziegler and Bluming, 1971).

The development of acute non-lymphocytic leukemia in Hodgkin's disease has now been reported in well over 100 cases. As Collins et al. (1977) reported this is quite unusual in nodular lymphoma, but should be

TABLE 13.10
Combination Chemotherapy in RCS

Drugs (mg/m²)	Days												
	0	1	8	15	22	29	36	43	50	57	64	71	85
Cyclophosphamide (IV)	1500												Next cycle
Vincristine (IV)		1.4	1.4	1.4									
Methotrexate (PO)[a]					120	120	120	120	120	120	120	120	
Leucovorin (PO)[b]					100	100	100	100	100	100	100	100	
Cytosine arabinoside (IV)[c]					300	←	←	←	←	←	←	←	

[a] Divided in 4 doses every 6 hours.
[b] Every 6 hours, 25 mg, beginning 6 hours after last dose of methotrexate.
[c] Sixteen hours after first dose of methotrexate, increasing each dose with 150 mg/m² as tolerated.

kept in mind when a patient with this disorder develops anemia, leuko-penia and thrombocytopenia unrelated to treatment several years after the established diagnosis. Another five cases were recently reported from the NCI (O'Donnell et al., 1978).

REFERENCES

Abrams, H. L., Takahashi, M., and Adams, D. F. Usefulness and accuracy of lymphangiography in lymphoma. Cancer Chemother. Rep., 52: 157–170, 1968.

Anderson, T., Bender, R. A., Fisher, R. I., DeVita, V. T., Chabner, B. A., Berard, C. W., Norton, L., and Young, R. C. Combination chemotherapy in non-Hodgkin's lymphoma; results of long term follow up. Cancer Treat. Rep., 61: 1057–1066, 1977.

Berard, C. W. Discussion II; roundtable discussion of histopathologic classification. Cancer Treat. Rep., 61: 1037–1048, 1977.

Berd, D., Cornog, J., DeConti, R. C., Levitt, M., and Bertino, J. R. Long-term remission in diffuse histiocytic lymphoma treated with combination sequential chemotherapy. Cancer, 35: 1050–1054, 1975.

Bitran, J. D., Kinzie, J., Sweet, D. L., Variakojis, D., Griem, M. L., Golomb, H. M., Miller, J. B., Oetzel, N., and Ultmann, J. E. Survival of patients with localized histiocytic lymphoma. Cancer, 39: 342–346, 1977.

Bloomfield, C. D., Kersey, J. H., Bruning, R. D., and Gajl-Peczalska K. J. Prognostic significance of lymphocytic surface markers and histology in adult non-Hodgkin's lymphoma. Cancer Treat. Rep., 61: 963–970, 1977.

Blum, R. H., and Carter, S. K. Adriamycin; a new anticancer drug with significant clinical activity. Ann. Intern. Med., 80: 249–259, 1974.

Blum, R. H., Carter, S. K., and Agre, K. A clinical review of bleomycin—a new antineoplastic agent. Cancer, 31: 903–914, 1973.

Bonadonna, G., Pizzetti, F., Musumeci, R., Valagussa, P., Banfi, A., and Veronesi, U. Staging laparotomy in non-Hodgkin's lymphomata. Br. J. Cancer, 31 (suppl. II): 252–260, 1975.

Brace, K., O'Connell, M. J., Vogel, V., and Schantz, A. Total body radiation therapy for disseminated lymphosarcoma; results of pilot study. Cancer Chemother Rep., 58: 401–405, 1974.

Brereton, H. D., Longo, D. L., Kirkland, L. R., Johnson, R. E., Young, R. C., and DeVita, V. T. Randomized prospective trial comparing combination chemotherapy (CRX) with total body irradiation (TBI) plus CRX in non-Hodgkin's lymphomas. Proc. Am. Soc. Clin. Oncol., 19: 327, 1978.

Brill, N. E., Baehr, G., and Rosenthal, N. Generalized giant follicle hyperplasia of lymph nodes and spleen. J.A.M.A., 84: 668–671, 1925.

Bunn, P. A., Jr., and DeVita, V. T., Jr. Central nervous system involvement in patients with histiocytic lymphoma, diffuse type; reply. Blood, 51: 178–179, 1978.

Burgess, N., Jr., Dockerty, M. B., and Remine, W. H. Sarcomatous lesions of the stomach. Ann. Surg., 173: 758–765, 1971.

Bush, R. S., Gospodarowicz, M., Sturgeon, J., and Alison, R. Radiation therapy of localized non-Hodgkin's lymphoma. Cancer Treat. Rep., 61: 1129–1136, 1977.

Canellos, G. P., DeVita, V. T., Young, R. C., Chabner, B. A., Schein, P. S., and Johnson, R. E. Therapy of advanced lymphocytic lymphoma; a preliminary report of a randomized trial between combination chemotherapy (CVP) and intensive radiotherapy. Br. J. Cancer, 31 (suppl. II): 474–480, 1975.

Carbone, P. P. Non-Hodgkin's lymphoma; recent observations on natural history and intensive treatment. Cancer, 30: 1511–1516, 1972.

Carter, S. K. An overview of the status of the nitrosoureas in other tumors. Cancer Chemother. Rep., 4: 35–46, 1973.

Castellino, R. A., Goffinet, D. R., Blank, N., Parker, B. R., and Kaplan, H. S. The role of radiography in the staging of non-Hodgkin's lymphoma with laparotomy correlation. Radiology, *110:* 329–338, 1974.

Chabner, B. A., Johnson, R. E., Chretien, P. B., Schein, P. S., Young, R. C., Canellos, G. P., Hubbard, S. H., Anderson, T., Rosenoff, S. H., and DeVita, V. T. Percutaneous liver biopsy, peritoneoscopy and laparotomy; an assessment of relative merits in the lymphomata. Br. J. Cancer, *31* (suppl. II): 242–247, 1975.

Chaffey, J. T., Hellman, S., Rosenthal, D. S., and Moloney, W. L. Total-body irradiation in the treatment of lymphocytic lymphoma. Cancer Treat. Rep., *61:* 1149–1152, 1977.

Chaoul, H., and Lange, K. Ueber Lymphogranulomatose und ihre Behandlung mit Roentgenstrahlen. Munch. Med. Wochenschr., *70:* 725–727, 1923.

Collins, A. J., Bloomfield, C. D., Peterson, B. A., and McKenna, R. W. Acute non lymphocytic leukemia in patients with nodular lymphoma. Cancer, *40:* 1748–1754, 1977.

Cox, J. D., Laugier, A. J., and Gerard-Marchant, R. Apparently localized and regionally advanced malignant lymphoreticular tumors in the adult; early course following irradiation. Cancer, *29:* 1043–1051, 1972.

Dessauer, F. Eine neue Anordnung zur Roentgenstrahlung. Arch. Phys. Med. Techn., *2:* 218, 1907.

DeVita, V. T., Jr., Canellos, G. P., Chabner, B., Schein, P., Hubbard, S. P., and Young, R. C. Advanced diffuse histiocytic lymphoma, a potentially curable disease. Results with combination chemotherapy. Lancet, *1:* 248–250, 1975.

Dick, F., Bloomfield, C. D., and Brunning, R. D. Incidence, cytology and histopathology of non-Hodgkin's lymphomas in the bone marrow. Cancer, *33:* 1382–1398, 1974.

Dorfman, R. F. Pathology of the non-Hodgkin's lymphomas; new classifications. Cancer Treat. Rep., *61:* 945–951, 1977.

Editorial. Follicular lymphomas. Lancet, *1:* 1088–1089, 1974.

Filly, R. A., Marglin, S., and Castellino, R. A. The ultrasonographic spectrum of abdominal and pelvic Hodgkin's disease and non-Hodgkin's lymphomas. Cancer, *38:* 2143–2148, 1976.

Garrett, T. J., Gee, T. S., Dowling, M. D., Lee, B. J., Middleman, M. P., Clarkson, B. D., and Young, C. W. Cyclophosphamide L2 protocol; a combination chemotherapeutic regimen for advanced non-Hodgkin's lymphoma. Cancer Treat. Rep., *61:* 7–16, 1977.

Goffinet, D. R., Warnke, R., Dunnick, N. R., Castellino, R., Glatstein, E., Nelson, T. S., Dorfman, R. F., Rosenberg, S. A., and Kaplan, H. S. Clinical and surgical (laparotomy) evaluation of patients with non-Hodgkin's lymphomas. Cancer Treat. Rep., *61:* 981–992, 1977.

Greenlaw, R. H., Weinstein, M. B., Brill, A. B., McBain, J. K., Murphy, L., and Kniseley, R. M. 67-Ga-citrate imaging in untreated malignant lymphoma; preliminary report of cooperative group. J. Nucl. Med., *15:* 404–407, 1974.

Hellman, S., Chaffey, J. T., Rosenthal, D. S., Moloney, W. C., Canellos, G. P., and Skarin, A. T. The place of radiation therapy in the treatment of non-Hodgkin's lymphomas. Cancer, *39:* 843–851, 1977.

Herman, T. S., and Jones, S. E. Systematic re-staging in the management of non-Hodgkin's lymphomas. Cancer Treat. Rep., *61:* 1009–1015, 1977.

Heublein, A. C. A preliminary report on continuous irradiation of the entire body. Radiology, *18:* 1051–1062, 1932.

Hoogstraten, B., Owens, A. K., Lenhard, R. E., Glidewell, O. J., Leone, L. A., Olson, K. B., Harley, J. B., Townsend, S. R., Miller, S. P., and Spurr, C. L. Combination chemotherapy in lymphosarcoma and reticulum cell sarcoma. Blood, *33:* 370–378, 1969.

Horn, N. L., Ray, G. R., and Kriss, J. P. Gallium-67 citrate scanning in Hodgkin's disease and non-Hodgkin's lymphoma. Cancer, *37:* 250–257, 1976.

Jacobs, D. S. Primary gastric malignant lymphoma and pseudolymphoma. Am. J. Clin. Pathol., *40:* 379–394, 1963.

Jacobson, L. O., Spurr, C. L., Guzman-Barron, E. S., Smith, T., Lushbaugh, C., and Dick, G. F. Nitrogen mustard therapy; studies on the effect of methyl-bis-(β-chloroethyl)amine hydrochloride on neoplastic disorders and allied disorders of the hemopoietic system. J.A.M.A., *132:* 263-271, 1946.

Jaffe, E. S., Shevach, E. M., Frank, M. M., Berard, C. W., and Green, S. Nodular lymphoma; evidence for origin from follicular B lymphocytes. N. Engl. J. Med., *290:* 813-819, 1974.

Johnson, R. E. Management of generalized malignant lymphomata with "systemic" radiotherapy. Br J. Cancer, *31* (suppl. II): 450-455, 1975.

Johnson, R. E., DeVita, V. T., Kun, L. E., Chabner, B. R., Chretien, P. B., Berard, C. W., and Johnson, S. K. Patterns of involvement with malignant lymphoma and implications for treatment decision making. Br. J. Cancer, *31* (suppl. II): 237-241, 1975.

Jones, S. E., Fuks, Z., Bull, M., Kadin, M. E., Dorfman, R. F., Kaplan, H. S., Rosenberg, S. A., and Kim, H. Non-Hodgkin's lymphomas; IV. Clinicopathologic correlation in 405 cases. Cancer, *31:* 806-823, 1973a.

Jones, S. E., Fuks, Z., Kaplan, H. S., and Rosenberg, S. A. Non-Hodgkin's lymphomas; V. Results of radiotherapy. Cancer, *32:* 682-691, 1973b.

Jones, S. E., Rosenberg, S. A., Kaplan, H. S., Kadin, M. E., and Dorfman, R. F. Non-Hodgkin's lymphomas; II. Single agent chemotherapy. Cancer, *30:* 31-38, 1972.

Jones, S. E., Tobias, D. A., and Waldman, R. S. Computed tomographic scanning in patients with lymphoma. Cancer, *41:* 480-486, 1978.

Kaplan, J., Mastrangelo, R., and Peterson, W. D., Jr. Childhood lymphoblastic lymphoma; a cancer of thymus-derived lymphocytes. Cancer Res., *34:* 521-525, 1974.

Koziner, B., Ellman, L., and Aisenberg, A. C. Lymphoma presenting as bone marrow failure. Cancer, *35:* 1426-1429, 1975.

Kundrat, H. Uber lymphosarkomatosis. Wien. Klin. Wochenschr., *6:* 211-213 and 234-239, 1893.

Law, I. P., Dick, F. R., Blom, J., and Bergevin, P. R. Involvement of the central nervous system in non-Hodgkin's lymphoma. Cancer, *36:* 225-231, 1975.

Leech, J. H., Glick, A. D., Waldron, J. A., Flexner, J. M., Horn, R. G., and Collins, R. D. Malignant lymphomas of follicular center cell origin in man; I. immunologic studies. J Natl. Cancer Inst., *54:* 11-21, 1975.

Lenhard, R. E., Jr., Prentice, R. L., Owens, A. H., Jr., Bakemeier, R., Horton, J. H., Shnider, B. I., Stolbach, L., Berard, C. W., and Carbone, P. P. Combination chemotherapy of the malignant lymphomas; a controlled clinical trial. Cancer, *38:* 1052-1059, 1976.

Levi, J. A., O'Connell, M. J., Murphy, W. L., Sutherland, J. C., and Wiernik, P. H. Role of 67-gallium citrate scanning in the management of non-Hodgkin's lymphoma. Cancer, *36:* 1690-1701, 1975.

Levine, G. D., and Dorfman, R. F. Nodular lymphoma; an ultrastructural study of its relationship to germinal centers and a correlation of light and electron microscopic findings. Cancer, *35:* 148-164, 1975.

Loehr, W. J., Mujahed, Z., Zahn, D., Gray, G. F., and Thorbjarnarson, B. Primary lymphoma of the gastrointestinal tract; a review of 100 cases. Ann. Surg., *170:* 231-238, 1969.

Lowenbraun, S., DeVita, V. T., and Serpick, A. A. Combination chemotherapy with nitrogen mustard, vincristine, procarbazine and prednisone in lymphosarcoma and reticulum cell sarcoma. Cancer, *25:* 1018-1025, 1970.

Luce, J. K., Gamble, J. F., Wilson, H. E., Monto, R. W., Isaacs, B. L., Palmer, R. L., Coltman, C. A., Hewlett, J. S., Gehan, E. A., and Frei, E., III. Combined cyclophosphamide, vincristine, prednisone therapy of malignant lymphoma. Cancer, *28:* 306-317, 1971.

Lukes, R. J., and Collins, R. D. A functional approach to the classification of malignant lymphoma. Recent Results Cancer Res., *46:* 18-30, 1974a.

Lukes, R. J., and Collins, R. D. Immunologic characterization of human malignant lymphomas. Cancer, *34:* 1488-1503, 1974b.

Lukes, R. J., and Collins, R. D. New approaches to the classification of the lymphomata. Br. J. Cancer, *31* (suppl. II): 1–28, 1975.

Lukes, R. J., and Tindle, B. H. Immunoblastic lymphadenopathy; a hyperimmune entity resembling Hodgkin's disease. N. Engl. J. Med., *292:* 1–8, 1975.

Lukes, R. J., Butler, J. J. and Hicks, E. B. Natural history of Hodgkin's disease as related to its pathologic picture. Cancer, *19:* 317–344, 1966.

McKelvey, E. M. Review of CHOP-HOP combination chemotherapy in malignant lymphoma. Proc. Am. Soc. Clin. Oncol., *19:* 415, 1978.

McKelvey, E. M., Gottlieb, J. A., Wilson, H. E., Haut, A., Talley, R. W., Stephens, R., Lane, M., Gamble, J. F., Jones, S. E., Grozea, P. E., Gutterman, J., Coltman, C., Jr., and Moon, T. E. Hydroxyl daunomycin (Adriamycin) combination chemotherapy in malignant lymphoma. Cancer, *38:* 1484–1493, 1976.

Medinger, F. G., and Craver, L. F. Total body irradiation, with review of cases. A.J.R., *48:* 651–671, 1942.

Mendelson, D., Block, J. B., and Serpick, A. A. Effect of large intermittent intravenous doses of cyclophosphamide in lymphoma. Cancer, *25:* 715–720, 1970.

Moran, E. E., Ultmann, J. E., Ferguson, D. J., Hoffer, P. B., Ranniger, K., and Rappaport, H. Staging laparotomy in non-Hodgkin's lymphoma. Br. J. Cancer, *31* (suppl. II): 228–236, 1975.

Mukherji, B., Yagoda, A., Lee, B. J., III, and Krakoff, I. H. A clinical study of the natural history of lymphosarcoma and reticulum cell sarcoma. Eur. J. Cancer, *10:* 497–505, 1974.

Murphy, S. B., Frizzera, G., and Evans, A. E. A study of childhood non-Hodgkin's lymphoma. Cancer, *36:* 2121–2131, 1975.

Naqvi, M. S., Burrows, L., and Kark, A. E. Lymphoma of the gastrointestinal tract; prognostic guides based on 162 cases. Ann. Surg., *170:* 221–231, 1969.

O'Donnell, J., Brereton, H., Greco, F., Gralnick, H., Gallagher, R., Peng, J., and Johnson, R. Acute myelocytic leukemia (AML) and acute myeloproliferative syndrome (AMPS) after therapeutic irradiation for non-Hodgkin's syndrome. Proc. Am. Assoc. Cancer Res., *19:* 60, 1978.

Patchefsky, A. S., Brodovsky, H. S., Menduke, H., Southard, M., Brooks, J., Nicklas, D., and Hoch, W. S. Non-Hodgkin's lymphomas; a clinicopathologic study of 293 cases. Cancer, *34:* 1173–1186, 1974.

Peckham, M. J. Aetiologic leads in the malignant lymphomas. Clin. Haematol., *311:* 3–37, 1974.

Peters, M. V., Bush, R. S., Brown, T. C., and Reid, J. The place of radiotherapy in the control of non-Hodgkin's lymphomata. Br. J. Cancer, *31* (suppl. II): 386–401, 1975

Pinkel, D., Johnson, W., and Aur, R. J. A. Non-Hodgkin's lymphoma in children. Br. J. Cancer, *31* (suppl. II): 298–323, 1975.

Pinkel, D., Hustu, H. O., Aur, R. J. A., Smith, K., Borella, L. D., and Simone, J. Radiotherapy in leukemia and lymphoma of children. Cancer, *39:* 817–824, 1977.

Portlock, C. S., and Rosenberg, S. A. Combination chemotherapy with cyclophosphamide, vincristine and prednisone in advanced non-Hodgkin's lymphomas. Cancer, *37:* 1275–1282, 1976.

Portlock, C. S., and Rosenberg, S. A. Chemotherapy of the non-Hodgkin's lymphomas; the Stanford experience. Cancer Treat. Rep., *61:* 1049–1055, 1977.

Portlock, C. S., and Rosenberg, S. A. No initial therapy in the management of advanced (stages III and IV) non-Hodgkin's lymphomas with favorable histologies. Proc. Am. Soc. Clin. Oncol., *19:* 366, 1978.

Portlock, C. S., Rosenberg, S. A., Glatstein, E., and Kaplan, H. S. Treatment of advanced non-Hodgkin's lymphomas with favorable histologies; preliminary results of a prospective trial. Blood, *47:* 747–756, 1976.

Quasim, M. M. Total body irradiation in non-Hodgkin lymphoma. Strahlentherapie, *149:* 364–367, 1975.

Rappaport, H. Tumors of the Hematopoietic System. *In* Atlas of Tumor Pathology, Sect. 3, Fasc. 8, p. 13. Armed Forces Institute of Pathology, Washington D.C., 1966.

Rappaport, H., Winter, W. J., and Hicks, B. J. Follicular lymphoma; a re-evaluation of its position in the scheme of malignant lymphoma, based on a survey of 253 cases. Cancer, *9:* 792–821, 1956.

Rodriguez, V., Cabanillas, F., Burgess, M. A., McKelvey, E. M., Valdivieso, M., Bodey, G. P., and Freireich, E. J. Combination chemotherapy ("CHOP-Bleo") in advanced (non-Hodgkin) malignant lymphoma. Blood, *49:* 325–333, 1977.

Rosenberg, S. A., and Kaplan, H. S. Clinical trials in the non-Hodgkin's lymphomata at Stanford University; experimental design and preliminary results. Br. J. Cancer, *31* (suppl. II): 456–464, 1975.

Rosenberg, S. A., Diamond, H. D., and Craver, L. F. Lymphosarcoma; the effects of therapy and survival in 1269 patients in a review of 30 years experience. Ann. Intern. Med., *53:* 877–897, 1960.

Rosenberg, S. A., Diamond, H. D., Jaslowitz, B., and Craver, L. F. Lymphosarcoma; a review of 1269 cases. Medicine, *40:* 31–84, 1961.

Rosenberg, S. A., Dorfman, R. F., and Kaplan, H. S. The value of sequential bone marrow biopsy and laparotomy and splenectomy in a series of 127 consecutive untreated patients with non-Hodgkin's lymphoma. Br. J. Cancer, *31* (suppl. II): 221–227, 1975.

Roulet, F. Das primare Retothelsarkom den Lymphknoten. Virchows Arch. Pathol. Anat., *277:* 15–47, 1930.

Rudders, R. A. Treatment of advanced malignant lymphoma with bleomycin. Blood, *40:* 317–332, 1972.

Schechter, J. P., Jones, S. E., Woolfenden, J. M., Lilien, D. L., and O'Mara, R. E. Bone scanning in lymphoma. Cancer, *38:* 1142–1148, 1976.

Schein, P. S., Chabner, B. A., Canellos, G. P., Young, R. C., Berard, C., and DeVita, V. T. Potential for prolonged disease-free survival favoring combination chemotherapy of non-Hodgkin's lymphoma. Blood, *43:* 181–189, 1974.

Schein, P. S., DeVita, V. T., Hubbard, S., Chabner, B. A., Canellos, G. P., Berard, C., and Young, R. C. Bleomycin, Adriamycin, cyclophosphamide, vincristine, and prednisone (BACOP) combination chemotherapy in the treatment of advanced diffuse histiocytic lymphoma. Ann. Intern. Med., *85:* 417–422, 1976.

Schein, P. S., O'Connell, M. J., Blom, J., Hubbard, S., Magrath, I. T., Bergevin, P., Wiernik, P. H., Ziegler, J. L., and DeVita, V. T. Clinical antitumor activity and toxicity of streptozotocin (NSC 85998). Cancer, *34:* 993–1000, 1974.

Schultz, D. R., and Yunis, A. A. Immunoblastic lymphadenopathy with mixed cryoglobulinemia; a detailed case study. N. Engl. J. Med., *292:* 8–12, 1975.

Sexauer, J. M., Penner, J. A., and Nishiyama, R. H. Staging of lymphocytic lymphoma. South. Med. J., *67:* 1297–1300, 1975.

Skarin, A. T., Rosenthal, D. S., Moloney, W. C., and Frei, E., III. Combination chemotherapy of advanced non-Hodgkin's lymphoma with bleomycin, Adriamycin, cyclophosphamide, vincristine and prednisone (BACOP). Blood, *49:* 759–770, 1977.

Smith, J. L., Jr., and Helwig, E. B. Malignant lymphoma of the stomach; its diagnosis, distinction and biologic behavior (abstr.). Am. J. Pathol., *34:* 553, 1958.

Spivak, S. D. Procarbazine. Ann. Intern. Med., *81:* 795–800, 1974.

Sweet, D. L., Golomb, H. M., Ultmann, J. E., Bitran, J. D., Lester, E. P., and Miller, J. B. Central nervous system involvement in patients with histiocytic lymphoma, diffuse type (letter to the editor). Blood, *51:* 177–178, 1978.

Symmers, D. Giant follicular lymphadenopathy with or without splenomegaly. Arch. Pathol., *26:* 603–647, 1938.

Teschendorf, W. Uber Bestrahlung des ganzen menschlichen Korpus bei Blutkrankheiten. Strahlentherapie, *16:* 720, 1927.

Tietjen, G. W., and McAllister, F. F. Spontaneous regression of gastric reticulum cell sarcoma. N.Y. State J. Med., *74:* 680–683, 1974.

Tranum, B. L., Haut, A., Rivkin, S., Weber, E., Quagliana, J. M., Shaw, M., Tucker, W. G., Smith, F. E., Samson, M., and Gottlieb, J. A phase II study of methyl CCNU in the treatment of solid tumors and lymphomas; a Southwest Oncology Group Study. Cancer, *35:* 1148–1153, 1975.

Vinciguerra, V., and Silver, R. T. The importance of bone marrow biopsy in the staging of patients with lymphosarcoma. Blood, *41:* 913–920, 1973.

Virchow, R. Weisses Blut. Neue Notizen aus dem Gebiete der Natur und Heilkunde, *36:* 151–155, 1845.

Warnke, R. A., Kim, H., Fuks, Z., and Dorfman, R. F. The coexistence of nodular and diffuse patterns in nodular non-Hodgkin's lymphomas. Cancer, *40:* 1229–1233, 1977.

Wollner, N., Burchenal, J. H., Lieberman, P. H., Exelby, P., D'Angio, G., and Murphy, M. L. Non-Hodgkin's lymphoma in children; a comparative study of two modalities of therapy. Cancer, *37:* 123–134, 1976.

Yagoda, A., Mukherji, B., Young, C., Etcubanas, E., Lamonte, C., Smith, J. R., Tan, C. T. C., and Krakoff, I. H. Bleomycin, an antitumor antibiotic; clinical experience in 274 patients. Ann. Intern. Med., *77:* 861–870, 1972.

Ziegler, J. L., and Bluming, A. Z. Intrathecal chemotherapy in Burkitt's lymphoma. Br. Med. J., *3:* 508–512, 1971.

Chapter 14

Gastrointestinal Tract

PATRICK R. BERGEVIN, M.D.

ESOPHAGUS

Cancer of the esophagus predominates in males and is frequently associated with heavy alcohol consumption and tobacco smoking. Patients with achalasia or esophageal stricture may also be more at risk for the development of this carcinoma. Most are poorly differentiated squamous cell carcinomas. Adenocarcinoma uncommonly may occur and in the terminal third of the esophagus usually represents extension from a primary gastric carcinoma. The tumor is usually quite extensive at the time of diagnosis with involvement through the wall of the esophagus into adjacent tissues via lymphatics and blood vessels. Perhaps the lack of a serosal covering of the esophagus allows earlier local extension of the cancer. Cervical, mediastinal and abdominal lymph nodes are frequently involved, depending upon the location of the carcinoma. Roughly 10% of the tumors involve the cervical esophagus, with 40% in the upper half and 50% in the lower half of the thoracic esophagus. The liver and lungs are the most frequent sites of distant metastasis.

Cure of esophageal carcinoma is rare by either surgery or radiotherapy or a combination of the two modalities. Palliation for only a few months is the rule. The 5-year survival in most series is only about 5–10%. It is clear that the morbidity and mortality of surgery are less for carcinomas below the aortic arch (Sweet, 1954). For lesions at the cardioesophageal junction, partial esophagogastrectomy, pyloroplasty and regional node dissection with esophagogastric anastamosis through a thoracoabdominal approach is often performed. Tumors at higher levels in the esophagus are often treated by esophagogastrostomy or jejunostomy above an unresectable tumor, or preoperative radiation therapy is given, followed by resection and then immediate or staged reconstruction with a colonic segment. Serial esophageal bougienage and/or permanent peroral implantation of a wide diameter plastic prosthesis have been advocated for the maintenance of swallowing and in addition to block a fistula track (Palmer, 1973). Although gross tumor regression follows radiation therapy in 50–80% of patients, cure is the exception. Tumor may involve much of the esophagus, although extended radiotherapy or surgical resection have not made an appreciable difference in survival. Local recurrence even within the irradiated volume is common. It is generally accepted that radiotherapy for carcinoma of the cervical esophagus produces less functional impairment than does surgery, as well as an at least comparable cure rate (Pearson, 1969). The fixation of tumor to large vessels and trachea and the consequent threat of perforation, together with the generally poor condition of these frequently elderly patients, are obstacles to control by radiotherapy. In addition, there is no acceptable evidence of an increase in survival induced by either pre- or postoperative radiotherapy. The results of chemotherapy have been rather dismal, although the recent addition of bleomycin and methyl-GAG to the oncologist's armamentarium may serve to increase the palliation of these unfortunate patients. Falkson (1971) reported on the treatment of 21 patients with far-advanced esophageal cancer with methyl-GAG, in which 10 patients had objective measurable tumor shrinkage.

STOMACH

In 1977 it was estimated that 14,000 patients would die from gastric cancer and over 23,000 new cases would be diagnosed. However, for reasons which are not altogether clear, the incidence and mortality rates from gastric cancer in the United States have declined markedly during the past 20 years, in contrast to Japan, where 54% of all malignancies arise from the stomach. Various etiologic factors are proposed, including exposure to benzpyrenes and nitrosamines, asbestos contamination of polished rice in Japan, atrophic gastritis and immunodeficiency.

Prolla et al. (1969) have summarized the Japanese experience with the early detection of gastric cancer by mass screening with barium studies, occasionally supplemented by endoscopy. Resectability of lesions and thereby 5-year survival have been increased by this means. This mass survey approach is impractical in the United States because of the much lower incidence; however, frequent examination of high risk patients such as those with pernicious anemia, chronic atrophic gastritis and gastric polyps is indicated.

Adenocarcinoma comprises the bulk of gastric cancers and tends to be located in the antrum and pyloric region, although it may be multicentric in origin or extensively infiltrate the stomach wall, leading to the so-called linitis plastica type of carcinoma. The overall cure rate of stomach cancer is still only about 13% despite aggressive surgery, since the disease has usually spread to regional nodes and adjacent organs at the time of diagnosis. Nevertheless, palliative resection even in the presence of liver or lung metastases should be performed if possible to eliminate or reduce the incidence of obstruction, bleeding, perforation, fistulization, aspiration pneumonia and starvation. Those factors which favor survival in resected cases include: noninvolvement of nodes with tumor, tumor in the body or antrum of the stomach (away from the cardia) and well-differentiated tumors infiltrated with immune cells.

Responses to 5-fluorouracil are generally less than 25%, with an average duration of response of 4–5 months (Comis and Carter, 1974). Mitomycin C offers an 18% response rate, BCNU an 18% response rate and Adriamycin a 25–36% response rate. There are little data on the efficacy of the alkylating agents. The combination of 5-fluorouracil and methyl-CCNU allowed a 40% response rate in the study of Mittelman et al. (1976). Dramatic results with the combination of 5-fluorouracil, Adriamycin and mitomycin C were reported by Woolley et al. (1977). A 48% response rate in advanced gastric carcinoma was seen with this regimen with a median duration of response in excess of 11 months. The combination of BCNU and 5-fluorouracil allowed a 41% response rate in one study, with an increase in survival over patients treated with 5-fluorouracil alone (Kovach et al., 1974). Radiotherapy results suggest only a palliative effect. Survival may be enhanced, however, by the addition of 5-fluorouracil to radiotherapy. In a controlled double-blind study (Moertel et al., 1969), 48 patients with locally unresectable gastric carcinoma received radiotherapy at a total dosage of 3750 R over 4 weeks. Half the patients received 5-fluorouracil, 45 mg/kg by intravenous injection in 3 or 4 divided doses at the onset of radiotherapy and the other half received a placebo. The mean survival of the placebo group was 5.9 months and that of the 5-fluorouracil-treated group was 14 months.

LIVER

Hepatocellular carcinoma (hepatoma) comprises the bulk of primary liver tumors (roughly 90%) with the remainder including intrahepatic bile duct carcinoma and various mixed liver cell carcinomas. Hepatoma predominates in males and reaches its peak incidence in the sixth decade. The most common presenting features are hepatomegaly, abdominal pain and weight loss. Jaundice is uncommon at the time of diagnosis. A decided majority of hepatomas in most series are associated with chronic liver disease, particularly postnecrotic cirrhosis but also with nutritional cirrhosis, in which the hepatoma diffusely involves the liver in most cases. The tumor is often disseminated at the time of diagnosis, with involvement predominantly of regional nodes and lungs. The portal or hepatic veins are frequently involved with tumor, leading to thrombosis. The average survival time from diagnosis to death is less than six months.

α-1-Fetoprotein (AFP), an embryonic α-1-globulin, is detectable in 40–100% of hepatoma patients, depending on the geographic location of the patient and the sensitivity of the assay employed. African and Far Eastern patients with hepatoma appear to have a higher incidence of AFP (Smith and O'Neill, 1971). The level of AFP in the serum correlates well with the presence of tumor and is thus a useful marker for response to therapy and for detection of early relapse, e.g. postsurgical excision (Purtilo et al., 1973). The carcinoembryonic antigen (CEA) assay may also be positive. Hepatic angiography as a diagnostic tool is more sensitive than scanning procedures and, in addition, is useful in staging patients for possible hepatic lobectomy. Patients with solitary hepatomas may be cured or their survival extended by surgical excision of the tumor. However, the great majority of patients have multicentric involvement of the liver or disseminated tumor and are not surgical candidates. Radiotherapy has not been particularly effective.

The use of 5-fluorouracil in the treatment of hepatoma has given mixed results (Kennedy et al., 1977; Link et al., 1977). The combination of BCNU and 5-fluorouracil was reported by Moertel (1977) to give 7/19 responses with 3 patients in complete response for 3, 4 and 6 years. Cochrane et al. (1977) reported promising results with a combination of cyclophosphamide, vincristine, methotrexate and 5-fluorouracil. In 1973 Tormey et al. reported long survivals with the combination of Adriamycin and bleomycin in all 3 of their treated patients with hepatoma. This was followed by the report of Olweny et al. (1975) in which all 11 evaluable African cases treated with Adriamycin responded with 3 patients achieving a complete response. The median survival for Olweny's 11 patients was 8 months; patients who achieved complete remission survived 8, 9 and 13 months. Vogel et al. (1977) also reported good results with Adriamycin in patients from Zambia and the United States. Cady and Oberfield (1974a) have reported their results with arterial infusion chemotherapy of hepatoma in 18 patients, utilizing mainly 5-FUDR, and obtained an increase in median survival to 16.5 months, although 5 patients died as a result of complications arising from the therapy.

GALLBLADDER

Primary adenocarcinoma of the gallbladder is the fifth most common malignant tumor of the gastrointestinal tract. In excess of 6000 persons die of this disease in the United States each year. The tumor predominates in females with a sex ratio of 2–4 to 1 and peak incidence in the age group 60–70 years. Persons of Latin-American extraction may have an increased incidence of the tumor compared to other groups.

The association of gallbladder cancer with cholelithiasis is well established. There is no question that the elective excision of diseased gallbladders would reduce by a considerable degree the later development of cancer. Frozen section examination of suspicious lesions in the gallbladder at the time of surgery would allow the surgeon to extend the operation for possible cure if cancer is found. Unfortunately most patients with gallbladder cancer present with advanced disease with extension to the liver and nodes along the common bile duct and even direct extension to adjacent abdominal organs and abdominal wall, such that curative resection is usually impossible. Few 5-year survivors are seen. The roles of chemotherapy and radiotherapy have not been well defined but may offer some palliation (Treadwell and Hardin, 1976).

EXTRAHEPATIC BILE DUCTS

Primary adenocarcinoma of the extrahepatic bile ducts is an uncommon lesion with a very poor prognosis. The disease has been linked etiologically with cholelithiasis, choledocholithiasis and sclerosing cholangitis. Because of early spread to regional nodes and liver, surgical cures are uncommon (Yarbrough, 1973). Nevertheless, palliative procedures to relieve jaundice or to correct duodenal obstruction should be offered.

AMPULLA OF VATER

Patients with primary adenocarcinoma of the ampulla of Vater usually present with jaundice and often with guaiac positive stools. The upper gastrointestinal (GI) series often reveal an ulcerated duodenal mass, and cytology from duodenal drainage is often positive. Resection of the tumor together with pancreaticoduodenectomy is attempted for cure, with long term results being more favorable than with tumors of the head of the pancreas. Bypass palliative procedures are indicated for obstructive jaundice or duodenal obstruction (Wilson and Block, 1974).

PANCREAS

Since the 1940s there has been an increase in the incidence of carcinoma of the pancreas in this country, at a rate of 15% per 10-year period, accounting for approximately 9–10% of all persons diagnosed with tumors of the gastrointestinal tract. Adenocarcinoma of the pancreas presently ranks as the fourth most common cause of death by cancer. Possible etiologic factors include exposure to industrial chemicals and association with diabetes mellitus and calcific pancreatitis (Mainz and Webster, 1974). Adenocarcinoma of the pancreas is predominantly a disease of elderly males and arises mainly in the head of the gland (75%), presenting with abdominal pain, weight loss and jaundice in most instances. Carcinomas of the body and tail present with abdominal and back pain and weight loss and frequently have involved contiguous viscera before symptoms have occurred. Regional lymph nodes and liver are the most common metastatic sites. An enlarged, palpable and nontender gallbladder (Courvoisier's sign) will be found in approximately 60% of patients with carcinoma of the head of the pancreas. A widened duodenal loop on upper gastrointestinal series is significant but rarely presents until the tumor is advanced. Diabetes mellitus is found in a number of patients. Steatorrhea, venous and arterial thrombotic episodes and emotional disturbances have also been described in patients with pancreatic cancer.

75-Selenomethionine scanning of the pancreas or celiac arteriography may serve to demonstrate pancreatic carcinoma but are not generally very useful diagnostic tests. A negative scan or arteriogram would not rule out the smaller lesions which have the highest chance of resectability. Duodenal aspiration following administration of pancreatic secretagogue may provide diagnostic cytology in up to 70% of cases. By means of endoscopic retrograde choledochopancreatography, it may be possible to differentiate pancreatic cancer from chronic pancreatitis. Ultrasonography and computerized axial tomography are occasionally useful noninvasive techniques for the diagnosis as well as monitoring of pancreatic carcinoma. CEA assays (see section on colorectal cancer) appear to correlate well with development of progressive disease.

The mean survival from diagnosis is still less than 1 year, and even with extensive surgery the salvage rate is low. In selected cases either a radical total pancreatectomy or a Whipple procedure in which the tail of the pancreas is retained can be performed for tumors of the head of the pancreas (Remine et al., 1970; Monge et al., 1964). Radical surgery is less often possible in cancer of the body and tail since diagnosis is so frequently delayed. Patients with biliary obstruction may be palliated by a bypass procedure. Five-year survivals of 10–20% have been reported after "curative" surgery, although these figures are less than the operative mortality rate of many series. Gastrojejunostomy may be required for gastric retention secondary to duodenal obstruction, or may be performed prophylactically at the time of initial surgery to eliminate the necessity for a second operation in the terminal stages of the disease.

Conventional radiotherapy at doses of 3000–4000 R is of little benefit for patients with unresectable pancreatic adenocarcinoma. Increased radiation at 6000 R, however, did increase 2-year survival to 24% in the series of Haslam et al. (1973). Combined therapy with 4000 R + 5-fluorouracil in patients with unresectable disease allowed a longer survival (median 28 weeks) than 6000 R alone (median 17 weeks) and was as effective as 6000 R + 5-fluorouracil in the study of Moertel et al. (1976). The effectiveness of this combined therapy suggests that it be used as adjuvant treatment after "curative" resections.

Useful chemotherapeutic agents include 5-fluorouracil, mitomycin and streptozotocin although responses are few and are only of a few months duration.

SMALL INTESTINE

Adenocarcinoma of the small intestine is a relatively rare tumor of the gastrointestinal tract. The relative immunity of the small bowel to development of malignant changes has been discussed by Wilson et al. (1974) and may be related to: (a) the rapid transit time of small bowel contents which may in turn decrease exposure to carcinogens; (b) a difference in bacterial population of the small bowel, which possibly results in formation of fewer carcinogenic compounds from bile or other substances than in the colon; (c) the presence of protective enzymes such as the benzpyrene hydrolase, which can detoxify potential carcinogens; and (d) a high concentration of immunoglobulin A, which may result in a greater neutralization of potentially immunogenic viruses. Patients with familial polyposis and Gardner's syndrome have an increased risk of developing malignant changes in a small bowel adenomatous polyp. An increasing number of cases of adenocarcinoma developing in an area of regional enteritis are being reported.

Most patients are in the age group 50–70 years and present with abdominal pain, bleeding, obstruction or weight loss. Small bowel barium studies, occasionally supplemented by celiac and superior mesenteric arteriography, will make the presumptive diagnosis in most cases. Most of these tumors are located in the duodenum and jejunum. Surgery is the treatment of choice and usually entails removal of a generous segment of bowel to permit resection of potentially involved mesentery and node drainage areas. Tumors of the duodenum generally also require pancreatectomy. Cecal tumors usually require in addition a standard right hemicolectomy. Unfortunately, the majority of tumors have already spread to regional nodes or liver at the time of diagnosis. Nevertheless, palliative resection to relieve obstruction or to control bleeding is beneficial to patients in whom resection cannot be done. The roles of radiotherapy and chemotherapy are uncertain but short term palliation may be offered with these modalities.

COLON AND RECTUM

The incidence of colorectal cancer is increasing in the United States, with over 100,000 new cases diagnosed and over 50,000 deaths each year, representing about 15% of all the malignant neoplasms. There is no definite etiologic factor, although diet may play a large role. A low incidence of colorectal cancer is associated with the consumption of a high bulk, unrefined diet. The amount of crude fiber in the diet affects transit time and stool bulk. Intestinal transit time is prolonged following ingestion of a refined diet, allowing the opportunity for prolonged contact of the mucosal surface with potential dietary carcinogens. The role of carcinogenic substances is further strengthened by the observation that patients who have undergone ureterosigmoidostomy have a greatly increased risk of colon cancer, with tumor formation usually exactly at the site of ureteral entrance into the colon (Lowenfels, 1973).

Many adenocarcinomas of the colon and rectum arise from adenomatous polyps, predominantly those polyps greater than 1.5–2.0 cm in diameter. It is generally recommended that all polyps within reach of sigmoidoscopy should be excised regardless of size. The larger polyps (over 1.5–2.0 cm in diameter) are associated with at least a 10-fold increase of carcinoma and should be excised if the patient is in good condition, even if laparotomy is necessary. If the stalk of the polyp has been invaded at its base by carcinoma, then the risk of dissemination is high and a standard cancer operation must be performed (Leffall and Chung, 1974).

Multiple familial polyposis is a hereditary condition with the appearance early in life of large numbers of adenomatous polyps of the colon and rectum. If left untreated, nearly all affected patients will eventually develop carcinoma, which is usually multiple and presumably of multicentric origin. Early total colectomy with ileoproctostomy and fulguration of remaining polyps in the rectal segment is the preferred treatment. Another hereditary condition, Gardner's syndrome (multiple colorectal polyps, soft tissue and bony tumors, dental abnormalities and other anomalies), is treated as the patient with multiple familial polyposis. Peutz-Jeghers' syndrome is a hereditary disorder characterized by melanin spots on the buccal mucosa, lips and digits associated with polyps of the entire gastrointestinal tract, especially the small bowel. These polyps are hamartomas and are not prone to malignant change. Hyperplastic polyps of the colon and rectum are very common but are not associated with the development of adenomas or carcinomas.

The patient with ulcerative colitis has a greatly increased risk of developing carcinoma, which is frequently multifocal, infiltrating and associated with a very poor prognosis. This increased risk begins to rise after 10 years of colitis and is particularly associated with colitis involving the entire colon with chronic exacerbations. In high risk patients, a subtotal colectomy with ileorectal anastomosis is often done as a prophylactic measure.

The patient with colorectal cancer commonly presents with rectal bleeding, obstruction, abdominal pain or evidence of distant metastases. Early detection centers concentrate on several diagnostic methods which if diligently applied will undoubtedly increase the cure rate of these patients. Frequent determination of occult blood in the stool, exfoliative cytology, periodic proctosigmoidoscopy or colonoscopy and barium enemas in selected patients will allow an earlier diagnosis in the majority.

The primary treatment of adenocarcinoma of the colon is surgery. A hemicolectomy with as complete resection of the mesentery of the cancer bearing bowel segment as possible is performed. The surgeon attempts to minimize cancer cell contamination of the tumor bed, adjacent viscera and abdominal wall. Cancer emboli through vascular channels are minimized by early ligation or limited manipulation of the tumor (Stearns and Schottenfeld, 1971). Prophylactic bilateral oophorectomy may be indicated, especially in postmenopausal females, since metastatic tumor in the ovaries occurs in a significant number of these patients. Adenocarcinoma of the rectum is treated by an anterior or anteroposterior resection, depending on the distance of the tumor from the anal verge. Lesions within 6–7 cm of the anus are most commonly treated with anteroposterior resection, while higher lesions require an anterior resection, or occasionally a pull-through procedure is done to preserve the sphincter. Preoperative radiotherapy for rectal cancer has improved survival rates in several series (Rodriguez-Antunez et al., 1973; Urdaneta-Lafee et al., 1972; Brady et al., 1974). Brady et al. (1974) observed a significant reduction in the incidence of positive regional nodes following preoperative radiotherapy of cancer of the sigmoid colon and rectum. The 5-year survival for the radiotherapy group was 40% vs. 27.5% for the surgery only group. Preoperative radiotherapy may also improve the resectability rate by decreasing the tumor bulk. Postoperative radiotherapy of colorectal cancer may offer significant palliation in nonresectable cases (Whiteley et al., 1970). Palliative resections are indicated to relieve obstruction, hemorrhage, and rectal drainage, even in the presence of liver and lung metastases.

CEA, a glycoprotein present in a wide variety of carcinomas, is similar to antigens normally present in the fetal circulation. It is a useful biochemical test in following the course of disease. The specificity of the test is hampered by the fact that antigen is present in a variety of benign disorders, such as heavy smokers, alcoholic cirrhosis and ulcerative colitis. However, malignant may be differentiated from nonmalignant processes in part by the amount of CEA in the serum. A negative assay does not exclude the diagnosis of early cancer, although it makes highly unlikely the diagnosis of widespread metastatic cancer. In one study, the CEA was elevated in only one-half of patients with resectable gastrointestinal cancer; thus the CEA is not a sensitive screening tool (Dykes and King, 1972). Preoperatively, an undetectable CEA in a patient with known colonic cancer suggests a localized tumor with a good prognosis. An elevated CEA in such patients correlates with extensive metastatic disease and a poor prognosis. Postoperatively, an elevated CEA usually indicates residual or metastatic tumor (Dhar et al., 1972). Serial serum CEA determinations have some value in following the course of gastrointestinal cancer after surgery or chemotherapy, but interpretation of results must be made in the context of the overall clinical picture.

"Second look" surgery in colorectal cancer has been useful in determining extent of residual tumor and resection of same where possible. In the study reported by Gunderson and Sosin (1974), 75 patients with rectal carcinoma with complete bowel wall penetration and/or positive regional nodes at the time of initial curative resection had planned single or multiple reoperations: distant metastases alone were uncommon. Peritoneal seeding was rare. Local failure and/or regional node metastases occurred as some component in the majority of patients. It was suggested that postoperative radiotherapy might be a useful adjuvant in view of this rather high incidence of local regional failures.

Over the past 20 years, survival statistics compiled by the American Cancer Society have indicated little change in the 5-year survival (approximately 35%) of patients who have been operated upon for curative resection of colorectal carcinoma, particularly when nodal metastases were present. From 39 to 68% of reported large bowel carcinomas at surgery already have regional node metastases (DePyster and Gilchrist, 1969) and 15% have liver metastases (Moertel and Reitemeier, 1969). Utilizing the Duke classification, the 5-year survival for Stage A (confined to mucosa and submucosa) is 61–81%, for Stage B (invasion through muscularis without nodal metastases) 25–64%, and for Stage C (metastases to regional nodes) 6–28%.

Moertel and Reitemeier (1969) at the Mayo Clinic reviewed 484 untreated patients with colorectal carcinoma who had a median survival of 7 months from the time the cancer was proved to be incurable. Patients with only regional node spread had a median survival of 12 months, while those with hepatic metastases had a median survival of 5 months. Pestana et al. (1964), in a review of the Mayo Clinic experience, noted no difference in survival between right and left colon carcinoma (median survival 10.9 and 10.4 months, respectively, but the median survival for rectal carcinoma was only 8.8 months from the time of diagnosis of inoperable cancer. The length of survival was related to the grade of malignancy: patients with low grade carcinoma survived twice as long as those with grade four lesions.

Early data on the efficacy of 5-fluorouracil given intravenously for the treatment of advanced colorectal cancer comes from Ansfield et al. (1962) and Curreri et al. (1958), who utilized a 5-day course of the drug at doses generally of 15 mg/kg/day for 5 days by direct intravenous injection, with additional half doses given to the point of toxicity. With this regimen a response rate of approximately 25% was seen, although toxicity was marked, with diarrhea, stomatitis, nausea and vomiting reported in a large number of patients. Equivalent results with the weekly administration of 5-fluorouracil at 15–20 kg/kg/week by direct intravenous injection were obtained by Jacobs et al. (1971) with a marked reduction in drug toxicity, although the responses seen generally lasted less than 6 months. Horton et al. (1970) compared weekly 5-fluorouracil given by direct intravenous injection in various malignancies at doses of 7.5, 15 and 20 mg/kg and obtained objective responses in colorectal cancer in 1/25, 5/25, and 5/17, respectively. The time to onset of remission was similar at 15 and 20 mg/kg but was significantly longer at 7.5 mg/kg, and the toxicity of the 20 mg/kg dose was prohibitive. Moertel and Reitemeier (1969) noted that an optimal response is achieved by treating patients to the point of mild to moderate toxicity. Kung et al. (1966) investigated the use of 5-fluorouracil given orally, postulating that since the drug would reach a high concentration in the portal system, it might be of greater benefit to the patient with liver metastases. They found that the toxicity was no different than that encountered when the drug was given intravenously on a weekly basis. Lahiri et al. (1971) used 5-fluorouracil orally in patients with advanced colorectal cancer at a dose of 15 mg/kg/day for 6 days, then a weekly maintenance at the same dose. There were 11/14 responses and toxicity was mild. After administration of oral 5-fluorouracil, peak plasma levels occur rapidly but are generally lower than those seen after intravenous administration of comparable doses. The drug is more extensively metabolized after oral administration, and there is more variability in absorption than with a comparable intravenous dose. The use of 5-fluorouracil as an oral preparation, therefore, still remains experimental. Baker et al. (1973) showed that a continuous 120-hour intravenous infusion of 5-fluorouracil at a dosage of 30 mg/kg/day was superior in rate of remission with a decrease in severity of toxicity when compared to the conventional 5-day course of the drug given by direct intravenous injection. In this randomized study of disseminated colorectal cancer, the response rate for the 120-hour infusion was 44% and that for the conventional "loading dose" of 5-fluorouracil was only 22%. The duration of remission in both groups however was equal. In no reported study has it been clearly demonstrated that 5-fluorouracil by oral or intravenous administration can prolong survival in patients with advanced colorectal cancer. The patient with more clinically indolent disease, as evidenced by a longer interval from the diagnosis of the primary lesion to diagnosis of recurrent or metastatic disease appears more likely to respond than the patient with a more aggressive tumor.

Response rates with other standard single agent chemotherapy are no better than with that seen with 5-fluorouracil (Carter, 1976). Moertel (1973) has reviewed his experience with the nitrosoureas: of 137 patients with advanced gastrointestinal carcinoma treated with BCNU, the overall response rate was only 12%, these responses were maintained for a median duration of only two months. Randomized comparisons of BCNU and 5-fluorouracil in major gastrointestinal carcinomas revealed the inferiority of BCNU in terms of rate, completeness and duration of response. The overall response rate to CCNU was 9%. In a small series randomizing patients between 5-fluorouracil and methyl-CCNU, an equal response with the latter drug was seen, and further trials with this agent in combination with other active drugs seems indicated. Results with several other agents, including mitomycin C, bleomycin, Adriamycin, hexamethylmelamine, streptozotocin, ICDT and L-asparaginase have been disappointing to date. Falkson et al. (1974) reported on the use of 5-fluorouracil, vincristine, ICDT and BCNU in the treatment of colorectal cancer, with a response rate of 42.8% versus 25% with 5-fluorouracil alone. There was no significant impact on the median duration of remission, however. Moertel et al. (1975) compared methyl-CCNU, 5-fluorouracil and vincristine with 5-fluorouracil alone. The three-drug combination gave a response rate of 43.5% versus 19.5% with 5-fluorouracil alone, again with no impact on survival over that of 5-fluorouracil alone. No increased response with addition of BCNU, CCNU, mitomycin C, cyclophosphamide, hexamethylmelamine, vinblastine, cytosine arabinoside or actinomycin D to 5-fluorouracil has been noted. Various other two, three- and four-drug combinations have given results no better than that of either drug when used alone. Results in early adjuvant chemotherapy utilizing 5-fluorouracil given intravenously and/or intraluminally for limited to prolonged courses show no definite improvement in survival in patients with regional node metastasis (Wooley et al., 1976).

Pelvic perfusion of 5-fluorouracil in patients with locally recurrent or inoperable rectal or sigmoid carcinoma thought to be limited to the pelvis has given generally poor results (Ryan et al., 1967; Yount and Hurley, 1963). Infusion of 5-fluorouracil into the hepatic artery for control of liver metastases has allowed objective response rates exceeding 50% in several series. Moreover, there is often prolongation in survival over patients treated with conventional systemic therapy (Ansfield et al., 1971; Cady and Oberfield, 1974b), but the complications of hepatic infusion, including liver damage and failure, septicemia, arterial occlusions, hemorrhage and catheter leakage have limited the usefulness of this mode of therapy.

The role of immunotherapy in colorectal carcinoma is extensively being investigated. Mavligit et al. (1978) studied the use of 5-fluorouracil vs. BCG plus 5-fluorouracil in patients with Dukes' C (regional node) involvement; both treatment arms were equivalent regarding disease free interval and survival and both were significantly better than historical controls.

ANUS

The currently accepted therapeutic procedures for epidermoid lesions in the anal area range from wide local excision to anteroposterior resection with or without radical groin dissection, depending upon the extent of disease and the presence of nodal involvement. Radiotherapy and chemotherapy, particularly with bleomycin or methotrexate may be useful palliative measures.

REFERENCES

Ansfield, F. J. Schroeder, J. M. and Curreri, A. R. Five-year clinical experience with 5-fluorouracil. J.A.M.A., *181:* 295–299, 1962.

Ansfield, F. J., Ramirez, G., Skibba, J. L., Bryan, G. T., Davis, H. L. and Wirtanen, G. W. Intrahepatic arterial infusion with 5-fluorouracil. Cancer, *28:* 1147–1151, 1971.

Baker, L. H., Seifert, P., Reed, M. L., and Vaitkevicius, V. K. Evaluation of prolonged infusion of 5-fluorouracil vs. bolus 5-fluorouracil in treatment of advanced colorectal carcinoma. Proc. Am. Soc. Clin. Oncol., abstr. 86, 1973.

Brady, L. W., Antoniades, J., Prasvinichai, S., Torpie, R. J., Asbell, S. O., and Glassburn, J. R. Preoperative radiation therapy. Cancer, *34:* 960–964, 1974.

Cady, B., and Oberfield, R. A. Arterial infusion chemotherapy of hepatoma. Surg. Gynecol. Obstet., *138:* 381–384, 1974a.

Cady, B., and Oberfield, R. A. Regional infusion chemotherapy of hepatic metastases from carcinoma of the colon. Am. J. Surg., *127:* 220–227, 1974b.

Carter, S. K. Current protocol approaches in large bowel cancer. Semin. Oncol., *3:* 433–443, 1976.

Cochrane, A. M. G., Murray-Lyon, I. M., Brinkley, D. M., and Williams, R. Quadruple chemotherapy versus radiotherapy in treatment of primary hepatocellular carcinoma. Cancer, *40:* 609–614, 1977.

Comis, R. L., and Carter, S. K. A review of chemotherapy in gastric cancer. Cancer, *34:* 1576–1586, 1974.

Curreri, A. R., Ansfield, F. J., Mclver, F. A., et al. Clinical studies with 5-fluorouracil. Cancer Res., *18:* 478–484, 1958.

Davis, H. L., Ramirez, G., and Ansfield, F. J. Adenocarcinomas of stomach, pancreas, liver and biliary tracts. Cancer, *33:* 193–197, 1974.

DePeyster, F. A., and Gilchrist, R. K. Pathology and manifestations of cancer of the colon and rectum. *In* Diseases of the Colon and Anorectum, edited by R. Turell, pp. 428–452. W. B. Saunders, Philadelphia, 1969.

Dhar, P., Moore, T., Zamcheck, N., and Kupchik, H. Z. Carcinoembryonic antigen (CEA) in colonic cancer. J.A.M.A., *221:* 31–35, 1972.

Dykes, P. W., and King, J. Progress report; carcinoembryonic antigen (CEA). Gut, *13:* 1000–1013, 1972.

Falkson, G. Methyl-GAG (NSC-32946) in the treatment of esophagus cancer. Cancer Chemother. Rep., *55:* 209–212, 1971.

Falkson, G., van Eden, E. B., and Falkson, H. C. Fluorouracil, imidazole carboxamide dimethyl triazeno, vincristine and bis-chloroethyl nitrosourea in colon cancer. Cancer, *33:* 1207–1209, 1974.

Gunderson, L. L., and Sosin, H. Areas of failure found at reoperation (second or symptomatic look) following "curative surgery" for adenocarcinoma of the rectum. Cancer, *34:* 1278–1292, 1974.

Haslam, J. B., Cavanaugh, P. J., and Stroup, S. L. Radiation therapy in the treatment of unresectable adenocarcinoma of the pancreas. Cancer, *32:* 1341–1345, 1973.

Horton, J., Olson, K. B., Sullivan, J. et al. 5-Fluorouracil in cancer; an improved regimen. Ann. Intern. Med., *73:* 897–900, 1970.

Jacobs, E. M., Reeves, W. J., Wood, D. A., Pugh, R., Braunwald, J., and Bateman, J. R. Treatment of cancer with weekly intravenous 5-fluorouracil. Cancer, *27:* 1302–1305, 1971.

Kennedy, P. S., LeHane, D. E., Smith, F. E., and Lane, M. Oral fluorouracil therapy of hepatoma. Cancer, *39:* 1930–1935, 1977.

Kung, C. L., Hall, T. C., Piro, A. J., et al. A clinical trial of oral 5-fluorouracil. Clin. Pharmacol. Ther., *7:* 527–533, 1966.

Kovach, J. S., Moertel, C. G., Schute, A. J. Hahn, R. G., and Reitemeier, R. J. A controlled study of combined 1,3-bis-(2-chloroethyl)-1-nitrosourea and 5-fluorouracil therapy for advanced gastric and pancreatic cancer. Cancer, *33:* 563–567, 1974.

Lahiri, S. R., Boileu, G., and Hall, T. C. Treatment of metastatic colorectal carcinoma with 5-fluorouracil by mouth. Cancer, *28:* 902–906, 1971.

Leffall, L. D., and Chung, E. B. Surgical management of colorectal polyps. Cancer, *34:* 940–947, 1974.

Link, J. S., Bateman, J. R., Paroly, W. S., Durkin, W. J., and Peters, R. L. 5-Fluorouracil in hepatocellular carcinoma; report of twenty-one cases. Cancer, *39:* 1936–1939, 1977.

Lowenfels, A. B. Etiological aspects of cancer of the gastrointestinal tract. Surg. Gynecol. Obstet., *137:* 291–298, 1973.

Mainz, D., and Webster, P. D. Pancreatic carcinoma; a review of etiologic considerations. Am. J. Dig. Dis., *19:* 459–464, 1974.

Mavligit, G. M., Gutterman, J. V., Malahy, M. A., Burgess, M. A., McBride, C. M., Jubert, A., and Hersh, E. M. Systemic adjuvant immunotherapy and chemoimmunotherapy in patients with colorectal cancer (Dukes' C class): Prolongation of disease-free interval and survival. *In* Immunotherapy of Cancer: Present Status of Trials in Man, edited by W. D. Terry and D. Windhorst, pp. 597–604. Raven Press, New York, 1978.

Mittelman, J. A., Bakemeier, R. F., Engstrom, P., and Hanley, J. Sequential and combination chemotherapy of advanced gastric cancer. Cancer, *38:* 678–682, 1976.

Moertel, C. G. Therapy of advanced gastrointestinal cancer with the nitrosoureas. Cancer Chemother. Rep., *4:* 27–34, 1973.

Moertel, C. G. Gastrointestinal cancer, treatment with fluorouracil-nitrosourea combinations. J.A.M.A., *235:* 2135–2136, 1977.

Moertel, C. G., and Reitemeier, R. J. Advanced Gastrointestinal Cancer; Clinical Management and Chemotherapy. Harper & Row, New York, 1969.

Moertel, C. G., Childs, D. S., Reitemeier, R. J., Colby, M. Y., and Holbrook, M. A. Combined 5-fluorouracil and supervoltage radiation therapy of locally unresectable gastrointestinal cancer. Lancet, *2:* 865–867, 1969.

Moertel, C. G., Schutt, A. J., Hahn, R. G., and Reitemeier, R. J. Therapy of advanced colorectal cancer with a combination of 5-fluorouracil, methyl-1,3-cis-(2-chloroethyl)-1-nitrosourea and vincristine. J. Natl. Cancer Inst., *54:* 69–71, 1975.

Moertel, C. G., Lokich, J. J., Schein, P. S., et al. An evaluation of high dose radiation and combined radiation and 5-fluorouracil (5FU) therapy for locally unresectable pancreatic carcinoma. Proc. Am. Soc. Clin. Oncol., *17:* 244, 1976.

Monge, J. J., Judd, E. S., and Gage, R. P. Radical pancreaticoduodenectomy. Ann. Surg., *160:* 711–722, 1964.

Olweny, C. L. M., Toya, T., Mbidde, E. K., Muwerga, J., Kyalwazi, S. K., and Cohen, H. Treatment of hepatocellular carcinoma with Adriamycin; preliminary communication. Cancer, *36:* 1250–1257, 1975.

Palmer, E. D. Peroral prosthesis for the management of incurable esophageal carcinoma. Amer. J. Gastroenterol., *59:* 487–498, 1973.

Pearson, J. G. The value of radiotherapy in the management of esophageal cancer. Am. J. R., *105:* 500–513, 1969.

Pestana, C., Reitemeier, R. J., Moertel, C. G., Judd, E. S., and Dockerty, M. B. The natural history of carcinoma of the colon and rectum. Am. J. Surg., *108:* 826–833, 1964.

Prolla, J. C., Kobayashi, S., and Kirsner, J. B. Gastric cancer; some recent improvements in diagnosis based upon the Japanese experience. Arch. Intern. Med., *124:* 238–246, 1969.

Purtilo, D. T., Kersey, J. H., Hallgren, H. M., Fox, K. R., and Yunis, E. J. Alpha-fetoprotein; diagnostic and prognostic use in patients with hepatomas. Am. J. Clin. Pathol., *59:* 295–299, 1973.

Remine, W. H., Priestly, J. T., Judd, E. S., et al. Total pancreatectomy. Ann. Surg., *172:* 595–604, 1970.

Rodriguez-Antunez, A., Chernak, E. S., Jelden, G. L., and Hunter, T. W. Preoperative irradiation of carcinoma of the rectum. Radiology, *108:* 689–690, 1973.

Ryan, R. F., Schramel, R. J., and Creech, D. Value of perfusion in pelvic surgery. Dis. Colon Rectum, *6:* 297–300, 1967.

Smith, J. B., and O'Neill, R. T. Alpha-fetoprotein; occurrence in germinal cell and liver malignancies. Ann. Intern. Med., *51:* 767–771, 1971.

Stearns, M. W., and Schottenfeld, D. Techniques for the surgical management of colon cancer. Cancer, *28:* 165–169, 1971.

Sweet, R. H. Late results of surgical treatment of carcinoma of the esophagus. J.A.M.A., *155:* 422–425, 1954.

Tormey, D. C., Bergevin, P., Blom, J., and Petty, W. Preliminary trials with a combination of Adriamycin (NSC-123127) and bleomycin (NSC-125066) in adult malignancies. Cancer Chemother. Rep., *57:* 413–418, 1973.

Treadwell, T. A., and Hardin, W. J. Primary carcinoma of the gallbladder; the role of adjunctive therapy in its treatment. Am. J. Surg., *132:* 703–706, 1976.

Urdaneta-Lafee, N., Kligerman, M. M., and Knowlton, A. H. Evaluation of palliative irradiation in rectal carcinoma. Radiology, *104:* 673–677, 1972.

Vogel, C. L., Bagley, M. C., Brooker, R. J., Anthony, P. P., and Ziegler, J. L. A phase II study of Adriamycin (NSC-123127) in patients with hepatocellular carcinoma from Zambia and the United States. Cancer, *39:* 1923–1929, 1977.

Whiteley, H. W., Searns, M. W., Leaming, R. H., and Deddish, M. R. Palliative radiation therapy in patients with cancer of the colon and rectum. Cancer, *25:* 343–346, 1970.

Wilson, S. M., and Block, G. E. Periampullary carcinoma. Arch. Surg., *108:* 539–544, 1974.

Wilson, J. M., Melvin, D. B., Gray, G. F., and Thorbjarnarson, B. Primary malignancies of the small bowel; a report of 96 cases and review of the literature. Ann. Surg., *180:* 175–179, 1974.

Woolley, P. V., MacDonald, J. S., and Schein, P. S. Chemotherapy of malignancies of the gastrointestinal tract. Prog. Gastroenterol., *3:* 671–692, 1977.

Yarbrough, D. R. Primary carcinoma of the extrahepatic bile ducts. Am. J. Surg., *125:* 723–725, 1973.

Yount, L. J., and Hurley, J. D. Pelvic perfusion for carcinoma of the colon. Am. J. Surg., *105:* 102–107, 1963.

Chapter 15

Renal Cell Carcinoma

CHARLES F. MILLER, M.D. and RICHARD A. MISKOFF, M.D., A.B.

INCIDENCE

The incidence of malignant neoplasms of the kidney varies between 1.2% and 3.0% (Bennington, 1973; King, 1967) of all human cancers. Of the malignant kidney neoplasms, renal adenocarcinoma represents 83.4–89.0%. Males predominate with an occurrence rate of at least twice that of females (Bennington and Kadijian, 1967; Holland and Frei, 1973). Renal adenocarcinoma is decidedly rare in children (about 1% of renal adenocarcinoma), but rapidly increases in frequency with advancing age. Some authors report a decrease after the sixth and seventh decades (King, 1967; Holland and Frei, 1973), whereas Bennington (1973) noted a steady rise in incidence into the eighth decade.

Familial occurrence of hypernephroma is rare. It has been reported most frequently in siblings (Brinton, 1960; Riches, 1963; Rusche, 1953; Klinger, 1968) with one reported case of occurrence in a mother and daughter (Steinberg et al., 1972). There is a definite increase in occurrence of hypernephroma in association with von Hippel-Lindau's disease (Kernohan et al., 1931; Christoferson et al., 1961).

ETIOLOGY

The cause of renal adenocarcinoma is unknown. Many carcinogens have been identified in experimental animals (Bennington, 1973); however, exposure of man to many of these agents is not common. A possible carcinogen in man may be dimethylnitrosoamine, an ingredient in tobacco. Several studies (Bennington and Laubscher, 1968; Bennington et al., 1968) have shown a positive correlation between tobacco use and hypernephroma. These findings have been supported by Kolonel (1976) who also reported an increased risk of renal cancer from occupational exposure to cadmium. A suggested synergism between cigarette smoking and cadmium exposure has also been noted.

A viral etiology has been considered based on viral related adenocarcinoma of the kidney in the frog (Lucke, 1952), chicken (Carr, 1960) and other animals (King, 1967). Both DNA and RNA viruses have induced renal neoplasms in experimental animals (King, 1967).

Estrogens have been shown to induce renal tumors in the male syrian golden hamster (Kirkman and Bacon, 1952). The part this plays in the etiology of human renal cell carcinoma is unknown, but is most likely of little significance since the incidence of the neoplasm is higher in males.

Radiation to experimental animals has been associated with a significant increase in renal tumors (Rosen et al., 1961); however, this relationship does not seem to be borne out in man. Thorotrast, a radioactive colloidal suspension of thorium dioxide, has been used in the past for retrograde pyelographic studies. This material appears to be responsible for the induction of human renal tumors which usually appear 15–30 years after exposure (King, 1967). Most of these, however, have been squamous cell carcinomas of the renal pelvis. In some instances granules of the unaltered thorotrast have been found in both the malignant and normal kidneys as long as 30 years after receiving the agent. Kantor (1977) points out, however, that no controlled studies have been performed and the residual thorotrast might also be found in patients without any history of malignant renal changes.

PATHOLOGY

Renal cancer can be divided into three major types depending upon the cell of origin (Carter, 1968).

1. Renal adenocarcinoma which arises from the proximal tubular epithelium (Oberling et al., 1960)

2. Transitional cell carcinoma and squamous cell carcinoma which arise from the epithelial lining of the pelvicalyceal system

3. Wilm's tumor which arises from immature parenchymal tissue.

Renal adenocarcinoma can be further subdivided into cell types:

1. Medullary
2. Tubular
3. Cystic
4. Papillary.

Additional subdivision of renal adenocarcinoma include cell type (clear or granular) and morphology (stage of differentiation); however, with the exception of the rare sarcomatoid pattern (Farrow et al., 1968), which has a poor prognosis, there appears at present to be little agreement relating histologic type to prognosis (Skinner et al., 1971; Foot et al., 1951; Riches, 1964).

One histologic feature which may be important in prognosis is the appearance of lymphoid and/or plasma cell infiltration in the tumor as reported by Kiely et al. (1972). In his series of 112 patients, the presence of lymphocytes was directly related to an increased 5-year tumor-free interval.

Renal adenocarcinoma also has several characteristic histochemical features (Bennington, 1973), based on intracellular substances:

1. Positive periodic acid-Schiff (PAS) reaction which demonstrates intracytoplasmic glycogen that is removed by diastase digestion

2. Positive oil red O, Sudan IV and percholoric acid napthaquinone on frozen section which stains renal lipids that are completely removed by prior treatment with xylene or chloroform with methyl alcohol.

3. Positive Sudan black which stains phospholipids that are not removed by prior treatment with xylene or chloroform with methyl alcohol.

A controversial subject in the pathology of renal tumors is the relationship of renal adenoma to renal adenocarcinoma. The male predominance in adenomas is similar to that in renal adenocarcinoma; the increased incidence of adenoma in kidneys with adenocarcinoma and the often seen histologic similarity between adenoma and adenocarcinoma (Holland and Frei, 1973) makes differentiation between the two extremely difficult. The rather arbitrary distinction on the basis of size has evolved between these two entities. The rarity of metastasis in renal tumors under 3 cm serves as the basis for labeling them adenomas. Also, a lesion greater than 3 cm has an increased incidence of metastasis and is, therefore, labeled adenocarcinoma. This reasoning is obviously faulty, especially when one tries to classify a renal tumor less than three centimeters that has metastasized. Confusing as it may seem, this does indirectly establish the renal adenoma as a possible premalignant lesion.

Metastases occur via the venous and lymphatic route as well as by direct extension. Venous invasion is probably related to prognosis and will be discussed below in the section on staging. Metastases can occur in any organ and are seen frequently in bone, lung and liver. A somewhat unique metastatic site, which may mimic a primary lung carcinoma, is the endobronchial area (Caplan, 1959). Therefore, in the appropriate patient with pulmonary symptoms bronchoscopic examination may be helpful for diagnosis and evaluation.

STAGING

Staging is important in renal carcinoma from two aspects: (1) intelligent surgical approach, and (2) prognosis. A workable staging system has been proposed by Robson et al. (1963):

Stage 1: Tumor confined to the kidney

Stage 2: Perirenal fat involvement, but confined within Gerota's fascia

Stage 3: A. Gross renal vein or inferior vena cava involvement
B. Lymphatic involvement
C. Vascular plus lymphatic involvement

Stage 4: A. Adjacent organs other than adrenals involved
B. Distant metastasis.

Based on Robson's study of 88 patients, length of survival was directly related to stage. His study has been criticized (Holland, 1973) because his patients underwent a more thorough preoperative evaluation and a more radical surgical approach than patients in most other series and thus more advanced disease may have been more effectively ruled out. Table 15.1 is a compilation of the relationship of stage to prognosis of the major series to date. Although results vary which may affect preoperative evaluation, all series reflect a direct relationship of increasing stage to poor prognosis. The only exception to this was Skinner's series (Skinner et al., 1971) in which Stage 3 did better than Stage 2.

PRESENTATION

Renal cell carcinoma can present either with local or systemic manifestations. The classic presentation of hematuria, pain and tumor mass occurs in only about 10–15% of patients. Hematuria is the most common

TABLE 15.1

Relationship of Stage to Prognosis in Renal Adenocarcinoma (5-Year Survival of 920 Patients)[a]

	Mean (%)	Range (%)
Stage 1	60	46[4]–66[2]
Stage 2	46	37[4]–64[2]
Stage 3	29	9[4]–51[1]
Stage 4	7	2.9[5]–12[3]

[a] Skinner et al. (1971)[1]; Holland (1973)[2]; Arvola and Lilius (1972)[3]; Flocks and Kadesky (1958)[4]; Cox et al. (1970)[5].

presenting symptom occurring about 60% of the time. If clots are formed and pass down the ureter, then hematuria may be accompanied by pain. Flank mass may be palpated 20–50% of the time and depends on the size and location within the kidney. This triad usually are late manifestations and, therefore, signal a poor prognosis. Varicocele, which usually occurs on the left, is a grave prognostic sign indicating possible tumor thrombus of the left internal spermatic vein. The systemic manifestations are discussed below.

COMPLICATIONS

The major direct complications of renal adenocarcinoma include hemorrhage, thrombosis, obstruction, arteriovenous malformation and tumor compression of the renal artery with resultant hypertension. These complications may be responsible for a high association between renal adenocarcinoma and cardiovascular disease such as high output failure and vascular catastrophe (Gordon, 1963). Aside from these direct effects there have been reported several indirect effects of renal adenocarcinoma.

Raised erythropoietin levels have been found in patients with renal tumors; however, actual erythrocytosis occurred only in 8–10% of the patients in Murphy's series (Murphy et al., 1970). In this series erythropoietin levels fell to normal in patients whose renal carcinoma was resected in which no metastatic disease was found. Metastatic renal carcinomas, on the other hand, had both elevated levels of erythropoietin prior to nephrectomy and afterwards.

The anemia of chronic disease with low serum iron and transferrin levels is a frequent finding in renal cell carcinoma. Resolution of this anemia has been reported with resection of the tumor (Greenberg and Cheger, 1971; Bowman and Martinez, 1968).

Hypercalcemia unassociated with bone metastasis has been reported by several authors (Buckle et al., 1970; Munson et al., 1965; Blair et al., 1973). They all found evidence of ectopic hyperparathyroidism with evidence of increased levels of parathyroid-like hormone both in the serum and in tumor extracts. The metastatic deposits also appeared to secrete a PTH-like substance.

Aside from hypertension caused by direct effects of the tumor, such as renal artery compression and arteriovenous fistula, hyper-reninemia has been demonstrated although most of these cases have been hemangiopericytomas (Eddy and Sanchez, 1971; Lee, 1971).

Hepatic dysfunction manifested by abnormal liver function tests in association with hypernephroma has been reported (Utz et al., 1970) and appears to occur about 40% of the time. Return of the liver function abnormalities to normal after nephrectomy has occurred often and implies a favorable prognosis.

Hepatomegaly also occurs frequently, and liver biopsy may show a nonspecific reactive hepatitis manifested by Kupfer-cell proliferation, fatty changes in hepatic cells and portal triaditis (Utz et al., 1970).

Peripheral neuropathy, mostly in the form of motor neuron disease, occurs rarely in renal adenocarcinoma (Lloyd and Chakrabart, 1973; Buchanan and Mulamud, 1973). Of interest is the fact that often after nephrectomy the neurological manifestations become worse before improving.

Fever and weight loss are also seen in renal cell carcinoma not infrequently. These signs appear to be toxic systemic manifestations. The fever is thought to be a result of tumor necrosis and resorption of pyrogen (Rawlins et al., 1970). Renal cell carcinoma should be considered in patients with FUO.

TREATMENT

Surgery

The primary treatment of renal cell carcinoma is surgical resection. Controversy exists concerning the correct surgical approach. Some surgeons believe that a radical approach utilizing a thoracoabdominal incision affords the patient a better chance for a long term survival. Robson (1963) demonstrated a 66% 10-year survival for patients who underwent radical nephrectomy as opposed to 22% for those treated by simple nephrectomy. A more recent study by Middleton and Presto (1973) revealed a 40% 10-year survival utilizing radical nephrectomy compared to a historical control of 18% treated by a simple nephrectomy. A large study by Skinner et al. (1971) with 309 patients showed no statistical relationship between simple and radical nephrectomy when compared by stage. Skinner cautions, however, that patient selection probably played a major role and a conclusion based on his data is not justifiable. Even simple nephrectomy sometimes is not advisable when the patient has either an absent or a hypoplastic kidney on the opposite side. To prevent the problem of renal failure in this unusual circumstance a partial nephrectomy is sometimes possible.

Nephrectomy in the face of metastatic disease may relieve many of the problems attendant to renal cell carcinoma such as fever, pain, infection and hematuria. Although reported, rarely has removal of the primary tumor resulted in regression of the metastatic disease (Middleton, 1967; Mathias, 1971).

A recent review of the literature (Bloom, 1973) revealed that there have been only 40 documented cases of spontaneous regresssion of metastatic adenocarcinoma of the kidney. In 38 of the 40 cases regression occurred in the lungs. A possible hormonal basis may be involved because of the predominance of spontaneous regression in males (79%).

Surgery on metastatic lesions may be beneficial to the patient and afford an increase in survival especially if there is only a single metastasis or if there has been a long disease-free interval after the diagnosis. Marcove et al. (1972) reviewed the literature and found that in patients with a solitary metastasis there was a 3-year survival of 45% and a 5-year survival of 34%. Surgical removal had not been carried out on these patients. It was his conclusion that this may represent a slower growing tumor which should be treated vigorously with surgical extirpation. He also introduced the concept of cryosurgery for metastatic bone lesions as an acceptable way of removing tumor without having to sacrifice a limb. More recently, Katzenstein et al. (1978) have recommended resection of unilateral pulmonary metastases in conjunction with radical nephrectomy. This aggressive surgical approach to patients with limited metastatic disease is also supported by Klugo et al. (1977) who recommend resection of any solitary metastasis. This approach has been criticized by Montie et al. (1977b) whose data suggest that nephrectomy is indicated only in patients who have bony metastases.

Radiotherapy

A controversial and as yet unresolved question in the treatment of renal cell carcinoma is the role of radiotherapy. Riches et al. (1951), utilizing a large series of patients, demonstrated that postoperative irradiation was superior to nephrectomy alone at both the 5- and 10-year survival levels. Flocks and Kaderky (1958) also demonstrated the value of radiotherapy, especially the 10-year survival in preoperatively irradiated individuals. Recently a randomized study conducted in the Netherlands (van der Werf-Messing, 1973) demonstrated that preoperative irradiation did not improve 5-year survival. She did show, however, that residual growth was higher in the nonirradiated group suggesting that perhaps preoperative irradiation may render otherwise inoperable cases operable.

A controlled trial by Finney (1973) comparing surgery alone to surgery plus postoperative radiation failed to reveal a statistically significant difference in survival. Radiotherapy conferred no advantage in preventing local recurrence. Also, there were several deaths due to radiation-induced hepatitis.

Radiation of metastatic renal carcinoma can many times produce effective palliation and relief of pain. Response to radiation may be slow (Riches, 1964; Vaeth, 1973). More recent reviews (Bissada, 1977) have emphasized the relative radioresistance of renal cell carcinoma. Our present recommendation is that neither preoperative nor postoperative radiation therapy is useful in the routine management of renal carcinoma.

Chemotherapy

Treatment of renal adenocarcinoma with hormonal manipulation and/ or cytotoxic agents is disappointing; however, few medical centers have had an opportunity to evaluate this tumor because of its relative infrequency. The poor response to cytotoxic agents has resulted in an increased interest in hormonal therapy. The classic experiment utilizing the prolonged administration of diethylstilbestrol to induce kidney tumors in syrian golden hamsters (Kirkman and Bacon, 1952) has served as the prototype of subsequent clinical studies. This experiment demonstrated that testosterone and medroxyprogesterone could prevent induction of kidney tumors. Diethylstilbestrol (DES) may also deserve clinical trial based on Soloway and Myers' (1973) data of effectiveness of DES on spontaneous renal tumors in mice.

A more recent review of the literature of hormonal therapy in the treatment of renal adenocarcinoma is by Bloom (1973) who recorded 272 cases from 10 medical centers noting an overall objective response rate of 15% with a range of 6–33%, with subjective responses in 50% of the cases. Better results were achieved in men than in women. Progestins and testosterone were used either alone or in combination. The largest series reviewed by Bloom was his own group of 80 patients revealing a 16% objective response with remissions lasting 2–35 months. Again, male response was superior. Survival was only increased in those patients responding to hormone therapy. It is difficult to assess the optimum dosage of hormone and the frequency of administration. In one study of 23 patients, Samuels et al. (1968) noted no response to oral medroxyprogesterone in 7 patients, but three objective responses to parenteral medroxyprogesterone in 16 patients using either 100 mg/day or 400 mg/ week. Bloom (1973) obtained similar results using medroxyprogesterone orally 100 mg, 3 times a day. The optimal dosage for testosterone has not been studied. Testosterone has been administered in a variety of ways. Bloom (1973) used testosterone propionate 100 mg daily 5 times a week, later reduced to 3 times a week. Talley (1973) used a variety of agents including testosterone proprionate 100 mg, 3 times a week, testosterone cyclopentyl propionate 200 mg IM weekly or fluoxymesterone 30 mg daily PO.

It appears that many of the response rates to hormonal agents reported in earlier studies were overestimated. The results of published studies from 1971 through 1977 show a much lower remission rate of 8 of 416 or 1.8% responses (Hrushesky and Murphy, 1977). This is only slightly greater than the rate of spontaneous regressions reported by Montie et al. (1977a). This discrepancy probably stems from the much stricter criteria applied in recent years to definition of objective response. These same authors do report a somewhat more encouraging response rate of

17% in a small group of patients with metastatic disease treated by nephrectomy and medroxyprogesterone. Two patients achieved complete regression of all metastatic disease surviving 11 and 23 months. Thus, the use of progestational agents in combination with radical surgery may be considerably better than when used in patients whose tumor load has not been reduced.

The experience with cytotoxic agents in the treatment of renal cell carcinoma has been limited and disappointing. Earlier reviews (Talley, 1973; Lokich and Harrison, 1975) only demonstrated that almost no chemotherapeutic agents have had adequate clinical trials. Hrushesky and Murphy (1977) have recently summarized and updated chemotherapy of renal cell carcinoma. From their data it is clear that vinblastine is the most active single agent, with an overall objective response rate of 25% in 125 patients. The highest response rates are correlated with the highest weekly doses of this drug. Table 15.2 lists the few other agents reported to have some minimal activity for hypernephroma. The activity of dibromodulcitol is based on preliminary phase II studies (Carter and Wasserman, 1975) and has not been confirmed.

A recent report showed no objective responses to cis-diamminedichloro-platinum in 23 patients with metastatic disease (Rodrigues and Johnson, 1978). This is somewhat surprising since this drug is known to have activity in many other genitourinary tumors. Wong et al. (1977) reported no objective responses in 17 patients treated with vindesine sulfate, a derivative of vinblastine. Other negative studies have shown little activity for piperazinedione (Pasmantier et al., 1977), thio-tepa, and CCNU (Hahn et al., 1977); many of these reports can be criticized, however, because of the small number of patients in each study. The large majority of chemotherapeutic agents have simply not received adequate clinical trial as single agents.

The use of combination chemotherapy in this tumor has not proved to be very beneficial either. Using CCNU and vinblastine, Merrin et al. (1975) found only a 16% response rate; Davis and Manalo (1978) obtained

TABLE 15.2
Chemotherapeutic Agents with Activity in Renal Cell Carcinoma[a]

Drug	Response Rate (%)
Vinblastine	24
Dibromodulcitol	20
Nitrogen Mustard	11
MeCCNU	9
5-Fluorouracil	11
Hydroxyurea	11
Bleomycin	9

[a] Modified from Hrushesky and Murphy (1977).

a 24% response with the same combination. Johnson et al. (1975) found no objective responses using vincristine and hydroxyurea. Similar results, less than 20% objective responses, have been obtained using CCNU, bleomycin and steroids with or without adriamycin (Richards et al., 1977). The addition of hormonal therapy to chemotherapy has not shown any improvement in objective response in several studies (Alberto and Senn, 1974; Lokich and Harrison, 1975). These trials were, however, very limited in the number of agents examined. Essentially no useful trials have been reported using adjuvant chemotherapy in early stage hypernephroma. From information presently available, vinblastine is the most obvious candidate for an adjuvant therapy study.

Because of the paucity of effective drugs, we feel that patients with advanced renal cell carcinoma should be treated under a protocol study. For those patients in whom this is not feasible, our recommendation is a trial of vinblastine in the highest tolerable doses. Because of newer results showing little if any objective response from progestational agents, these cannot be recommended as initial therapy, but may provide some symptomatic palliation in patients unresponsive to vinblastine. Much further work needs to be done to evaluate both older and new chemotherapeutic agents in renal cell carcinoma. Routine adjuvant chemotherapy and/or hormone therapy cannot be recommended at the present time.

The use of immunotherapy in renal carcinoma is exceedingly limited. This is somewhat surprising in view of past emphasis on spontaneous regression of metastases, which may imply that these tumors may be dependent on immune mechanisms. Nonspecific immunotherapy with BCG has been utilized in a small number of patients with metastatic disease (Minton et al., 1976). Treatment was relatively ineffective except that one patient did obtain a prolonged complete remission. Montie et al. (1977a) used transfer factor in a similar group of patients, but obtained no objective responses. No significant results have been reported to date using immunotherapy in an adjuvant setting.

REFERENCES

Alberto, P., and Senn, H. J Hormonal therapy of renal carcinoma alone and in association with cytostatic drugs. Cancer, 33: 1226–1229, 1974.

Arvola, I., and Lilius, H. G. Prognosis of renal adenocarcinoma in a central hospital. Ann. Chir. Gynaecol. Fenn., 61: 223–226, 1972.

Bennington, J. L. Cancer of the kidney—etiology, epidemiology and pathology. Cancer, 32: 1017–1029, 1973.

Bennington, J., Ferguson, B. R., and Campbell, P. B. Epidemiologic studies of carcinoma of the kidney; II. Association of renal adenocarcinoma with smoking. Cancer, 21: 821–823, 1968.

Bennington, J. L., and Kadijian, R. M. Renal Carcinoma. W. B. Saunders, Phildadelphia, 1967.

Bennington, J. L., and Laubscher, F. A. Epidemiologic studies of carcinoma of the kidney— association of renal adenocarcinoma with smoking. Cancer, 21: 1069–1071, 1968.

Bissada, N. K. Renal cell adenocarcinoma. Surg. Gynecol. Obstet., *145:* 97–103, 1977.

Blair, A. J., Jr., Hawker, C. D., and Utiger, R. D. Ectopic hyperparathyroidism in a patient with metastatic hypernephroma. Metabolism, *22:* 147–154, 1973.

Bloom, H. J. G. Hormone induced and spontaneous regression of metastatic renal cancer. Cancer, *32:* 1066–1071, 1973.

Bowman, H. S., and Martinez, E. J. Fever, anemia and hyperhaptoglobinemia—an extra renal triad of hypernephroma. Ann. Intern. Med., *68:* 613–620, 1968.

Brinton, L. F. Hypernephroma; familial occurrence in one family. J.A.M.A., *173:* 888–890, 1960.

Buchanan, D. S., and Mulamud, N. Motor neuron disease with renal cell carcinoma and postoperative neurologic remission. Neurology, *23:* 891–894, 1973.

Buckle, R. M., McMillan, M., and Mallinson, C. Ectopic secretion of parathyroid hormone by renal adenocarcinoma in a patient with hypercalcemia. Br. Med. J., *4:* 724–726, 1970.

Caplan, H. Solitary endobronchial metastasis from carcinoma of the kidney. Br. J. Surg., *46:* 624–625, 1959.

Carr, J. G. Kidney carcinoma of the fowl induced by the MH_2 reticuloendothelioma virus. Br. J. Cancer, *14:* 77–82, 1960.

Carter, R. L. The pathology of renal cancer. J.A.M.A., *204:* 129–130, 1968.

Carter, S. K., and Wasserman T. H. The chemotherapy of urologic cancer. Cancer, *36:* 729–747, 1975.

Christoferson, L. A., Gustafson, M. B., and Peterson, A. G. Von Hipple-Lindau's disease. J.A.M.A., *178:* 280–282, 1961.

Cox, C. E., Lacy, S. S., Montgomery, W. G., and Boyce, W. H. Renal adenocarcinoma: 28-year review, with emphasis on rationale and feasibility of preoperative radiotherapy. J. Urol., *104:* 53–61, 1970

Davis, T. E., and Manalo, F. B. Combination chemotherapy of advanced renal cell cancer with CCNU and vinblastine. Proc. Am. Soc. Clin. Oncol., *19:* 316, 1978.

Eddy, R. L., and Sanchez, S. A. Renin-secreting renal neoplasm and hypertension with hypokalemia. Ann. Intern. Med., *75:* 725–729, 1971.

Farrow, G. W., Harrison, E. G., and Utz, D. C. Sarcomas and sarcomatoid and mixed malignant tumor of the kidney in adults—Parts I, II, and III. Cancer, *22:* 545–563, 1968.

Finney, R. An evaluation of postoperative radiotherapy in hypernephroma treatment—a clinical trial. Cancer, *32:* 1332–1340, 1973.

Flocks, R. H., and Kadesky, M. C. Malignant neoplasms of the kidney; an analysis of 353 patients followed five years or more. J. Urol., *79:* 196–201, 1958.

Foot, N. C., Humphreys, G. A., and Whitmore, W. F. Renal tumors; pathology and prognosis in 295 cases. J. Urol., *66:* 190–200, 1951.

Gordon, D. A. The extra renal manifestation of hypernephroma. Can. Med. Assoc. J., *88:* 61–67, 1963.

Greenberg, P. L., and Cheger, W. B. The anemia of chronic disorder due to renal cell carcinoma; ferrokinetic and morphologic documentation of its surgical correction. Am. J. Med. Sci., *261:* 265–267, 1971.

Hahn, D. M., Schimpff, S. C., Ruckdeschel, J. C., and Wiernik, P. H. Single agent therapy for renal cell carcinoma; CCNU, vinblastine, thiotepa, or bleomycin. Cancer Treat. Rep., *61:* 1585–1587, 1977.

Holland, J. F., and Frei, E., III. Cancer Medicine. Lea & Febiger, Phildadelphia, 1973.

Holland, J. M. Cancer of the kidney–natural history and staging. Cancer, *32:* 1030–1042, 1973.

Hrushesky, W. J., Murphy, G. P. Current status of the therapy of advanced renal cell carcinoma. J. Surg. Oncol., *9:* 277–288, 1977.

Johnson, D. E., Rodrigues, L., Holoye, P. Y., and Samuels, M. L. Combination vincristine (NSC-67574) and hydroxyurea (NSC-32065) for metastatic renal carcinoma. Cancer Chemother. Rep., *59:* 1159–1160, 1975.

Kantor, A. F. Current concepts in the epidemiology and etiology of primary renal cell carcinoma. J. Urol., *117:* 415–417, 1977.

Katzenstein, A., Purvis, R., Gmelich, J., and Askin, F. Pulmonary resection for metastatic renal adenocarcinoma. Cancer, *41:* 712–723, 1978.

Kernohan, J. W., Woltman, H. W., and Adson, A. W. Intramedullary tumors of the spinal cord; a review of 51 cases with an attempt at histologic classification. Arch. Neurol. Psychiatry, *25:* 679–701, 1931.

Kiely, E., Creally, M., and Creally, J. On the significance of lymphoid cell infiltration in hypernephroma. Ir. J. Med. Sci., *141:* 108–111, 1972.

King, J. S. Renal Neoplasia. Little, Brown & Co., Boston, 1967.

Kirkman, H., and Bacon, R. L. Estrogen-induced tumors of the kidney; I. Incidence of renal tumors in intact and gonadectomized male golden hamsters treated with diethylstilbestrol. J. Natl. Cancer Inst., *13:* 745–755, 1952.

Klinger, M. Renal cell carcinoma in siblings; a case report. J. Am. Geriatr. Soc., *16:* 1042–1052, 1968.

Klugo, R. C, Detmers, M., Stiles, R. E., Talley, R. W., and Cerny, J. C. Aggressive versus conservative management of stage IV renal cell carcinoma. J. Urol., *118:* 244–246, 1977.

Kolonel, L. N. Association of cadmium with renal cancer. Cancer, *37:* 1782–1787, 1976.

Lloyd, G. H. T., and Chakrabart, A. K. Relapsing peripheral neuropathy in association with renal carcinoma. J Indian Med. Assoc., *60:* 200–205, 1973.

Lokich, J. J., and Harrison, J. H. Renal cell carcinoma; natural history and chemotherapeutic experience. J. Urol., *114:* 371–374, 1975.

Lucke, B. Kidney carcinoma in the leopard frog; a virus tumor. Ann. N.Y. Acad. Sci., *54:* 1093–1109, 1952.

Marcove, R. C., Sadreich, J. , Hwos, A. G., and Grabstald, H. Cryosurgery in the treatment of solitary or multiple bone metastasis from renal cell carcinoma. J. Urol., *108:* 540–547, 1972.

Mathias, D. B. A case of spontaneous regression of pulmonary metastasis arising from hypernephroma following nephrectomy. Br. J. Urol., *43:* 65–68, 1971.

Merrin, C., Mittleman, A., Fanous, N., Wajsman, A., and Murphy, G. P. Chemotherapy of advanced renal cell carcinoma with vinblastin and CCNU. J. Urol., *113:* 21–23, 1975.

Middleton, R. G. Surgery for metastatic renal cell carcinoma. J. Urol., *97:* 973, 1967.

Middleton, R. G., and Presto, A. J., III. Radical thoraco-abdominal nephrectomy for renal cell carcinoma. J. Urol., *110:* 36–37, 1973.

Minton, J. P., Pennline, K., Nawrocki, J. F., Kibbey, W. E., and Dodd, M. C. Immunotherapy of human kidney cancer. Proc. Am. Soc. Clin. Oncol., *17:* 301, 1976.

Montie, J. E., Bukowski, R. M., Deedhar, S. D., Hewlett, J. S., Stewart, B. H., and Straffon, R. A. Immunotherapy of disseminated renal cell carcinoma with transfer factor. J. Urol., *117:* 553–556, 1977a.

Montie, J. E., Stewart, B. H., Straffon, R. A., Banowsky, L. H. W., Hewitt, C. B., and Montague, D. K. The role of adjunctive nephrectomy in patients with metastatic renal cell carcinoma. J. Urol., *117:* 272–275, 1977b.

Munson, P. L., Tashjian, A. H., Jr., and Levine, L. Evidence for parathyroid hormone in nonparathyroid tumors associated with hypercalcemia. Cancer Res., *25:* 1062–1067, 1965.

Murphy, G. P., Kenny, G. M., and Mirand, E. A. Erythropoietin levels in patients with renal tumors or cysts. Cancer, *26:* 191–194, 1970.

Oberling, C., Riviere, M., and Haguenau, F. Ultrastructure of the clear cells in renal carcinoma and its importance for the demonstration of their renal origin. Nature, *186:* 402–403, 1960.

Pasmantier, M. W., Coleman, M., Kennedy, B. J., Eagan, R., Carolla, R., Weiss, R., Leone, L., and Silver, R. T. Piperazinedione in metastatic renal carcinoma. Cancer Treat. Rep., *61:* 1731–1732, 1977.

Rawlins, M. D., Luff, R. H., and Cranston, W. I. Pyrexia in renal carcinoma. Lancet, *1:* 1371–1373, 1970.

Richards, F., Muss, H. B., White, D. R., Cooper, M. R., and Spurr, C. L. CCNU, bleomycin, and methyl-prednisolone with or without Adriamycin in renal cell carcinoma; a randomized trial. Cancer Treat. Rep., *61:* 1591–1593, 1977.

Riches, E. On carcinoma of the kidney. Ann. R. Coll. Surg. Engl., *32:* 201–208, 1963.

Riches, E. Tumors of the kidney and suprarenals; I. Tumor of the kidneys and suprarenals in adults. Br. J. Radiol., *37:* 124–128, 1964.

Riches, E. W., Griffiths, I. H., and Thackray, A. C. New growths of the kidney and ureter. Br. J. Urol., *23:* 297–356, 1951.

Robson, C. J., Churchill, B. M., and Anderson, W. The results of radical nephrectomy for renal cell carcinoma. J. Urol., *89:* 37–42, 1963.

Rodrigues, L. H., and Johnson, D. E. Clinical trial of cis-platinum (NSC-119875) in metastatic renal cell carcinoma. Urology, *11:* 344–346, 1978.

Rosen, V. J., Castanera, T. J., Kimeldorf, D. J., and Jones, D. C. Neoplasm in the irradiated and non-irradiated Sprague-Dawley rat. Am. J. Pathol., *38:* 359–369, 1961.

Rusche, C. Silent adenocarcinoma of the kidney with solitary metastases occurring in brothers. J. Urol., *70:* 146–151, 1953.

Samuels, M. L., Sullivan, P., and Howe, C. D. Medroxyprogesterone acetate in the treatment of renal cell carcinoma (hypernephroma). Cancer, *22:* 525–532, 1968.

Skinner, D. G., Colvin, R. B., Vermillion, C. D., Pfister, R. C., and Leadbetter, W. F. Diagnosis and management of renal cell carcinoma. A clinical and pathologic study of 309 cases. Cancer, *28:* 1165–1177, 1971.

Soloway, M. S., and Nyers, G. H., Jr. The effect of hormonal treatment on a transplantable renal cortical adenocarcinoma in syngeneic mice. J. Urol., *109:* 356–361, 1973.

Steinberg, S. M., Brodovsky, H. S., and Goepp, C. E. Renal carcinoma in mother and daughter. Cancer, *29:* 222–225, 1972.

Talley, R. W. Chemotherapy of adenocarcinoma of the kidney. Cancer, *32:* 1062–1065, 1973.

Utz, D. C., Warren, M. M., Gregg, J. A., Ludwig, J., and Kelalu, P. P. Reversible hepatic dysfunction associated with hypernephroma. Mayo Clin. Proc., *45:* 161–169, 1970.

Vaeth, J. M. Cancer of the kidney—radiation therapy and its indications in non-Wilm's tumor. Cancer, *32:* 1053–1055, 1973.

van der Werf-Messing, B. Carcinoma of the kidney. Cancer, *32:* 1056–1061, 1973.

Wong, P. P., Yagoda, A., Currie, V. E., and Young, C. W. Phase II study of vindesine sulfate in the therapy for advanced renal cell carcinoma. Cancer Treat. Rep., *61:* 1727–1729, 1977.

Chapter 16

Urinary Bladder

CHARLES F. MILLER, M.D.

Carcinoma of the urinary bladder is the most common malignancy of the urinary tract. Thirty thousand new cases were estimated to occur in 1977, with an attendant 10,000 deaths; this accounts for almost 3% of cancer deaths in the United States for that year. The male to female ratio is 3:1, and the peak incidence for this neoplasm is between 50 and 70 years of age. Over the past 25 years there has occurred an unaccountable 35% decreased incidence in females (American Cancer Society, 1977). The worldwide incidence of transitional cell carcinoma is highest in the urbanized countries of western Europe and the United States; lowest rates are found in Japan and Chile. The incidence is also increased in lower socioeconomic classes, but is two times higher in American whites than in blacks (Seidman et al., 1976).

The incidence of squamous cell bladder carcinoma is very high in Egypt and other parts of the middle east, but this is specifically related to the high incidence of schistosomiasis infections in these areas (Oyasu and Hopp, 1974).

ETIOLOGY

Although the basic pathogenesis of bladder cancer remains unknown, it is one of the few human tumors which has been clinically related to several specific carcinogens.

A partial list of agents which have been implicated in producing bladder cancer in man is presented in Table 16.1*A*.

Because of occupational exposure, workers in certain industries are at increased risk of developing bladder carcinoma; these industries are listed in Table 16.1*B*.

The association between aromatic amines and bladder cancer in both animals and men has been well established (Wendel et al., 1974; Oyasu and Hopp, 1974). Cole et al. (1971) have demonstrated an increased risk

TABLE 16.1
Etiology

A. *Carcinogenic agents for human bladder cancer*
   Cigarettes
   Aromatic amines
   Cyclophosphamide
   Cyclamates, saccharine
   Instant coffee
   Phenacitin
   Nitrosoamines
   Schistosomiasis (squamous cell)
B. *Industries with increased risk of bladder cancer*
   Textile
   Dye
   Printing
   Rubber
   Cable
   Plastics
   Pitch, Tar
   Gas
   Aluminum

in heavy cigarette smokers. Several reports have implicated prolonged cyclophosphamide therapy in inducing bladder tumors (Ansell and Castro, 1975; Wall and Clauson, 1975). Cyclamates, saccharin, phenacetin (Jackson and Baetcke, 1976), nitrosoamines (Radomoski and Hearn, 1976), abnormal tryptophan metabolism (Yoshida et al., 1970) and prior pelvic radiation in the female as well as females with a prior history of cancer of the uterine cervix (Prout, 1974; Newell et al., 1975) have all been linked to bladder tumors. An increased risk has been noted in aluminum workers (Wigle, 1977).

A. B. Miller (1977) has shown that intake of instant coffee may also be an important risk factor in bladder cancer. Other increased risk factors are chronic cystitis, urethral strictures and urinary retention (Prout, 1974). This implicates a carcinogen(s) in the urine that produce(s) cancer only under conditions of prolonged contact with the urothelium. Indeed, animals exposed to 2-naphthylamine—a known bladder carcinogen—did not develop bladder tumors when the urinary stream was diverted, but tumors developed in the ureters and renal pelvis which were still exposed to the carcinogen on a chronic basis (Scott and Boyd, 1953). Weissman et al. (1978) have reviewed recent developments in experimental bladder tumors and point out that chronic bladder irritation produces an unstable urothelium. This has the potential to develop hyperplastic, and subsequently malignant, clones at many sites and different times. The continuous exposure of the human bladder to presently unknown carcinogens could easily account for the frequent recurrences and multifocality of transitional cell carcinoma in man.

Infection with Schistosoma hematobium is closely associated with squamous cell carcinoma of the bladder in Africa and the Middle East. This appears to be a distinctly different form of bladder neoplasm in that it generally arises in the vault of the bladder and makes its appearance at an earlier age. This is the most common type of cancer in Egyptian males (Elsebai, 1977).

HISTOLOGY

The vast majority of bladder cancers in the United States are transitional cell carcinomas—94%; only about 5% are squamous cell carcinoma and less than 1% are adenocarcinomas. The degree of differentiation exhibited by these neoplasms is quite variable. Superficial papillomas are histologically benign, but 50–65% will recur locally and 5–15% may later develop invasive carcinoma (Bagshaw et al., 1972). Squamous cell and adenocarcinoma may be very well differentiated, but clinically act like highly malignant, anaplastic tumors (Prout, 1972). Mixtures of transitional cell carcinoma and squamous cell carcinoma can occur, but the usual pattern is islands of squamous metaplasia in a predominantly transitional cell cancer (Pugh, 1973). Transitional cell carcinomas are a very diverse group of neoplasms. Their differentiation ranges from low grade carcinoma in situ to highly anaplastic invasive tumors. Variations in grade may occur within a single tumor. The histologic grading system adopted by the American Joint Committee (1977) is based on the degree of differentiation a tumor exhibits. Well differentiated lesions are placed in Grades 1 and 2, while the more poorly developed and anaplastic tumors are in Grades 3 and 4. The Union Internationale Contre le Cancer (UICC) (1974) also uses four classes, but begins with a Grade 0 which is limited only to superficial benign papillomas. It is obviously important for the clinician to be aware of the system that is being used by his pathology consultant, as the clinical behavior of a papilloma is entirely different from a grade 1 papillary carcinoma. Table 18.2 gives a comparison of the two grading systems. DeMeester et al. (1975) pointed out the basically benign nature of inverted papillomas which may be mistaken for low grade transitional cell carcinomas.

Carcinoma in situ can occur as a papillary or macular lesion; in the latter case it cannot be identified by visual inspection. It is practically always a transitional cell cancer, frequently characterized by a marked degree of anaplasia and multifocal occurrence (Farrow et al., 1977). It can precede, accompany or follow true invasive carcinoma.

Several investigators have called attention to multifocal in situ disease frequently associated with high grade invasive transitional cell carcinoma;

TABLE 16.2

AJC and UICC Grading Systems

AJC System	
Grade	Description
1	Well differentiated transitional cell carcinoma
2	Moderately well differentiated transitional cell carcinoma
3	Poorly differentiated transitional cell carcinoma
4	Very poorly differentiated transitional cell carcinoma

UICC System	
0	No evidence of anaplasia (i.e., papilloma)
1	Low grade malignancy
2	Medium grade malignancy
3	High grade malignancy

in these studies squamous cell disease was never associated with in situ cancer (Skinner et al., 1974; Pugh, 1973). Seemayer et al. (1975) have pointed out that commonly there will be silent intraductal prostatic invasion associated with in situ carcinoma. The distal ureters may also show evidence of in situ change. Soto and associates (1977) suggest there may actually be two forms of bladder cancer: One type which develops in a local restricted area, and theoretically has a much lower predisposition for metastases, and a second, more diffuse and more malignant tumor which develops in multiple sites throughout a generally abnormal urothelium and is usually associated with extensive carcinoma in situ. Cooper et al. (1973) have made the point that histologic grade is adequately related to prognosis for very well differentiated or very poorly differentiated lesions, but is unreliable for tumors of intermediate grade. This supports Jewett's (1973) statement that prognosis after therapy is better related to stage than histologic grade. Undoubtedly, these problems have contributed to the failure to agree on a grading system.

New approaches to bladder cancer include DNA labeling studies which have shown a correlation between increasing grade of malignancy and rapid tumor doubling times (Hainau and Dombernowski, 1974). Koss (1977) has evaluated ultrastructural changes in premalignant and malignant bladder cells, and Falor and Ward (1978) have correlated chromosomal abnormalities with recurrence in very early transitional cell carcinoma. The value of these new techniques to the clinician is as yet unproved, but they hold the potential of markedly increasing our ability to predict which early tumors will be more malignant and thus require more aggressive treatment.

CLASSIFICATION

The classification of bladder cancer is currently in an unsettled state. The Marshall (1952) modification of Jewett and Strong's (1946) original system is most commonly utilized in the United States. It is based on a positive correlation between the depth of tumor invasion into the bladder wall and the incidence of metastases and prognosis. Dissatisfaction with this system has been expressed because of poor correlation between clinical and surgical staging (Prout, 1972). The UICC (1974) and the American Joint Committee (1977) have both developed similar TNM classification of bladder cancer that are achieving a wider acceptance. The TNM system provides a more accurate description of the extent of disease and can also be correlated with the World Health Organization (WHO, 1973) histopathologic grading system.

Table 16.3 gives a comparative description of the two systems. Stage 0 (TIS) includes carcinoma in situ, and in Marshall's system, also superficial papillomas. The main point is that the neoplastic cells are limited to the mucosa and are not invasive. Stage A (T_1) implies that tumor has invaded the submucosa and is limited to that level. Stage B_1 (T_2) is defined as superficial muscle invasion less than one-half the thickness of the bladder wall musculature, while B_2 (T_{3A}) lesions exhibit deeper muscle invasion. Stage C (T_{3B}) has tumor extending into the perivesical fat; D_1 lesions imply tumor involving pelvic lymph nodes (N_{1-3}) or invasion of adjacent pelvic organs by local extension (T_4). D_2 disease has metastatic tumor in nodes outside the pelvis (N_4) or in distant viscera (M_1). Richie and associates (1975) have recently questioned the significance of differentiating B_1 from B_2 lesions, and have demonstrated an equally poor 5-year survival rate of 40% for both B_1 and B_2 patients. This may only reflect the difficulty in interpreting depth of invasion from a small biopsy specimen, but it could also mean that any muscle invasion implies a poor prognosis. Prout (1977a) also supports this concept and states that patients with even superficial muscle involvement have a decreased survival. Skinner (1977) criticizes both staging systems described above.

TABLE 16.3
Current Classifications of Bladder Cancer[a]

Stage		Description
Marshall	UICC	
0	TIS	Carcinoma in situ
A	T_1	Tumor invasion into submucosa
B_1	T_2	Tumor invasion into superficial muscle
B_2	T_{3A}	Tumor invasion into deep muscle
C	T_{3B}	Tumor invasion into perivesical fat
D	T_4	Tumor invasion into adjacent organs
D_1	N_{1-3}	Tumor involving pelvic lymph nodes
D_2	N_4	Tumor involving nodes outside of the pelvis or distant visceral
	M_1	organs

[a] Modified from Skinner (1977).

He points out that they offer little assistance in the clinical management of patients, and histologic differentiation of tumor is not taken into account. While none of the classification systems are entirely satisfactory, hopefully one will eventually be adopted to facilitate comparison and exchange of information.

NATURAL HISTORY

Bladder cancer can present clinically as variable a picture as it does histologically. Gross hematuria is the presenting symptom in three-fourths of invasive carcinoma (Prout, 1974). This bleeding may be light or so heavy that the patient passes clots. Bleeding may be intermittent, thus it is important that the first episode of hematuria be thoroughly investigated. A third of these patients may have symptoms of chronic cystitis—frequency, dysuria, urgency, nocturia—either alone or in conjunction with intermittent hematuria. Cystitis symptoms may be of many months duration and are usually indicative of carcinoma in situ rather than invasive tumors (Utz and Zineke, 1974). Other associated symptoms include weight loss, fever, suprapubic and flank pain. Whitmore (1977) pointed out that hydronephrosis may be present in up to one-third of patients at diagnosis. These symptoms are usually related to extensive disease and imply a relatively poor prognosis. Interestingly, complete or partial outlet obstruction is extremely rare. Patients may also rarely present with metastatic symptoms of bone pain, pulmonary or liver involvement. Kerr (1976) as well as other authors have shown that papillary, well differentiated lesions tend to cause symptoms early, while solid, invasive ones do not. Indeed, carcinoma in situ probably remains asymptomatic for many months, with patients coming to a urologist only on the basis of asymptomatic microscopic hematuria (Farrow et al., 1977).

As mentioned earlier, the number of patients with benign papillomas who develop true transitional cell carcinoma is relatively small (5–15%); presently, there is no way to predict which patients are at risk for this change. Any associated mucosal atypia or abnormal urine cytology may assist in this regard. Carcinoma in situ carries a very high risk of developing invasive cancer (Melamed et al., 1964; Althausen et al., 1976). The occurrence of in situ disease in conjunction with overt carcinoma implies a diffusely abnormal urothelium and high risk of recurrence regardless of stage (Skinner et al., 1974; Farrow et al., 1977). Hendry et al. (1974) and Gowing (1960) noted a 20% incidence of urethral in situ disease in patients dying of bladder cancer. Ten percent of patients with bladder cancer subsequently develop tumors in the upper tracts (Linker and Whitmore, 1975). Transitional cell carcinoma originating in the renal pelvis or ureters generally has a poorer prognosis than equivalent tumors in the bladder (Pfister, 1976). The natural history of overt transitional cell carcinoma is most significantly affected by the stage of the tumor at initial presentation. Table 16.4 lists overall survival according to stage. Other factors influencing survival are grade, size, location and number of the tumors (Barnes et al., 1977a) and, obviously, treatment.

Stage 0 or A tumors with grade 1 histology have a 5-year survival equal to the general population, while grade 2 histology in the same stage produced a significantly lower rate (Barnes, 1977a). In general, the stage and grade of tumors are well correlated and increasing grade/stage are related to shorter survival (Caldwell, 1970). An early report from the National Bladder Cancer Collaborative Group A (1977a) describes a 33% one-year recurrence rate for superficial tumors completely removed by transurethral resection (TUR). Tumor size, grade and stage did not affect recurrence, but the number of initial tumors did. Survival in recurrent tumors is also affected by grade and stage, and if tumor(s) recur within 3 years in a higher grade or stage than the initial neoplasm, more aggressive treatment is indicated (Barnes et al., 1977b).

For patients in more advanced Stages B_1, B_2, C, survival is relatively poor. Prior studies have used mostly clinical staging procedures, and it is clear that many patients were understaged. The incidence of pelvic nodal metastases may be as high as 60% in clinically staged B_2 and C patients (Bagshaw et al., 1972). The majority of patients in these stages (B_1, B_2, C) die of distant metastases from their tumor, implicating any degree of muscle invasion as already having disseminated tumor (Whitmore, 1977). The internal chain of the external iliac nodes is the first site of lymphatic drainage for the bladder and also the first site of pelvic metastasis. Next most common sites of distant tumor spread are periaortic nodes, liver, lungs and bone. The incidence of metastases increases with increasing depth of invasion of the bladder wall (Prout, 1974).

DIAGNOSIS

In any patient presenting with gross or microscopic hematuria or with symptoms of cystitis not responsive to initial conservative treatment, a

TABLE 16.4
Survival in Transitional Cell Carcinoma Related to Stage of Tumor at Diagnosis

Stage	5-Year Survival (%)
0	80
A	70
B_1	50
B_2 C	20–30
D_1	15
D_2	0

bladder tumor must be ruled out. Besides history and physical, the work-up should include urine cultures for acid fast bacteria as well as common pathogens, a routine blood count, renal and hepatic function tests, and a chest x-ray. Urologic investigations should include an intravenous pye-logram, urine cytology, cystography, and cystoscopy with biopsy (Pfister, 1976). If evidence of a tumor is found on any study prior to cystoscopy, further staging procedures should perhaps be undertaken to determine the extent of the disease prior to initial cystoscopy. This will be discussed further under staging. Urine cytology is positive only in high grade or invasive tumors. There is a very high false negative rate when the tumor is superficial or low grade (Flanagan and Miller, 1978). The incidence of false positive examinations is acceptably low, but cytologic alterations mimicking malignancy can be produced by chronic cystitis, benign pros-tatic hypertrophy, renal calculi and chemotherapy effects (Frable et al., 1977). Obviously, the symptoms of bladder tumors are not specific, and can be caused by a large number of different pathologic entities. The differential diagnosis includes all forms of cystitis, including tuberculous cystitis which may be extremely difficult to diagnose. Disease at any point in the urinary tract may produce hematuria; it is especially impor-tant to rule out medical diseases of the kidneys and, in males, prostatic lesions. Likewise tumors of other pelvic organs including the ovaries, uterus, and rectum must be looked for. Occasionally, nonmalignant disease of these organs, such as endometriosis, Crohn's disease or diver-ticulitis may masquerade by producing bladder symptoms. A small per-centage of bladder tumors may be partially calcified when first discovered (Miller and Pfister, 1974). Attempts to identify premalignant changes in bladder urothelium have recently begun (Friedell, 1977). Most of these studies are still investigational, however O'Flynn and Mullaney (1974) reported a 25% incidence of squamous cell carcinoma developing in patients with long standing vesical leukoplakia. Because neither close cystoscopic follow-up, nor urinary diversion predicted or prevented de-velopment of the cancer, they recommend total cystectomy as treatment of choice for this disorder.

STAGING

The staging of bladder cancer is the most important step for planning management of the individual patient. Frequently, the investigations utilized in diagnosis, bimanual palpation and cystoscopic biopsy, may already have established the stage in superficial tumors Stage 0, A. Frequently carcinoma in situ will produce symptoms of cystitis or micro-hematuria and positive cytology; in this case multiple random biopsies of the bladder mucosa must be done in order not to miss the diagnosis. Our recommendations for staging of bladder tumors are listed in Table 16.5.

TABLE 16.5
Diagnostic and Staging Workup for Bladder Tumors

Urine cultures
Urine cytology
Serum and urinary carcinoembryonic antigen
Complete blood count
Chest x-ray
Liver and renal function tests
Intravenous pyelogram
Cystogram
Pelvic sonogram
Radioisotopic scans—liver, bone and brain
Bimanual palpation (under anesthesia)
Cystoscopy and biopsy
Lymphangiography[a]
Pelvic angiography[a]
Computerized axial tomography of pelvis[a]

[a] See text.

Obviously these investigations need to be selectively applied. Patients with only carcinoma in situ would not require such extensive metastatic evaluations. Most other patients will require those procedures down to and including cystoscopy and biopsy. For patients with papillomas and superficial carcinomas this is probably adequate for initial staging; if the biopsy specimen shows a higher stage lesion, however, further evaluation for extent of disease is indicated. Changes in carcinoembryonic antigen (CEA) levels, while not specific for diagnosis or staging, may be of value in following individual patient response to treatment (Wahren et al., 1975). While Jewett (1973) still believes a 90% accuracy can be achieved between clinical and pathological staging, others do not (Prout, 1972; Murphy, 1978). Whitmore (1977) has pointed out that a significant number of patients with clinical Stage B and C disease are understaged on the basis of findings at the time of surgery. Because of these difficulties many institutions have been evaluating more extensive diagnostic studies prior to deciding on definitive treatment. Lymphangiography (LAG) alone appears to have a low accuracy (48%) in predicting which patients have pelvic nodal metastases (Farah and Cerny, 1978). However, Winterberger et al. (1978) have demonstrated a much greater accuracy with pelvic angiography in combination with LAG. They correctly diagnosed 80% of Stage C and 95% of Stage D lesions preoperatively using a combination of angiography and lymphography. Accuracy for Stage B lesions was only 45%, but still better than clinical assessment alone. Computerized tomography is now available in many centers and may prove very valuable in preoperative staging. Its efficacy needs to be established in clinical trials, but it has the potential of replacing sonography, lymphangiography and angiography. Pelvic lymphadenectomy is usually performed as an integral part of total cystectomy, but can be done as a staging procedure in lesser operations. Because of the high incidence of occult Stage D_1 disease, we feel surgical staging, in conjunction with treatment, is indicated in all patients who demonstrate tumor invasion of bladder musculature. The presence of obvious metastatic disease, Stage D_2, naturally contradicts the previous statement.

MANAGEMENT

The management of bladder cancer is most influenced by stage at initial presentation. Most urologists feel that transurethral resection (TUR) and frequent cystoscopic follow-up is adequate for benign papillomas. Solitary superficial carcinomas, Stage 0, A, are probably best treated by TUR and fulguration. The very high rate of recurrence, however, demands close follow-up. Usually patients are evaluated at 3-month intervals for the first 2 years and then every 6 months over the subsequent three years (Prout, 1972). Follow-up includes cystoscopy with biopsy of any suspicious areas of mucosa, and cytology of bladder washings. High grade, multiple lesions or associated areas of carcinoma in situ increase the likelihood of early recurrence. Skinner et al. (1974) suggest that patients exhibiting multiple areas of carcinoma in situ at diagnosis are best treated by total cystectomy, especially if the lesions are in a high pathologic grade. Recurrent tumor in a higher grade or stage within the first three years should probably also be managed by total cystectomy (Barnes et al., 1977b). Van der Werf-Messing (1973) reported equivalent survival of patients with large superficial transitional cell carcinomas with radiation therapy alone. External radiation therapy can be recommended as a therapeutic alternative in patients with large or multiple superficial tumors or who are otherwise not amenable to TUR.

The use of intravesical thiotepa has been recommended as both treatment and for the prevention of recurrence of small, multiple superficial bladder tumors (Veenema, 1968). Approximately one-third of patients have a complete response to thio-TEPA, with disappearance of all tumors, one-third have a partial response and one-third have no benefit. The prophylactic value of this agent to prevent recurrence is currently being evaluated in a prospective trial by the National Bladder Cancer Collaborative Group A (1977b). An earlier report showed the addition of urokinase to thiotepa instillations was more efficacious in preventing recurrence (Hisazumi et al., 1975). Intravesical bleomycin produced a somewhat higher response rate, but also had a high incidence of cystitis complications (Bracken et al., 1977). Izbicki et al. (1976) reported a complete remission in two-thirds of patients treated with intravesical Adriamycin. The large question of prophylaxis, however, still remains unanswered; if intravesical chemotherapy can be shown to prevent the development of more invasive disease it will indeed be a therapeutic breakthrough. The use of intravesical formalin has been shown to be very effective in controlling massive hematuria from bladder tumors and other causes (Servadio and Nissenkorn, 1976). This therapy should be used only in the patient whose hematuria is massive and cannot be controlled by other more conventional means.

The use of segmental bladder resection has a very limited applicability. Generally, it is recommended only for the treatment of solitary, primary lesions which are located so as to allow adequate tumor-free margins and will not require reimplantation of a ureter (Prout, 1974, 1977b). Utz et al. (1973) and Brannon et al. (1978) both report respectable 5-year survival rates of 40–60% and 30–35% for Stage B_2 and C lesions, respectively. Peress et al. (1977) recently described a 54% recurrence rate in Stage A high grade tumors treated by partial cystectomy. It appears if proper criteria are met partial cystectomy is a useful treatment for certain solitary, low grade bladder tumors. The treatment of bladder tumors which have invaded the muscularis (Stage B_1, B_2) or the perivesical fat (Stage C) is presently somewhat controversial. In the past, B_1 cancers were considered to have a much lower incidence of dissemination than B_2 lesions and could be adequately treated by TUR. More recently evidence has accumulated that any degree of muscle invasion implies a high risk of dissemination (Skinner, 1977; Whitmore, 1977) and should be treated the same as Stage C tumors (Galleher et al., 1977). Treatment of locally invasive transitional cell carcinoma has varied; radiation therapy alone (Birkhead et al., 1976), surgery alone (Cordonnier, 1974; Pearse et al., 1978) and various combinations of the two have been utilized. Radiotherapy and surgery, when used alone, provide essentially equivalent survival rates in B_2 and C lesions (Bagshaw et al., 1972; Caldwell, 1977). Many investigators have now reported increased survival in patients treated with a combination of pre-operative radiation followed by cystectomy (van der Werf-Messing, 1975; Miller, 1977; Whitmore et al., 1977; Galleher et al., 1977; Prout, 1977b). Specifically, improved survival was noted in those patients who had a reduction in the stage of their tumor by radiotherapy; low dose radiation preoperatively is probably as effective as high dose, with fewer complications (Whitmore et al., 1977); postoperative radiation led to a high rate of late recurrence and is not indicated as a surgical adjuvant treatment (L. S. Miller, 1977). It can reasonably be used when gross or microscopic disease remains following a primary operative procedure (Bagshaw et al., 1972). All of the combined treatment studies have shown a disappointingly high incidence of failure due to metastatic disease. This only serves to emphasize that many patients have distant micrometastases when initially evaluated, and are not curable by localized treatment. The need for effective systemic adjuvant therapy in these patients is all too clear.

Patients who have disease spread to the pelvic organs or nodes at diagnosis (D_1) have a poor prognosis. The best 5-year survival for this group of patients is less than 20%. Whitmore et al. (1977) have shown a combination of radiation and surgery to be somewhat better than cystectomy alone, and these patients should probably be given this slight benefit. Patients with distant metastatic disease (D_2) have no hope for cure and treatment should be palliative for control of symptoms. All Stage D patients would obviously benefit from effective chemotherapy. The present role of chemotherapy in bladder cancer is unclear. Table 16.6 lists the average response rates of various drugs used as single agents in treating transitional cell carcinoma of the bladder. Cyclophosphamide (Merrin et al., 1975) and cis-diamminedichloroplatinum (Merrin, 1978) are the two agents with the highest activities. Reports cite a 60% response rate using a combination of these two agents (Yagoda and Grabstald, 1977). Other combination studies have not been as efficacious. Cross et al. (1976) reported only a 35% response rate for Adriamycin and 5-fluorouracil together; this was not significantly different from Adriamycin alone. Yagoda et al. (1977) also found the combination of Adriamycin and Cytoxan to be no better than either agent alone. A combination of Adriamycin and VM-26 likewise showed no added activity (Rodriguez et al., 1977). Al-Sarraf et al. (1977) reported 2 of 4 patients responding to a combination of 5-fluorouracil and vinblastine. Preliminary reports of multidrug combinations are somewhat more encouraging. Sternberg et al. (1977) noted 9 of 12 patients responding to a three-drug regimen of cis-diamminedichloroplatinum (DDP), cyclophosphamide and Adriamycin. Troner and Hemstreet (1978) noted 4 of 9 patients responding to the same regimen. Williams et al. (1978) reported 62.5% responses with cis-diamminedichloroplatinum, Adriamycin and 5-fluorouracil. Reviews of the status of bladder cancer chemotherapy have recently been presented (deKerrion, 1977; Murphy, 1977; Yagoda, 1977). Although complete re-

TABLE 16.6
Drugs with Activity Against Bladder Carcinoma

Agent	Objective Response (%)
Adriamycin	25
Bleomycin	30
Cyclophosphamide	40
cis-Diamminedichloroplatinum	50
5-Fluorouracil	30
Methotrexate	25
Mitomycin C	40
VM-26	25

sponses have been few, and duration of any responses have been relatively short, almost all trials have been in patients with very far advanced disease. Adjuvant chemotherapy trials are now in progress and hopefully will show even better effects in patients with only microscopic tumor burdens. Although there is still much need for improvement, currently we would recommend chemotherapy for patients with metastatic bladder carcinoma with a combination of the two most active agents, cyclophosphamide and cis-platinum, which can be expected to provide a partial remission in approximately 50% of patients. Obviously, these drugs should be given only by a clinician who is familiar with their use and is able to provide appropriate support for any toxicities encountered.

IMMUNOTHERAPY

Currently almost nothing has been reported regarding immunotherapy of bladder cancer. Intravesical and intradermal BCG has been used in patients with multiple recurrent superficial cancers resistant to intravesical chemotherapy. Early follow-up showed no recurrence of tumors in seven patients followed from four to 11 months (Eidinger and Morales, 1976). Evidence of altered immunity in transitional cell carcinoma has been well demonstrated (Elhilali et al., 1978). Cell-mediated immunity as measured by skin reactivity to primary (DNCB) and recall antigens is frequently suppressed in bladder cancer patients. The percentage of suppressed patients increases with increasing stage of the tumor (Bean, 1977). Initial reactivity to DNCB is associated with better prognosis (Elhilali et al., 1978).

Also, Hakala et al. (1976) have shown that suppressed cell-mediated cytotoxicity can be enhanced in bladder cancer patients by either removing the primary tumor or administering BCG as a nonspecific immuno stimulant.

The clinical relevance of all these findings is eagerly awaited.

REFERENCES

Al-Sarraf, M., Amer, M. H., and Vaitkevicius, V. K. Chemotherapy and survival in patients with urinary bladder cancer. Proc. Am. Assoc. Cancer Res., 18: 116, 1977.

Althausen, A., Daly, J. J., and Prout, G. R., Jr. A retrospective study on the prognostic import of flat carcinoma in situ associated with papillary, low stage carcinoma of the bladder. J. Urol., 116: 575–580, 1976.

American Cancer Society. Cancer statistics. CA, 27: 26–41, 1977.

American Joint Committee for Cancer Staging and End Results Reporting. Manual for Staging of Cancer, pp. 113–118, American Joint Committee, Chicago, 1977.

Ansell, I. D., and Castro, J. E. Carcinoma of the bladder complicating cyclophosphamide therapy. Br. J. Urol., 47: 413–418, 1975.

Bagshaw, M., Caldwell, W. L., Grabstald, H., and Wizenberg, M. Rx of bladder cancer; complex and controversial. CA, 23: 81–91, 1972.

Barnes, R. W., Dick, A. L., Hadley, H. L., and Johnston, O. L. Survival following transurethral resection of bladder carcinoma. Cancer Res., 37: 2895–2897, 1977a.

Barnes, R., Hadley, H., Dick, A., Johnston, O., and Dexter, J. Changes in grade and stage of recurrent bladder tumors. J. Urol., *118:* 177–178, 1977b.

Bean, M. A. Some immunologic considerations relevant to the study of human bladder cancer. Cancer Res., *37:* 2879–2884, 1977.

Birkhead, B. M., Conley, J. G., and Scott, R. M. Intensive radiotherapy of locally advanced bladder cancer. Cancer, *37:* 2746–2748, 1976.

Bracken, R. B., Johnson, D. E., Rodriguez, L., Samuels, M. L., and Ayala, A. Treatment of multiple superficial tumors of the bladder with intravesical bleomycin. Urology, *9:* 161–163, 1977.

Brannon, W., Ochsner, M. G., Fuselier, H. A., and Landry, G. R. Partial cystectomy in the treatment of transitional cell carcinoma of the bladder. J. Urol., *119:* 213–215, 1978.

Caldwell, W. L. Cancer of the Urinary Bladder, pp. 23–42. Warren H. Green, St. Louis, 1970.

Caldwell, W. L. The role of irradiation in the management of clinical stage B_1 (grades II and III) and stages B_2 and C bladder cancer. Cancer Res., *37:* 2759–2763, 1977.

Cole, P., Monson, R. R., Haning, H., and Friedell, G. H. Smoking and cancer of the lower urinary tract. N. Engl. J. Med., *284:* 129–134, 1971.

Cooper, E. H., Anderson, C. K., Steele, L., and O'Boyle, P. Assessment of bladder cancer. Cancer, *32:* 1263–1266, 1973.

Cordonnier, J. J. Simple cystectomy in management of bladder carcinoma. Arch. Surg., *108:* 190–191, 1974.

Cross, R. J., Glashan, R. W., Humphrey, C. S., Robinson, M. R., Smith, P. H., and Williams, R. E. Treatment of advanced bladder cancer with adriamycin and 5-fluorouracil. Br. J. Urol., *48:* 609–615, 1976.

deKernion, J. B. The chemotherapy of advanced bladder carcinoma. Cancer Res., *37:* 2771–2774, 1977.

DeMeester, L. G., Farrow, G. M., and Utz, D. C. Inverted papillomas of the urinary bladder. Cancer, *36:* 505–513, 1975.

Elhilali, M. M., Brosman, S. A., Vescera, C., Paul, J. G., and Fahey, J. L. The effects of treatment on delayed cutaneous hypersensitivity responses (DNCB, castor oil, and recall antigen) in patients with genitourinary cancer. Cancer, *41:* 1765–1770, 1978.

Eidinger, D., and Morales, A. Discussion paper: Treatment of superficial bladder cancer in man. Ann. N.Y. Acad. Sci., *277:* 239–240, 1976.

Elsebai, I. Parasites in the etiology of cancer—bilharziasis and bladder cancer. CA, *27:* 100–106, 1977.

Falor, W. H., and Ward, R. M. Prognosis in early carcinoma of the bladder based on chromosomal analysis. J. Urol., *119:* 44–48, 1978.

Farah, R. N., and Cerny, J. C. Lymphangiography in staging patients with carcinoma of the bladder. J. Urol., *119:* 40–41, 1978.

Farrow, G. M., Utz, D. C., Rife, C. C., and Green, L. F. Clinical observations on sixty-nine cases of in situ carcinoma of the urinary bladder. Cancer Res., *37:* 2794–2798, 1977.

Flanagan, M. J., and Miller, A., III. Evaluation of bladder washing cytology for bladder cancer surveillance. J. Urol., *119:* 42–43, 1978.

Frable, W. J., Paxon, L., Barksdale, J. A., and Koontz, W. W. Current practice of urinary bladder cytology. Cancer Res., *37:* 2800–2805, 1977.

Friedell, G. H. Introduction: Recognition of "early" bladder cancer and premalignant epithelial changes. Cancer Res., *37:* 2792–2793, 1977.

Galleher, E. P., Young, J. D., Campbell, E. W., Jr., Wizenberg, M. J., Jacobs, J. A., and Millstein, D. I. Pre-cystectomy radiation for carcinoma of the bladder; 17-year experience. J. Urol., *118:* 179–183, 1977.

Gowing, N. F. C. Urethral carcinoma associated with cancer of the bladder. Br. J. Urol., *32:* 428–439, 1960.

Hainau, B., and Dombernowski, P. Histology and proliferation in human bladder tumors; autoradiography study. Cancer, *33:* 115–126, 1974.

Hakala, T. R., Lange, P. H., Elliott, A. Y., and Fraley, E. E. Changes in cell-mediated cytotoxicity during the clinical course of patients with bladder carcinoma. J. Urol., *115:* 268–273, 1976.

Hendry, W. F., Gowing, N. F. C., and Wallace, D. M. Surgical treatment of urethral tumors associated with bladder cancer. Proc. R. Soc. Med., *67:* 304–307, 1974.

Hisazumi, H., Uchibayashi, T., Naito, K., Misaki, T., and Miyazaki, K. The prophylactic use of thio-TEPA and urokinase in transitional cell carcinoma of the bladder; a preliminary report. J. Urol., *114:* 394–398, 1975.

Izbicki, R. M., Pontes, E., and Vaitkevicius, V. K. Adriamycin bladder instillation. Proc. Am. Soc. Clin. Oncol., *17:* 311, 1976.

Jackson, C. D., and Baetcke, K. P. Causative agents in the induction of bladder cancer. Ann. Clin. Lab. Sci., *6:* 223–232, 1976.

Jewett, H. J. Cancer of the bladder—diagnosis and staging. Cancer, *32:* 1072–1074, 1973.

Jewett, H. J., and Strong, G. H. Infiltrating carcinoma of the bladder; relation of depth of penetration of the bladder wall to incidence of local extension and metastases. J. Urol., *55:* 336–372, 1946.

Kerr, W. K. Clinical features of bladder cancer. Third International Symposium on Detection and Prevention of Cancer, pp. 479–480, Marcel Dekker, New York, 1976.

Koss, L. G. Some ultrastructural aspects of experimental and human carcinoma of the bladder. Cancer Res., *37:* 2824–2835, 1977.

Linker, D. G., and Whitmore, W. F., Jr. Ureteral carcinoma in situ. J. Urol., *113:* 777–780, 1975.

Marshall, V. F. The relation of the preoperative estimate to the pathologic demonstration of the extent of vesical neoplasms. J. Urol., *68:* 714–723, 1952.

Melamed, M. R., Vousta, N. G., and Grabstald, H. Natural history and clinical behavior of in situ carcinoma of the human urinary bladder. Cancer, *17:* 1533–1545, 1964.

Merrin, C. Treatment of advanced bladder cancer with cis-diamminedichloroplatinum II (NSC-119875); a pilot study. J. Urol., *119:* 493–495, 1978.

Merrin, C., Cartagena, R., Wajsman, Z., Baumgartner, G., and Murphy, G. P. Chemotherapy of bladder carcinoma with cyclophosphamide and Adriamycin. J. Urol., *114:* 884–887, 1975.

Miller, A. B. The etiology of bladder cancer from the epidemiological viewpoint. Cancer Res., *37:* 2939–2942, 1977.

Miller, L. S. Bladder cancer; superiority of preoperative irradiation and cystectomy in clinical stage B_2 and C. Cancer, *39:* 973–980, 1977.

Miller, S. W., and Pfister, R. C. Calcification in uroepithelial tumors of the bladder; report of five (5) cases and survey of the literature. A.J.R., *121:* 827–831, 1974.

Murphy, G. P. Chemotherapy of bladder cancer; current progress. N.Y. State J. Med., *77:* 1889–1895, 1977.

Murphy, G. P. Developments in preoperative staging of bladder tumors. Urology, *11:* 109–115, 1978.

National Bladder Cancer Collaborative Group A. Surveillance, initial assessment and subsequent progress of patients with superficial bladder cancer in a prospective longitudinal study. Cancer Res. 37: 2907–2910, 1977a.

National Bladder Cancer Collaborative Group A. The role of intravesical thiotepa in the management of superficial bladder cancer. Cancer Res., *37:* 2916–2917, 1977b.

Newell, G. R., Krementz, E. T., and Roberts, J. D. Excess occurrence of cancer of the oral cavity, lung and bladder following cancer of the cervix. Cancer, *36:* 2155–2158, 1975.

O'Flynn, J. D., and Mullaney, J. Vesical leukoplakia progressing to carcinoma. Br. J. Urol., *46:* 31–37, 1974.

Oyasu, R., and Hopp, M. L. The etiology of cancer of the bladder. Surg. Gynecol. Obstet., *138:* 97–108, 1974.

Pearse, H. D., Reed, R. R., and Hodges, C. V. Radical cystectomy for bladder cancer. J. Urol., *119:* 216–218, 1978.

Peress, J. A., Waterhouse, K., and Cole, A. T. Complications of partial cystectomy in patients with high grade bladder carcinoma. J. Urol., *118:* 761–762, 1977.

Pfister, R. R. Endoscopy and the detection of genitourinary carcinoma. Cancer, *37:* 471–474, 1976.

Prout, G. R., Jr. Bladder carcinoma. N. Engl. J. Med., *287:* 86–90, 1972.

Prout, G. R., Jr. The bladder. In Cancer Medicine, edited by J. F. Holland and E. Frei III, pp. 1670–1680. Lea & Febiger, Philadelphia, 1974.

Prout, G. R., Jr. Bladder carcinoma and a TNM system of classification. J. Urol., *117:* 583–590, 1977a.

Prout, G. R., Jr. The role of surgery in the potentially curative treatment of bladder carcinoma. Cancer Res., *37:* 2764–2770, 1977b.

Pugh, R. C. B. The pathology of cancer of the bladder. Cancer, *32:* 1267–1274, 1973.

Radomski, J. L., and Hearn, W. L. Nitrates, nitrites and the induction of bladder cancer from nitrosoamines. Proc. Am. Assoc. Cancer Res., *17:* 5, 1976.

Richie, J. P., Skinner, D. G., and Kaufman, J. J. Radical cystectomy for carcinoma of the bladder; 16 years experience. J. Urol., *113:* 186–189, 1975.

Rodriguez, L. H., Johnson, D. E., Holoye, P. Y., and Samuels, M. L. Combination VM-26 and Adriamycin for metastatic transitional cell carcinoma. Cancer Treat. Rep., *61:* 87–88, 1977.

Scott, W. W., and Boyd, H. L. A study of the carcinogenic effect of beta-naphthylamine on the normal and substituted isolated sigmoid loop bladder of dogs. J. Urol., *70:* 914–925, 1953.

Seemayer, T. A., Knaack, J., Thelmo, W. L., Wang, N., and Ahmed, M. N. Further observations on carcinoma in situ of the urinary bladder; silent but extensive intraprostatic involvement. Cancer, *36:* 514–520, 1975.

Seidman, H., Silverberg, E., and Holleb, A. I. A statistical comparison of black and white populations. CA, *26:* 2–13, 1976.

Servadio, C., and Nissenkorn, I. Massive hematuria successfully treated by bladder irrigation with formalin solution. Cancer, *37:* 900–902, 1976.

Skinner, D. G. Current stage of classification and staging of bladder cancer. Cancer Res., *37:* 2838–2842, 1977.

Skinner, D. G., Richie, J. P., Cooper, P. H., Waisman, J., and Kaufman, J. J. The clinical significance of carcinoma in situ of the bladder and its association with overt carcinoma. J. Urol., *112:* 68–71, 1974.

Sternberg, J. J., Bracken, R. B., Handel, P. B., and Johnson, D. E. Combination chemotherapy for advanced urinary tract carcinoma. J.A.M.A., *238:* 2282–2287, 1977.

Soto, E. A., Friedell, G. H., and Tiltman, A. J. Bladder cancer as seen in giant histologic sections. Cancer, *30:* 447–455, 1977.

Troner, M., and Hemstreet, G. Cyclophosphamide, Adriamycin and cis-platinum chemotherapy of metastatic transitional cell carcinoma of the bladder. Proc. Am. Assoc. Cancer Res., *19:* 161, 1978.

Union Internationale Contre le Cancer (UICC). TNM Classification of Malignant Tumors. Imprimerie G. de Buren SA, Geneva, 1974.

Utz, D. C., Schmitz, S. E., Fugelso, P. D., and Farrow, G. M. A clinicopathologic evaluation of partial cystectomy for carcinoma of the urinary bladder. Cancer, *32:* 1075–1077, 1973.

Utz, D. C., and Zineke, H. Masquerade of bladder cancer in situ as interstitial cystitis. J. Urol., *111:* 160–161, 1974.

Van der Werf-Messing, B. H. P. Carcinoma of the bladder treated by preoperative radiation followed by cystectomy. Cancer, *32:* 1084–1088, 1973.

Van der Werf-Messing, B. H. P. Carcinoma of the bladder $T_3N_xM_o$ treated by preoperative radiation followed by cystectomy. Cancer, *36:* 718–722, 1975.

Veenema, R. J. The role of thiotepa instillation in bladder cancer. Cancer, *206:* 2725–2727, 1968.

Wahren, B., Edsmyr, F., and Zimmerman, R. Measurement of urinary CEA-like substance. Cancer, *36:* 1490–1495, 1975.

Wall, R. L., and Clauson, K. P. Carcinoma of the urinary bladder in patients receiving cyclophosphamide. N. Engl. J. Med., *293:* 271–273, 1975.

Weissman, R. M., Coffey, D. S., and Jewett, H. J. Current concepts in the study of bladder cancer. Urol. Surv., *28:* 1–5, 1978.

Wendel, R. G., Hoegg, U. R., and Zavon, M. R. Benzidine; bladder carcinogen. J. Urol., *111:* 607–610, 1974.

Williams, S. D., Rohn, R. J., Donohue, J. P., and Einhorn, L. H. Chemotherapy of bladder cancer with cis-diamminedichloroplatinum (DDP), Adriamycin (ADR) and 5-fluorouracil. Proc. Am. Soc. Clin. Oncol., *19:* 316, 1978.

Whitmore, W. F., Jr. Introduction; assessment and management of deeply invasive and metastatic lesions. Cancer Res., *37:* 2756–2758, 1977.

Whitmore, W. F., Jr., Batata, M. A., Hilaris, B. S., Reddy, G. N., Unal, A., Ghoneim, M. A., Grabstald, H., and Chu, F. A comparative study of two preoperative radiation regimens with cystectomy for bladder cancer. Cancer, *40:* 1077–1086, 1977.

Wigle, D. T. Bladder cancer; possible new high risk occupation. Lancet, *2:* 83–84, 1977.

Winterberger, A. R., Wajsman, Z., Merrin, C., and Murphy, G. P. Eight years of experience with preoperative angiographic and lymphographic staging of bladder cancer. J. Urol., *119:* 208–212, 1978.

World Health Organization. International Histological Classification of Tumors. Histologic Typing of Urinary Bladder Tumors, edited by F. K. Mostofi. WHO, Geneva, 1973.

Yagoda, A. Future implications of phase 2 chemotherapy trials in ninety-five patients with measurable advanced bladder cancer. Cancer Res., *37:* 2775–2780, 1977.

Yagoda, A., and Grabstald, H. Diamminedichloride platinum II (DDP) and cyclophosphamide (CTX) in the treatment of advanced bladder cancer. Proc. Am. Soc. Clin. Oncol., *18:* 336, 1977.

Yagoda, A., Watson, R. C., Grabstald, H., Barzell, W. E., and Whitmore, W. F., Jr. Adriamycin and cyclophosphamide in advanced bladder cancer. Cancer Treat. Rep., *61:* 97–99, 1977.

Yoshida, O., Brown, R. R., and Bryan, G. T. Relationship between tryphophan metabolism and heterotopic recurrence of human urinary bladder tumors. Cancer, *25:* 773–778, 1970.

Chapter 17

Prostate

CHARLES F. MILLER, M.D.

INTRODUCTION AND EPIDEMIOLOGY

Malignant tumors of the prostate gland account for 17% of all male cancers and will cause over 20,000 deaths in 1977. In addition, it is estimated that 57,000 new cases of prostatic cancer will be diagnosed during that year making it the most common neoplasm in males over the age of 50, and second-most common to lung cancer for males of all ages (Cancer Statistics, 1977).

The age adjusted incidence rates for cancer of the prostate is 46 cases per 100,000 population per year, but this figure is markedly influenced by age—no cases being recorded below the age of 40 in most series. There are, however, rare case reports of prostatic adenocarcinoma developing in adolescents and even children (Chiu and Weber, 1974); the disease in these patients appears to be clinically much more aggressive than in adults. The incidence of the disease rises approximately 1.5% per year between the ages of 50 and 85, such that Scott and Mutchnik (1969) reported that over one-half of all males over 70 who underwent autopsy had evidence of this cancer. It is necessary, however, to distinguish between latent or incidental carcinoma found at autopsy or surgical resection and clinical disease. The incidence figures mentioned above include both types of cases, and while there is a 30% prevalence of all forms of prostatic tumors in 80-year-old patients, the amount of clinical disease is much lower at 0.8% (Wynder et al., 1971).

More to the point, the projected mortality rate for 1977 of 20,000 deaths is only one-third the estimated incidence of 57,000 cases. The risk of both latent and symptomatic prostatic cancer increases with increasing age (Franks, 1973).

In addition to age, race appears to be an important variable in prostatic cancer. The death and incidence rates are almost twice as high for U.S. blacks compared to whites (Seidman et al., 1976; Ernster et al., 1977). On

360

the other hand, the incidence of the disease among African blacks appears to be substantially different from a comparable group of U.S. blacks (Jackson et al., 1977). The disease incidence peaks a decade sooner in Nigerian blacks, and is also in a clinically more advanced stage when compared to a matched U.S. population. Also, while the incidence of incidental disease is essentially the same in the two populations studied, that of invasive carcinoma is much higher in U.S. blacks. The very low incidence of prostate cancer in oriental races has been noted for some time. Table 17.1 shows the relative age-adjusted mortality rates from cancer of the prostate from a number of countries. The highest rates occur primarily in northern European countries; in striking contrast to Sweden and Norway, Japan, Taiwan and the Philippines have less than one-eighth of the mortality from this disease. The United States has a mortality only slightly less than Sweden (Cancer Facts and Figures, 1975).

As yet there is no adequate explanation for these racial and geographic differences. Evaluation of hormone levels between various populations have failed to show significant differences between countries. The best explanation offered is that some environmental factors may be at work to account for the marked geographic variation in prostatic carcinoma (Hutchinson, 1976).

ETIOLOGY

In common with other malignant tumors, the underlying cause of prostatic cancer is unknown. Likewise, what factor or factors cause the disease to remain quiescent in the majority of men, and to be an aggressive, metastasizing tumor in others is entirely speculative. Viruses

TABLE 17.1
Age-adjusted Prostate Cancer Mortality by Country[a]

Country	Relative Mortality
Sweden	18
Switzerland	17
Norway	16
France	15
Austria	14
United States	14
Israel	7
Greece	6
Hong Kong	4
Singapore	3
Japan	2
Philippines	1
Taiwan	1

[a] Modified from "Cancer Facts and Figures, 1975," American Cancer Society, 1975.

have been implicated on the basis of immunologic and ultrastructure studies (Dmochowski and Horoszewicz, 1976; Dmochowski et al., 1977; McCombs, 1977). As in a number of other animal and human malignancies, evidence at present points toward C-type RNA viruses as playing a possible role in the causation of human prostatic cancer (Mickey et al., 1977), and some evidence supports the theory of venereal transmission of an infectious agent (Schuman et al., 1977), but further work is needed for confirmation.

Other possible etiologic theories include an alteration in hormonal balance, occupational exposure in rubber and cadmium workers, fertilizer and auto exhaust fume exposure and dietary effects (Hutchinson, 1976; Rotkin, 1977). Additional factors correlated with prostatic cancer are increased sexual drive and fertility, a history of venereal disease, and being married or divorced (Schuman et al., 1977).

In preliminary investigations Rotkin (1977) has reported a correlation between prostatic cancer and delayed and repressed sexual development and expression, and early cessation of sexual activity. He cites this as evidence of an endogenous factor, perhaps hormonally mediated, which may promote biochemical changes very early in adolescence which could eventually lead to invasive prostatic carcinoma. This is all the more intriguing in view of the tumor's known hormone responsiveness and the fact that most prostate cancers develop during the period of decreasing androgen secretion by the body. Socioeconomic status, urban versus rural environment, and pre-existence of benign prostatic hypertrophy (BPH) have not been clearly shown to have a positive correlation with prostatic cancer (Ernster et al., 1977). In the case of BPH, there are conflicting reports as to whether or not it increases the risk of prostatic carcinoma. However, it is clear that prior surgical resection of the prostate does not protect against subsequent malignant development (DeWys, 1976). Much further work is needed to clarify the reasons underlying the wide demographic and epidemiological variations in prostatic carcinoma. It is not known what contributions are made by genetic and environmental factors and what, if any, interactions occur between them.

CLASSIFICATION

In the United States, the most widely used classification for staging prostatic carcinoma is based on the original system proposed by Whitmore (1963). As shown in Table 17.2 this system divides the disease into four stages, with important subclassifications as noted. *Stage A* is clinically inapparent disease, found incidentally during pathologic examination of the gland either at autopsy or after surgical resection. The important point is that there is no clinical evidence, either by history, physical examination or laboratory evaluations, of prostatic cancer. This has been divided into stage A_1 and A_2 lesions. A_1 lesions are histologically well differentiated and limited to only one focus or a small number of resected chips. Stage A_2 should be used when the lesion is poorly differentiated or diffusely involves the gland. A_2 lesions have a much poorer prognosis than Stage A_1 (Fergusson, 1965; Scott and Mutchnik 1969). This poorer prognosis for some Stage A cancers may also be due in part to the known multicentricity of these lesions (McNeal, 1968). *Stage B* is clinically obvious disease that is confined to the prostate gland. B_1 lesions are limited to less than one lobe of the gland, while Stage B_2 requires more than one lobe to be involved. The poorer clinical course for this subclass of patients has been previously documented (Hanash et al., 1972). *Stage C* is clinically obvious disease that manifests local extension beyond the prostatic capsule, including seminal vesical or bladder neck invasion. *Stage D* is metastatic disease: D_1 lesions imply metastasis limited to the pelvic lymph nodes, while D_2 includes disease in any nodes or parenchymal tissue outside the pelvis. A TNM classification has been available since 1968 and recently updated (UICC, 1974), but has not received wide acceptance. As seen in Table 17.3, overall survival rates for Stage B and C patients are relatively poor. This is especially true for

TABLE 17.2
Staging Classification for Prostatic Carcinoma[a]

Stage			Percent at Clinical Diagnosis
A		*Incidental carcinoma, clinically silent, found at autopsy or surgery*	—
	A_1	Well differentiated lesions, limited to only a few foci	
	A_2	Poorly differentiated lesions usually with diffuse histologic involvement	
B		*Clinical disease, limited to the prostate gland*	10
	B_1	A discrete nodule, involving less than one lobe of the gland	
	B_2	Large lesions involving more than one lobe of the gland	
C		*Clinical disease, with extra capsular extension*	40
D		*Metastatic disease*	50
	D_1	Metastasis confined to the regional (pelvic) nodes	
	D_2	Metastasis beyond pelvis, including periaortic nodes or any parenchymal spread	

[a] Modified from Murphy (1974).

TABLE 17.3
Prostatic Carcinoma: 5-Year Survival by Clinical Stage

Stage	5-Year Survival (%)
A	75
B	60
C	30–40
D	15

Stage B lesions when most of these patients have usually undergone some form of radical treatment with a curative intent. Because of definite inadequacies relating Whitmore's classification to prognosis Ray et al. (1976) have proposed a modified TNM system which they correlated with operative staging. The results of their study and others (Flocks, 1965; Dahl et al., 1974) confirm that clinical staging frequently underestimates the actual extent of disease in many Stage B and C patients. Twenty percent of Stage B and 60% of Stage C patients were found to have tumor involving their pelvic nodes (Ray et al., 1976). This no doubt accounts for the relatively poor survival of these patients in prior studies. It is also clear that lymphangiography alone is inadequate for accurate assessment of regional node metastasis because of the high incidence of false positive and false negative studies (Loening et al., 1977). These radiographic studies should be used in conjunction with lymphadenectomy for accurate staging of patients.

HISTOLOGICAL GRADING

Histologically, adenocarcinomas represent more than 99% of all primary malignancies of the prostate with less than 1% being sarcomas or carcinosarcomas (Schmidt and Welch, 1976). The morphology of prostatic carcinoma definitely appears to influence prognosis and the problems associated with grading have recently been reviewed by Mostofi (1976). While no general consensus regarding a standard grading system has been reached, hopefully one will be adopted in the near future. For the present, it can only be said that the less differentiation and greater degree of anaplasia exhibited by the tumor, the poorer the prognosis (Mostofi, 1975). Frequently there may be a marked variation in the grade of tumor cells found in a single cancerous gland. In this case most investigators feel that prognosis is best correlated with the least differentiated section of the tumor. Features that appear most highly correlated with a poor prognosis include nuclear anaplasia (Harada et al., 1977), indistinct tumor cell borders, and lack of lymphocytic infiltration (Epstein and Fatti, 1976). Recently Sinha and others (1977) have attempted to correlate tumor morphology with hormone responsiveness. Their data suggest that it may be possible to predict the degree of hormonal responsiveness of a tumor from the initial biopsy. This assumption awaits confirmation by other investigators. It would seem that a system which takes both clinical stage and histologic grade of the tumor into account would be the most accurate in predicting prognosis (Table 17.4). Obviously this would be the most useful to the practicing clinician.

NATURAL HISTORY

Clearly, there are two distinct clinical facets of prostatic carcinoma, and although histologically inseparable, their natural histories are vastly

TABLE 17.4
Factors Affecting Prognosis of Prostatic Cancer

1. Histologic differentiation
2. Stage
3. Age
4. Clinical symptoms
5. Race

different. Most latent or unsuspected Stage A cancers are never associated with metastatic disease or a decrease in life expectancy. These can be considered a benign lesion and, indeed, by definition are not clinically diagnosable. The small subgroup of tumors which are undifferentiated and diffusely involve the prostate gland (Stage A_2) are probably better considered as in the next higher stage (B_1). The vast majority, if not all, of stage B patients are asymptomatic and are diagnosed by digital rectal examination with the finding of a "stony hard" nodule usually involving less than one lobe of the gland. The natural history of these small, asymptomatic lesions (Stage B_1) is variable (Whitmore, 1973). Some can remain limited to the prostate for long periods of time, but many do eventually metastasize and go on to kill the patient if left untreated. This is in contrast to the larger B_2 lesion which is frequently poorly differentiated and associated with a much worse prognosis. Patients with Stage C lesions frequently present with symptoms of obstruction or prostatism—frequency, dysuria, hesitancy and sometimes hematuria. The usual finding on physical examination is a large indurated mass extending outside the prostatic capsule which can involve the seminal vesicles or bladder neck. Prout (1973a) feels that obstructive symptoms from carcinoma are usually of short duration. This is in contrast to patients who have benign prostatic hypertrophy who will give a long history of gradually worsening urinary obstruction. Stage D patients, besides having localized symptoms, may also present solely with symptoms of metastatic disease. The most common presentation is bone pain associated with osteoblastic lesions. The most common sites of involvement in descending order of frequency are pelvis, spine, long bones and skull. Occasionally, patients may present with symptoms secondary to an anemia caused by replacement of the marrow with tumor. Other presentations can occur—pulmonary metastasis, skin, nodal, liver involvement—but are unusual (Murphy, 1976). The rate of detection of early prostatic cancer is very poor. Stage B lesions make up no more than 10% of clinically detected cases in most series. This implies either that rectal examinations are not being done or the acumen of most examiners is not sufficient for early detection of small lesions (Gittes, 1976). While Whitmore (1973) feels that many Stage A lesions may not pass through a clinical Stage B or C before becoming metastatic, presently the only way to detect localized lesions earlier is by frequent and thorough rectal examinations. These should be strongly encouraged in all males over 40. Newer diagnostic techniques are being evaluated at present including ultrasonography (Watanabe et al., 1975) and computerized tomography, which may allow more patients to be detected earlier while their disease is still in a curable state. One additional factor contributing to the difficult diagnosis of early lesions is that prostatic cancer develops in the outer, peripheral section of the gland. This allows for early lymphatic spread to the obturator and iliac nodes.

The serum acid phosphatase (SAP) has been used for many years as an indicator of advanced prostatic carcinoma. While very useful, its accuracy and specificity are less than satisfactory (Prout, 1973a). Even using various methods of measuring different isoenzymes the test may still yield a false negative rate of as much as 30% in patients with D_2 disease (Gittes and Chu, 1976). The recent introduction of specific radioimmune assay (RIA) techniques to measure the prostatic fraction of acid phosphatase is a very promising development (Choe et al., 1977). Foti et al. (1977) reported a diagnostic accuracy ranging from 50% for Stage A disease to 96% in Stage D patients using an RAI procedure. The application of this technique in evaluating bone marrow acid phosphatase may prove to be an even more sensitive indicator of prostatic carcinoma (Pontes et al., 1975).

Bruce et al. (1977) showed a high correlation between bone marrow acid phosphatase elevation and blood borne metastasis. If these results are confirmed, these tests may help provide an accurate method for screening patients both for early primary disease and for the quicker detection of recurrent or metastatic illness. A word of caution is necessary about frequency of false positive acid phosphatase measurements. These are not uncommon and can be caused by prior prostatic massage, prostatic infarcts, Paget's disease, bone tumors, hemolytic anemia and other miscellaneous conditions (Yam, 1974).

Other biochemical alterations reported in patients with adenocarcinoma of the prostate include changes in the lactic dehydrogenase (LDH) isoenzyme pattern (Grayhack, et al., 1977; Wood et al., 1973), and a shift in testosterone metabolism from primarily reductive to mostly oxidative (Morfin et al., 1977); variable elevations can be seen in serum alkaline phosphatase, usually associated with bony or liver involvement; the carcinoembryonic antigen level is likewise too variable to be of general prognostic or diagnostic significance (Murphy, 1976).

DIAGNOSIS

Once a prostatic lesion has been identified, the primary aim is to obtain histologic confirmation of the nodule. In a comprehensive review, Hudson and Stout (1966), found that over half of all prostatic nodules proved to be malignant. The procedure for biopsy will vary between urologists and with the actual location of the lesion. Perineal punch biopsy is perhaps the easiest technique and yields better than an 80% accuracy (Gittes and Chu, 1976); other procedures include transrectal, open rectal, open perineal and transurethral approaches (Murphy, 1976). If the initial biopsy is negative, it is vitally important that the patient receive close follow-up and rebiopsy if there is any change in the clinical features of the lesion. The serial measurement of prostatic acid phosphatase isoenzyme may prove to be of value in following these patients.

Stage B lesions account for only about 10% of clinically diagnosed prostatic cancer. The overall 5-year survival of 60% is not impressive, and for large lesions (Stage B_2) the survival falls to only 20% (Hanash et al., 1972). Whitmore (1973) feels that not all prostatic cancer may pass through a clinical Stage B, implying some tumors may go from clinically unapparent diseases directly to locally extensive (Stage C) or metastatic lesions (Stage D). This could be an additional reason for the very small percentage of tumors diagnosed at this early, and potentially curable, stage. It appears that the poor survival of some Stage B patients in earlier series is due to the high incidence of unsuspected regional node metastases, and much wider local extension of the tumor than is expected. Many investigators have reported pelvic nodes involved in as many as 25% of clinical Stage B patients (Castellino et al., 1973; Ray et al., 1976; Loening et al., 1977).

Stage C lesions account for up to 40% of clinical presentations and have a median survival of 2½ years (Whitmore, 1973). More recent investigations have demonstrated regional node metastasis in over 50% of these patients (Gittes and Chu, 1976). While most patients with Stage C disease progress rapidly to Stage D and die of their tumors, a few do not (Arnheim, 1948), and this small fraction of patients are potentially curable by radical surgery with or without radiation therapy. Essentially one-half of all patients with clinical prostatic carcinoma have Stage D disease at the time of diagnosis. Five-year survival in these patients approximates 15%, and death is usually due to metastases although a minority of patients die from other causes primarily because of the high association of cardiovascular disease in this age group. Besides regional and para-aortic nodes, the most common site of metastasis is bone; other less frequent sites of metastasis include bone marrow, lungs, liver and central nervous system (Catane et al., 1976; Varkarakis et al., 1974).

STAGING

After a diagnosis of prostatic cancer has been established an accurate staging work-up is required. Standard investigations (see Table 17.5)

TABLE 17.5
Staging Work-up for Prostatic Carcinoma

1. Routine blood count and serum chemistries
2. Total and prostatic serum acid phosphatase
3. LDH isoenzymes
4. Serum alkaline phosphatase
5. Carcinoembryonic antigen (CEA)
6. Chest x-ray
7. Metastatic bone survey
8. Intravenous pyelogram (IVP)
9. Pedal lymphangiogram
10. Bone scan
11. Bone marrow biopsy and acid phosphatase
12. Pelvic lymphadenectomy[a]

[a] Provided no evidence of dissemination has been found in prior tests.

include palpation of the gland, chest and metastatic bone x-rays, bone scan, serum chemistries to include alkaline and acid phosphatases, renal and liver function tests; other chemical measurements that may be of value include LDH isoenzymes and a carcinoembryonic antigen level. We also feel that a bone marrow aspiration and biopsy for cytology and acid phosphatase should be included in the initial evaluation. Providing there is no evidence of Stage D disease found during the initial staging, most larger centers are proceeding to lymphangiogram and pelvic lymphadenectomy for more definitive staging (Bruce, 1977; Ray et al., 1976; Loening et al., 1977; and Dahl et al., 1974). As mentioned earlier, a large percentage of these patients will be found to have Stage D disease at operative staging which will influence the choice of subsequent treatment. Prout (1973b) believes an elevated serum acid phosphatase is justification for including a patient in Stage D; he does not, however, describe his approach to such a patient with clinical Stage B disease. We believe an operative staging procedure is still indicated in these patients, because of a possible false positive acid phosphatase examination. In general, unless there is grossly obvious evidence of metastatic disease, all clinical Stage B and C patients should undergo operative staging of their tumor (DeWys, 1976).

Depending on the findings at surgery, some authors recommend a radical prostatectomy combined with total pelvic lymphadenectomy. This will be discussed further under treatment and management.

MANAGEMENT

The clinical management of patients with prostatic carcinoma is based on the stage of the disease at the time of diagnosis. As discussed previously, Stage B and C should be surgically confirmed because of the unreliability of the lymphangiogram.

Stage A. It is generally agreed that patients who are found to have Stage A_1 disease at TURP, require no other specific treatment than follow-up observation. However, if the disease is poorly differentiated, anaplastic, or involves more than a few of the resected prostatic chips, the prognosis is considerably worse and several authors have recommended treating these patients similar to Stage B patients (Bloom and Hendry, 1973).

Stage B. Patients with Stage B disease, limited to less than one lobe of the prostate, are usually treated with radical prostatectomy, which can be performed at the time of the staging lymphadenectomy. This therapy can provide survival rates almost equivalent to the age adjusted standards (Gilbertson, 1971; Belt and Schroeder, 1972). For those patients unable or unwilling to undergo an operative procedure, radical radiation therapy appears to provide as good a survival. Pistenma et al. (1976) reported 5- and 10-year survival rates of 71% and 45%, respectively, with approximately 7000 rads by external beam to the prostate area; these results compare favorably to those achieved by radical surgery alone (Jewitt et al., 1968).

Hilaris et al. (1974), have shown almost as good results using interstitial radiation therapy. Bagshaw et al. (1977) recently reported an 86% disease-free survival at 2 years with local and extended field radiation in 37 patients who had a negative laparotomy. Adjuvant hormonal therapy has not increased the survival in these patients (Hill et al., 1974; Bailar and Byar, 1970). The same approach can be used in Stage B_2 patients, however, the disadvantages of surgery such as temporary and sometimes permanent incontinence must be weighed against the side effects of the radiation such as proctitis and incontinence. The incidence of positive regional nodes in these patients is greater than in B_1 patients and if radiation therapy is to be used it should be administered through extended fields to include the regional lymphatics (Perez et al., 1977; Taylor, 1977).

Stage C. Well over half of all patients with locally advanced disease will have regional nodal metastasis. For the minority of patients with negative laparotomy findings, a radical prostatectomy perhaps followed by extended field radiation seems a reasonable approach (Bloom and Hendry, 1973). For most patients with positive nodes, however, extended field radiation presently offers the best hope for controlling the disease. McGowan (1977) reported 5-year survival of 40% in these patients using radiation alone. Bagshaw (1977) reported a disease-free survival of 71% at two years for a series of patients similarly treated. He also points out the very high incidence of bony metastasis in patients who have periaortic as well as pelvic nodes involved with tumor. This implies that these patients already have disease spread to parenchymal organs and are in need of systemic therapy at the time of diagnosis. On the basis of the

Veterans Administration studies (Bailar and Byar, 1970), hormonal therapy should not be instituted in Stage C patients until they become symptomatic. Hormonal therapy will be discussed more extensively under Stage D disease.

Stage D₁. These patients have clinical Stage B or C disease, but have positive nodes on staging laparotomy. Since staging laparotomies have only recently been introduced in this disease, long term treatment results and survival data are lacking. Surgery or extended field radiation may be adequate treatment for some patients (Bagshaw et al., 1977), but a considerable number are at risk for developing further metastatic disease. Studies to determine the value of adjuvant chemotherapy in these patients are definitely indicated.

Stage D₂. This group of patients accounts for roughly 50% of all newly diagnosed prostatic cancer patients. Therapy options are presently only of a palliative nature and consist of radiation therapy, hormonal manipulation, or chemotherapy. For patients with disseminated disease, the role of radiation is limited to providing relief of specific symptoms—i.e., urethral obstruction or bony pain. Usually good symptomatic control can be achieved for varying periods of time.

The role of hormonal therapy for prostatic cancer has been well known since the original report of Huggins and Hodges in 1941. It is clear from the Veterans Administration Cooperative Urological Research Group (VACURG) studies (1967) that estrogen treatment in older males is not innocuous. While 5.0 mg of diethylstilbesterol (DES) a day did reduce the deaths from prostatic cancer, this was overshadowed by the increase in cardiovascular mortality. A second study showed 1.0 mg/day of DES was as good as 5.0 mg/day in preventing cancer deaths, but without the increased risk of heart disease (Blackard, 1975). It is not clear, however, if 1.0 mg/day of DES is sufficient to depress plasma testosterone concentration to castration levels (Beck et al., 1978), or whether this is even necessary to control tumor growth (Catalona and Scott, 1978). Likewise, there is no clear answer about combining estrogens with orchiectomy or even about the optimum dose of estrogens to be used (Catalona and Scott, 1978). Since 70–80% of patients with metastatic prostatic carcinoma will respond, at least to some degree, to hormonal therapy (Breudler, 1969), we feel all symptomatic patients should receive an initial trial of hormonal manipulation. Because of fewer adverse side effects, orchiectomy is the first treatment of choice. If a subjective or objective remission occurs, further therapy should be held until relapse occurs.

The management of hormonal failure is a controversial one. While most patients receive no benefit from further hormonal treatment, a small percentage do, and in this group of patients an additional trial of DES 1.0–3.0 mg/day appears warranted (Ferguson, 1972). While a very few patients may benefit from further surgical hormone manipulation (adrenalectomy or hypophysectomy) most do not, and this form of therapy is not generally recommended (Grayhack, 1969). The greatest need is a method to predict which patients will respond to hormonal therapy. Much work is currently underway on androgen receptors in prostatic carcinoma and their relationship to hormonal responsiveness, but no information of clinical value is yet available (Menon et al., 1977). For those patients who fail hormonal therapy, chemotherapy is the treatment of choice. Scott and others (1976) reported clearly superior survival in patients who responded to treatment with either cyclophosphamide or 5-fluorouracil compared with supportive treatment alone.

The National Prostatic Cancer Project is currently sponsoring a number of different chemotherapy protocols for patients with advanced disease (Johnson et al., 1977). Early results show that a number of agents do have activity in advanced prostatic carcinoma (see Table 17.6). The most promising reports of high response rates have come with combination chemotherapy.

Perloff et al. (1977) reported a 43% objective response rate using the combination of cis-diamminedichloroplatinum and Adriamycin; initial reports of 40% response rate with the nitrosourea CCNU are also very encouraging (Tejada et al., 1977). By preference patients should be entered on various protocol studies, as further information on activity of drugs and combinations is badly needed. If such studies are not available, or if the patient does not qualify, a therapeutic trial with cyclophosphamide or 5-fluorouracil is indicated. Currently we favor using Adriamycin and cis-diamminedichloroplatinum as our treatment of choice. Obviously, these drugs are extremely toxic and should only be given under the direction of a clinician who is familiar with their administration.

IMMUNOTHERAPY

Huus et al. (1975) correlated the cellular immunity status of prostatic cancer patients with the extent of disease. Others (Schellhammer et al.,

TABLE 17.6

Chemotherapeutic Agents with Activity in Adenocarcinoma of the Prostate

Drug	Overall Response Rate (%)[a]
Cyclophosphamide	46
5-Fluorouracil	36
Estramustine	30
DTIC	48
Procarbazine	29
CCNU	40
Adriamycin	29
cis-Diamminedichloroplatinum	40

[a] Includes both objective remission and stable disease.

1976) have been unable to correlate abnormalities of the immune status with prognosis and survival in individual patients. Ablin (1975) recently reviewed the status of immunotherapy in prostatic cancer; although a rare favorable response has been reported, in general the results have been disappointing. However, it should be kept in mind that most trials have been in patients who have failed all other modes of therapy; immunotherapy trials in patients with minimal residual disease such as Stage D_1 may be more rational. Presently there is no indication for the routine use of the various forms of immunostimulation.

REFERENCES

Albin, R. J. Immunotherapy for prostatic cancer. Oncology, *31:* 177–202, 1975.

Arnheim, F. K. Carcinoma of the prostate—a study of the post mortem findings in one hundred and seventy-six cases. J. Urol., *60:* 599–603, 1948.

Bagshaw, M. A., Pistenma, D. A., Ray, G. R., Freiha, F. S., and Kempson, R. I. Evaluation of extended-field radiotherapy for prostatic neoplasm: 1976. Cancer Treat. Rep., *61:* 297–306, 1977.

Bailar, J. C., III, and Byar, D. P. Veterans Administration Cooperative Urological Research Group: Estrogen treatment for cancer of the prostate; early results with three (3) doses of diethylstilbestrol and placebo. Cancer, *26:* 257–261, 1970.

Beck, P. H., McAnich, J. W., Gobel, J. L., and Stutzman, R. E. Plasma testosterone in patients receiving diethylstilbestrol. Urology, *11:* 157–160, 1978.

Belt, E., and Schroeder, F.H. Total perineal prostatectomy for carcinoma of the prostate. J. Urol., *107:* 91–96, 1972.

Blackard, C. E. The Veteran's Administration Cooperative Urological Research Group studies of carcinoma of the prostate; a review. Cancer Chemother. Rep., *59:* 225–227, 1975.

Bloom, H. J. G., and Hendry, W. F. Treatment of prostatic cancer. In Modern Trends in Oncology—1, Part 2: Clinical Progress, edited by R. W. Raven, pp. 143–179. Butterworth, London, 1973.

Breudler, H. Therapy with orchiectomy or estrogens or both. J.A.M.A., *210:* 1074–1075, 1969.

Bruce, A. W., O'Cleireachain, F., Morales, A., and Awad, S. A. Carcinoma of the prostate; a critical look at staging. J. Urol., *117:* 319–322, 1977.

Cancer Facts and Figures, 1975. American Cancer Society, New York, 1975.

Castellino, R. A., Ray, G., Blank, N., Govan, D., and Bagshaw, M. Lymphangiography in prostatic carcinoma. J.A.M.A., *223:* 877–881, 1973.

Catalona, W. J., and Scott, W. W. Carcinoma of the prostate; a review. J. Urol., *119:* 1–8, 1978.

Catane, R., Kaufman, J., West, C., Merrin, C., Tsukada, Y., and Murphy, G. P. Brain metastases from prostatic carcinoma. Cancer, *38:* 2583–2587, 1976.

Chiu, C. L., and Weber, D. L. Prostate carcinoma in young adults. J.A.M.A., *230:* 724–726, 1974.

Choe, B. K., Pontes, E. J., McDonald, I., and Rose, N. R. Immunochemical studies of prostatic acid phosphatase. Cancer Treat. Rep., *61:* 201–204, 1977.

Dahl, D. S., Wilson, C. S., Middleton, R. G., and Bourne, H. H. Pelvic lymphadenectomy for staging localized prostatic carcinoma. J. Urol. *112:* 245–246, 1974.

Del Regato, J. A. Radiotherapy in the conservative treatment of operable and locally inoperable carcinoma of the prostate. Radiology, *88:*761–766, 1967.

DeWys, W.D., Bauer, M., Colsky, J., Cooper, R. A., Creech, R., and Carbone, P. P. Comparative trial of Adriamycin and 5-fluorouracil in advanced prostatic cancer—progress report. Cancer Treat. Rep., *61:* 325–328, 1977.

DeWys, W. W. Perspectives and overview (on prostatic cancer). Semin. Oncol., *3:* 189–192, 1976.

Dmochowski, L., and Horoszewicz, J. S. Viral oncology of prostatic cancer. Semin. Oncol., *3:* 141–150, 1976.

Dmochowski, L., Ohtsuki, Y., Seman, G., Maruyama, K., Knesek, J. E., East, J. L., Bowen, J. M., Yoshida, H., and Johnson, D. E. Search for oncogenic viruses in human prostate cancer. Cancer Treat. Rep., *61:* 119–127, 1977.

Epstein, N. A., and Fatti, L. P. Prostatic carcinoma, some morphologic features affecting prognosis. Cancer, *37:* 2455–2465, 1976.

Ernster, V. L., Winkelstein, W., Jr., Selvin, S., Brown, S. M., Sacks, S T., Austin, D. F., Mandel, S. A., and Bertolli, T. A. Race, socioeconomic status and prostatic cancer. Cancer Treat. Rep., *61:* 187–191, 1977.

Fergusson, J. D. The doubtfully malignant prostate. Br. J. Surg., *51:* 746–750, 1965.

Fergusson, J. D. Sequential management in advanced disease. In Endocrine Therapy in Malignant Disease, edited by B. A. Stoll, W. B. Saunders, Philadelphia, 1972.

Flocks, R. H. Clinical cancer of the prostate; a study of 4000 cases. J.A.M.A., *193:* 559–562, 1965.

Foti, A. G., Cooper, J. F., Herschman, H., and Malvaez, R. R. Detection of prostatic cancer by solid phase radioimmunoassay of serum prostatic acid phosphatase. N. Engl. J. Med., *297:* 1357–1361, 1977.

Franks, L. M. Etiology, epidemiology and pathology of prostate cancer. Cancer, *32:* 1092–1095, 1973.

Gilbertson, V. A. Cancer of the prostate gland. Results of early diagnosis and therapy undertaken for cure of the disease. J.A.M.A., *215:* 81–84, 1971.

Gittes, R. F., and Chu, T. M. Detection and diagnosis of prostatic cancer. Semin. Oncol., *3:* 123–130, 1976.

Grayhack, J. T. Adrenalectomy and hypophysectomy for carcinoma of the prostate. J.A.M.A., *210:* 1075–1076, 1969.

Grayhack, J. T., Wendel, E. F., Lee, C., and Oliver, L. Analysis of prostatic fluid in prostatic disease. Cancer Treat. Rep., *61:* 205–210, 1977.

Hanash, K. A., Utz, D. C., Cook, E. N., Taylor, W. F., and Titus, J. L. Carcinoma of the prostate—a 15-year follow-up. J. Urol., *61:* 723–729, 1972.

Harada, M., Mostofi, F. K., Corle, D. K., Byar, D. P., and Trump, B. F. Preliminary studies of histologic prognosis in cancer of the prostate. Cancer Treat. Rep., *61:* 223–225, 1977.

Hilaris, B. S., Whitmore, W. F., Jr., Batata, M. A., and Grabstald, H. Radiation therapy and pelvic node dissection in the management of cancer of the prostate. A.J.R., *121:* 832–838, 1974.

Hill, D. R., Crews, O. E., Jr., and Walsh, P. C. Prostate carcinoma; radiation treatment of the primary and regional lymphatics. Cancer, *34:* 156–160, 1974.

Hudson, P. B., and Stout, A. P. Prostatic cancer; XVI. Comparison of physical examination and biopsy for detection of curable lesions. N.Y. State Med. J., *66:* 351–355, 1966.

Huggins, C., and Hodges, D. V. The effect of castration, of estrogen and of androgen injection on serum phosphatases in metastatic carcinoma of the prostate. Cancer Res., *1:* 293–297, 1941.

Hutchinson, G. B. Epidemiology of prostate cancer. Semin. Oncol., *3:* 151–159, 1976.

Huus, J. C., Kursh, E. D., Poor, P., and Persky, L. Delayed cutaneous hypersensitivity in patients with prostatic adenocarcinoma. J. Urol., *114:* 86–87, 1975.

Jackson, M. A., Ahluwalia, B. S., Herson, J., Haeshmat, M. Y., Jackson, A. G., Jones, G. W., Kapoor, S. K., Kennedy, J., Kovi, J., Lucas, A. O., Nkposong, E. O., Olisa, E., and Williams, A. O. Characterization of prostatic carcinoma among blacks; a continuation report. Cancer Treat. Rep., *61:* 167–172, 1977.

Jewett, H. J., Bridge, R. W., and Gray, G. F., Jr. Palpable nodule of prostatic cancer. J.A.M.A., *203:* 403–406, 1968.

Johnson, D. E., Scott, W. W., Gibbons, R. P., Prout, G. R., Schmidt, J. D., Chu, T. M., Gaeta, J., Saroff, J., and Murphy, G. P. National randomized study of chemotherapeutic agents in advanced prostatic carcinoma; a progress report. Cancer Treat. Rep., *61:* 317–323, 1977.

Loening, S. A., Schmidt, J. D., Brown, R. C., Hawtrey, C. E., Fallon, B., and Culp, D. A. A comparison between lymphangiography and pelvic node dissection in the staging or prostatic cancer. J. Urol., *117:* 752–756, 1977.

McCombs, R. M. Role of oncornaviruses in carcinoma of the prostate. Cancer Treat. Rep., *61:* 131–132, 1977.

McGowan, D. G. Radiation therapy in the management of localized carcinoma of the prostate. Cancer, *39:* 98–103, 1977.

McNeal, J. E. Regional morphology and pathology of the prostate. Am. J. Clin. Pathol., *49:* 347–357, 1968.

Menon, M., Tananis, C. E., McLoughlin, M.G., and Walsh, P. C. Androgen receptors in human prostatic tissue; a review. Cancer Treat. Rep., *61:* 265–271, 1977.

Merrin, C. Treatment of advanced carcinoma of the prostate (Stage D) with infusion of cis-diamminedichloroplatinum (CPDD) and mannitol. Proc. Am. Assoc. Cancer Res., *18:* 100, 1977.

Mickey, D. D., Stone, K. R., Stone, M. P., and Paulson, D. F. Morphologic and immunologic studies of human prostatic carcinoma. Cancer Treat. Rep., *61:* 133–138, 1977.

Morfin, R. F., Leav, I., Charles, J. F., Cavazos, L. F., Ofner, P., and Floch, H. H. Correlative study of the morphology and C19 steroid metabolism of benign and cancerous human prostate tissue. Cancer, *39:* 1517–1534, 1977.

Mostofi, F. K. Grading of prostatic carcinoma. Cancer Chemother. Rep., *59:* 111–117, 1975.

Mostofi, F. K. Problems of grading carcinoma of the prostate. Semin. Oncol., *3:* 161–168, 1976.

Munsie, W.J., and Foster, E. A. Unsuspected very small foci of carcinoma of the prostate in transurethral resection specimens. Cancer, *21:* 692–698, 1968.

Murphy, G.P. Prostate Cancer, American Cancer Society, New York, 1974.

Murphy, G. P. The diagnosis of prostate cancer. Cancer, *37:* 589–596, 1976.

Perez, C. A., Bauer, W., Garza, R., and Royce, R. K. Radiation therapy in the definitive treatment of localized carcinoma of the prostate. Cancer, *40:* 1425–1433, 1977.

Perloff, M., Ohnuma, T., Holland, J. F., Kennedy, B. J., and Mills, R. C. Adriamycin and diamminedichloroplatinum in advanced prostatic carcinoma. Proc. Am. Soc. Clin. Oncol. *18:* 333, 1977.

Pistenma, D. A., Gray, G. R., and Bagshaw, M. A. The role of megavoltage radiation therapy in the treatment of prostatic cancer. Semin. Oncol., *3:* 115–122, 1976.

Pontes, J. E., Alcorn, S. W., Thomas, A. J., Jr., and Pierce, J. M., Jr. Bone marrow acid phosphatase in staging prostatic carcinoma. J. Urol., *114:* 422–424, 1975.

Prout, G. R., Jr. Diagnosis and staging of prostatic carcinoma. Cancer, *32:* 1096–1103, 1973a.

Prout, G. R., Jr. Prostate gland. In Cancer Medince, edited by J. F. Holland and E. Frei III, pp. 1680–1695. Lea & Feibiger, Philadelphia, 1973b.

Ray, G. R., Pistenma, D. H., Castellino, R. A., Kempson, R. L., Maeres, E., and Bagshaw, M. A. Operative staging of apparently localized carcinoma of the prostate; Results in fifty unselected cases. Cancer, *38:* 73–83, 1976.

Rotkin, I. D. Studies in the epidemiology of prostatic cancer; expanded sampling. Cancer Treat. Rep., *61:* 173–180, 1977.

Schellhammer, P. F., Bracken, R. B., Bean, M. A., Pinsky, C. M., and Whitmore, W. F., Jr. Immune evaluation of skin testing. Cancer, *38:* 149–156, 1976.

Schmidt, J. D., and Welch, M. J., Jr. Sarcoma of the prostate. Cancer, *37:* 1908–1912, 1976.

Schuman, L. M., Mandel, J., Backard, C., Bauer, H., Scarlett, J., and McHugh, R. Epidemiologic study of prostatic cancer; preliminary report. Cancer Treat. Rep., *61:* 181–186, 1977.

Scott, R., and Mutchnik, D. L. Carcinoma of the prostate in elderly men; incidence, growth characteristics and clinical significance. J. Urol., *101:* 602–607, 1969.

Scott, W. W., Gibbons, R. P., Johnson, D. E., Prout, G. R., Schmidt, J. D., Saroff, J., and Murphy, G. P. The continued evaluation of the effects of chemotherapy in patients with advanced carcinoma of the prostate. J. Urol., *116:* 211–213. 1976.

Seidman, H., Silverberg, E., and Holleb, A. I. Cancer statistics, 1976; a comparison of white and black populations. CA, *26:* 2–13,1976.

Sinha, A. A.., Blackard, C. E., and Seal, U. S. A critical analysis of tumor morphology and hormone treatments in the untreated and estrogen-treated responsive and refractory human prostate carcinoma. Cancer, *40:* 2836–2850, 1977.

Taylor,W. J. Radiation oncology; cancer of the prostate. Cancer, *39:* 856–861, 1977.

Tejada, F., Broder, L. E., Cohen, M. H., and Simon, R. Treatment of metastatic prostatic cancer with 5-fluorouracil (5FU) vs. 1-(2-chloroethyl)-3-cyclohexyl-1-nitrosourea (CCNU). Proc. Am. Soc. Clin. Oncol., *18:* 269, 1977.

UICC, Commission on Clinical Oncology of the Union Internationale Contre le Cancer. TNM Classification of Malignant Tumors, Ed. 2. International Union Against Cancer, Geneva, 1974.

Varkarakis, M. J., Winterberger, A. R., Gaeta, J., Moore, R. H., and Murphy, G. P. Lung metastases in prostatic carcinoma; clinical significance. Urology, *3:* 447–452, 1974.

Veterans Administration Cooperative Urological Research Group. Treatment and survival of patients with cancer of the prostate. Surg. Gynecol. Obstet., *124:*1011–1017, 1967.

Watanabe, H., Igari, D., Tanahashi, Y., Harada, K., and Saitoh, M. Transrectal ultrasonotomography of the prostate. J. Urol., *114:* 734–739, 1975.

Whitmore, W. F., Jr. The rationale and results of ablative surgery for prostatic cancer. Cancer, *16:* 1119–1132,1963.

Whitmore, W. F., Jr. The natural history of prostatic cancer. Cancer, *32:* 1104–1112, 1973.

Wood, D. C., Varela, V., Palmquist, M., and Weber, F. Serum lactic dehydrogenase and isoenzyme changes in clinical cancer. J. Surg. Oncol., *5:* 251–257, 1973.

Wynder, E. L., Mabuchi, K., and Whitmore, W. F. Epidemiology of cancer of the prostate. Cancer, *38:* 344–360, 1971.

Yam, L. T. Clinical significance of human acid phosphatases. Am. J. Med., *56:* 604–613, 1974.

Chapter 18

Germinal Cell Tumors of Testicle

JOHANNES BLOM, M.D.

Testicular tumors comprise less than 1% of all tumors and about 10% of all genitourinary tumors in men. Table 18.1 lists the histologic types of testicular tumors and their relative incidences.

GERMINAL CELL TUMORS

The incidence of testicular cancer in the United States is approximately 2 per 100,000 males per year and is responsible for about 0.6% of all male cancer deaths. It is primarily a tumor of young adults with the maximum incidence between 20 and 40 years of age, accounting for approximately 12% of all cancer deaths and thus constituting the fourth most common cause of death from neoplasia in this age group. Testis tumors are less common in Asiatics and in blacks in comparison to Caucasians. About 60% occur on the right side and in 1–2% the tumor is bilateral. They may occur simultaneously or successively, sometimes after a tumor-free interval of many years (Lefevre et al., 1975).

Testicular tumors in children, which are less common than in adults, were reviewed by Giebink and Ruymann in 1974. Approximately 65% are of germ cell and 35% of non-germ cell origin. Forty percent of the germ cell tumors are embryonal carcinoma, 27% teratomas and 21% teratocarcinomas. Seminomas are extremely rare. Sabio et al. (1974) reviewed eight pediatric cases of embryonal carcinoma seen at the Mayo Clinic from 1961 to 1971. The staging and therapeutic approach to pediatric cases is similar to that in adults. The prognosis appears better in children under 2 years of age than in older ones.

The etiology is unknown. A history of trauma is given in about 25% of cases; however, no connection between the trauma and the onset of the tumor has been established (Borski, 1973; Mostofi, 1973). Men with cryptorchidism have a 10–14 times greater incidence of testicular malignancies than the remainder of the male population (Mostofi, 1973). These

TABLE 18.1
Testicular Tumors

I.	Germinal tumors		95%
	a. Seminomas,	30–70%	
	b. Embryonal carcinomas,	30–40%	
	c. Teratomas,	9%	
	d. Choriocarcinomas,	1–2%	
	e. Teratocarcinomas,	15%	
II.	Nongerminal tumors		5%
	a. Interstitial cell (Leydig), 1%		
	b. Fibromas		
	c. Angiomas		
	d. Neurofibromas		
	e. Masculinizing (feminizing) androblastomas		
	f. Tumors of the tubules of the rete testis		
	g. Lymphomas		
	h. Leukemic infiltrates		
	i. Metastatic tumors		

tumors are predominantly seminomas. Surgical correction after the age of 6 does not alter the incidence of malignancy significantly (Dow and Mostofi, 1967). Cryptorchidism per se may not be the cause of the increased tumor incidence, but rather an abnormal testis may be the cause of both maldescendence and increased tumor incidence. About 50% of surgically corrected or uncorrected undescended testes lose their spermatogenic function. Since the number of spermatogonia seems to drop sharply at about the first year of age, surgical correction might best be performed prior to this time (Myers and Kelalis, 1973), provided that biopsy of the undescended testicle reveals normal histology. According to these authors early orchiopexy does nothing to alter the malignant potential, but may save testicular function, although the procedure itself may be damaging to the organ.

CLASSIFICATION

Anatomically the testicle consists of germ cells, supporting tissue and endocrine cells. Tumors can arise from all three structures; however, 96% of the tumors are of germ cell etiology. The most widely used classification of germ cell tumors is that by Dixon and Moore (1952) with some modifications (Table 18.2).

Because of the frequent presence of a mixture of tumor elements, careful study of multiple sections at different levels of the pathologic material is essential. Metastatic elements often differ from the primary tumor, and different metastases may be of different cell types (Mackenzie, 1966).

TABLE 18.2
Germinal Cell Tumors

1. Seminoma
2. Embryonal carcinoma with or without seminoma
3. Teratoma with or without seminoma
4. Teratoma with embryonal carcinoma or choriocarcinoma
5. Choriocarcinoma with or without embryonal carcinoma

Seminoma is thought to arise from the germ cell; it is composed of large uniform cells with clear cytoplasm which resemble primordial germ cells. The tumor is of relatively low malignancy and is highly radiosensitive. In about 10% of the cases areas of anaplastic and pleomorphic seminoma cell changes can be found which are sometimes difficult to differentiate from embryonal elements. Maier et al. (1968b) have pointed out that these anaplastic seminomas are equally radiosensitive, but are more aggressive with greater tendency toward early metastasis. These findings were confirmed by Johnson et al. (1975) when they analyzed 7 cases found among 218 cases of seminoma at M. D. Anderson Hospital. Seminoma comprises from 30 to 70% of the testicular tumors; it is most commonly seen in the third and fourth decades and has rarely been observed under the age of 10. The rare spermatocytic seminoma occurs mostly in the over-50 age group.

Embryonal carcinoma is a germ cell tumor derived from a totipotential germ cell. It is composed of cells with an anaplastic epithelial appearance and a variable pattern of acinar, tubular, papillary, solid and/or reticular structure. It comprises about 30–40% of the testicular tumors and is most commonly seen in the 15–30-year-old age group.

Teratoma is a complex tumor showing elements of more than one germ layer in various stages of maturation, sometimes in arrangements suggestive of organ formation. They are found in about 9% of patients with testicular tumors, mostly in the first 3 decades of life.

Choriocarcinoma is a highly malignant tumor composed of cytotrophoblastic and syncytiotrophoblastic cells. It is often mixed with embryonal carcinoma or other elements and is very rare in its pure form. It is most common in the second and third decades of life.

Teratocarcinoma is a mixture of teratomatous and carcinomatous elements and comprises about 15% of the testicular germ cell tumors.

NATURAL HISTORY

Initially, symptomatology is mostly limited to the testicle, often mimicking results of trauma and infection which have delayed the diagnosis of malignant tumor for an average of 6 months in many cases. Endocrine manifestations and occasionally metastatic involvement, particularly in choriocarcinoma with spread to the lungs, may herald the presence of a testicular tumor. More than 85% of the patients who are to die from their disease do so within 2 years from the time of diagnosis, from generalized metastasis.

METASTASIS

Knowledge of the methods of spread of testicular tumors is essential for the understanding of the symptomatology and for the proper treatment planning. Usually the tunica albuginea acts as a barrier to scrotal invasion; however, after penetration the tumor may extend along the cord, which makes for an unfavorable prognosis. Scrotal incisions or needle biopsies of testicular tumors are contraindicated because of possible scrotal implantation of tumor cells. Inguinal incision allows radical orchiectomy with a high ligation of the cord that may be involved with tumor. In addition, needle or open testicular biopsies for suspected tumor must be condemned because results may be misleading considering the great variability of testicular tumor pathology.

Spread is via the lymphatics; however, in addition choriocarcinoma tends to invade blood vessels with early hematogenous spread, usually to the lungs, but also to the liver and brain. The lymphatics accompany the spermatic cord through the internal inguinal ring. On the right side they drain into lymph nodes, lateral, anterior or medial to the inferior vena cava from the level of the renal vein above to the aortic bifurcation below. On the left side the drainage is to lymph nodes lateral to the aorta from the level of the renal vein above to the aortic bifurcation below. Crossover, particularly with right-sided tumors and node involvement, is a common occurrence as demonstrated with lymphangiography.

Iliac lymph nodes are infrequently areas of primary spread. Inguinal nodes are usually only involved after previous inguinal surgery, with scrotal wall involvement, with involvement of the epididymis, or with cryptorchidism. From the retroperitoneal space, lymph drainage is via the thoracic duct so that the left supraclavicular nodes may become involved early in the course of the disease (Ray et al., 1974). Buck et al. (1972) found on routine biopsy of nonpalpable left supraclavicular nodes tumor in 4 of 25 patients with Stage II disease. Fifteen patients with Stage I disease had no evidence of tumor in these nodes. Spread to the mediastinum may occur through reflux from above or via lymphatics that communicate directly with retroperitoneal nodes.

STAGING

Based on the characteristics of spread of testicular tumors, patients should be carefully staged before proper treatment can be instituted. In addition to a careful history and physical examination, liver function tests should be obtained, although early liver involvement is not common. Tomograms of the lungs in addition to standard roentgenograms are indicated to demonstrate early lung involvement, which is particularly common in choriocarcinoma. Gallium-67 citrate total body scans have also been helpful (Bailey et al., 1973). Patterson et al. (1976), found it particularly helpful in the evaluation and follow-up of patients with seminoma, and less consistent in embryonal carcinoma. Additional scans of liver, bones and brain may on occasion demonstrate the presence of metastatic disease. Urinary human chorionic gonadotrophin (HCG) titers may be elevated in addition to serum α-fetoprotein (Talerman and Haije, 1974) and carcinoembryonic antigen. Recently developed techniques of measuring these markers by double antibody radioimmunoassay using an antibody generated against the β subunit of HCG have greatly increased sensitivity so that now serum levels can be obtained (Cochran et al., 1975). Serial serum levels may be helpful in monitoring disease activity during therapy, and during remission status (Perlin et al., 1976; Lange et al., 1976). Excretory urograms and inferior vena cavograms are usually not very helpful. Although the accuracy of the bilateral pedal lymphangiogram has been reported as 7% falsely positive and 25% falsely negative (Maier and Schamber, 1972), it may give a clear outline of the nodes up to the renal vessels, not infrequently demonstrating crossover. In 5% of the patients it may show drainage to the right supraclavicular area, indicating a right-sided thoracic duct with the possibility of right supraclavicular node involvement. It serves as a good reference for the radiotherapist to position the treatment fields and for the surgeon as a guide to lymphadenectomy. The results of therapy can be observed on serial follow-up films as long as contrast material remains visible. Some testicular lymph channels may run to an eschelon node situated close to the renal pelvis, before draining into the lumbar para-aortic chain. These nodes are not filled with pedal lymphangiography, but may be visualized with spermatic cord lymphangiography. However, because of the minimal additional benefit of this study in the frequent postorchiectomy status of the patient when lymphangiography is contemplated, the bilateral pedal lymphangiogram will usually be performed. The value of this study has recently been reviewed by Wilkinson and MacDonald (1975), Fuchs and Girod (1975), and by Safer et al. (1975). Ultrasonography and computerized axial tomography of the abdominal area are useful adjunctive studies (Kreel, 1976) and according to some investigators more reliable than the lymphangiogram. Various staging systems have been described; two of these are currently used most widely and are outlined in Table 18.3.

TREATMENT

Surgery, radiation therapy and chemotherapy, singly or in combinations form the modes of therapy for the various stages and histologic

TABLE 18.3
Staging Systems[a]

Stage I or A:	Tumor confined to testis and adnexae
Stage II or B:	Lymph node involvement, limited to below the diaphragm, including cord and scrotum
Stage III or C:	Metastases above the diaphragm or visceral organs
Stage 1A:	Tumor confined to one testis
Stage 1B:	As in 1A but patient found to have histologic evidence of metastasis to iliac or para-aortic lymph nodes at time of retroperitoneal lymph node dissection
Stage 2:	Clinical or radiographic evidence of metastasis to femoral, inguinal, iliac or para-aortic lymph nodes; no demonstrable metastases above the diaphragm or to visceral organs
Stage 3:	Clinical or radiographic evidence of metastasis above the diaphragm or other distant metastasis to body organs

[a] Boden and Gibb (1951) and Maier et al. (1968a).

types of testicular cancer. The necessity of prompt transinguinal exploration of a testicle suspected to harbor a malignancy or of a tender, swollen testicle that has not responded to conservative treatment after about 2 weeks has been alluded to earlier. Prior to the availability of modern staging methods, 3–5-year survival figures ranging from 5 to 49% have been reported with orchiectomy alone (Vechinski et al., 1965). This procedure will control the disease at the primary site in almost all cases.

Approximately 30–35% of patients with seminoma will have lymphatic metastasis which can be demonstrated with approximately 90% accuracy with lymphangiography. Comparative studies of retroperitoneal lymphadenectomy following orchiectomy and the combination of lymphadenectomy and postoperative radiation therapy have established the value of radiation therapy alone for treatment of Stage I and II seminoma. Local recurrences after 2000 rads in 2 weeks to clinically positive nodes have been described (Maier et al., 1968b), but none after at least 3000 rads, unless reseeding occurred from other distant metastases. Doornbos et al. (1975), found 2500 rads adequate for prophylactic irradiation and 3500 rads for metastatic disease, regardless of size. For Stage I patients doses varying from 2000 to 3000 rads and for Stage II patients doses from 3000 to 4000 rads to the ipsilateral inguino-iliac, and bilateral para-aortic lymph nodes plus 2000–3000 rads to mediastinal and left supraclavicular lymph node areas will yield 5- and 10-year survival rates of close to 90% (Maier et al., 1968a, 1968b; Maier and Sulak, 1973a). Stage III disease is radio-curable in only a small percentage of patients and should, therefore, be treated with chemotherapy in addition to radiation therapy. Fortunately the number of patients with Stage III seminoma is small and the experience with chemotherapy accordingly; however, alkylating agents, particularly chlorambucil, have been found to be effective (Mackenzie,

1966). Maier et al. (1968a) and Maier and Sulak (1973a) have shown that anaplastic seminoma is more aggressive, that a greater percentage of patients present with Stage III disease, but that these tumors are radiosensitive. With careful staging the survival figures, stage for stage, are comparable to those of classical seminoma. This was recently confirmed by Johnson et al. (1975).

Choriocarcinoma spreads early via the blood stream and often presents as a rapidly progressive tumor with extensive pulmonary metastasis, frequently causing dyspnea and hemoptysis. It is rarely amenable to surgery and/or radiation therapy alone. Unfortunately it lacks the responsiveness of the female choriocarcinoma to chemotherapeutic agents. However, with newer drug combinations responses have become more frequent (Samuels et al., 1975a; Wittes et al., 1976).

The common approach to Stage I and II nonseminomatous tumors is bilateral retroperitoneal lymph node dissection. Postoperative radiation therapy for clinical Stage I patients whose retroperitoneal lymph nodes were histologically negative for tumor probably does not enhance the prospects of a cure. The role of postoperative radiation therapy in Stage II patients who had all abnormal nodes resected is highly controversial. Positive lymph node metastases above the renal pedicle usually preclude resection, unless the thoraco-abdominal approach is utilized which allows for better exposure of that area (Skinner and Leadbetter, 1971). The incision begins over the 10th rib in the posterior axillary line and is carried to the inguinal area near the lateral border of the rectus muscle. A modified technique combining the advantages of transabdominal and retroperitoneal operations has been described by Fraley et al. (1977). Although retroperitoneal lymph node dissection is an extensive operation, side effects in reported series have been tolerable. Absence of ejaculation, which occurs in the majority of patients, should be explained prior to surgery. Potency and experience of orgasm are uneffected (Kedia et al., 1975). Two- to five-year survival after bilateral lymph node dissection in Stage I embryonal carcinoma is fairly uniform and varies from 66 to 94% with only a small number of patients in the higher and lower categories. For Stage II disease, usually with postoperative radiation therapy, these figures vary from 29 to 66% with only Staubitz et al. (1973, 1974) reporting an 83% (10 of 12 patients) 5-year survival. The number of patients with other than embryonal carcinoma is not sufficient for reliable figures, but generally the presence of chorionic elements worsens the survival. According to Maier and Sulak (1973b), a positive urinary chorionic gonadotrophin titer worsens the prognosis for all histologic types.

In all series most relapses occur in the first 2 years. Maier and Sulak (1973b) in the Walter Reed Army Medical Center series of 503 nonseminoma patients found no statistically significant difference in survival between unilateral and bilateral lymphadenectomy with positive nodes; with either procedure the 5-year survival was approximately 45%. When the lymph nodes were negative for metastases there was improved survival for the bilateral operation, approximately 95% at 5 years versus 75% for the unilateral operation. This probably reflects that all retroperitoneal lymph nodes were truly free of metastases with the bilateral operation, whereas the decreased survival for the unilateral lymphadenectomy with negative nodes indicates metastasis via crossover lymphatics and an incomplete resection. The presence of node metastasis, whether completely removed or not, increases the risk of further spread and lowers the survival. Staubitz et al. (1973, 1974) in a series of 72 nonseminoma patients from the Roswell Park Memorial Institute reported a 3-year survival of 93% for patients with Stage I disease and of 75% for those with Stage II disease; the 5-year survival figures were 86% and 70%, respectively. They performed a bilateral retroperitoneal lymphadenectomy in 65 patients, 20 of whom had metastatic nodes, and excluded 7 patients because they were inoperable with disease above the renal pedicle but without evidence of disease above the diaphragm; thus, they were still Stage II patients. If these patients are included in the Stage II group, the figures are 55% and 50%, essentially identical to other reported series. MacKay and Sellers (1966) from the Ontario Cancer Foundation Clinics reported on a group of 827 patients which was similar in composition and in survival probabilities to the Walter Reed Army Medical Center series; however, 95% of their patients were treated by orchiectomy and radiation therapy, while the Walter Reed patients underwent radical lymphadenectomy, followed by radiation therapy. Questions which remain to be answered are whether radiation therapy can replace the retroperitoneal lymph node dissection and whether postlymphadenectomy radiation in patients with no residual disease prolongs the survival. However, more important is whether more patients can be salvaged with postoperative adjuvant chemotherapy, which becomes more promising with the introduction of highly effective drug combinations which will be described below. Postoperative radiation therapy compromises the use of these regimens.

CHEMOTHERAPY

Mackenzie (1966) and Golbey (1970) have indicated that alkylating agents such as melphalan and chlorambucil are the most effective agents in seminoma. For the nonseminomatous testicular tumors, actinomycin D has long been recommended as the single most effective agent.

Curreri and Ansfield (1960) and Parker et al. (1960) published the first clinical experiences with mithramycin. They found it extremely toxic and minimally effective, but Curreri and Ansfield suggested further evaluation in testicular tumors. Kofman and Eisenstein (1963) (Table 18.4) explored

TABLE 18.4

Mithramycin in Nonseminomatous Metastatic Testicular Tumors

Author	Schedule	No. of Patients	Response[a] CR	PR	Improved
Kofman and Eisenstein (1963)	0.050 mg/kg daily for 5 days, or lesser dosage	7	1		3
Brown and Kennedy (1965)	0.050 mg/kg daily for 5 days	11			7
	0.025 mg/kg in 8-hour infusion	1			
Ream et al. (1968)	0.025 mg/kg in 24-hour infusion	26	2	7	
Kennedy (1970)	0.025–0.050 mg/kg for 5 days or to toxicity	21	6		4
	0.050 mg/kg q.o.d. for 5 days	23	5		5
Hill et al. (1972)	0.025 mg/kg in 24-hour infusion	74	5	14	

[a] CR and PR, complete and partial response, respectively.

it further and found activity in embryonal cancers. Subsequent studies (Table 18.4) have confirmed its usefulness in testicular tumors, particularly embryonal carcinoma (Kennedy et al., 1965). Pitts (1970) in a summary of the experience with mithramycin in 1160 patients found 11% complete responders and 26% partial responders in 305 evaluable patients with testicular tumors. In 74 patients treated in a cooperative study group, 5 (7%) obtained a complete response and 14 (19%) a partial response (Hill et al., 1972). In doses of 0.025 mg/kg of body weight given daily for 10 days or 0.050 mg/kg given every other day for 10 days to be repeated after clearance of toxicity—usually in 3–4 weeks, the side effects have been tolerable. It is essential, however, that white blood cell counts, platelet counts, liver function studies and coagulation studies such as clotting time, prothrombin time and fibrinogen levels be performed regularly, by preference 3 times per week and the drug administration interrupted when the values become progressively abnormal. There does not seem to be a cross-resistance between actinomycin D and mithramycin.

Li et al. (1960) were the first to report on combination therapy with methotrexate, chlorambucil and actinomycin D (Table 18.5); of 23 patients so treated, 12 had a response, 7 of which were complete or "near complete" which was not further defined by the authors. Nine patients were treated with chlorambucil and actinomycin D and one obtained a complete response and one a temporary regression. Several variations of this triple therapy regimen have been described.

Mackenzie (1966) reviewed the experience at Memorial and James Ewings Hospitals and concluded that actinomycin D alone was as effective as combinations with actinomycin D. Thirty-six of 72 previously untreated patients responded to Li's triple therapy, 10 of whom had a complete response; 13 of 24 responded to actinomycin D plus chlorambucil with 5 complete responders and 8 of 12 responded to actinomycin D alone, with 4 complete responders.

Golbey (1970) outlined the more recent approach to the treatment of testicular tumors at Memorial Hospital. He advocated actinomycin D plus chlorambucil for patients with nonseminomatous tumors who had positive nodes at lymphadenectomy. In case the response to these two drugs is incomplete he recommended adding methotrexate and vincristine. Postoperative radiation therapy is not utilized unless there is residual disease. He has observed, like others, that abdominal nodes do not regress as readily and completely with chemotherapy as pulmonary metastases. Maintenance treatment is continued for 3 years because at Memorial Hospital no relapses have been observed beyond that period of time. Chabner et al. (1972) and Blom (1974) described recurrence 8 and 7½ years after a complete remission.

TABLE 18.5
Combination Treatment Regimens for Nonseminomatous Metastatic Testicular Tumors

Author	Drugs and Schedule	No. of Patients	Response[a] CR	Response[a] CR + PR	Total Responses
Li et al. (1960)	Methotrexate 5.0 mg PO for 16–25 days Chlorambucil 10.0 mg PO for 16–25 days Actinomycin D 0.5 mg IV day 3–7, 12–16, 21–25	23	7		12
	Chlorambucil Actinomycin D	9	1		2
Mackenzie (1966)	Li's regimen	72	10	36	
	Chlorambucil Actinomycin D	24	5	13	
	Actinomycin D	12	4	8	
Silvay et al. (1973)	Actinomycin D 0.0075–0.015 mg/kg IV for 3 days Vinblastine 0.025–0.05 mg/kg IV for 3 days Bleomycin 0.4 mg/kg IV for 3 days Repeat courses every 7–14 days for 2–3 courses	16		8	15
Mendelson and Serpick (1970)	5-Fluorouracil 7.5 mg/kg IV for 5 days Cyclophosphamide 7.5 mg/kg IV on day 1 and 4 Methotrexate 0.75 mg/kg IV on day 1 and 4 Vincristine 0.025 mg/kg IV on day 1 and 4	17	5	7	12
Blom and Brodovsky (1976)	Actinomycin D 0.4–0.6 mg/m² IV on day 1 thru 5	42	5	9	
	Actinomycin D 0.4–0.6 mg/m² IV on day 1 thru 5 Vincristine 1 mg/m² IV on day 1 and 8 Bleomycin 15 mg/m² IV on days 1, 8 and 15 Courses repeated every 3 weeks	42	8	29	

[a] CR and PR, complete and partial response, respectively.

Jacobs (1970) reviewed the experience in several institutions including his own from 1958 to 1968 with several multiple drug regimens. Results were not dramatically different but complete responses can be obtained with a variety of regimens, however, long term survival, even of complete responders, is less than 10%. The first randomized study in which actinomycin D was compared with actinomycin D, vincristine plus bleomycin was completed by members of the Eastern Cooperative Oncology Group (Blom and Brodovsky, 1976). Five of 42 patients treated with actinomycin D and 8 of 42 patients treated with the combination had a complete remission (Table 18.5). The median survival was 44 and 39 weeks, respectively.

A new promising combination is actinomycin D, vinblastine and bleomycin (Silvay et al., 1973). These investigators from Memorial Sloan Kettering Cancer Center administered actinomycin D 0.0075–0.015 mg/kg of body weight, vinblastine 0.025–0.05 mg/kg and bleomycin 0.4 mg/kg IV. for 3 days and repeated this course every 7–14 days for 2 or 3 courses (Table 18.5). Eight of 16 evaluable patients had objective and subjective remissions, lasting from 1 to 5+ months, 6 of these 8 patients had regressions of 75% or greater; 7 had responses of lesser degree. One patient had no response. Hematologic toxicity was tolerable. Mucocutaneous toxicity was often severe and dose limiting. Wittes et al. (1976) reported on further experience with this regimen at this center. Although only 7 of 47 patients obtained a complete remission, these complete responders were from a group of 13 who had not received any prior therapy and a group of 5 who had had only actinomycin D. Remissions continued at 14, 15, 17, 20 and 21 months. One patient failed and died 17 months after beginning therapy and one failed at 16 months.

Mendelson and Serpick (1970) reported 5 complete and 2 partial responses in 17 patients, 15 with embryonal and 2 with teratocarcinoma, who were treated with 5-fluorouracil, cyclophosphamide, methotrexate and vincristine (Table 18.5). The median duration of complete response was 9 months. The toxicity was described as mild.

Samuels and Howe (1970) at the M. D. Anderson Hospital have used vinblastine and vinblastine plus melphalan since 1962 and vinblastine plus bleomycin since August 1970 (Table 20.6). Four of 21 patients treated with vinblastine had a complete response and 7 had a partial response. Two of 11 patients treated with vinblastine plus melphalan had a complete response and two had a partial response. Median duration was 5+ months for the single drug treatment and 7+ months for the combination. The addition of the melphalan did not enhance the response nor prolong the duration significantly. Sixteen of 50 patients treated with vinblastine and bleomycin obtained a complete response (Samuels et al., 1973). The complete plus partial response rate was 76%, higher than in studies

TABLE 18.6

Vinblastine Combination Treatment for Metastatic Testicular Tumors

Author	Drugs and Schedule	No. of Patients	Response[a]	
			CR	CR + PR
Samuels and Howe (1970)	Vinblastine 0.4–0.8 mg/kg in 2–3 daily doses	21	4	11
	Vinblastine 0.35–0.4 mg/kg Melphalan 0.5–1.0 mg/kg IV	11	2	4
Samuels et al. (1973)	Vinblastine 0.4–0.6 mg/kg IV in 2 daily doses Bleomycin 30 mg IM twice weekly	50	16	38
Spigel and Coltman (1974)	Vinblastine 0.4 mg/kg Bleomycin 15.0 mg/m^2 IV twice weekly	11	5	9
Samuels et al. (1975a)	Vinblastine 0.4 mg/kg in 2 daily doses Bleomycin 30 mg 24-hour infusion for 5 days	23	9	17

[a] CR and PR, complete and partial response, respectively.

published heretofore (Table 18.6). Spigel and Coltman (1974) reported 5 complete and 4 partial responses in 11 patients treated with a regimen similar to Samuels': vinblastine 0.4 mg/kg divided in two daily doses and bleomycin 15 mg/m^2 twice weekly intravenously (Table 18.6). In 1975 Samuels et al. reported 9 complete and 8 partial responses in 23 patients with Stage III disease who received treatment with vinblastine 0.4 mg/kg in two fractions on days 1 and 2 plus continuous intravenous bleomycin, 30 mg daily for 5 days (Samuels et al., 1975b). Although these results were similar to their previous ones, they were remarkable because 12 patients had received prior therapy and almost all patients had advanced, bulky disease, in whom complete responses were only approximately 15% with the previous intermittent bleomycin program. These same authors (1975a) summarized their experience with 82 Stage III patients, 70 of whom were evaluable. Twenty-two patients had a complete response with a mean survival of 100+ weeks, with the longest at 172+ weeks and 11 alive beyond 2 years with no evidence of disease. The 31 partial responses had a mean duration of 36 weeks with only 8 patients living. Clearly the purpose of our treatment should be to obtain a complete remission and to find effective maintenance regimens that are relatively well tolerated. Toxicity, particularly hematologic, is considerable, and requires meticulous and aggressive treatment with appropriate antibiotics in patients with leukopenia and the use of platelet transfusions in patients with thrombocytopenia. Twenty-four patients who relapsed on the bleomycin-vinblastine regimen or who had never responded to this, plus 11 previously untreated patients were treated by the same investigators with a five-drug program, consisting of bleomycin, cyclophosphamide, vincristine, methotrexate and 5-fluorouracil (BleoCOMF) (Table 18.7). Three of 7 patients who had not responded to previous therapy obtained a complete remission and 4 of 11 previously untreated patients (Table 18.8).

Of the newer agents, Adriamycin holds some promise with 65% regressions in 20 patients for a median duration of 3 months, reported by Italian investigators (Monfardini et al., 1972). Higby et al. (1974) reported promising results with cis-diamminedichloroplatinum II (DDP), particularly in patients with abdominal and hepatic disease. Investigators at

TABLE 18.7
BleoCOMF in Metastatic Testicular Tumors[a]

Bleomycin	30 mg IM twice weekly for 4 doses
Cyclophosphamide	200 mg/m^2 PO daily for 14 doses
Vincristine	2 mg IV on days 1 and 7
Methotrexate	15 mg/m^2 IV twice weekly for 4 doses
5-Fluorouracil	400 mg/m^2 IV daily for 5 doses

[a] Repeated every 4–6 weeks depending on the blood counts.

Memorial Sloan Kettering Cancer Center (Cvitkovic et al., 1975) have incorporated DDP in their VAB regimen and changed to continuous 24-hour infusion of bleomycin—the VAB II program (Table 18.9). Seven of 24 evaluable patients had a complete remission and 12 a partial remission. In the VAB III program cyclophosphamide was added to the regimen and the dose of cis-platinum was increased to 120 mg/m^2 which required mannitol diuresis to prevent renal damage. Eighteen of 26 evaluable patients had a complete response and 6 had a partial response. Responses began within 5–6 days. The VAB IV regimen is a slight modification of the VAB III (Table 18.10). Toxicity is mostly mucositis with minimal

TABLE 18.8
BleoCOMF Response

	No. of Patients	Response	
		Complete	Partial
Previous therapy	24	3	12
Complete response	5		4
Partial response	12		8
No response	7	3	
No previous therapy	11	4	3

TABLE 18.9
Combination Treatment Regimens in Testicular Tumors[a]

VAB	Vinblastine	0.025–0.05 mg/kg IV for 3 days
	Actinomycin D	0.0075–0.015 mg/kg IV for 3 days
	Bleomycin	0.4 mg/kg IV for 3 days

Repeat courses every 7–14 days for 2–3 courses.

VAB II	Vinblastine	0.06 mg/kg on day 1
	Actinomycin D	0.02 mg/kg on day 1
	Bleomycin	0.5 mg/kg daily for 7 days
	cis-Platinum	1 mg/kg on day 8

Maintenance: VLB, actinomycin D and bleomycin weekly with cis-platinum substituting for actinomycin D every third week.

VAB III	Vinblastine	4 mg/m^2 on day 1
	Actinomycin D	1 mg/m^2 on day 1
	Bleomycin	20 mg/m^2 in 24-hour infusion for 7 days
	Cyclophosphamide	600 mg/m^2 on day 1
	cis-Platinum	120 mg/m^2 on day 8 with mannitol diuresis

Maintenance:	Vinblastine	4 mg/m^2 every 3 weeks	
	Chlorambucil plus	4 mg/m^2 for 2 of every 3 weeks	
	Actinomycin D	1 mg/m^2	alternating every 3 weeks
	Adriamycin	45 mg/m^2	
	cis-Platinum	50 mg/m^2	

[a] Induction repeated after 2 maintenance cycles.

depression of the hemopoietic system. These results were updated in 1977 (Cvitkovic et al., 1977, and personal communication) (Table 18.11). The median follow-up for the VAB IV was 16 months with the longest 23 months. Overall toxicity has been moderate with no toxic deaths.

Einhorn et al. (1976) utilized cis-platinum 20 mg/m² daily for 5 days, based on the Higby experience, vinblastine 0.2 mg/kg on days 1 and 2 every 3 weeks, plus bleomycin 30 mg intravenously weekly for 12 weeks, given 6 hours after the second dose of vinblastine. Maintenance consisted of vinblastine every 4 weeks with BCG by scarification for all patients with a complete remission (Table 18.12). The results were updated in 1977 (Einhorn and Donohue, 1977). Thirty-five of 47 evaluable patients (74%) had a complete remission; 29 of these remained alive and disease-free from 6+ to 30+ months. There were 4 deaths in the early part of the study, but none in the past 2 years. Meticulous follow-up and aggressive treatment with antibiotics after proper cultures have been obtained is

TABLE 18.10
Modified VAB III Combination Treatment Regimen in Testicular Tumors[a]

VAB IV	Vinblastine	4 mg/m² on day 1
	Actinomycin D	1 mg/m² on day 1
	Bleomycin	30 mg/m² push on day 1
		20 mg/m² in 24-hour infusion day 1–6
	Cyclophosphamide	600 mg/m² on day 1
	cis-Platinum	120 mg/m² on day 7 with mannitol diuresis
Maintenance:		
	Vinblastine	4 mg/m² every 3 weeks
	Chlorambucil	4 mg/m² for 1 of every 3 weeks
	plus	
	Actinomycin D	1 mg/m²⎱ alternating every 3 weeks
	Adriamycin	30 mg/m²⎰

[a] Induction repeated after 2 maintenance cycles.

TABLE 18.11
Results with VAB Regimens

Response[a]	Regimen			
	I	II	III	IV
Adequately treated	68	50	93	52
CR	15 (22%)	30 (60%)	57 (61%)	29 (56%)
PR	17 (25%)	15 (30%)	23 (25%)	14 (27%)
MR	36 (53%)	5 (10%)	13 (14%)	9 (17%)
No prior chemotherapy				
CR	13/30 (43%)	16/25 (64%)	27/45 (60%)	
PR	8/30 (26%)	9/25 (36%)	13/45 (29%)	
CR relapse rate	6/15 (40%)	13/30 (43%)	15/57 (26%)	4/29 (14%)

[a] CR, PR, and MR, complete, partial, and minor response, respectively.

TABLE 18.12
Combination Treatment—Einhorn Regimen

cis-Platinum	20 mg/m^2 in 15 min. daily for 5 doses	Every 3 weeks
Vinblastine[a]	0.2 mg/kg on day 1 and 2	
Bleomycin	30 mg weekly for 12 doses, 6 hours after VLB	

Total 3–4 courses

Maintenance with monthly vinblastine for 2 years with BCG 1, 2, and 3 weeks after vinblastine for the first 4 months and subsequently 1 and 3 weeks thereafter.

[a] VLB dose reduced to 0.15 mg/kg for 2 doses for patients who had prior radiation therapy.

necessary when patients develop fever. Only 3 of these 35 complete remissions have relapsed, all within 9 months of the initiation of the chemotherapy. Five of 12 patients with a partial remission were made disease-free after surgical removal of residual disease. Three of these 5 patients had only benign teratomatous elements and have remained disease-free from 9+ to 24+ months after surgery. Similar good results with combination chemotherapy and surgery for residual disease were reported by Bains et al. (1978).

Samson and Stephens (1978) reported for the Southwest Oncology Group with a slightly modified Einhorn regimen—32 complete and 17 partial remissions in 57 evaluable patients. Three of 32 patients with a complete remission and 8 of 17 with a partial remission relapsed. Median duration of the complete remissions was 20+ weeks with a range of 4+ to 60+ weeks.

Merrin et al. (1976, 1977) from Roswell Park Memorial Institute have used a combination of bleomycin, vinblastine, cis-platinum, Adriamycin, cyclophosphamide and actinomycin D, followed by reductive surgery. In 8 of 16 patients only benign tumors were found at surgery, indicating the effectivenss of this multisequential treatment in patients with far advanced disease.

TREATMENT OUTLINE

There is no controversy that Stage I and II seminoma is curable with radiation therapy. The dose may vary from 2000 to 3000 rads in 2–3 weeks with usually the higher dose for Stage II disease to the inguinal nodes on the involved side and the retroperitoneal nodes. Large lymph node masses may be boosted to 4000 rads in 4 weeks. The mediastinum and left supraclavicular area are included as a prophylaxis, usually 2000 rads in 2 weeks after a 4-week rest period, although not all investigators consider this necessary (Ytredal and Bradfield, 1972). For Stage III disease chlorambucil 0.15 mg/kg per day is indicated with or without local radiation therapy. However, the above described combinations with bleomycin and cis-platinum have also had excellent results in a limited number of patients with seminoma and would, therefore, be preferable, particularly in patients with extensive disease. Treatment of nonseminomatous tumors is much more controversial, particularly Stage II disease. Patients with clinical Stage I disease will usually undergo bilateral retroperitoneal lymph node dissection and no further therapy if all nodes and markers are negative. Stage II disease is variously treated with either preoperative radiation therapy, bilateral retroperitoneal lymphadenectomy followed by further radiation therapy (Maier and Mittemeyer, 1977) with or without chemotherapy for 2–3 years or retroperitoneal lymph node dissection followed by radiation therapy or retroperitoneal lymph node dissection followed by chemotherapy for 2–3 years. Three years adjuvant chemotherapy is chosen by some investigators because recurrences after this period of time are rare (Golbey, 1970). However, the number of relapses after 2 years is also very small. Preoperative radiation also exposes Stage I patients, who are cured with retroperitoneal node dissection alone in approximately 80% of the cases. Patients who relapse after radiation therapy tolerate the intensive chemotherapy necessary to cure these patients very poorly and can tolerate frequently only minor doses, insufficient for cure. The combination of actinomycin D and chlorambucil is often chosen because of the possibility of seminomatous admixtures for which alkylating agents are more effective. Unfortunately there are few data available from nonrandomized studies (Vugrin et al., 1978) and none from randomized studies to compare the value of these treatments. In an interesting study by Ansfield et al. (1969), 13 patients clinically free of disease received Li's (1960) triple therapy after the orchiectomy for periods up to 1 year. Two patients died after a tumor-free period of 3 and 6 months, one from brain metastasis. Three of the remaining 11 patients had positive lymph nodes, 2 had negative nodes and 6 had no node dissection. All 11 patients were still free of disease from 30 to 89 months (Ansfield, personal communication).

The value of intensive adjuvant chemotherapy with the VAB III or Einhorn regimens in Stage II patients after radical node dissection remains to be studied. However, if with close follow-up after lymphadenectomy relapsing patients are treated early when they may have minimal disease, the complete response rate is 100% (Einhorn, personal communication). Exposing all patients after lymphadenectomy to these intensive treatments may then not be necessary.

Possibly extensive clinical staging, as outlined before, plus selective retroperitoneal lymph node biopsies might give a sufficiently reliable stage, so that Stage I patients may not need to undergo further radical lymphadenectomy, thus sparing these patients sterility and that Stage II patients with a limited number of small nodes may be cured with postoperative radiation therapy (Tyrrell and Peckham, 1976), or with intensive chemotherapy or total lymph node dissection.

Stage II disease with large, inoperable, abdominal masses, Stage III disease, all stages of choriocarcinoma and probably Stage II patients who have residual elevation of α-fetoprotein and/or HCG after radical lymph node dissection are best treated with one of the vinblastine-bleomycin-cis-platinum-containing regimens, by preference in centers familiar with these intensive treatments and where further data can be gathered on the treatment of these relatively rare tumors.

In selected cases with Stage III disease, particularly when this is limited to one or two pulmonary lesions or when there are one or two residual pulmonary lesions after chemotherapy, excision of these lesions or whole lung radiation to 1500–2000 rads with local boosts have on several occasions led to prolonged disease-free survival (Woodhead et al., 1971; Cox et al., 1972; Van der Werf-Messing, 1973; Wharam et al., 1974). As benign teratomas are now found more frequently in these patients with residual disease after intensive treatment with these newer drug combinations (Merrin et al., 1975; Einhorn and Donohue, 1977; Bains et al., 1978), surgical exploration is preferable over radiation therapy which can then be limited to patients who have truly minimal residual disease.

The determination of serum markers preorchiectomy and if positive, postorchiectomy and postretroperitoneal node dissection, is strongly recommended. The value of these markers during chemotherapy and follow-up has been alluded to earlier.

REFERENCES

Ansfield, F. J., Korbitz, B. C., Davis, Jr., H. L., and Ramirez, G. Triple drug therapy in testicular tumors. Cancer, 24: 442–446, 1969.

Bailey, T. B., Pinsky, S. M., Mittemeyer, B. T., Borski, A. A., and Johnson M. A new adjuvant in testis tumor staging: Gallium-67 citrate. J. Urol., 110: 307–310, 1973.

Bains, M. S., McCormack, P. M., Cvitkovic, E., Golbey, R. B., and Martini, N. Results of combined chemo-surgical therapy for pulmonary metastases from testicular carcinoma. Cancer, 41: 850–853, 1978.

Blom, J. Late recurrence of testicular tumor. J. Urol., 112: 211, 1974.

Blom, J., and Brodovsky, H. S. Comparison of the treatment of metastatic testicular tumors with actinomycin D or actinomycin D, bleomycin, and vincristine (abstr.). Proc. Am. Soc. Clin. Oncol., 17: 290, 1976.

Boden, G., and Gibb, R. Radiotherapy and testicular neoplasms. Lancet, 2: 1195–1197, 1951.

Borski, A. A. Diagnosis, staging and natural history of testicular tumors. Cancer, 32: 1202–1205, 1973.

Brown, J. H., and Kennedy, B. J. Mithramycin in the treatment of disseminated testicular neoplasms. N. Engl. J. Med., 272: 111–117, 1965.

Buck, A. S., Schamber, D. T., Maier, J. G., and Lewis, E. L. Supraclavicular node biopsy and malignant testicular tumors. J. Urol., 107: 619–621, 1972.

Chabner, B. A., Canellos, G. P., Olweny, C. L. M., and DeVita, V. T. Late recurrence of testicular tumor. N. Engl. J. Med., 287: 413, 1972.

Cochran, J. S., Walsh, P. C., Parker, J. C., Nicholson, T. C., Madden, J. O., and Peters, P. C. The endocrinology of human chorionic gonadotropin-secreting testicular tumors; new methods in diagnosis. J. Urol., *114*: 549–555, 1975.

Cox, J. D., Gingerelli, F., Ream, N. W., and Maier, J. G. Total pulmonary irradiation for metastases from testicular carcinoma. Radiology, *105*: 163–167, 1972.

Curreri, A. R., and Ansfield, F. J. Mithramycin-human toxicology and preliminary therapeutic investigation. Cancer Chemother. Rep., *8*: 18–22, 1960.

Cvitkovic, E., Wittes, R., Golbey, R., and Krakoff, I. H. Primary combination chemotherapy (VAB II) for metastatic or unresectable germ cell tumors (abstr.). Proc. Am. Soc. Clin. Oncol., *16*: 174, 1975.

Cvitkovic, E., Hayes, D., and Golbey, R. 1976. Primary combination chemotherapy (VAB III) for metastatic or unresectable germ cell tumors (abstr.). Proc. Am. Soc. Clin. Oncol. *17*: 296, 1976.

Cvitkovic, E., Cheng, E., Whitmore, W. F., and Golbey, R. B. Germ cell tumor chemotherapy update (abstr.). Proc. Am. Soc. Clin. Oncol., *18*: 324, 1977.

Dixon, F. J., and Moore, R. A. Tumors of the male sex organs. Atlas of Tumor Pathology, Fascicles 31b and 32. Armed Forces Institute of Pathology, Washington, D. C., 1952.

Doornbos, J. F., Hussey, D. H., and Johnson, D. E. Radiotherapy for pure seminoma of the testis. Radiology, *116*: 401–404, 1975.

Dow, J. A., and Mostofi, F. K. Testicular tumors following orchiopexy. South. Med. J., *60*: 193–195, 1967.

Einhorn, L. H., and Donohue, J. cis-Diamminedichloroplatinum, vinblastine and bleomycin combination chemotherapy in disseminated testicular cancer. Ann. Intern. Med., *87*: 293–298, 1977.

Einhorn, L. H., Furnas, B. E., and Powell, N. Combination chemotherapy of disseminated testicular carcinoma with cis-platinum diamine chloride (CPDD), vinblastine (VLB), and bleomycin (Bleo) (abstr.). Proc. Am. Soc. Clin. Oncol., *17*: 240, 1976.

Fraley, E. E., Markland, C., and Lange, P. H. Surgical treatment of Stage I and Stage II nonseminomatous testicular cancer in adults. Urol. Clin. North Am., *4*: 453–463, 1977.

Fuchs, W. A., and Girod, M. Lymphography as a guide to prognosis in malignant testicular tumours. Acta Radiol., *16*: 305–312, 1975.

Giebink, G. S., and Ruymann, F. B. Testicular tumors in childhood. Am. J. Dis. Child., *127*: 433–438, 1974.

Golbey, R. B. The place of chemotherapy in the treatment of testicular tumors. J. A. M. A., *213*: 101–106, 1970.

Higby, D. J., Wallace, H. J., Albert, D. J., and Holland, J. F. Diaminodichloroplatinum; a phase I study showing responses in testicular and other tumors. Cancer, *33*: 1219–1225, 1974.

Hill II, G. J., Sedransk, N., Rochlin, D., Bisel, H., Andrews, N. C., Fletcher, W., Schroeder, J. M., and Wilson, W. L. Mithramycin (NSC 24559) therapy of testicular tumors. Cancer, *30*: 900–908, 1972.

Jacobs, E. M. Combination chemotherapy of metastatic testicular germinal cell tumors and soft part sarcomas. Cancer, *25*: 324–332, 1970.

Johnson, D. E., Gomez, J. J., and Ayala, A. G. Anaplastic seminoma. J. Urol., *114*: 80–82, 1975.

Kedia, K. R., Markland, C., and Fraley, E. E. Sexual function following high retroperitoneal lymphadenectomy. J. Urol., *114*: 237–239, 1975.

Kennedy, B. J., Griffen, W. O., and Lober, P. Specific effect of mithramycin in embryonal carcinoma of the testis. Cancer, *18*: 1631–1636, 1965.

Kennedy, B. J. Mithramycin therapy in advanced testicular neoplasms. Cancer, *26*: 755–766, 1970.

Kofman, S., and Eisenstein, R. Mithramycin in the treatment of disseminated cancer. Cancer Chemother. Rep., *32*: 77–96, 1963.

Kreel, L. The EMI whole body scanner in the demonstration of lymph node enlargement. Clin. Radiol., *27*: 421–429, 1976.

Lange, P. H., McIntire, K. R., Waldmann, T. A., Hakala, T. R., and Fraley, E. E. Serum alpha-fetoprotein and human chorionic gonadotropin in the diagnosis and management of nonseminomatous germ-cell testicular cancer. N. Engl. J. Med., *295*: 1237–1240, 1976.

Lefevre, R. E., Levin, H. S., Banowsky, L. H., Straffon, R. A., Stewart, B. H., and Hewitt, C. B. Bilateral testicular tumors of germ cell origin. J. Urol., *114*: 556–559, 1975.

Li, M. C., Whitmore, Jr., W. F., Golbey, R., and Grabstald, H. Effects of combined drug therapy on metastatic cancer of the testis. J. A. M. A., *174*: 1291–1299, 1960.

MacKay, E. H., and Sellers, A. H. A statistical review of malignant testicular tumours based on the experience of the Ontario Cancer Foundation Clinics, 1938–1961. Can. Med. Assoc. J., *94*: 889–899, 1966.

Mackenzie, A. R. Chemotherapy of metastatic testis cancer; results in 154 patients. Cancer, *19*: 1369–1376, 1966.

Maier, J. G., and Mittemeyer, B. Carcinoma of the testis. Cancer, *39*: 981–986, 1977.

Maier, J. G., and Schamber, D. T. The role of lymphangiography in the diagnosis and treatment of malignant testicular tumors. A.J.R., *114*: 482–491, 1972.

Maier, J. G., and Sulak, M. H. Radiation therapy in malignant testis tumors; I. Seminoma. Cancer, *32*: 1212–1216, 1973a.

Maier, J. G., and Sulak, M. H. Radiation therapy in malignant testis tumors; II. Carcinoma. Cancer, *32*: 1217–1226, 1973b.

Maier, J. G., Mittemeyer, B. T., and Sulak, M. H. Treatment and prognosis in seminoma of the testis. J. Urol., *99*: 72–78, 1968a.

Maier, J. G., Sulak, M. H., and Mittemeyer, B. T. Seminoma of the testis; analysis of treatment success and failure. A.J.R., *102*: 596–602, 1968b.

Mendelson, D., and Serpick, A. A. Combination chemotherapy of testicular tumors. J. Urol., *103*: 619–623, 1970.

Merrin, C., Baumgartner, G., and Wajsman, Z. Benign transformation of testicular carcinoma by chemotherapy. Lancet, *1*: 43–44, 1975.

Merrin, C., Takita, H., Weber, R., Wajsman, Z., Baumgartner, G., and Murphy, G. P. Combination radical surgery and multiple sequential chemotherapy for the treatment of advanced carcinoma of the testis (stage III). Cancer, *37*: 20–29, 1976.

Merrin, C., Takita, H., Beckley, S., and Kassis, J. Treatment of recurrent and widespread testicular tumor by radical reductive surgery and multiple sequential chemotherapy. J. Urol., *117*: 291–295, 1977.

Monfardini, S., Bajetta, E., Musumeci, R., and Bonadonna, G. Clinical use of adriamycin in advanced testicular cancer. J. Urol., *108*: 293–296, 1972.

Mostofi, F. K. Testicular tumors—epidemiologic, etiologic, and pathologic features. Cancer, *32*: 1186–1201, 1973.

Myers, R. P., and Kelalis, P. P. Cryptorchidism reassessed. Mayo Clin. Proc., *48*: 94–97, 1973.

Parker, G. W., Wiltsie, D. S., and Jackson, Jr., C. B. The clinical evaluation of PA-144 (mithramycin) in solid tumors of adults. Cancer Chemother. Rep., *8*: 23–26, 1960.

Paterson, A. H. G., Peckham, M. J., McCready, V. R. Value of gallium scanning in seminoma of the testis. Br. Med. J., *1*: 1118–1121, 1976.

Perlin, E., Engeler, Jr., J. E., Edson, M., Karp, D., McIntire, K. R., and Waldmann, T. A. The value of serial measurement of both human chorionic gonadotropin and alpha-fetoprotein for monitoring germinal cell tumors. Cancer, *37*: 215–219, 1976.

Pitts, N. Clinical data accumulated by Pfizer for NDA for mithramycin, Nov. 5, 1970.

Proceedings of the Chemotherapy Conference on (1) Mithramycin (Mithracin): Development and Application and (2) Symposium on the Theory of Testicular Neoplasms, edited by S. K. Carter and M. A. Friedman. Cancer Therapy Evaluations Branch, National Cancer Institute, Bethesda, Md.

Ray, B., Hajdu, S. I., and Whitmore, Jr., W. F. Distribution of retroperitoneal lymph node metastases in testicular germinal tumors. Cancer, *33*: 340–348, 1974.

Ream, N., Perlin, C., Wolter, J., and Taylor, S. Mithramycin therapy in disseminated germinal testicular cancer. J.A.M.A., *204*: 1030–1036, 1968.

Sabio, H., Burgert, Jr., E. O., Farrow, G. M., and Kelalis, P. P. Embryonal carcinoma of the testis in childhood. Cancer, *34*: 2118–2121, 1974.

Safer, M. L., Green, J. P., Crews, Jr., Q. E., and Hill, D. R. Lymphangiographic accuracy in the staging of testicular tumors. Cancer, *35*: 1603–1605, 1975.

Sampson, M. K., and Stephens R. L. Vinblastine (VLB), bleomycin (BLEO) and cis-diamminedichloroplatinum II (DDP) in disseminated testicular cancer (abstr.). Proc. Am. Assoc. Cancer Res., *19*: 12, 1978.

Samuels, M. L., and Howe, C. D. Vinblastine in the management of testicular cancer. Cancer, *25*: 1009–1017, 1970.

Samuels, M. L., Johnson, D. E., and Holoye, P. Y. The treatment of stage 3 metastatic germinal cell neoplasia of the testis with bleomycin combination chemotherapy (abstr.). Proc. Am. Assoc. Cancer Res. *14*: 23, 1973.

Samuels, M. L., Johnson, D. E., and Holoye, P. Y. Continuous intravenous bleomycin (NSC-125066) therapy with vinblastine (NSC-49842) in stage III testicular neoplasia. Cancer Chemother. Rep., *59*: 563–570, 1975a.

Samuels, M. L., Holoye, P. Y., and Johnson, D. E. Bleomycin combination chemotherapy in the management of testicular neoplasia. Cancer, *36*: 318–326, 1975b.

Silvay, O., Yagoda, A., Wittes, R., Whitmore, W., and Golbey, R. Treatment of germ cell carcinomas with a combination of actinomycin D, vinblastine, and bleomycin (abstr.). Proc. Am. Assoc. Cancer Res., *14*: 68, 1973.

Skinner, D. G. and Leadbetter, W. F. The surgical management of testis tumors. J. Urol., *100*: 84–93, 1971.

Spigel, S. C., and Coltman, Jr., C. A. Vinblastine (NSC 49842) and bleomycin (NSC 125066) therapy for disseminated testicular tumors. Cancer Chemother. Rep., *58*: 213–216, 1974.

Staubitz, W. J., Early, K. S., Magoss, I. V., and Murphy, C. P. Surgical treatment of nonseminomatous germinal testes tumors. Cancer, *32*: 1206–1211, 1973.

Staubitz, W. J., Early, K. S., Magoss, I. V., and Murphy, G. P. Surgical management of testis tumor. J. Urol., *111*: 205–208, 1974.

Talerman, A., and Haije, W. G. Alpha-fetoprotein and germ cell tumors; a possible role of yolk sac tumor in production of alpha-fetoprotein. Cancer, *34*: 1722–1726, 1974.

Tyrrell, C. J., and Peckham, M. J. The response of lymph node metastases of testicular teratoma to radiation therapy. Br. J. Urol., *48*: 363–370, 1976.

Van der Werf-Messing, B. The treatment of pulmonary metastases of malignant teratoma of the testis. Clin. Radiol., *24*: 121–123, 1973.

Vechinski, T. O., Jaeschke, W. H., and Vermund, H. Testicular tumors—an analysis of 112 consecutive cases. A.J.R., *95*: 494–514, 1965.

Vugrin, D., Cvitkovic, E., Whitmore, W., Jr., and Golbey, R. B. Prophylactic chemotherapy of testicular germ cell carcinomas (nonseminomas) stage II following orchiectomy and retroperitoneal dissection. Am. Soc. Clin. Oncol., *19*: 352, 1978.

Wharam, M. D., Phillips, T. L., and Jacobs, E. M. Combination chemotherapy and whole lung irradiation for pulmonary metastases from sarcomas and germinal cell tumors of the testis. Cancer, *34*: 136–142, 1974.

Wilkinson, D. J., and MacDonald, J. S. A review of the role of lymphography in the management of testicular tumours. Clin. Radiol., *26:* 89–98, 1975.

Wittes, R. E., Yagoda, A., Silvay, O., Magill, G. B., Whitmore, W., Krakoff, I. H., and Golbey, R. B. Chemotherapy of germ cell tumors of the testis; I. Induction of Remissions with vinblastine, actinomycin D, and bleomycin. Cancer, *37:* 637–645, 1976.

Woodhead, D. M., Johnson, D. E., Pohl, D. R., and Robison, J. R. Aggressive management of advanced testicular malignancy; experience with 147 patients. Milit. Med., *136:* 634–638, 1971.

Ytredal, D. O., and Bradfield, J. S. Seminoma of the testicle; prophylactic mediastinal irradiation versus periaortic and pelvic irradiation alone. Cancer, *30:* 628–633, 1972.

Chapter 19

Gynecologic Malignancies

WILLIAM M. PETTY, M.D., and ROBERT C. PARK, M.D.

CERVICAL CANCER

Before the pap smear was widely used for detecting cervical neoplasms, cancer of the uterus (cervix and endometrium combined) was the leading cause of cancer deaths in women. Cervical cancer is now decreased to the sixth most common cancer in women. The incidence of cervical cancer was formerly 5 times that of endometrial cancer. Today its incidence is actually less than that of endometrial cancer (Silverberg and Holleb, 1974).

Squamous cell carcinoma is the main histologic cell type, accounting for more than 90% of cervical cancer. Cervical adenocarcinoma occurs approximately 5% of the time; this histologic type will be discussed separately when indicated. Table 19.1 depicts the staging system for cervical cancer as recommended by the International Federation of Gynecology and Obstetrics (FIGO).

Both early onset of intercourse and intercourse with multiple partners are associated with an increased incidence of squamous cell carcinoma. The role of herpes progenitalis, that is, herpesvirus type 2 (HV-2), in causing cervical cancer is being studied. Rawls et al. (1970) found that 83% of patients with invasive squamous cell carcinoma of the cervix had antibodies to HV-2 and about one-third of the patients with carcinoma in situ had antibodies to HV-2. This level was higher than in either higher or lower socioeconomic controls. They feel that herpesvirus may act as a carcinogen in some cases of squamous cell cancer. On the other hand, Amstey et al. (1973) discovered that 28 patients with intraepithelial neoplasia of the cervix had HV-2 smears only after the neoplastic diagnosis was made. Twenty-four of these patients had a primary type herpes infection, so they report that HV-2 infections occur more commonly after atypical changes have occurred. This suggests a greater susceptibility of atypical epithelium to HV-2 infection. Aurelian et al. (1971) have actually

TABLE 19.1
Carcinoma of the Cervix Uteri (FIGO)

Stage	Description
0	Carcinoma in situ, intraepithelial carcinoma
I	The carcinoma is strictly confined to the cervix (extension to the corpus should be disregarded)
IA	Microinvasive carcinoma (early stromal invasion)
IB	All other cases of Stage I; occult cancer should be marked "occ"
II	The carcinoma extends beyond the cervix, but has not extended to the pelvic wall. The carcinoma involves the vagina, but not as far as the lower third
IIA	No obvious parametrial involvement
IIB	Obvious parametrial involvement
III	The carcinoma has extended to the pelvic wall. On rectal examination, there is no cancer-free space between the tumor and the pelvic wall. The tumor involves the lower third of the vagina. All cases with a hydronephrosis or nonfunctioning kidney are included
IIIA	No extension to the pelvic wall
IIIB	Extension to the pelvic wall and/or hydronephrosis or nonfunctioning kidney
IV	The carcinoma has extended beyond the true pelvis or has clinically involved the mucosa of the bladder or rectum. A bullous edema as such does not permit a case to be allotted to Stage IV
IVA	Spread of the growth to adjacent organs
IVB	Spread to distant organs

isolated HV-2 from cervical tumor cells. The relationship between HV-2 and cervical carcinoma remains to be further elucidated.

The relationship of invasive squamous cell cancer to identifiable precursors is important in population screening. Carcinoma in situ of the cervix is the most common precursor of invasive cancer. Abell (1973) estimates that 85–90% of cancers arise from carcinoma in situ. Not all have an in situ phase. Some infiltrate into the cervical stroma after the cancerous change takes place in the parabasal cells (Abell, 1973). Cervical pap smears may not accurately reflect the degree of epithelial abnormality in these cases since cancer is not present on the surface of these invasive lesions.

Treatment of low stages of invasive cancer can be accomplished by either pelvic radiotherapy or radical hysterectomy. Greater than 90% 5-year survivals and comparably low 2–3% major morbidity rates are reported in treatment of Stage I disease with either radiotherapy (Fletcher, 1971; Easley and Fletcher, 1971) or surgery (Park et al., 1973). With either modality a well organized approach to treatment and compulsive, meticulous attention to detail are essential to achieve the highest cure rates with lowest morbidity rates.

Both radiotherapy and surgery are used for Stage II A cervical cancer. Radiotherapy is the treatment of choice for cervical cancer above Stage

II A. Recurrent cancer postoperatively or symptomatic unirradiated metastases are best controlled with radiotherapy. The patient with cervical cancer involving the bladder or rectum with no lateral spread may be treated by primary exenterative surgery as well as by radiotherapy. Central pelvic cancer recurrences post radiotherapy may be cured by pelvic exenteration.

Presently, chemotherapy is used for palliation of cervical cancer and is being evaluated as an adjunct to radiotherapy. Hreshchyshyn (1968, 1975b) and Piver et al. (1974) have reported improved radiotherapy effectiveness in patients who received adjunctive hydroxyurea when undergoing radiotherapy. Malkasian et al. (1968a) found lower response rates in patients treated with both 5-fluorouracil and radiotherapy than in those treated with radiotherapy alone.

Single drugs and multiple drug combinations are used in widely disseminated and recurrent carcinoma. Objective responses to cyclophosphamide, methotrexate, 5-fluorouracil (Livingston and Carter, 1970), hexamethylmelamine (Stolinsky and Bateman, 1973), and Adriamycin (Barlow et al., 1973) as single agents occur in 20–25% of patients. Barlow et al. (1973) found that the response rate to bleomycin and to a combination of Adriamycin and bleomycin was less than to Adriamycin alone. They concluded that Adriamycin is more effective than bleomycin in cervical carcinoma. Tormey et al. (1973) reported a patient with a complete response to Adriamycin-bleomycin.

Although the results of systemic chemotherapy are generally not encouraging, Piel et al. (1973) used methotrexate and bleomycin and reported that 3 of 8 patients had complete responses and 2 had partial responses. Piver et al. (1978) reported the use of multiple regimens of Adriamycin, bleomycin, cyclophosphamide, vincristine, and 5-fluorouracil in 100 patients with carcinoma of the cervix and vagina. The overall response rate was 9%. But in the small series of 7 patients with a 5-day regimen of cyclophosphamide, Adriamycin and 5-fluorouracil, 1 patient had a complete response and 3 had a partial response. They therefore found that Adriamycin in conjunction with cyclophosphamide gave the best response rate.

Solidoro et al. (1966) compared chemotherapy tumor response to prior radiotherapy response. They found that patients who had no control of pelvic tumor by radiotherapy had no response to cyclophosphamide. Almost one-half of the patients who responded to radiotherapy with even temporary pelvic control did respond to chemotherapy. They found that none of the patients with pelvic or abdominal-pelvic disease had chemotherapy responses. All the responders had either disseminated tumor or pulmonary metastasis.

The subjective response rate to alkylating agents, 5-fluorouracil or methotrexate is twice the objective response rate. Smith (1969a) reported that 50% of patients with pain had excellent pain control for at least 3 months with cyclophosphamide. None of the patients who obtained pain relief required cordotomy.

Intra-arterial pelvic infusions of single and combination agent chemotherapy have been attempted. Response rates are greater than 50% to methotrexate (Hodgkinson and Boyce, 1965; Masterson and Nelson, 1965), alkylating agents (Frick et al., 1965), or multiple agents (Cavanagh et al., 1965). Intermittent methotrexate and vincristine have also been used (Averette et al., 1970). Some decrease in pain from the tumor is reported. Except for a patient reported by Bateman et al. (1966) who had enough tumor shrinkage to undergo a pelvic exenteration and survived 10 years afterward, it is felt this procedure does not give significant palliation or prolongation of survival time.

CHORIOCARCINOMA—GESTATIONAL TROPHOBLASTIC DISEASE

Gestational choriocarcinoma is a tumor which arises from placental tissue and is composed of cytotrophoblast and syncytiotrophoblast without the evidence of chorionic villi. Approximately one-half of the cases follow delivery of a hydatidiform mole, a generally unaggressive placental neoplasm which contains distended, grapelike chorionic villi. The remaining cases of gestational choriocarcinoma occur following normal pregnancies, ectopic pregnancies or abortions. Five hundred to 750 cases of malignant trophoblastic disease are estimated to occur yearly in the United States (Hammond and Parker, 1970). Choriocarcinoma arising primarily from the ovary, without preceding pregnancy, behaves like an embryonal carcinoma of the ovary and should be treated as such. It is discussed under ovarian carcinoma.

A hydatidiform mole which invades the uterine musculature, i.e., an invasive mole or chorioadenoma destruens, can cause fatal hemorrhage or sepsis. So chorioadenoma destruens must also be considered a potentially lethal disease. Often the endometrial cavity of the uterus will not contain any choriocarcinoma or chorioadenoma destruens when the neoplasm presents. This makes a histologic diagnosis impossible by uterine curettage. When a histologic diagnosis of choriocarcinoma or chorioadenoma destruens cannot be made on uterine curettings the more general diagnosis of malignant trophoblastic disease should be made.

Human chorionic gonadotropin (HCG) is produced by malignant trophoblastic disease as it is by the normal placenta. Measurement of HCG in serum allows careful monitoring of the tumor since HCG production is proportional to the volume of tumor present.

Urine pregnancy tests can accurately measure HCG titers to as low as 1000 IU per liter. However, 25–30% of patients with active trophoblastic disease will have HCG titers below this level (Hammond and Parker, 1970), so the more sensitive tests, including radioimmunoassay (RAI) or β subunit assays are required to adequately evaluate these patients. RAI tests for HCG cross-react with luteinizing hormone (LH) because of the similarity of these hormones. A β subunit assay, specific for HCG and not affected by LH, has been developed by Vaitukaitis et al. (1972).

The diagnosis of malignant trophoblastic disease is infrequently made histologically from a uterine dilatation and curettage specimen. More commonly it is made by a positive HCG titer in a patient with symptoms of bleeding or pain from a metastatic site and a history of prior pregnancy. The lungs and vagina are the most common metastatic sites; the pelvis, central nervous system, gastrointestinal tract, and liver are less commonly involved. Patients with metastatic CNS lesions may present with paralysis, convulsions, mental changes, or headaches.

Patients at highest risk for development of malignant trophoblastic disease are those who have delivered hydatidiform moles. Forty percent of patients with positive titers at 60 days after evacuation of a mole developed choriocarcinoma or an invasive mole (Delfs, 1959). Treatment is given after evacuation of a hydatidiform mole if: (1) metastasis is found by physical examination or x-ray, (2) an increasing HCG titer indicates proliferation of residual tissue, (3) a stable HCG titer indicates lack of trophoblastic tissue regression, or (4) an HCG titer is persistent at 6–8 weeks, unless a rapid fall is occurring and very close follow-up is possible.

Prophylactic Chemotherapy

Goldstein (1971) has studied the use of prophylactic chemotherapy at the time of delivery of a hydatidiform mole to prevent trophoblastic disease, as initially proposed by Lewis et al. (1966). Three patient groups were given chemotherapy for 5 consecutive days. One received methotrexate, 0.3 mg/kg/day, intramuscularly, another received actinomycin D, 9 μg/kg/day intravenously and the third received actinomycin D, 12 μg/kg/day intravenously. The mole was evacuated on the third day of the 5-day course of drugs. No subsequent metastatic trophoblastic disease occurred in any group. However, evidence of persistent nonmetastatic trophoblastic disease, i.e., tumor clinically confined to the uterus, was found in each group. The high dose actinomycin D group had the lowest incidence of persistent nonmetastatic trophoblastic disease in the uterus. In a later study, Goldstein (1974) reported that only 2 patients developed nonmetastatic trophoblastic disease of 100 who received high dose actinomycin D prophylactically. In contrast, of 100 patients who did not receive prophylactic treatment, 4 developed metastatic trophoblastic disease and 12 developed nonmetastatic trophoblastic disease. He suggested the use of prophylactic chemotherapy in high risk or poor follow-up patients but emphasized that prophylactic chemotherapy is not a substitute for close follow-up. Because prophylactic methotrexate has been associated with several deaths and high dose actinomycin D appears the most effective regimen, high dose actinomycin D appears to be the preferred drug regimen if prophylactic treatment is used.

The prophylactic use of chemotherapy with termination of a molar pregnancy is controversial. All patients followed closely after evacuation of a hydatidiform mole and who later developed trophoblastic disease have survived following appropriate therapy (C. B. Hammond, unpublished data).

Nonmetastatic Trophoblastic Disease

If the patient has no further desire for childbearing then a hysterectomy may be an appropriate means of treatment. Most women desire to maintain their reproductive potential, however, so curative chemotherapy is more commonly used. Nonmetastatic trophoblastic disease is curable from 93 to 100% of the time with single-agent methotrexate (Hammond et al., 1967) or actinomycin D (Goldstein et al., 1972). Methotrexate is usually administered at the rate of 0.3–0.4 mg/kg (maximum 25 mg) per day intramuscularly daily for 5 days. Actinomycin D is given at the rate of 10–12 μg/kg per day, intravenously daily for 5 days. The next course of either drug is started after bone marrow recovery is documented—usually 10–14 days after the onset of the previous course.

The patient is followed with weekly β subunit serum HCG, complete blood count with differential count and platelet count, and physical examination. A chest x-ray should be obtained before each course of drugs to exclude new pulmonary metastases which would indicate drug resistance.

Treatment continues until the patient's HCG titer has reached normal levels. More recently, patients have been treated one course past a normal HCG titer if it is felt the patient can safely tolerate an additional course. This is to ensure adequacy of treatment since several patients have had persistent disease despite achieving normal HCG titers and presumably therefore having no further tumor (C. B. Hammond, personal communication).

If the tumor becomes resistant to the chemotherapeutic agent being used then the other agent should be considered for use. If the patient is unable to use the other drug (e.g., liver or renal impairment) or her tumor becomes resistant to both drugs then a hysterectomy should be considered.

Metastatic Trophoblastic Disease

Metastatic trophoblastic disease has good and poor prognostic factors which may alter treatment. Patients with an initial HCG titer greater than 100,000 IU or with a duration of disease greater than 4 months, have a worse prognosis (Hertz et al., 1961). The presence of brain and liver metastases are also poor prognostic factors.

Hammond et al. (1973) using single agent methotrexate or actinomycin D cured 70 of 71 patients who had metastatic trophoblastic disease without the above poor prognostic factors. Either drug may be used with a comparable response rate and is used as described above under non-metastatic trophoblastic disease. Actinomycin D is used if evidence of hepatic injury is present because methotrexate is more hepatotoxic. Patients with HCG titers which are not falling or which are rising or who have evidence of new metastases under treatment should be changed from one drug to the other.

Hammond et al. (1973) initially treated patients with poor prognosis metastatic disease with single agent actinomycin D and chlorambucil was used if tumor resistance or progression occurred. Only 1 of 7 patients survived who were treated in this manner. He then used the above triple therapy initially. Methotrexate was given at 15 mg IM per day, actinomycin D 0.5 mg IV per day, and chlorambucil 10 mg PO per day. All are given daily for 5 days and then repeated after the bone marrow has recovered from toxicity. He changed to actinomycin D when drug toxicity occurred. This gave better results. Seven of 10 patients survived. He therefore recommends initial use of triple therapy in patients with poor prognosis disease. When brain or liver metastases are present, low dose irradiation of that organ at the onset of chemotherapy is also recommended to prevent fatal hemorrhage.

Follow-up Guidelines for All Patients

Patients are considered to be in complete remission when 3 weekly normal HCG titers have occurred. HCG titers should be obtained monthly the first 6 months after remission and bimonthly the next 6 months. Pregnancy should be prevented the first year so that any recurrence can be promptly determined.

Oral contraceptive agents should be considered for fertility control if there is no contraindication to their use. These drugs depress serum LH so that the nonspecific HCG radioimmunoassay titers will not be falsely elevated. Because they are effective contraceptive agents, the difficult problem of differentiating early pregnancy from recurrent neoplasm may be avoided.

ENDOMETRIAL CANCER

Adenocarcinoma of the uterine endometrium classically occurs in the postmenopausal, obese, hypertensive, diabetic female who has been infertile, with late menopause or excessive bleeding at the time of menopause. Patients may exhibit all, several, or none of these characteristics.

Abnormal uterine bleeding is the most common sign of uterine cancer. The abnormal bleeding presents as increased frequency or amount of flow in the menstruating female and as postmenopausal bleeding in the postmenopausal female.

Since the endometrium is a hormone responsive tissue, patients with constant or hyperestrogen states have been studied for endometrial cancer. Significant numbers of patients with estrogen-producing ovarian tumors, ovarian or hepatic abnormalities giving rise to high or constant estrogen levels, or patients who are taking oral estrogen preparations develop endometrial cancer. No causal relationship has been proven.

Different estrogen metabolism may occur in patients with this tumor. Estrogen metabolism studies indicate that androstenedione is a major precursor for estrogen in postmenopausal women. Women with endometrial cancer exhibit a significantly increased conversion of androstenedione to estrone (Hausknecht and Gusberg, 1973).

Benign endometrial conditions which precede carcinoma have been studied in an effort to determine precancerous lesions. Hertig and Sommers (1949) studied prior dilatation and curettage specimens of patients with endometrial carcinoma. Seventeen of 32 patients had cystic hyperplasia 6–13 years before the carcinoma. On the other hand, adenomatous hyperplasia occurred in 19 of 32 patients just 3–5 years before the cancer was discovered. Gusberg and Kaplan (1963) found that 12% of patients with adenomatous endometrial hyperplasia later developed adenocarcinoma. These studies suggest that adenomatous hyperplasia is sometimes a precursor to endometrial cancer. The staging of endometrial cancer is depicted in Table 19.2.

Surgery and Radiotherapy

Hysterectomy alone is effective treatment for Stage I endometrial cancer which is moderately well differentiated and invades less than one half the uterine wall (Keller et al., 1974). A combination of radiotherapy (external, internal, or both) and surgery give the best patient survival rates when the tumor is anaplastic or deeply invasive. Radiotherapy significantly reduces both vaginal and pelvic recurrences. Adjunctive progesterone therapy for a 14-week period of time has not been shown to increase survival in Stage I disease (Lewis et al., 1974).

Stage II adenocarcinoma may be treated by radical surgery, radiotherapy alone, or combined radiotherapy and simple surgery. The latter approach allows removal of the central tumor and detection of lymph node metastases out of the pelvic radiotherapy field. Postoperative radiotherapy may then be given to these untreated areas. Whether operative removal of large nodal metastases increases survival rates is not known. Advanced cancers (Stages III and IV) have the best chance of cure if treated by radiotherapy alone if the tumor is localized to the pelvic area.

TABLE 19.2
Carcinoma of the Corpus Uteri (FIGO)

Stage	Description
0	Carcinoma in situ. Histologic findings are suspicious of malignancy; cases of Stage 0 should not be included in any therapeutic statistics
I	The carcinoma is confined to the corpus
IA	The length of the uterine cavity is 8 cm or less.
IB	The length of the uterine cavity is more than 8 cm. It is desirable that the Stage I cases be subgrouped with regard to the histologic type of the adenocarcinoma as follows: GI—Highly differentiated adenomatous carcinoma G2—Differentiated adenomatous carcinoma with partly solid areas G3—Predominantly solid or entirely undifferentiated carcinoma
II	The carcinoma has involved the corpus and the cervix but has not extended outside the uterus
III	The carcinoma has extended outside the uterus but not outside the true pelvis
IV	The carcinoma has extended outside the true pelvis or has obviously involved the mucosa of the bladder or rectum. A bullous edema as such does not permit a case to be allotted to Stage IV
IVA	Spread of the growth to adjacent organs
IVB	Spread to distant organs

Chemotherapy

Chemotherapy has been used for disseminated or recurrent carcinoma. Cytotoxic drugs have been evaluated as single agents in very few patients. Alkylating agents, purine and pyrimidine antagonists, and antitumor antibiotics have been used with little success (Masterson and Nelson, 1965; Frick et al., 1965). Malkasian et al. (1968a) indicated a low response rate and a short response duration, 38% for 3 months, 29% for 4 months, for patients treated with 5-fluorouracil.

In collected series reviewed by the National Cancer Institute (NCI), only cyclophosphamide, 5-fluorouracil and Adriamycin had been adequately evaluated to be considered as possibly active (DeVita et al., 1976). Further study of Adriamycin as a single agent was carried out by the Gynecologic Oncology Group and definite activity was documented (Thigpen et al., 1979). Combination chemotherapy has been tried in relatively small numbers of patients. Adriamycin + cyclophosphamide yielded 6 responses in 8 patients (Lloyd et al., 1975; Muggia et al., 1974). Two other combinations have been tested at Mt. Sinai School of Medicine, including cyclophosphamide + Adriamycin + 5-fluorouracil and melphalan + 5-fluorouracil (Bruckner, et al., 1977; Cohen et al., 1977). Both were highly active in small numbers of patients, but results are clouded by the inclusion of progestin (Megace). A number of clinical trials are currently underway utilizing cytoxic agents in the treatment of this disease. At the present time, however, data are too early to evaluate.

Hormone Therapy

Progesterone is more frequently effective than cytotoxic chemotherapy. Overall response rates are 30–35%. Several factors are associated with a higher probability of response. Younger, perimenopausal women frequently respond whereas older, postmenopausal women rarely respond to progesterone. Smith (1969b) has found that the site of metastasis or recurrence does not influence the frequency of response. However, others have found that pulmonary and osseous metastases respond more frequently than pelvic recurrences (Kelley and Baker, 1961; Kennedy, 1968). Well differentiated lesions respond better than poorly differentiated lesions. Late recurrences may respond better than early ones.

Patients who respond to progesterone have longer average survivals than do nonresponders. Smith et al. (1966) indicate that 8 patients who had an objective remission for 9 months survived for more than 2 years. The average survival rates were 25.4 months for responders and 6.6 months for nonresponders (Smith, 1969b). Kennedy (1968) found similar results. Smith (1969b) reported that 3 of 6 patients who had early and complete responses to progesterone had their progesterone stopped after 4 years. None had a recurrence. These results suggest that patients who respond to progesterone may have an increased length of survival and, indeed, may have complete abolition of tumor.

A subjective response to progesterone occurs frequently with or without an objective response. This is manifested by an improved sense of well being, increased appetite and weight gain. Kennedy (1968) found a mean survival rate of 14.1 months in patients with a subjective response and only 3.7 months in patients with no subjective response. Whether this indicates that progesterone has an unmeasurable tumor effect is not known.

A histologic response to progesterone is usually found within 2–4 weeks of therapy (Trelford, 1970; Varga and Henriksen, 1965). Objective clinical responses are perceptible only after 2–3 months of treatment, however. Treatment should be continued as long as an objective or subjective response occurs.

The effects of progesterone on endometrial cancer may be direct or indirect. The antiestrogenic action of progesterone may directly effect the tumor. Other direct effects on endometrial cancer are thought to occur (Taylor et al., 1971).

Medroxyprogesterone acetate (Depo-Provera), 500–1000 mg deep IM every 1–2 weeks; hydroxyprogesterone (Delalutin), and megestrol acetate (Megace), 120–180 mg daily by mouth, are progesterone compounds used in endometrial carcinoma. Treatment should be continued for 12–16 weeks before considering it a failure.

When response to a progestational agent fails, an increase in dosage of drug or changing to a different form of progesterone may be useful. Adding additional chemotherapy such as an alkylating agent to the progesterone may induce an additional remission.

FALLOPIAN TUBE CARCINOMA

Fallopian tube carcinoma is the rarest gynecologic malignancy. It accounts for approximately 0.3% of all gynecologic cancer. The most common presenting symptoms are low abdominal pain and abnormal vaginal bleeding or discharge. A pelvic mass, usually lateral, is the most common physical finding. The classical finding of hydrops tubae profluens, sudden relief of abdominal pain associated with a gush of fluid from the vagina and disappearance of a pelvic mass, is less common. This triad occurs more commonly with a hydrosalpinx than fallopian tube carcinoma. Yellow colored or bloody fluid suggests early tubal cancer.

Tubal cancer has occurred in women from ages 18 to 80 (Gusberg and Frick, 1978b). It most frequently occurs in women in their sixth decade. A history of infertility or not carrying pregnancies to term occurs in over half the patients.

No standard staging system exists. Schiller and Silverberg (1971) have correlated 5-year survival without disease with the initial tumor extent histologically. In tumor limited to the tubal mucosa survival was 82%, with submucosal or muscular invasion but no serosal involvement 53%, with serosal involvement 16%, with extension to the ovary or endometrium 8%, and with extragenital spread 9%. An average survival rate of several series is 25%. Fifty percent of patients die of their disease within 2 years of diagnosis.

Surgical removal of the uterus, tubes, and ovaries is the treatment of choice. Postoperative irradiation may be beneficial (Dodson et al., 1970). Phelps and Chapman (1974) reported an excellent 90% survival rate: 8 of 9 patients who had pelvic tumor only and received postoperative radiotherapy. They recommend both the use of radioactive colloids and pelvic irradiation since cancer recurrence is predominantly intraperitoneal. None of 6 patients survived who had tumor spread to the abdominal cavity despite having received both radiotherapy and chemotherapy.

Hanton et al. (1966) found that nitrogen mustard, 5-fluorouracil, thio-TEPA, and cyclophosphamide did not cause any significant tumor regression. However, Tururen (1969) reported encouraging results with cyclophosphamide as did Boronow (1973) with melphalan (Alkeran). Dodson et al. (1970) reported a 2-year survivor with extra-abdominal metastases who received melphalan after surgery and radiotherapy. Synthetic progestational preparations have been used in combination with alkylating agents, however, the efficacy of these regimens is unproven.

OVARIAN CANCER

Ovarian malignancy is the leading cause of gynecologic cancer deaths, although it is only the third most common gynecologic malignancy. The low overall 5-year survival rate of 20–30% occurs largely because so many patients are diagnosed only in late stages of the disease when symptoms first appear and curability is low. The common symptoms of ovarian neoplasm include abdominal discomfort, vague gastrointestinal complaints, increasing abdominal girth from ascites or abdominal mass, and unexplained weight loss. Early ovarian carcinoma is usually identified as an asymptomatic mass found at the time of pelvic examination.

One percent of women develop ovarian cancer. Eighty to 90% of primary ovarian cancers are epithelial tumors. They are serous, mucinous, endometrioid, mesonephric, and undifferentiated types histologically. The less common types of ovarian cancer are discussed later. Refer to Table 19.3 for staging of this tumor.

Epithelial Tumors

Each histologic type of epithelial tumor is classified into (1) benign tumor, (2) tumor of low malignant potential which has proliferating

TABLE 19.3
Carcinoma of the Ovary (FIGO)

Stage	Description
I	Growth limited to the ovaries
IA	Growth limited to one ovary; no ascites
	i. No tumor on the external surface; capsule intact.
	ii. Tumor present on the external surface, or capsule(s) ruptured, or both
IB	Growth limited to both ovaries; no ascites
	i. No tumor on the external surface; capsule intact
	ii. Tumor present on the external surface, or capsule(s) ruptured, or both
IC	Tumor either Stage IA or Stage IB, but with ascites[a] present or with positive peritoneal washings
II	Growth involving one or both ovaries with pelvic extension
IIA	Extension and/or metastases to the uterus and/or tubes
IIB	Extension to other pelvic tissues
IIC	Tumor either Stage IIA or Stage IIB, but with ascites present or with positive peritoneal washings
III	Growth involving one or both ovaries with intraperitoneal metastases outside the pelvis, or positive retroperitoneal nodes, or both. Tumor limited to the true pelvis with histologically proven malignant extension to small bowel or omentum
IV	Growth involving one or both ovaries with distant metastases. If pleural effusion is present, there must be positive cytology to allot a case to Stage IV. Parenchymal liver metastases equals Stage IV

Special Category—Unexplored cases that are thought to be ovarian carcinoma

[a] Ascites is peritoneal effusion which, in the opinion of the surgeon, is pathologic, or clearly exceeds normal amounts, or both.

epithelial activity and nuclear abnormalities but no infiltrative destructive growth, and (3) carcinoma, by FIGO. The tumors of low malignant potential correspond to Grade I tumors of earlier literature and tumor deaths are less common than with true carcinoma. Five-year survival rates are 95–100% with Stage I borderline tumors and 75% in Stages III and Stage IV. Tumor related mortalities do occur 10 and 15 years after diagnosis. Surgical removal is the only proven effective treatment.

Patients with true ovarian carcinoma have a much poorer survival rate. The survival rate correlates strongly with both the stage of disease and tumor differentiation. Van Orden et al. (1966) clearly document markedly worsened survival rates in patients with increased stages of tumor and with more anaplastic grades of tumor. Mucinous adenocarcinomas tend to be of lower stage and lower histologic grade than papillary serous adenocarcinomas, but the stage and histologic grade of a tumor are better prognostic factors than is the actual histologic type (Decker et al., 1975; Gallager, 1975; Day et al., 1975).

Treatment of ovarian cancer is an individualized integration of surgery, radiotherapy, and chemotherapy. The importance of each modality varies with the extent of disease. Operative removal of the maximal amount of tumor possible is imperative in improving survival. Survival rates in Stage II and Stage III carcinomas with complete tumor removal are twice that of patients with incomplete removal (Aure et al., 1971). Survival is improved if maximal tumor can be removed so that residual tumor masses are no more than 1.5 cm (Griffiths, 1975) or 2 cm (Delclos and Smith, 1973). Long and Sala (1963) report improved survival in patients with cancer confined to the pelvis but involving intestines or bladder by completely resecting the involved areas. The use of postoperative radiotherapy (Munnell, 1968) or chemotherapy (Hreshchyshyn, 1973) is essential to improve the patient survival rate from maximal tumor resection.

Omentectomy or omental biopsy should be performed at the time of operation. The omentum is one of the earliest sites to be involved with metastatic cancer (Hreshchyshyn et al., 1967) and metastases may be present though not clinically obvious. Because detection of abdominal metastases will alter staging and may alter one's therapeutic approach, omentectomy is becoming more widely advocated.

Ovarian cancer may metastasize early to para-aortic lymph nodes and also to the undersurface of the diaphragm. These areas must be evaluated to ensure proper determination of extent of tumor. Rosenoff et al. (1975) found that 6 of 7 patients thought to be Stage I or II at the time of operation actually had subdiaphragmatic implantations which were identified by using the peritoneoscope (laparoscope). These patients then had more extensive disease than suspected which would possibly alter the type of treatment they might receive.

Each stage of tumor is unique as far as current knowledge of effective therapy and so each will be considered separately. Stage I ovarian cancer can be treated surgically by removal of the ovary only, if the patient is young and has a strong desire to preserve her child bearing potential and if the tumor is a well differentiated cancer which is totally intracystic and not ruptured. Otherwise minimal standard therapy consists of a careful exploration of the pelvis and abdomen using laparoscopy for the under-surface of the diaphragms if necessary, plus a total hysterectomy, bilateral salpingooophorectomy, and omental biopsy or removal. Within Stage I ovarian cancer, survival depends upon extent of tumor within that stage. Malkasian (1975) has found that if Stage I carcinoma is histologically intracystic, the 5-year survival is 90%; extracystic, 68%; adherent to other structures, 50%; and ruptured at the time of surgery, 58%.

The role of radiotherapy in ovarian carcinoma has been reviewed by Perez and Bradford (1972). External whole pelvis radiotherapy alone does not appear to improve survival (Munnell, 1968; Delclos and Quinlan, 1969) in Stage I ovarian cancer. The latter reported that tumor recurred outside the pelvis in all of their patients with recurrences. Whole pelvic and abdominal radiotherapy is as effective as any other form of therapy however (Rutledge, 1976; Dembo et al., 1978).

The intraperitoneal use of radioactive gold (^{198}Au) or more recently chromic phosphate (^{32}P) is also useful. Elkins and Keetel (1956) reported a 90% 4-year survival in patients treated with ^{198}Au whose cancer was confined to the ovary. Burns et al. (1967) found that survival rates in patients with early ovarian cancer are similar with the use of intraperi-toneal gold and external strip irradiation. ^{32}P has shown an increased survival rate from 80% to 92% for Stage I patients (Hilaris and Clark, 1971) and to 94% for Stage IA patients (Piver, 1972).

For patients treated with ^{198}Au or ^{32}P Pezner et al. (1978) reported 5-year actuarial survivals of 95% for Stage IAi, 82% for IAii, 73% for IB, 67% for IC, 67% for IIA, 67% for IIB without gross residual ovarian cancer, 25% for IIB with gross residual tumor, and 50% for III with minimal or no gross residual tumor. Addition of pelvic radiotherapy did not affect survival of patients with Stage I and IIA tumors. So they concluded that postoperative radiocolloid appears to provide the greatest chance of survival with the least chance of complication.

The Gynecologic Oncology Group is completing a study randomizing patients with Stage IA and IB ovarian carcinoma to no further treatment, external radiotherapy of the pelvis, or melphalan chemotherapy. Hresh-chyshyn (1975a) reported and R. C. Park substantiated (personal com-munication, 1978) a trend for melphalan therapy to be more effective than pelvic radiotherapy or no therapy.

So, to date, postoperative treatment of women with Stage I ovarian carcinoma, excluding Stage IAi, seems to be best by treatment of the entire peritoneal cavity of the pelvis and abdomen with either whole abdominal and pelvic radiotherapy, intraperitoneal use of a radioactive colloid, or the systemic use of an alkylating agent.

Stage II carcinoma of the ovary has been treated with postoperative radiotherapy and chemotherapy with 5-year survivals ranging from 19% to 67%. The Gynecologic Oncology Group, Radiation Therapy Oncology Group and Eastern Cooperative Oncology Group are currently studying prospectively the effect of whole abdominal and pelvic radiotherapy vs. pelvic radiotherapy and melphalan vs. melphalan alone in an attempt to determine the best therapeutic approach.

Stage III carcinoma of the ovary is most importantly treated with operative removal of all gross tumor if possible. Postoperative treatment with whole abdominal and pelvic radiotherapy by either open field or strip technique has been studied by Delclos and Quinlan (1969). They found increased survivals in patients who received both pelvic and abdominal radiotherapy plus an additional 2000 rads of irradiation to the pelvis.

The limiting factors to this radiotherapy is dose tolerance of the kidneys and the liver. They must be partially shielded from the irradiation or fatal injury to the kidneys or to the liver (Wharton, et al., 1974) may occur. Therapeutic levels of irradiation cannot be given to large tumor masses overlying the kidneys or liver. This limits the usefulness of radiotherapy. Delclos and Smith (1975) found that postoperative irradiation is not effective when gross residual tumor masses remain and feel that irradiation has no place in the management of gross ovarian masses. In this situation, they prefer a chemotherapeutic approach.

Chemotherapy is useful in epithelial carcinomas of the ovary which are not completely removed. Li and Hsu (1970) have summarized response rates with single chemotherapeutic agents. Alkylating agents, which give up to 30–50% response rates, are most important in treating ovarian cancer. Cyclophosphamide (Beck and Boyer, 1968), thio-TEPA (Wallach et al., 1970), chlorambucil (Masterson and Nelson, 1965), and melphalan (Smith and Rutledge, 1970) induce similar response rates. Melphalan causes little alopecia, or hemorrhagic cystitis. It is given orally only 5 days per month and so is commonly used. High dose intravenous cyclophosphamide is no more effective than oral melphalan and it is unacceptably toxic (Young et al., 1974).

Both response and survival rates correlate directly with the dose of alkylating agent given (Hreshchyshyn, 1973). Patients who respond to treatment have approximately a 6-month longer survival than nonresponders (Frick et al., 1965). Smith et al. (1972) reported 103 patients with unresectable tumor who responded well to chemotherapy and underwent a second exploratory laparotomy. Twenty-three had no evidence of residual tumor and chemotherapy was stopped. Twenty-two patients survived 2 years and 17 are living over 5 years from the onset of therapy. This suggests that chemotherapy can cause long term remissions and possibly cure a small number of patients with unresectable ovarian cancer.

Other effective chemotherapeutic agents in ovarian cancer include 5-fluorouracil (DeVita et al., 1976), methotrexate (DeVita et al., 1976), Adriamycin (DeVita et al., 1976), hexamethylmelamine (Legha et al., 1976) and cis-platinum diammine. These agents are being employed with some success either with alkylating agents in prospective trials in an attempt to improve response rates or as secondline chemotherapeutic agents.

Several groups have compared the use of alkylating agents to combination drug regimens. Greenspan and Fieber (1962) reported that although their 70% response rate with thio-TEPA plus methotrexate may not be better than the best single alkylating agent series, the degree and persistence of regression appeared improved. Li and Hsu (1970) similarly reported that a combination of 5-fluorouracil and chlorambucil does not significantly improve the remission or long term survival rate over chlorambucil alone but it slightly improves survival at 2 years. Smith et al. (1972) reported no increased response rate and survival of patients treated with a combination of actinomycin D, 5-fluorouracil, and cyclophosphamide (Cytoxan) compared to patients treated with melphalan alone.

Young et al. (1975) reported preliminary results with a combination of hexamethylmelamine, cyclophosphamide, methotrexate and 5-fluorouracil which gave an 85% partial response rate. This combination has been tested against melphalan in a prospective study of 80 patients (Young et al., 1978). It shows a better response rate (76% vs. 54% with melphalan), more complete responses (33% vs. 16%) and longer overall survival (29 vs. 17 months). This is the first chemotherapy combination which is better than a single alkylating agent in advanced ovarian cancer.

Patients who failed to respond to one chemotherapeutic agent have had further chemotherapy. The overall response rates to second trial drugs is 6% (Stanhope et al., 1977). Greenspan and Fieber (1962) and Smith and Rutledge (1970) have observed poor response by treating with another alkylating agent. The latter obtained an excellent 39% response in 47 patients resistant to alkylating agents, by treating with actinomycin D, 5-fluorouracil, and cyclophosphamide. A recent Phase II trial of cyclophosphamide, hexamethylmelamine, Adriamycin and cis-platinum combination chemotherapy (CHAP) reports a 50% response rate in 22 patients (Kane et al., 1978).

Dysgerminoma

The dysgerminoma, which most commonly occurs in the second and third decades of life, metastasizes by direct extension to other pelvic organs and by lymphatic spread to para-aortic lymph nodes. Stage IA lesions of less than 10 cm, in young girls who want to preserve their fertility may be treated by a unilateral oophorectomy provided there is no ascites, and the tumor is well differentiated, and a pure dysgerminoma (Krepart et al., 1978). It is the most common type of ovarian tumor to metastasize to bone (Burns et al., 1969). Because it is the most radiosensitive ovarian tumor, postoperative radiotherapy is the treatment of choice for unresectable tumor, or metastatic sites and recurrences. Experiences with chemotherapy are limited. Smith and Rutledge (1970) report that none of 7 patients responded to alkylating agents. Two patients have responded to the combination of actinomycin D, 5-fluorouracil and cyclophosphamide (Krepart et al., 1978).

Granulosa Theca Cell Tumor

Granulosa theca cell tumors are estrogen-producing tumors which can be fatal. Granulosa cells are the more malignant component of this tumor. When analyzing 203 patients with granulosa theca cell tumors, Norris and Taylor (1968) found that invasion of the ovarian capsule and lymphatic invasion were associated with tumor persistence or recurrence. All 4 patients with capsular invasion of the ovary and gross extension had tumor persistence. Two of 7 patients with invasion of lymphatics had tumor persistence. Cellular atypism and mitotic rates did not have any prognostic significance. Most recurrences occurred more than 5 years after diagnosis. These tumors tend to be radioresponsive, so radiotherapy is recommended for recurrent tumor. Some responses have been reported to melphalan or vincristine, actinomycin D and cyclophosphamide (Cytoxan) (Wharton, 1976).

Malignant Teratoma, Embryonal Carcinoma

Malignant teratomas and embryonal carcinomas are uncommon. Radiotherapy has a limited role in persistent or recurrent disease. Li and Hsu (1970) report that a quadruple therapy of vincristine, actinomycin D, methotrexate, and chlorambucil is effective against germinal tumors. Barlow et al. (1973) report that Adriamycin has a high degree of antitumor activity against some of the unusual ovarian cancers such as malignant teratomas. The combination of vincristine, actinomycin D and cyclophosphamide (VAC) is the most effective proven regimen for embryonal carcinoma. Smith and Rutledge (1975) had 15 of 20 patients survive with

VAC. The combination of bleomycin, vinblastine and cis-platinum, similar to that used in testicular malignancies, appears promising in a small number of patients.

Metastatic Cancer

Ovarian cancer which is metastatic from another primary site constitutes approximately 10% of ovarian malignancies. Breast and gastrointestinal carcinoma are the most common primary sites. Ovarian metastases, from the gastrointestinal tract, particularly from the stomach, are known as Krukenberg tumors. Masterson and Nelson (1965) reported that 2 of 3 patients with Krukenberg tumors had dramatic objective responses to 5-fluorouracil.

SARCOMAS OF UTERUS

Uterine sarcomas are highly malignant neoplasms. Five-year survivals range from 0 to 30% in several series. Actual survival rates of the many histologic types are difficult to establish because these tumors are rare. Mixed mesodermal sarcomas and leiomyosarcomas are the most common histologic types (Edwards, 1969).

Presenting symptoms in 32 patients with carcinosarcoma have been described by Bartsich et al. (1967). Abnormal vaginal bleeding occurred most frequently. Abdominal pain and weight loss were more common than an abdominal mass. Taylor and Norris (1966) indicated that in 15 patients dying of leiomyosarcoma, all had involvement of pelvic or abdominal viscera, 80% had lung or pleural involvement, and 40% had para-aortic lymph node involvement. This suggests that direct, hematogenous, and lymphatic spread all occur.

Differentiation of sarcomas from benign, smooth muscle tumors is imperative. Taylor and Norris (1966) found that the number of mitotic figures in a smooth muscle tumor is the most reliable means of differentiating a leiomyoma from a leiomyosarcoma. The degree of cellular atypism or the number of giant cells are not as reliable. Thirty-one of 36 patients with 10 or more mitoses per 10 high power fields (HPF) had a recurrence or metastases of tumor. All patients with less than 10 mitoses per 10 HPF had a benign course. Kempson and Bari (1970) similarly found that tumors with greater than 10 mitoses per 10 HPF were malignant. They found that some metastasized which had 4–9 mitoses per HPF. Those with lower mitotic rates were benign.

Kempson and Bari (1970) also classified endometrial stromal tumors as benign or malignant by mitotic counts. All those metastasized which had mitotic counts of about 20 per 10 HPF. None metastasized with less than 5 mitoses per 10 HPF.

Kempson (1973) noted that sarcomas which have invaded beyond the uterus at the time of operation have an almost hopeless prognosis. Neoplasms with a high mitotic activity, marked anaplasia or blood vessel invasion also have a very poor prognosis.

Stimuli which lead to the formation of sarcomas are not known. Norris and Taylor (1965) indicated in their series that 12% of 144 patients with uterine sarcomas had a history of pelvic irradiation. They also reported that 30% of the mixed mesodermal sarcomas studied had a history of prior irradiation whereas none of their leiomyosarcomas had that history.

Operative removal of the tumor is essential to achieving cures. Mortel et al. (1974) found that no patient survived unless surgery was a part of the treatment.

The role of radiotherapy is less well defined. Mortel et al. (1974) reported that there is no evidence that radiotherapy influences prognosis either way. Edwards (1960), on the other hand, reported that 15 of 29 patients survived who were treated with both preoperative radium application and surgery; only 6 of 21 patients survived who were treated only surgically. Badib et al. (1969) reported improved survival and decreased recurrence rates in patients with Stage I uterine sarcomas who received both radiotherapy and surgery.

Chemotherapy of uterine sarcomas has had only minimal success to date. Malkasian et al. (1967) found no responses in 8 patients to alkylating agents but reported that 5 of 10 patients responded to high dose, intermittent 5-fluorouracil. They similarly had 4 of 9 patients respond to a combination of actinomycin D and radiotherapy. The responses were brief and they feel survival was not increased significantly.

A combination of vincristine, actinomycin D and cyclophosphamide (Cytoxan) (VAC), similar to that described by Donaldson et al. (1973), has been used successfully by Smith and Rutledge (1975). They reported 14 of 38 patients with pelvic sarcomas were without evidence of disease after the VAC regimen. Adriamycin presently shows much promise either in combination (Gottlieb et al., 1972) or as a single agent. Barlow et al. (1973) reported that 5 of 7 patients responded to Adriamycin alone.

VAGINAL CANCER

Primary neoplasms of the vagina constitute only 1% of all gynecologic malignancies, and squamous cell carcinoma accounts for 90% of all tumors. Less common are sarcoma botryoides and clear cell adenocarcinoma.

Squamous Cell Carcinoma

Squamous cell carcinoma of the vagina tends to spread locally and to metastasize slowly to regional nodes and later to distant sites. Cancer of the lower one third of the vagina metastasizes to inguinal nodes and lesions of the upper vagina to the deep pelvic nodes. See Table 19.4 for staging.

The importance of vaginal irritants in the etiology of vaginal cancer is not known. Vaginal carcinoma is commonly preceded by carcinoma of the cervix or vulva. Brown et al. (1971) report that 18 of 34 patients with in situ vaginal carcinoma had prior in situ or invasive carcinoma of the cervix. This emphasizes the importance of periodic examinations of patients with prior cervical cancer.

In situ carcinoma grossly may look like a pink blush on the vaginal epithelium or may have a granular or white appearance. Invasive carcinoma is nodular, ulcerative, exophytic, or endophytic. Vaginal bleeding is the most common symptom. Dyspareunia or dysuria may occur depending on the site of the lesion.

The proximity of the vagina to the bladder and rectum and the importance of the vagina in sexual functioning make treatment of vaginal carcinoma difficult. In situ carcinoma may be treated with intravaginal or interstitial radioactive sources or with wide excisions. Brown et al. (1971) indicate that radiotherapy of carcinoma in situ located in the upper vagina often fails because mucosal ridges cause decreased contact with the surface of the radiation source. Gray and Christopherson (1969) reported only one recurrence in 12 patients with upper vaginal lesions which were removed operatively.

Use of topical 5-fluorouracil (1–2%) has been reported by Woodruff et al. (1975). They record cures in 8 of 9 patients treated with this agent and followed for 6 weeks to 6 years. The one therapeutic failure was in a patient with a hyperkeratotic lesion. Therefore selection of therapeutic approach on an individual basis may be worthwhile.

Early invasive vaginal lesions are best treated by radiotherapy so that bowel, bladder, and vaginal integrity may be maintained. The use of interstitial needles when possible maintains vaginal pliability better than

TABLE 19.4
Carcinoma of the Vagina (FIGO)

Stage	Description
0	Carcinoma in situ; intraepithelial carcinoma
I	The carcinoma is limited to the vaginal wall
II	The carcinoma has involved the subvaginal tissue but has not extended to the pelvic wall
III	The carcinoma has extended to the pelvic wall
IV	The carcinoma has extended beyond the true pelvis or has involved the mucosa of the bladder or rectum. Bullous edema as such does not permit a case to be allotted to Stage IV
IVA	Spread of the growth to adjacent organs
IVB	Spread to distant organs

intravaginal sources. The operative approaches of anterior, posterior, or total pelvic exenteration, which would be needed to achieve adequate surgical margins, are not frequently used because of the obligatory removal of pelvic organs.

In late invasive disease, involving primarily the bladder or rectum, survivals are few by radiotherapy alone. Combined use of radiotherapy and surgery may improve results.

Chemotherapy reports are few for vaginal carcinoma. Malkasian et al. (1968b) reported that 5-fluorouracil responses were short lived. Two of 5 patients responded for 3 months and only 1 was responding at 4 months. One patient given Adriamycin responded and 1 patient given bleomycin did not respond (Barlow et al., 1973). One patient given intra-arterial methotrexate did not respond (Trussell and Mitford-Barberton, 1961). Piver et al. (1978) used multiple chemotherapeutic agents for carcinoma of the vagina and cervix. They found a 57% response rate to a combination of cyclophosphamide, Adriamycin and 5-fluorouracil. Generally, chemotherapy of squamous cell carcinoma of the vagina is similar to squamous cell carcinoma of the cervix.

Sarcoma Botryoides

Sarcoma botryoides of the vagina is the most common tumor of the urogenital tract in young girls (Daniel et al., 1959). Over half the reported cases occur before age 3.

Classifying sarcoma botryoides as an embryonal rhabdomyosarcoma or mixed mesodermal sarcoma is variable. Sutow et al. (1970) reported that children with botryoid sarcomas of different sites had better survival rates than those with embryonal or alveolar rhabdomyosarcomas. This suggests tumor differences between botryoid and embryonal rhabdomyosarcomas.

Sarcoma botryoides grossly appears to be a group of clear, fluid filled vesicles. It begins in the subepithelial layer of the vagina and expands within the limits of the vaginal wall before invading tissue surrounding the vagina. It tends to metastasize to regional lymph nodes and the lungs (Hilgers et al., 1970). The tumor tends to be multicentric with involvement of the vagina, cervix, uterus, and bladder. If this tumor is untreated, death usually occurs within one year.

Distant metastases occur late but most commonly involve the regional lymph nodes and lungs. Most treatment failures are due to local recurrences which usually present within one year.

Pelvic exenteration is effective treatment for this tumor (Hilgers et al., 1973). Rutledge and Sullivan (1967) reported 4 of 5 patients surviving with this treatment.

Adjunctive use of radiotherapy and chemotherapy with radical surgery may contribute to increased survivals. Grosfield et al. (1972) reported 2 of 3 girls with rhabdomyosarcoma extending from the primary site who survived after postoperative radiotherapy and chemotherapy. Actinomycin D and vincristine were started with the onset of radiotherapy and were continued in 9-week cycles for 1 year. Hilgers et al. (1973) used actinomycin D, Adriamycin, vincristine, and cyclophosphamide sequentially in 90-day courses repeated for 2 years. Radiotherapy is added if tumor is near a resection margin.

Significant palliation of embryonal rhabdomyosarcoma with radiotherapy and chemotherapy is reported (Nelson, 1968), so an aggressive approach to this tumor is worthwhile.

Clear Cell Adenocarcinoma

Adenocarcinoma of the vagina accounts for less than 5% of all vaginal cancers. There has been marked interest in this disease since 1970 when Herbst et al. (1971) demonstrated a high correlation between this tumor in young women and the administration of diethylstilbesterol (DES) to their mothers during pregnancy. A national registry for these tumors has been established by Herbst et al. (1972). Currently the disease remains relatively rare with less than 344 cases of DES-exposed children with vaginal or cervical adenocarcinoma recorded in the DES registry. However, many girls and young women have had intrauterine exposure to DES so the problem may become more prominent. Up to 90% of these exposed persons have benign vaginal adenosis, the significance of which is unknown at this time.

Most reported cases are in patients 14 to 25 years of age although a few have been in premenarchal children. Treatment is similar to squamous cell vaginal tumors. Both radiotherapy and radical surgery can be effective. There are no reported series of chemotherapy used to treat this tumor.

Any female who has had intrauterine exposure to DES should have a pelvic examination any time vaginal bleeding or discharge occurs. If asymptomatic, she should have a pelvic examination at the time of puberty since a significant number of clear cell adenocarcinomas occur then. Males receiving intrauterine exposure to DES have been found to have epididymal cysts, hypoplastic testes, or cryptorchidism in 30% of those examined (Gill et al., 1978).

VULVAR CANCER

Cancer of the vulva constitutes three to 5% of gynecologic malignancies. Squamous cell carcinoma is the most common histologic type. Adenocarcinoma, melanoma, and sarcoma occur less frequently.

Squamous Cell Carcinoma

Squamous cell carcinoma of the vulva must not be considered simply a skin cancer. It is an aggressive, frequently metastatic, potentially lethal cancer. FIGO staging is a TNM system. See Table 19.5 for details.

A Stage I tumor is a lesion of 2 cm or less in diameter confined to the vulva with no suspicious groin nodes and no evidence of distant metastases. Stage II cancer is a lesion greater than 2 cm in diameter confined to the vulva with no suspicious groin nodes or evidence of distant metastases. Stage III disease is tumor spread to the urethra, vagina, perineum, or anus with normal or suspicious nodes or tumor confined to the vulva with suspicious nodes. Stage IV includes any lesion with fixed or ulcerated lymph nodes, tumor fixed to bone, tumor metastatic as judged by palpable deep pelvic lymph nodes or other metastases or tumor infiltrating the mucosa of the upper urethra, bladder or rectum.

Symptoms are most commonly those of a vulvar mass, pruritis, dysuria, pain, bleeding, or a groin mass. Green et al. (1958a) found that young women with rapidly growing vulvar cancer frequently had a history of prior syphilis and speculated on the relationship of these two diseases. Saltzstein et al. (1956) reported 13 patients with vulvar cancer who had prior lymphogranuloma venereum, granuloma inguinale, or condyloma accuminata which suggests that these might be predisposing lesions.

The pattern of lymph node metastasis can be quite variable with vulvar cancer. Lymph node metastasis may occur on the same side of the lesion only, on the opposite side only, or on both sides (Green et al., 1958b).

Way and Hennigan (1966) reported 5 of 117 patients who had deep pelvic node metastases only. Rutledge et al. (1970), on the other hand,

TABLE 19.5
Carcinoma of the Vulva (FIGO)

Stage	Description
0	Carcinoma in situ, e.g., Bowen's disease, noninvasive Paget's disease
I	Tumor confined to the vulva, 2 cm or less in largest diameter. Nodes are not palpable or are palpable in either groin, not enlarged, mobile (not clinically suspicious of neoplasm)
II	Tumor confined to the vulva more than 2 cm in diameter. Nodes are not palpable, or are palpable in either groin, not enlarged, mobile (not clinically suspicious of neoplasm)
III	Tumor of any size with (1) adjacent spread to the urethra and any or all of the vagina, the perineum, and the anus; and/or (2) nodes palpable in either or both groins (enlarged firm, and mobile, not fixed but clinically suspicious of neoplasm)
IV	Tumor of any size (1) infiltrating the bladder, mucosa, or the rectal mucosa, or both, including the upper part of the urethral mucosa; and/or (2) fixed to the bone or other distant metastases

found no deep pelvic lymph node metastases unless Cloquet's node and the inguinal lymph nodes were affected.

The size and depth of the cancer may correlate with the frequency of lymph node metastases and so help in planning therapy. Wharton et al. (1974) found that none of 25 patients with lesions less than 2 cm in diameter and less than 5 mm of invasion had no evidence of lymphatic metastases. They suggest that conservative vulvectomy may be adequate treatment. However, Dipaola et al. (1975) reported that 4 of 22 patients with less than 5 mm of tumor invasion either had positive groin metastases or developed recurrence in the groin. Rutledge et al. (1970) report that 34% of patients with 2–8-cm lesions had positive nodes and 50% had positive nodes when lesions were greater than 8 cm in diameter. Taylor and Nathanson (1942) found a similar correlation with an even higher incidence of metastatic lymph nodes. To the contrary, Way and Hennigan (1966) found no correlation between the size of the primary lesion and the frequency of nodal metastasis. They did find that 65% of patients with anaplastic tumors had lymph node metastasis, whereas only 35% of patients with more differentiated tumors had metastases.

Radical vulvectomy and bilateral inguinal lymphadenectomy is the treatment of choice in the clinically operable patient. A deep pelvic lymph node dissection is considered if superficial nodes are positive or the tumor is near the clitoris where primary drainage is to the deep pelvic nodes. Way (1954) reported 86% 5-year survival of patients with negative lymph nodes and 48% 5-year survival of patients with lymph node metastasis to the inguinal lymph nodes. Two of nine patients with metastasis to deep pelvic nodes survived. Excision of primary tumor and lymph node metastases improves survival.

Radiotherapy is a less curative form of treatment. Tod (1949) reports a 5-year survival of 33% for early cases and 14% for late cases with radium implantation. Ellis (1949) feels that radiotherapy is not satisfactory for treating vulvar cancer because vulvar necrosis and subsequent morbidity occurred in one third of his patients.

Gusberg and Frick (1978a) treated 3 patients with the 22.5 million volt betatron. They obtained tumor control for 1 year or more and had no skin sloughs with this supervoltage irradiation. They feel that supervoltage is useful and without the serious morbidity of orthovoltage because the depth of maximum ionization is 2–6 cm below the skin surface. Electrocoagulation can achieve curative control of local disease (Berven, 1949).

The results of chemotherapeutic treatment of vulvar cancer are generally disappointing. Squamous cell carcinoma of the vulva has been treated with nitrogen mustard, Cytoxan, thio-TEPA, chlorambucil, alkeran, 6-mercaptopurine, 5-fluorouracil, mitomycin C and methotrexate with no lasting effect (Masterson and Nelson, 1965; Frick et al., 1965; Haffner and Frick, 1970). Suzuki et al. (1969) found that vulvar carcinoma responded better to bleomycin therapy than did any other type of female genital malignancy. They report that some vulvar carcinomas were cured with bleomycin only. Further evaluation of the use of bleomycin with vulvar carcinoma is needed.

Topical 5-fluorouracil cream has been used for a variety of cutaneous malignancies (Litwin et al., 1971). Woodruff et al. (1973) indicated that topical 5-fluorouracil cream was successful in 9 of 13 cases of vulvar squamous cell carcinoma in situ. Krupp and Bohm (1978) reported that 6 out of 8 in situ patients responded. However, Forney et al. (1977) reported none of 6 patients with vulvar carcinoma in situ responded to 5-fluorouracil.

Melanoma

Melanoma of the vulva, although a highly malignant disease, is associated with a significant number of patient survivals if the tumor is localized. Yackel et al. (1970) reported that 33% of their patients achieved 5-year survivals. Morrow and Rutledge (1972) reported that 6 of 8 patients with tumor localized to the vulva survived 5 years. Only 1 of 6 patients with tumor spread beyond the vulva survived 5 years, however. Fenn and Abell (1973) indicated that no survivals occurred among the 6 patients who had melanoma extending beyond the dermis. Chung et al. (1975) found that Clark's level could not be used on vulvar melanoma because of the lack of a well defined papillary dermis. They did find that survival correlated with the depth of invasion, however, and proposed a method of evaluating depth of invasion.

Radical surgical removal of the vulvar melanoma and the primary lymphatic drainage is the treatment of choice. Radical vulvectomy and inguinal lymphadenectomy, vaginectomy, urethral resection, pelvic exenteration and pelvic lymphadenectomy may be appropriate depending on location and extent of the tumor.

Chemotherapy may be useful in recurrent or metastatic melanoma and is discussed in Chapter 28.

Sarcomas and adenocarcinomas of the vulva are best treated with radical surgery.

REFERENCES

Abell, M. R. Invasive carcinomas of the uterine cavity. *In* The Uterus, edited by H. J. Norris, A. T. Hertig, and M. R. Abell, p. 413–456. Williams & Wilkins, Baltimore, 1973.

Amstey, M. S., Patten, S. F., and Turk, M. Herpesvirus cervicitis and neoplasia—a cytological review. Cancer, *32*: 1321–1324, 1973.

Aure, J. C., Hoeg, K., and Kolstad, P. Clinical and histological studies of ovarian carcinoma. Obstet. Gynecol., *37*: 1–9, 1971.

Aurelian, L., Strandberg, J. D., Melendez, L. V., and Johnson, L. A. Herpesvirus type 2 isolated from cervical tumor cells grown in tissue culture. Science, *174:* 704–707, 1971.

Averette, H. E., Weinstein, G. D., and Frost, P. Autoradiographic analysis of cell proliferation kinetics in human genital tissues. Am. J. Obstet. Gynecol., *108:* 8–17, 1970.

Badib, A. O., Vongtama, B., Kurohara, S. S., and Webster, J. H. Radiotherapy in the treatment of sarcomas of the corpus uteri. Cancer, *24:* 724–729, 1969.

Barlow, J. J., Piver, M. S., Chuang, J. T., Cortes, E. P., Ohnuma, T., and Holland, J. F. Adriamycin and bleomycin, alone and in combination, in gynecologic cancers. Cancer, *32:* 735–743, 1973.

Bartsich, E. G., O'Leary, J. A., and Moore, J. G. Carcinosarcoma of the uterus, a 50-year review of 32 cases (1917–1966). Obstet. Gynecol., *30:* 518–523, 1967.

Bateman, J. R., Hazen, J. G., Stolinsky, D. C., and Steinfield, J. C. Advanced carcinoma of the cervix treated by intra-arterial methotrexate. Am. J. Obstet. Gynecol., *96:* 181–187, 1966.

Beck, R., and Boyer, D. Treatment of 126 cases of advanced ovarian carcinoma with cyclophosphamide. Can. Med. Assoc. J., *98:* 539–541, 1968.

Berven, E. G. E. Carcinoma of the vulva—the treatment of cancer of the vulva symposium. Br. J. Radiol., *22:* 498–507, 1949.

Boronow, R. C. Chemotherapy for disseminated tubal cancer. Obstet. Gynecol., *42:* 62–66, 1973.

Brown, G. R., Fletcher, G. H., and Rutledge, F. N. Irradiation of "in-situ" and invasive squamous cell carcinomas of the vagina. Cancer, *28:* 1278–1283, 1971.

Bruckner, H. W., Deppe, G., and Cohen, C. J. Intensive combination chemotherapy of advanced endometrial adenocarcinoma with Adriamycin, cyclophosphamide, 5-fluorouracil and medroxyprogesterone acetate. Obstet. Gynecol., *50:* 10s–12s, 1977.

Burns, B. C., Jr., Rutledge, F. N., Smith, J. P., and Delclos, L. Management of ovarian carcinoma, surgery, irradiation, and chemotherapy. Am. J. Obstet. Gynecol., *98:* 374–386, 1967.

Burns, B. C., Jr., Underwood, P. B., Jr., and Rutledge, F. N. A review of carcinoma of the ovary at the University of Texas, M. D. Anderson Hospital and Tumor Institute at Houston. *In* Cancer of the Uterus and Ovary, p. 123–147. Yearbook Medical Publishers, Chicago, 1969.

Carter, S. K., Bakowski, M. T., and Hellmann, K. Chemotherapy of Cancer, pp. 163–166. John Wiley & Sons, New York, 1977.

Cavanagh, D., Martin, D. S., and Ferguson, J. H. Closed pelvic perfusion in advanced gynecologic cancer. South. Med. J., *58:* 549–557, 1965.

Chung, A. F., Woodruff, J. M., and Lewis, J. L., Jr. Malignant melamona; a report of 44 cases. Obstet. Gynecol., *45:* 638–646, 1975.

Cohen, C. J., Deppe, G., and Bruckner, H. W. Treatment of advanced adenocarcinoma of the endometrium with melphalan, 5-fluorouracil, and medroxyprogesterone acetate. Obstet. Gynecol., *50:* 415–417, 1977.

Daniel, W. W., Koss, L. G., and Brunschwig, A. Sarcoma botryoides of the vagina. Cancer, *12:* 74–84, 1959.

Day, T. G., Jr., Gallagher, H. S., and Rutledge, F. N. Epithelial carcinoma of the ovary; prognostic importance of histologic grade. Natl. Cancer Inst. Monogr., *42:* 15–18, 1975.

Decker, D. G., Malkasian, G. D., Jr., and Taylor, W. F. Prognostic importance of histologic grading in ovarian carcinoma. Natl. Cancer Inst. Monogr., *42:* 9–12, 1975.

Delclos, L., and Quinlan, E. J. Malignant tumors of the ovary managed with postoperative megavoltage irradiation. Radiology, *93:* 659–663, 1969.

Delclos, L., and Smith, J. P. Textbook of Radiotherapy, edited by G. H. Fletcher, Ed. 2. Lea & Febiger, Philadelphia, 1973.

Delclos, L., and Smith, J. P. Ovarian cancer with special regard to types of radiotherapy. Natl. Cancer Inst. Monogr., 42: 129–135, 1975.

Delfs, E. Chorionic gonadotropin determinations in patients with hydatidiform mole and choriocarcinoma. Ann. N.Y. Acad. Sci., 80: 125–139, 1959.

Dembo, A. J., Bush, R. S., Beal, F. A., Bean, H. A., Pringle, J. F., and Sturgeon, J. Increased survival following adjuvant radiation therapy in ovarian carcinoma stages I, II and asymptomatic III (abstr.). Proc. Am. Soc. Clin. Oncol., 19: 325, 1978.

DeVita, V. T., Jr., Wasserman, T. H., Young, R. C., and Carter, S. K. Perspectives on research in gynecologic oncology; treatment protocols. Cancer, 38: 509–525, 1976.

Dipaola, G. R., Gomez-Rueda, N., and Arrighi, L. Relevance of microinvasion in carcinoma of the vulva. Obstet. Gynecol., 45: 647–649, 1975.

Dodson, M. G., Ford, J. H., Jr., and Averette, H. E. Clinical aspects of fallopian tube carcinoma. Obstet. Gynecol., 36: 935–939, 1970.

Donaldson, S. S., Castro, J. R., Wilbur, J. R., and Jesse, R. H. Rhabdomyosarcoma of head and neck in children—combination treatment by surgery, irradiation, and chemotherapy. Cancer, 31: 26–35, 1973.

Easley, J. D., and Fletcher, G. H. Analysis of the treatment of stage I and stage II carcinomas of the uterine cervix. A.J.R., 111: 243–248, 1971.

Edwards, C. L. Undifferentiated tumors. In Cancer of the Uterus and Ovary, pp. 84–94. Yearbook Medical Publishers, Chicago, 1969.

Elkins, H. B., and Keetel, W. C. Radioactive gold in the treatment of ovarian carcinoma. A.J.R., 75: 1117–1123, 1956.

Ellis, F. Cancer of the vulva treated by radiation. Br. J. Radiol., 22: 513–520, 1949.

Fenn, M. E., and Abell, M. R. Melanomas of vulva and vagina. Obstet. Gynecol., 41: 902–911, 1973.

Fletcher, G. H. Cancer of the uterine cervix—Janeway Lecture, 1970. A.J.R., 111: 225–242, 1971.

Forney, J. P., Morrow, C. P., Townsend, D. E., and DiSaia, P. J. Management of carcinoma in situ of the vulva. Am. J. Obstet. Gynecol., 127: 801–806, 1977.

Frick, H. C., II, Atchoo, N., Adamsons, K., Jr., and Taylor, H. C., Jr. The efficacy of chemotherapeutic agents in the management of disseminated gynecologic cancer. Am. J. Obstet. Gynecol., 93: 1112–1121, 1965.

Gallager, H. S. Prognostic importance of histologic type in ovarian carcinoma. Natl. Cancer Inst. Monogr., 42: 13–14, 1975.

Gill, W. B., Schumacher, G. F. B., and Bibbo, M. Genital and semen abnormalities in adult males two and one half decades after in utero exposure to diethylstilbestrol. In Intrauterine Exposure to Diethylstilbestrol in the human, pp. 55–57. American College of Obstetricians and Gynecologists, Chicago, 1978.

Goldstein, D. P. Prophylactic chemotherapy of patients with molar pregnancy. Obstet. Gynecol., 38: 817–822, 1971.

Goldstein, D. P., Winig, P., and Shirley, R. L. Actinomycin D as initial therapy of gestational trophoblastic disease; a reevaluation. Obstet. Gynecol., 39: 341–345, 1972.

Goldstein, D. P. Prevention of gestational trophoblastic disease by use of actinomycin-D in molar pregnancies. Obstet. Gynecol., 43: 475–479, 1974.

Gottlieb, J. A., Baker, L. H., Quagliana, J. M., Luce, J. K., Whitecar, J. P., Sinkovics, J. G., Rivkin, S. E., Brownlee, R., and Frei, E., III. Chemotherapy of sarcomas with a combination of Adriamycin and dimethyl triazeno imidazole carboxamide. Cancer, 30: 1632–1638, 1972.

Gray, L. A., and Christopherson, W. M. In situ and early invasive carcinoma of the vagina. Obstet. Gynecol., 34: 226–230, 1969.

Green, T. H., Jr., Ulfelder, H., and Meigs, J. V. Epidermoid carcinoma of the vulva: analysis of 238 cases; Part I. Etiology and diagnosis. Am. J. Obstet. Gynecol., *75:* 834–847, 1958a.

Green, T. H., Jr., Ulfelder, H., and Meigs, J. V. Epidermoid carcinoma of the vulva: analysis of 238 cases; Part II. Therapy and end results. Am. J. Obstet. Gynecol., *75:* 848–864, 1958b.

Greenspan, E. M., and Fieber, M. Combination chemotherapy of advanced ovarian carcinoma with the antimetabolite, methotrexate, and the alkylating agent, thiotepa. J. Mt. Sinai Hosp., *29:* 48–62, 1962.

Grosfeld, J. L., Smith, J. P., and Clatworthy, H. W. Pelvic rhabdomyosarcoma in infants and children. J. Urol., *107:* 673–675, 1972.

Griffiths, C. T. Surgical resection of tumor bulk in the primary treatment of ovarian carcinoma. Natl. Cancer Inst. Monogr., *42:* 101–104, 1975.

Gusberg, S. B., and Frick, H. C., II. Cancer of the vulva. *In* Gynecologic Cancer, Ed. 5, pp. 100–119. Williams & Wilkins, Baltimore, 1978a.

Gusberg, S. B., and Frick, H. C., II. Cancer of the fallopian tube. *In* Gynecologic Cancer, Ed. 5, pp. 368–374. Williams & Wilkins, Baltimore, 1978b.

Gusberg, S. B., and Kaplan, A. L. Precursors of corpus cancer; IV. Adenomatous hyperplasia as stage 0 carcinoma of the endometrium. Am. J. Obstet. Gynecol., *87:* 662–678, 1963.

Haffner, W. H. J., and Frick, H. C., II. Intermittent intravenous methotrexate in the treatment of advanced epidermoid carcinoma of the cervix and vulvovagina. Cancer, *26:* 812–815, 1970.

Hammond, C. B., Hertz, R., Ross, G. T., Lipsett, M. B., and Odell, W. D. Primary chemotherapy for nonmetastatic gestational trophoblastic neoplasms. Am. J. Obstet. Gynecol., *98:* 71–78, 1967.

Hammond, C. B., and Parker, R. T. Diagnosis and treatment of trophoblastic disease; a report from the Southeastern Regional Center. Obstet. Gynecol., *35:* 132–143, 1970.

Hammond, C. B., Borchert, L. G., Tyrey, L., Creasman, W. T., and Parker, R. T. Treatment of metastatic trophoblastic disease; good and poor prognosis. Am. J. Obstet. Gynecol., *115:* 451–457, 1973.

Hanton, E. M., Malkasian, G. D., Jr., Dahlin, D. C., and Pratt, J. H. Primary carcinoma of the fallopian tube. Am. J. Obstet. Gynecol., *94:* 832–839, 1966.

Hausknecht, R. U., and Gusberg, S. B. Estrogen metabolism in patients at high risk for endometrial carcinoma; II. The role of androstenedione as an estrogen precursor in postmenopausal women with endometrial carcinoma. Am. J. Obstet. Gynecol., *116:* 981–984, 1973.

Herbst, A. L., Ulfelder, H., and Poskanzer, D. C. Adenocarcinoma of the vagina; association of maternal stilbestrol therapy with tumor appearance in young women. N. Engl. J. Med., *284:* 878–881, 1971.

Herbst, A. L., Kurman, R. J., Scully, R. E., and Poskanzer, D. C. Clear-cell adenocarcinoma of the genital tract in young females. N. Engl. J. Med., *287:* 1259–1264, 1972.

Hertig, A. T., and Sommers, S. C. Genesis of endometrial carcinoma; I. Study of prior biopsies. Cancer, *2:* 946–956, 1949.

Hertz, R., Lewis, J. L., Jr., and Lipsett, M. B. Five years' experience with the chemotherapy of metastatic choriocarcinoma and related trophoblastic tumors in women. Am. J. Obstet. Gynecol., *82:* 631–640, 1961.

Hilaris, B. S., and Clark, D. G. C. The value of postoperative intraperitoneal injection of radiocolloids in early cancer of the ovary. A.J.R., *112:* 749–754, 1971.

Hilgers, R. D., Malkasian, G. D., Jr., and Soule, E. H. Embryonal rhabdomyosarcoma (botryoid type) of the vagina. Am. J. Obstet. Gynecol., *107:* 484–502, 1970.

Hilgers, R. D., Ghavimi, F., D'Angio, G. J., Exelby, P., and Lewis, J. L., Jr. Memorial hospital experience with pelvic exenteration and embryonal rhabdomyosarcoma of the vagina. Gynecol. Oncol., *1:* 262–270, 1973.

Hodgkinson, C. P., and Boyce, C. R. Prolonged intra-arterial therapy for advanced pelvic malignancy. Cancer, *18:* 1536–1543, 1965.

Hreshchyshyn, M. M., Schueller, E. F., and Randall, C. L. Problems in management of patients with ovarian cancer. Clin. Obstet. Gynecol., *10:* 599–624, 1967.

Hreshchyshyn, M. M. Hydroxyurea with irradiation for cervical carcinoma—preliminary report. Cancer Chemother. Rep., *52:* 601–602, 1968.

Hreshchyshyn, M. M. Single-drug therapy in ovarian cancer; factors influencing response. Gynec. Oncol., *1:* 220–232, 1973.

Hreshchyshyn, M. M. Results of Gynecologic Oncology Group trials on ovarian cancer; preliminary report. Natl. Cancer Inst. Monogr., *42:* 155–165, 1975a.

Hreshchyshyn, M. M. Gynecologic Oncology Group reports I and II. Gynec. Oncol., *3:* 251–258, 1975b.

Kane, R., Andrews, T., Bernath, A., Curry, S., Dixon, R., Gottlieb, R., Harvey, H., Kukrika, M., Lipton, A., Mortel, R., Ricci, J., and White, D. Phase II trial of cyclophosphamide, Adriamycin and cis-platinum combination therapy (CHAP) in advanced ovarian carcinoma (abstr.). Proc. Am. Soc. Clin. Oncol., *19:* 320, 1978.

Keetch, W. C., Fox, M. R., Longnecker, D. S., and Latourette, H. B. Prophylactic use of radioactive gold in the treatment of primary ovarian cancer. Am. J. Obstet. Gynecol., *94:* 766–779,

Keller, D., Kempson, R. L., Levin, G., and McLennan, C. Management of the patient with early endometrial carcinoma. Cancer, *33:* 1108–1116, 1974.

Kelley, R. M., and Baker, W. H. Progestational agents in the treatment of carcinoma of the endometrium. N. Engl. J. Med., *264:* 216–222, 1961.

Kempson, R. L. Sarcomas and related neoplasms. *In* The Uterus, edited by H. J. Norris, A. T. Hertig, and M. R. Abell, pp. 298–319. Williams & Wilkins, Baltimore, 1973.

Kempson, R. L., and Bari, W. Uterine sarcomas; classification, diagnosis, and prognosis. Hum. Pathol., *1:* 331–349, 1970.

Kennedy, B. J. Progestogens in the treatment of carcinoma of the endometrium. Surg. Gynecol. Obstet., *127:* 103–114, 1968.

Krepart, G., Smith, J. P., Rutledge, F., and Delclos, L. The treatment for dysgerminoma of the ovary. Cancer, *41:* 986–990, 1978.

Krupp, P. J., and Bohm, J. W. 5-Fluorouracil topical treatment of in-situ vulvar cancer; a preliminary report. Obstet. Gynecol., *51:* 702–706, 1978.

Legha, S. S., Slavik, M., and Carter, S. K. Hexamethylmelamine; an evaluation of its role in the therapy of cancer. Cancer, *38:* 27–35, 1976.

Lewis, G. C., Jr., Slack, N. H., Mortel, R., and Bross, I. D. Adjuvant progesterone therapy in the primary definitive treatment of endometrial cancer. Gynecol. Oncol., *2:* 368–376, 1974.

Lewis, J., Jr., Gore, H., Hertig, A. T., and Goss, D. A. Treatment of trophoblastic disease with rationale for the use of adjunctive chemotherapy at the time of indicated operation. Am. J. Obstet. Gynecol., *96:* 710–722, 1966.

Li, M. C., and Hsu, K. Combined drug therapy for ovarian carcinoma. Clin. Obstet. Gynecol., *13:* 928–944, 1970.

Livingston, R. B., and Carter, S. K. Single Agents in Cancer Chemotherapy. IFI/Plenum, New York, 1970.

Litwin, M. S., Ryan, R. F., Reed, R. J., and Krementz, E. T. Topical chemotherapy of advanced cutaneous malignancy with 5-fluorouracil cream. J. Surg. Oncol., *3:* 351–365, 1971.

Lloyd, R. E., Jones, S. E., Salmon, S. E., et al. Phase II trial of Adriamycin and cyclophosphamide; a Southwest Oncology Group pilot study. Proc. Am. Assoc. Cancer Res., *16:* 265, 1975.

Long, R. T. L., and Sala, J. M. Radical pelvic surgery combined with radiotherapy in the treatment of locally advanced ovarian carcinoma. Surg. Gynec. Obstet., *117:* 201-204, 1963.

Masterson, J. G., and Nelson, J. H., Jr. The role of chemotherapy in the treatment of gynecologic malignancy. Am. J. Obstet. Gynecol., *93:* 1102-1108, 1965.

Malkasian, G. D., Jr., Mussey, E., Decker, D. G., and Johnson, C. E. Chemotherapy of gynecologic sarcomas. Cancer Chemother. Rep., *51:* 507-516, 1967.

Malkasian, G. D., Decker, D. G., Mussey, E., and Johnson, C. E. Observations on gynecologic malignancy treated with 5-fluorouracil. Am. J. Obstet. Gynecol., *100:* 1012-1017, 1968a.

Malkasian, G. D., Decker, D. G., Mussey, E., and Johnson, C. E. Chemotherapy of squamous cell carcinoma of the cervix, vagina, and vulva. Clin. Obstet. Gynecol., *11:* 367-381, 1968b.

Malkasian, G. D. Discussion; surgery in ovarian cancer. Natl. Cancer Inst. Monogr., *42:* 113-115, 1975.

Morrow, C. P., Creasman, W. T., DiSaia, P. J., Curry, S. L., and DePetrillo, A. D. Methotrexate, hydroxyura, and vincristine; chemotherapy in squamous carcinoma of the female genitalia. Gynecol. Oncol., *1:* 314-319, 1973.

Morrow, C. P., and Rutledge, F. N. Melanoma of the vulva. Obstet. Gynecol., *39:* 745-752, 1972.

Mortel, R., Koss, L. G., Lewis, J. L., Jr., and D'Urso, J. R. Mesodermal mixed tumors of the uterine corpus. Obstet. Gynecol., *43:* 248-252, 1974.

Munnell, E. W. The changing prognosis and treatment in cancer of the ovary. Am. J. Obstet. Gynecol., *100:* 790-805, 1968.

Muggia, F. M., Perloff, M., Chia, G. A., Juden Reed, L., and Escher, G. C. Adriamycin in combination with cyclophosphamide (NSC26271); a phase I and II evaluation. Cancer Chemother. Rep., *58:* 919-926, 1974.

Nelson, A. J., III. Embryonal rhabdomyosarcoma; report of twenty-four cases and study of the effectiveness of radiation therapy upon the primary tumor. Cancer, *22:* 64-68, 1968.

Norris, H. J., and Taylor, H. B. Post-irradiation sarcomas of the uterus. Obstet. Gynecol., *26:* 689-694, 1965.

Norris, H. J., and Taylor, H. B. Prognosis of granulosa-theca tumors of the ovary. Cancer, *21:* 255-263, 1968.

Park, R. C., Patow, W. E., Rogers, R. E., and Zimmerman, E. A. Treatment of stage I carcinoma of the cervix. Obstet. Gynecol., *41:* 117-122, 1973.

Perez, C. A., and Bradfield, J. S. Radiation therapy in the treatment of carcinoma of the ovary. Cancer, *29:* 1027-1037, 1972.

Peterson, O. Spontaneous course of cervical precancerous conditions. Am. J. Obstet. Gynecol., *72:* 1063-1071, 1956.

Pezner, R. D., Stevens, K. A., Jr., Tong, D., and Allen, C. V. Limited epithelial carcinoma of the ovary treated with curative intent by the intraperitoneal instillation of radiocolloids. Cancer, *42:* 2563-2571, 1978.

Phelps, H. M., and Chapman, K. E. Role of radiation therapy in treatment of primary carcinoma of the uterine tube. Obstet. Gynecol., *43:* 669-673, 1974.

Piel, I. J., Slayton, R. E., Perlia, C. P., and Wilbanks, G. D. Combination chemotherapy with bleomycin and methotrexate in recurrent and disseminated cervical carcinoma; a preliminary study. Gynecol. Oncol., *1:* 184-190, 1973.

Piver, M. S. Radioactive colloids in the treatment of stage IA ovarian cancer. Obstet. Gynecol., *40:* 42-44, 1972.

Piver, M. S., Barlow, J. J., Vongtoma, V., and Webster, J. Hydroxyurea and radiation therapy in advanced cervical cancer. Am. J. Obstet. Gynecol., *120:* 969-972, 1974.

Piver, M. S., Barlow, J. J., and Xynos, F. P. Adriamycin alone or in combination in 100 patients with carcinoma of the cervix or vagina. Am. J. Obstet. Gynecol., *131:* 311-313, 1978.

Rawls, W. E., Gardner, H. L., and Kaufman, R. L. Antibodies to genital herpesvirus in patients with carcinoma of the cervix. Am. J. Obstet. Gynecol., *107:* 710–716, 1970.

Rosenoff, S. H., Young, R. C., Anderson, T., Bagley, C., Chabner, B., Schein, P. S., Hubbard, S., and DeVita, V. T. Peritoneoscopy; a valuable staging tool in ovarian carcinoma. Ann. Intern. Med., *83:* 37–41, 1975.

Ross, G. T., Hammond, C. B., and Odell, W. D. Chemotherapy for nonmetastatic gestational trophoblastic neoplasm. Clin. Obstet. Gynecol., *10:* 323–329, 1967.

Rutledge, F., Smith, J. P., and Franklin, E. W. Carcinoma of the vulva. Am. J. Obstet. Gynecol., *106:* 1117–1130, 1970.

Rutledge, F., and Sullivan, M. P. Sarcoma botryoides. Ann. N.Y. Acad. Sci., *142:* 694–708, 1967.

Rutledge, F. Treatment of epithelial cancer of the ovary. *In* Gynecologic Oncology, edited by F. Rutledge, R. C. Boronow and J. T. Wharton, pp. 183–199. John Wiley & Sons, New York, 1976.

Saltzstein, S. L., Woodruff, J. D., and Novak, E. R. Postgranulomatous carcinoma of the vulva. Obstet. Gynecol., *7:* 80–90, 1956.

Schiller, H. M., and Silverberg, S. G. Staging and prognosis in primary carcinoma of the fallopian tube. Cancer, *28:* 389–395, 1971.

Silverberg, E., and Holleb, A. I. Cancer statistics 1974—worldwide epidemiology. CA, *24:* 2–21, 1974.

Smith, J. P., Rutledge, F., and Soffar, S. W. Progestins in the treatment of patients with endometrial adenocarcinoma. Am. J. Obstet. Gynecol., *94:* 977–984, 1966.

Smith, J. P., Rutledge, F., Burns, B. C., Jr., and Soffar, S. Systemic chemotherapy for carcinoma of the cervix. Am. J. Obstet. Gynecol., *97:* 800–807, 1967.

Smith, J. P. General discussion of treatment of distant metastasis from squamous cell carcinoma of the uterine cervix. *In* Cancer of the Uterus and Ovary, p. 345. Yearbook Medical Publishers, Chicago, 1969a.

Smith, J. P. Hormone therapy for adenocarcinoma of the endometrium. *In* Cancer of the Uterus and Ovary, pp. 73–83. Yearbook Medical Publishers, Chicago, 1969b.

Smith, J. P., and Rutledge, F. N. Chemotherapy in the treatment of cancer of the ovary. Am. J. Obstet. Gynecol., *107:* 691–703, 1970.

Smith, J. P., Rutledge, F., and Wharton, J. T. Chemotherapy of ovarian cancer; new approaches to treatment. Cancer, *30:* 1565–1571, 1972.

Smith, J. P., and Rutledge, F. Advances in chemotherapy for gynecologic cancer. Cancer Suppl., *36:* 669–674, 1975.

Solidoro, A. S., Esteves, L., Castellano, C., Valdivia, E., and Barriga, O. Chemotherapy of advanced cancer of the cervix; experience in 55 cases treated with cyclophosphamide. Am. J. Obstet. Gynecol., *94:* 208–213, 1966.

Stanhope, C. R., Smith, J. P., and Rutledge, F. Second trial drugs in ovarian cancer. Gynecol. Oncol., *5:* 52–58, 1977.

Stolinsky, D. C., and Bateman, J. R. Further experience with hexamethylmelamine (HSC-13875) in the treatment of carcinoma of the cervix. Cancer Chemother. Rep., *57:* 497–499, 1973.

Sutow, W. W., Sullivan, M. P., Reid, H. L., Taylor, H. G., and Griffith, K. M. Prognosis in childhood rhabdomyosarcoma. Cancer, *25:* 1384–1390, 1970.

Suzuki, M., Murai, A., Watanabe, T., and Nunokawa, O. Treatment of female genital carcinoma with the tumor antibiotic bleomycin. *In* Proceedings of the 6th International Congress of Chemotherapy. University of Tokyo Press, Tokyo, 1969.

Taylor, G. W., and Nathanson, I. T. Lymph node metastases; incidence and surgical treatment in neoplastic disease. *In* Gynecological Cancer, edited by S. B. Gusberg and H. C. Frick II, Ed. 4, pp. 119. Williams & Wilkins, Baltimore, 1970.

Taylor, H. B., and Norris, H. J. Mesenchymal tumors of the uterus; IV. Diagnosis and prognosis of leiomyosarcomas. Arch. Pathol., *82*: 40–44, 1966.

Taylor, R. W., Brush, M. G., King, R. J. B., and Witt, M. The uptake of oestrogen by endometrial carcinoma. Proc. R. Soc. Med., *64*: 407–408, 1971.

Thigpen, J. T., Buchsbaum, H. J., Mangan, C., and Blessing, J. A. A Gynecologic Oncology Group study. Cancer Treat. Rep. *62*: 21–28, 1979.

Tod, M. C. Radium implantation treatment of carcinoma of vulva. Br. J. Radiol., *22*: 508–512, 1949.

Tormey, D. C., Bergevin, P., Blom, J., and Petty, W. Preliminary trials with a combination of Adriamycin (NSC-123127) and bleomycin (NSC-125066) in adult malignancies. Cancer Chemother. Rep., *57*: 413–418, 1973.

Trelford, J. D. A discussion of the results of chemotherapy on gynecological cancer and the host's immune response. Proc. Natl. Cancer Conf., *6*: 365–385, 1970.

Trussell, R. R., and Mitford-Barberton, G. de B. Carcinoma of the cervix treated with continuous intra-arterial methotrexate and intermittent intramuscular Leukovorin. Lancet, *1*: 971–972, 1961.

Tururen, A. Diagnosis and treatment of primary tubal carcinoma. Int. J. Obstet. Gynecol., *7*: 292–300, 1969.

Vaitukaitis, J. L., Braunstein, G. D., and Ross, G. T. A radioimmunoassay which specifically measures human chorionic gonadotropin in the presence of human luteinizing hormone. Am. J. Obstet. Gynecol., *113*: 751–758, 1972.

Van Orden, D. E., McAllister, W. B., Zerne, S. R. M., and Morris, J. M. Ovarian carcinoma, problems of staging and grading. Am. J. Obstet. Gynecol., *94*: 195–202, 1966.

Varga, A., and Henriksen, E. Histologic observations on the effect of 17-alpha-hydroxyprogesterone-17-N-caproate on endometrial carcinoma. Obstet. Gynecol., *26*: 656–664, 1965.

Wallach, R. L., Kabakow, B., Blinick, G., and Antopol, W. Thio-TEPA chemotherapy for ovarian carcinoma. Obstet. Gynecol., *35*: 278–286, 1970.

Way, S. Results of a planned attack on carcinoma of the vulva. Br. Med. J., *2*: 780–782, 1954.

Way, S., and Hennigan, M. The late results of extended radical vulvectomy for carcinoma of the vulva. J. Obstet. Gynecol. Br. Commonw., *73*: 594–598, 1966.

Wharton, J. T., Gallager, S., and Rutledge, F. N. Microinvasive carcinoma of the vulva. Am. J. Obstet. Gynecol., *118*: 159–162, 1974.

Wharton, J. T., Delclos, L., Gallager, S., and Smith, J. P. Radiation hepatitis induced by abdominal irradiation with cobalt 60 moving-strip technique. A.J.R., *117*: 73–80, 1973.

Wharton, J. T. Treatment of ovarian cancers (germ cell and mesenchymal origin). *In* Gynecologic Oncology, edited by F. Rutledge, R. C. Boronow and J. T. Wharton, pp. 201–209. John Wiley & Sons, New York, 1976.

Woodruff, J. D., Julian, C., Puray, T., Mermut, S., and Katanama, P. The contemporary challenge of carcinoma in-situ of the vulva. Am. J. Obstet. Gynecol., *115*: 677–684, 1973.

Woodruff, J. D., Parmley, T., and Julian, C. Topical 5-fluorouracil in the treatment of vaginal carcinoma in situ. Gynec. Oncol., *3*: 124–132, 1975.

Yackel, D. B., Symmonds, R. F., and Kempers, R. D. Melanoma of the vulva. Obstet. Gynecol., *35*: 625–631, 1970.

Young, R. C., Canellos, G. P., Chabner, B. A., Schein, P. S., Hubbard, S. P., and DeVita, V. T., Jr. Chemotherapy of advanced ovarian carcinoma; a prospective randomized comparison of phenylalanine mustard with high dose cyclophosphamide. Gynecol. Oncol., *2*: 489–497, 1974.

Young, R. C., Chabner, B. A., Hubbard, S. P., Canellos, G. P., and DeVita, V. T., Jr. Preliminary results of trials of chemotherapy in advanced ovarian carcinoma. Natl. Cancer Inst. Monogr., *42*: 145–148, 1975.

Young, R. C., Chabner, B. A., Hubbard, S. P., Fisher, R. I., Bender, R. A., Anderson, T., and DeVita, V. T. Advanced ovarian adenocarcinoma; melphalan (PAM) vs. combination chemotherapy (Hexa-CAF) (abstr.). Proc. Am. Soc. Clin. Oncol., *19*: 393, 1978.

Chapter 20

Breast

DOUGLASS C. TORMEY, M.D., Ph.D., and PHILIP COHEN, M.D.

The treatment of carcinoma of the breast underwent dramatic changes at the end of the 19th century. Prior to that time the primary therapeutic modality employed was a simple mastectomy. Near the turn of the century many advances occurred almost simultaneously: better anesthesia, improved antisepsis, disease regressions associated with bilateral oophorectomy, the development of radiotherapy, and improved surgical techniques. The ensueing 20–30 years were concerned primarily with defining the patient populations which should receive these developing therapeutic approaches. In the early 1940s the usefulness of exogenous estrogen therapy in postmenopausal women with recurrent disease was first utilized. Following the introduction of nitrogen mustard in the mid-1940s chemotherapeutic agents became a part of the armamentarium for advanced disease. Since that time a variety of single agents have been shown to induce disease regression. In 1963, Greenspan first introduced combination chemotherapy which then gained wide acceptance in 1969 after Cooper's report. At the present time investigative approaches are utilizing all of these modalities as well as immunotherapy in the treatment of both primary and recurrent disease.

Carcinoma of the breast became the leading cause of cancer deaths among women in the United States during the 1940s (American Cancer Society, 1978; Seidman, 1972). Today it is the leading cancer killer of women between the ages of 15 and 75. The risk of an individual female developing the disease over her life time is approximately 1 in 14. Although the peak incidence occurs at around age 50 the risk of developing the disease increases throughout life and is higher in women within a familial kindred (Anderson, 1977; Lynch et al., 1976). The 1978 American Cancer Society estimate of new cases of breast carcinoma diagnosed was 91,000, with approximately 34,000 deaths. Breast cancer is a rare tumor among males accounting for about 1% of the total cases seen annually. Although self-examination appears to detect the majority of tumors, the role of mammography in suspected cases for diagnostic assessment and localization is important. The use of routine mammography for screening, albeit controversial, does appear to be of value in selected cases, especially those women over age 50 (Strax et al., 1973).

STAGING

The currently accepted staging system for a patient presenting with carcinoma of the breast is presented in Table 20.1. It is currently urged that the parameters of tumor size, tumor extension, and axillary involvement should be assessed at the operative table to provide information relevant to the surgical stage of the patient. The same information should also be recorded by the pathologist and is referred to as the pathologic stage. The overall stage of a patient is based on the greatest and most accurate information which is available. This is important from the standpoint that approximately 25% of patients with clinically uninvolved ipsilateral axillary nodes will have involved axillary nodes by histologic exam and will thereby have a poorer prognosis (Fisher et al., 1969). Similarly, about 50% of patients with clinically palpable ipsilateral axillary nodes will be found to have uninvolved nodes histologically and their prognosis may be improved accordingly.

PATHOLOGY

The Armed Forces Institutes of Pathology (AFIP) classification of the histologic types of breast cancer is shown in Table 20.2. Approximately 80% of the tumors are scirrhous infiltrating ductal carcinomas. This classification varies slightly from the World Health Organization (WHO) classification which is shown in Table 20.3. The variations in survival based on histologic type are minimal, however the presence of tumor in the ipsilateral axillary nodes, absence of sinus histiocytosis, and a poorly differentiated appearance of the tumor nuclei all appear to be associated with a relatively poor prognosis (Seidman, 1972; Fisher et al., 1969). Sites of disease dissemination from autopsy data are shown in Table 20.4 (Cutler, 1962).

SURVIVAL

The survival in untreated patients with breast carcinoma was reviewed by Bloom (1974). The mean survival of 1728 such patients was 3.3 years. The median survival across all stages of the disease today is approximately 8.3 years (Seidman, 1972). This apparent improvement is deceptive since the death rate from the disease has remained at 24–30 per 100,000 population since 1940 (Seidman, 1972). Bond (1967) has shown that the risk of dying from breast carcinoma is logarithmic for at least 15 years from the time of diagnosis. During this time interval the risk of

TABLE 20.1

Abbreviated American Joint Committee for Cancer TNM Classification of Breast Carcinoma[a]

Primary Tumor (T)

TX   Tumor cannot be assessed

T1S   Carcinoma in situ or Paget's disease of the nipple with no demonstrable tumor

T0   No demonstrable tumor in the breast

T1   Tumor $\leq$2 cm; T1a, without fixation to pectoral fascia and/or muscle; T1b, with fixation to pectoral fascia and/or muscle

T2   Tumor >2 cm but $\leq$5 cm; T2a, without fixation to pectoral fascia and/or muscle; T2b, with fixation to pectoral fascia and/or muscle

T3   Tumor >5 cm; T3a, without fixation to pectoral fascia and/or muscle; T3b, with fixation to pectoral fascia and/or muscle

T4   Tumor of any size with direct extension to chest wall or skin; T4a, with fixation to chest wall; T4b, with edema or extension to skin; T4c, both of above; T4d, inflammatory carcinoma

Note: The above clinical classifications may be altered by the post-surgical-pathologic information to the extent that T1b lesions may be further classified as: (i) tumor <0.5 cm, (ii) tumor 0.5–0.9 cm, (iii) tumor 1.0–1.9 cm.

Nodal Involvement (N)

NX   Regional lymph nodes cannot be clinically assessed

N0   No palpable homolateral axillary nodes

N1   Movable homolateral axillary nodes; N1a, nodes not considered to contain tumor; N1b, nodes considered to contain tumor

N2   Homolateral axillary nodes fixed to each other or to other structures

N3   Homolateral supraclavicular of infraclavicular nodes or arm edema

Note: The above clinical classification may be altered by the post-surgical-pathologic information to the extent that N1a is lymph nodes with only histologic growth, and N1b is gross metastatic carcinoma in lymph nodes with: (i) micrometastasis <0.2 cm, (ii) metastasis >0.2 cm in 1 to 3 nodes, (iii) metastasis to >3 nodes, (iv) any node positive >2 cm in diameter.

Distant Metastasis (M)

MX   Not assessed

M0   No distant metastases known

M1   Distant metastases including skin beyond the breast area with sites specified

Stage Groupings for Invasive Carcinoma

Stage I   T1a or T1b, N0 or N1a, M0

Stage II   T0, N1b, M0

            T2a or T2b, N0 or N1a or N1b, M0

Stage III   Any T3, N1 or N2, M0

Stage IV   T4, Any N, Any M

            Any T, N3, Any M

            Any T, Any N, M1

[a] From the *Manual for Staging of Cancer* (1977).

developing a second primary in the opposite breast ranges from 26% for comedo and lobular carcinomas to 17% for anaplastic ductular carcinomas, and to 14% for medullary carcinomas (Adair et al., 1974). Over the 30-year period from diagnosis the risk of developing a primary in the

TABLE 20.2
Armed Forces Institute of Pathology (AFIP) Classification of Breast Carcinoma

I. Noninfiltrating duct carcinoma
   1. Papillary (cribriform)
   2. Solid (comedo)
II. Infiltrating duct carcinoma
   1. Scirrhous
   2. Comedo
   3. Medullary
   4. Papillary
   5. Colloid
III. Paget's disease of the nipple
IV. Noninfiltrating lobular carcinoma
V. Infiltrating lobular carcinoma
VI. Rare carcinomas
   1. Sweat gland (apocrine)
   2. Adenoid cystic
   3. Tubular
   4. Inflammatory
   5. Metaplastic lesions
      a. Cartilage
      b. Spindle
      c. Squamous

TABLE 20.3
World Health Organization (WHO) Classification of Breast Carcinoma

I. Intraductal and intralobular noninfiltrating carcinoma
II. Infiltrating carcinoma
III. Special variants
   1. Medullary
   2. Papillary
   3. Cribriform (adenoid cystic)
   4. Mucous (colloid)
   5. Lobular
   6. Squamous
   7. Paget's
   8. Carcinoma in fibroadenoma

second breast drops from 3.8% in the first 5 years to 1.6% between 25 and 30 years (Adair et al., 1974). The 5-year survival figures for each clinical stage of the disease are: Stage I—85%, Stage II—66%, Stage III—41%, and Stage IV—10%. If these figures are altered to combine clinical staging with pathologic staging it is observed that the influence of histologically positive ipsilateral axillary nodes is an important determinant of overall risk of recurrence and subsequent survival (Table 20.5). The influence of pathologic type on 5-year survival ranges from 57% for lobular carcinomas to 89% for papillary carcinomas; however, these figures have not been corrected for prognostic factors such as the presence or absence of nodal involvement (Adair et al., 1974). The time from first recurrence of disease to death has been reported to be about 9 months (Fisher et al., 1968).

THERAPEUTIC APPROACHES—PRIMARY DISEASE

Patients presenting for the first time can be divided into those who are operable and those who are inoperable. This latter category generally includes patients with primary lesions which are fixed to the chest wall, are large and ulcerating, or are associated with extensive edema or inflammatory changes of the skin overlying the breast; or are associated with matted axillary nodes, or edema of the arm, or supraclavicular metastases; or have disseminated disease. Some surgeons also include patients with any skin ulcerations, subcutaneous "satellite" nodules, or axillary nodes more than 2 cm in transverse diameter. In those patients with metastatic disease at the time of presentation local therapy is directed at reducing the subsequent development of secondary local

TABLE 20.4
Breast Carcinoma Metastases—Autopsy Data[a]

Organ	Percent	Organ	Percent
Lymph nodes	87	Kidney	13
Lungs	58–78	Diaphragm	13–14
Brain	58	Spleen	13–23
Liver	54–59	Pancreas	12–13
Bone	43–48	Skin	11–38
Adrenals	31–44	Cervix/Uterus	11
Gastrointestinal tract	26	Peritoneum	9–20
Pleura	23–35	Thyroid	9
Heart	21–33	Other	12–13
Ovary	13–16		

[a] Adapted from Cutler (1962).

TABLE 20.5
Effect of Histologic Evidence of Ipsilateral Axillary Lymph Node Involvement upon Recurrence Rate and Survival of Clinical Stage I and II Patients with Breast Carcinoma[a]

Nodal Status	Recurrence Rate (%)		Survival	
	5-year	10-year	5-year	10-year
Negative nodes	21	24	56	65
Positive nodes				
1–3	53	65	62	38
≥4	80	86	31	13

[a] Adapted from Fisher (1974).

complications such as skin ulceration. This is usually accomplished with either radiotherapy to the primary lesion and/or a total, i.e., simple, mastectomy followed by treatment of the disseminated disease as outlined below.

Patients without disseminated disease but who have inoperable lesions are generally treated first by radiotherapy to the primary lesion. If the lesion becomes operable during the course of radiotherapy some physicians would then extirpate the lesion with a simple or modified radical mastectomy. This may be done after the completion of radiotherapy but in some centers the radiotherapy is interrupted in order to perform the operative procedure. In the latter instance the radiotherapy is usually completed postoperatively.

The cohort of patients which are primarily operable would include those in Stages I and II and those in Stage III which have T3a lesions. It should be noted that some patients who have T4b lesions manifested by less than 2 or 3 cm of skin ulceration are also considered operable by many physicians. With lesions greater than 5 cm in diameter some centers will perform preoperative radiotherapy. The most common approach, however, would be to perform an operative procedure as the initial therapeutic approach. The baseline procedure in this country is a Halsted radical mastectomy, however, a modified radical mastectomy is the more common operation. In the latter procedure all or a portion of the pectoralis muscles are left intact but the axillary contents are still dissected free along with the entire breast and nipple. Other procedures which are occasionally utilized include a total mastectomy (removal of the breast only) or a wedge resection of the lesion. A few physicians will perform an extended radical mastectomy by removing the second, third, and fourth costal cartilages in order to dissect the internal mammary nodes. A superradical mastectomy is rarely performed but would involve removal of a portion of the chest wall and the supraclavicular nodes. There is little information from which to choose the best procedure at the present time. Current randomized clinical trials are attempting to delineate the conditions under which these various operative procedures should be utilized.

The use of adjuvant therapy postoperatively continues to be the subject of extensive clinical investigation. Postoperative radiotherapy is frequently used for patients who receive an operative procedure less than a modified radical mastectomy, or have medial or central lesions and/or have histologically positive ipsilateral axillary lymph nodes. There are a number of prospective randomized clinical trials testing postoperative radiotherapy in patients who have received a radical mastectomy (Fisher, 1973). The utilization of postoperative radiotherapy will decrease the local recurrence rate from 15% to 8%, however, the decrease in the local recurrence rate is frequently associated with increased distant metastases as the first evidence of recurrence. This is not unexpected since Bruce et al. (1970) have shown that local and distant metastases tend to occur concomitantly. In addition no improvement in overall survival has been noted with the use of postoperative radiotherapy. A recent analysis of the pooled data from randomized trials testing postoperative radiotherapy suggests that survival may be decreased in the radiated groups (Stjernsward, 1974).

The use of prophylactic oophorectomies postoperatively has come under study in several centers and has yet to have its role defined (Fisher, 1973). Postoperative castration has been reported to increase the time to first recurrence, but not survival, in premenopausal patients who have positive axillary nodes at the time of mastectomy; it has not been shown to have any benefit for those patients who had negative axillary nodes. Similar information is available for patients in the postmenopausal age groups. The use of radiotherapeutic ovarian ablation has been suggested as a useful means for delaying the time to recurrence and prolonging survival in both pre- and postmenopausal patients in another study. This area continues to be under investigation and no firm guidelines have yet evolved. In view of the conflicting data it should be remembered that postoperative castration in premenopausal patients removes one means for assessing whether or not relapsed patients might respond to subsequent hormonal procedures.

The use of chemotherapy for patients at high risk of relapse following mastectomy has been tested in several centers (Fisher, 1973; Tormey, 1975). Cyclophosphamide given for less than 2 months postoperatively has yielded both beneficial and detrimental results in different studies. At the present time it would appear that the use of a combination of cyclophosphamide, methotrexate, and 5-fluorouracil for up to 1 year postoperatively in premenopausal patients with positive ipsilateral axillary nodes provides a distinct survival benefit to at least 4 years (Bonadonna et al., 1978). Although lengthening of the disease-free time was observed with such therapy in postmenopausal women no improvement was noted in overall survival. This area is currently under extensive investigation with single and combination chemotherapeutic as well as immunotherapeutic approaches.

THERAPEUTIC APPROACHES—FIRST RECURRENCE

Once a patient has developed a first recurrence of breast cancer therapy continues to be relatively well standardized. The initial therapy for the premenopausal patient is usually an oophorectomy. Those patients who respond to the oophorectomy and then relapse can then be selected for treatment by either adrenalectomy or hypophysectomy. Following failure to these endocrine ablative procedures patients are treated with androgens in some cancer clinics whereas others will proceed with chemotherapy.

For the patient >5 years postmenopausal the treatment of first recurrence continues to be the initial use of an exogenous estrogen such as diethylstilbesterol 5 mg t.i.d. For patients within 5 years of the menopause, especially with osseous lesions, many physicians prefer to use androgens instead of estrogens. Those patients responding to estrogen or androgen therapy are sometimes considered for an adrenalectomy or hypophysectomy at their next disease progression; following this some clinicians use the alternate androgen or estrogen whilst others turn to chemotherapy. The side effects of estrogen and androgen therapy are shown in Tables 20.6 and 20.7.

Despite this relatively well standardized therapeutic flow there is data to suggest that a response to exogenous hormones in postmenopausal patients has no predictive value for a response to subsequent ablative procedures (Dao and Nemoto, 1965). In most centers hormone procedures are abandoned in favor of chemotherapy in the presence of central nervous system involvement, lymphangitic pulmonary metastases, hepatic involvement manifested by jaundice or a very large liver, bone marrow involvement manifested systemically, or if the patient fails to respond to the first hormone manipulation.

The use of chemotherapy as an adjunct to hormone manipulation for the treatment of first recurrent breast cancer is currently undergoing test in several centers. Most of these trials are based on Van Dyk and Falkson's observation that the addition of postoperative cyclophospha-

TABLE 20.6

Side Effects of Testosterone Propionate in Patients with Advanced Breast Cancer[a]

Side Effect	Treated > 6 Weeks (48 Patients)		Treated >3 Months (33 Patients)	
	+ Effect	Incidence (%)	+ Effect	Incidence (%)
Feeling of well being	27	56	26	78
Appetite increase	31	64	25	75
Weight gain	28	58	24	72
Hirsutism	34	70	30	92
Hoarseness	36	75	31	93
Acne	30	63	26	78
Libido increase	32	67	27	81
Hair loss	9	18	9	27
Flushing	33	69	27	81
Erythrocytosis	20	41	18	54
Edema	16	33	15	45
Congestive failure	2	4	1	3
Nausea	9	18	8	24
Vomiting	3	6	2	6
Drowsiness	3	6	2	6
Hypercalcemia	4	8	2	6

[a] Adapted from Kennedy (1965).

TABLE 20.7

Side Effects of Diethylstilbestrol in Patients with Advanced Breast Cancer[a]

Side Effect	Treated > 6 Weeks (45 Patients)		Treated > 3 Months (30 Patients)	
	+ Effect	Incidence (%)	+ Effect	Incidence (%)
Nausea	31	69	20	67
Vomiting	16	36	7	23
Pigmentation	21	47	18	60
Skin rash	4	9	3	10
Mastodynia	15	33	12	40
Vaginal bleeding	8	18	7	23
Vaginal discharge	6	13	5	17
Incontinence	18	40	15	50
Edema	17	38	14	47
Congestive failure	1	2	1	3
Drowsiness	2	4	1	3
Hypercalcemia	2	4	0	—

[a] Adapted from Kennedy (1965).

mide appeared to double the 5-year survival rate for premenopausal patients who undergo oophorectomy as treatment for their first recurrent disease (Van Dyk and Falkson, 1971). They also reported that the systemic treatment of a first recurrent breast cancer should be instituted as soon after the diagnosis of recurrence as possible. Those patients in whom treatment was delayed for more than two months after their recurrence had been diagnosed experienced a significantly lower 5-year survival fraction than those who were treated within 2 months of recurrence.

THERAPEUTIC APPROACHES—CHEMOTHERAPY

Breast cancer responds to a variety of chemotherapeutic agents given singly (Table 20.8). These responses tend to be 4–6 months in duration, and very few complete responses are obtained (Broder and Tormey, 1974).

A landmark in the chemotherapy of breast cancer was the work by Greenspan published in 1963 and 1966 and the report by Cooper in 1969 in which 60–90% response rates were observed utilizing combinations of drugs. The best known combination is that reported by Cooper which included cyclophosphamide, vincristine, methotrexate, 5-fluorouracil, and prednisone. Other groups have used similar combinations of these drugs and have also obtained response rates greater than 50% (Broder and Tormey, 1974). Current investigations have been designed to ascertain first, whether all five drugs are needed in the combination to obtain this high response rate; and second, if the response rate can be improved by changes in drug scheduling or by substitution of other drugs. Three to five drug combinations have been tested against sequential use of the

TABLE 20.8

Single Agent Therapy in Advanced Breast Carcinoma[a]

Drug	No. of Patients Evaluable	No. of Patients Responding	Percent Responding
ALKYLATING AGENTS			
Cyclophosphamide	529	182	34
Nitrogen mustard	92	32	35
Phenylalanine mustard	86	20	23
Chlorambucil	54	11	20
Thio-TEPA	162	48	30
ANTIMETABOLITES			
5-Fluorouracil	1236	324	26
Methotrexate	356	120	34
6-Mercaptopurine	44	6	14
Cytosine arabinoside	64	6	9
Hydroxyurea	16	2	12
VINCA ALKALOIDS			
Vincristine	226	47	21
Vinblastine	95	19	20
ANTIBIOTICS			
Adriamycin	221	81	37
Mitomycin C	60	23	38
Other antibiotics (acti-nomycin D, mithramy-cin, streptonigrin, bleo-mycin, daunomycin)	99	13	13
SYNTHETICS			
BCNU	76	16	21
CCNU	155	18	12
MCCNU	33	2	6
Hexamethylmelamine	39	11	28
Imidazole carboxamide	29	2	7
Dibromodulcitol	22	6	27
Procarbazine	21	1	5

[a] Adapted from Broder and Tormey (1974). Abbreviations: BCNU = 1,3-bis(2-chloro-ethyl)-1-nitrosourea, CCNU = 1-(2 chloroethyl)-3-cyclohexyl-1-nitrosourea, and MCCNU = 1-(2-chloroethyl)-3-(4-methylcyclohexyl)-1-nitrosourea.

same agents given singly and have provided higher response rates with longer survivals (Tormey and Neifeld, 1977). In general the use of three to five drug combination chemotherapy yields response rates ranging from 50 to 85%, which is twice the level obtained with single agents. The survival of the patients who exhibit a response ranges from 13 to 24 months (Tormey and Neifeld, 1977). The patients who do not respond to the combination have a median survival of 4–9 months. Combination chemotherapy thus appears to mark a significant improvement in the outlook for patients who present with metastatic disease. Reviews of the multiplicity of approaches to combination chemotherapy appeared in 1974 and 1977 (Broder and Tormey, 1974; Tormey and Neifeld, 1977).

OTHER THERAPEUTIC APPROACHES

Recently, considerable investigative interest has developed in the use of "antihormones." The steroid synthesis inhibitor, aminoglutethimide, is being evaluated as an alternative to ablative therapy. Preliminary results suggest it may be associated with a response rate approximating that of adrenalectomy. The "antiestrogen" class of drugs, e.g., nafoxidine and tamoxifen, appear to block the effects of estrogens on target tissues by binding to the estrogen receptor protein and are associated with response rates of approximately 25–35%. Drugs such as L-dopa appear to be potent prolactin inhibitors and are being evaluated for their capability to substitute for the use of hypophysectomy.

MARKERS IN BREAST CANCER

There is currently one major hormone marker being evaluated extensively for its prognostic importance in breast cancer. In order for a tumor's growth to be either dependent upon or sensitive to estrogen the tumor must be capable of binding estrogen to a cytoplasmic receptor, the estrogen binding protein (EBP). The presence of the EBP in the tumor appears to be associated with a 45–60% chance of responding to appropriate hormone procedures, whereas its absence appears to be associated with less than a 10% chance of responding (McQuire et al., 1975).

Other biochemical markers of disease activity are also under investigation. Significant numbers of breast cancer patients have abnormal blood or urine levels of carcinoembryonic antigen (CEA), human chorionic gonadotrophin (HCG), L-fucose, polyamines, pseudouridine, methylated nucleosides, and Regan's isoenzyme. The usefulness of these and other tests in predicting the effects of therapeutic manipulations are under evaluation.

COMPLICATIONS OF BREAST CARCINOMA

Breast cancer can metastasize to virtually any organ site (Table 22.4). Because of problems related to diagnosis and clinical management, some of these sites are considered separately below.

Bone and Bone Marrow

One of the most common sites of breast cancer metastasis is bone. When major weight-bearing bones are involved with cortex-eroding lesions, e.g., vertebral column, pelvic acetabulae, or femoral necks, many physicians suggest early radiotherapy to the involved sites. The predilection for osseous involvement is also associated with hypercalcemia in up to 30% of patients during their disease. A special circumstance is the development of hypercalcemia within the first 2 weeks of initiating therapy with exogenous hormones. In this setting the hormone should be withdrawn until normocalcemia returns, after which it may be reinstituted at lower doses (e.g., 5 mg of diethylstilbesterol per day) and the dose escalated in 25–30% increments every 3–7 days until the projected therapeutic levels are obtained.

The high incidence of bone marrow involvement with metastatic breast carcinoma has not been appreciated. In one study approximately 50% of the patients with metastatic disease had bone marrow involvement (Ingle et al., 1978). All but one of the patients with bone marrow involvement had bone cortex involvement. Bone marrow aspirates were often negative when bone marrow biopsies were positive. Tumor cells in the bone marrow can evoke an intense sclerotic reaction which can lead to pancytopenia. On the other hand mild to moderate bone marrow infiltration can cause a marked leukemoid reaction or occasionally a leukoerythroblastic blood picture. In the setting of marked cytopenias secondary to tumor involvement of the bone marrow (WBC <2,500; platelets <75,000) combination chemotherapy should be instituted at relatively low dosages, e.g., at 25% of the usual dosage. On this type of regimen many of the patients will show a gradual bone marrow tumor cell lysis with replacement of the fibrous reaction by normal bone marrow elements (Ingle et al., 1977). Such a normalization of the bone marrow with improvement of peripheral blood counts occurs slowly over many months. Drug dosages should be increased as peripheral blood counts improve.

Soft Tissue

Local and/or regional skin and soft tissue recurrence is quite common (from 5 to 40% of patients) and most frequently involves the chest wall in the area of the original mastectomy site. Although many physicians have treated initial cutaneous recurrences with local excision and/or local radiotherapy, evidence from Bruce et al. (1970) indicates that the time from mastectomy to the first local/regional recurrence and to distant metastasis is equivalent, suggesting the disseminated nature of the disease at the time of "local/regional" recurrence. Because of this observation we feel that local/regional cutaneous or soft tissue recurrence is an indication for systemic treatment with an endocrine manipulation and/or chemotherapy.

Central Nervous System

Metastatic involvement of the brain occurs in approximately 20% of patients with breast carcinomas. The symptoms are those of generalized increased intracranial pressure with or without associated neurologic deficits, the nature of which depends on the location of the metastatic lesion. Because of the high proportion of multiple brain lesions in these patients, and since the presence of CNS disease is almost invariably associated with dissemination to other organ sites, craniotomy with resection of the metastatic tumor mass is generally not indicated. Treatment usually involves the use of osmotic diuretics, high dose glucocorticoids (e.g., 8–12 mg dexamethasone daily in divided doses), cranial radiotherapy (4000–6000 R), and the use of systemic chemotherapy, including agents that cross the blood brain barrier.

Diffuse involvement of the leptomeninges with tumor occurs in approximately 10% of patients with metastatic breast carcinoma. The commonest initial symptoms of meningeal carcinomatosis are headache, low back pain, and dysaesthesias of the legs. Lower extremity weakness, depressed tendon reflexes, sensory abnormalities, and sphincter dysfunction are also commonly seen. Cranial nerve involvement and deterioration of mental function are generally late stages in the course of the syndrome.

The early peripheral symptoms of carcinomatous meningitis are similar to those of spinal epidural compression from metastatic breast carcinoma. It is important to differentiate between these two entities since the latter is quite amenable to radiotherapy of the involved spinal segments. Myelography may be helpful in establishing a diagnosis of epidural compression and must be performed in suspected cases but may be negative in the face of positive neurologic findings, in which case local radiation therapy is still indicated. Isolated spinal epidural compression generally occurs adjacent to roentgenographically involved vertebral bodies.

Forty percent of the patients with carcinomatous meningitis have histologic involvement of the spinal leptomeninges and cauda equina. Isolated forms of meningeal carcinomatosis involving the spine alone have been reported. Coexisting CNS mass lesions are seen in 25% of patients with meningeal carcinomatosis. The "classic" cerebrospinal fluid (CSF) findings of high protein, low sugar, mononuclear pleocytosis, and tumor cells on cytological examination are seen in only 30% of the patients. In the presence of suggestive symptomatology, therefore, repeat lumbar punctures with CSF examinations for malignant cells are often necessary to establish a diagnosis. The use of a Millipore filter or cytocentrifuge increases the yield of finding abnormal cells in the CSF. The prognosis for patients with meningeal carcinomatosis is poor. In recent series the median survival for patients with breast cancer was less than 6 weeks from the time of diagnosis of the meningeal involvement. Currently used treatment modalities involve the use of craniospinal radiation, intrathecal methotrexate, or a combination of the two modalities. The diagnosis, clinical course and treatment of carcinomatous meningitis have been reviewed by Little et al. (1974) and Olson et al. (1974).

Pulmonary

Pulmonary metastases are seen in approximately 50–70% of autopsied patients with metastatic breast carcinoma, and can be nodular and/or lymphangitic. Metastases may be so small as to be undetectable on routine chest x-ray examination—in such cases whole lung tomograms may disclose metastatic foci. The presence of a single, isolated pulmonary lesion does not preclude surgical removal of the pulmonary lesion, especially in patients with a long disease-free interval from mastectomy (>5 years). However, the disseminated nature of the disease at the time of the discovery of an apparently isolated metastatic focus, plus recent advances in adjuvant chemotherapy, would argue in favor of systemic treatment for these patients following resection of the lesion.

Lymphangitic carcinomatosis of the lungs is secondary to a rapid growth and dissemination of tumor cells through the peribronchial and perivascular lymphatics that penetrate the pleural lymphatic network, and occurs particularly commonly in patients with prior pleural or mediastinal tumor involvement. Its diagnosis is often heralded by the appearance of Kerley B lines on chest roentgenograms and/or frequent coughing. Its clinical appearance can be abrupt and rapidly progressive with chest pain, cough, and severe dyspnea with hypoxia. Symptomatic treatment should include the use of oxygen, nebulizers, and intermittent positive pressure breathing (IPPB). Because there is often an associated damage to the pulmonary microvascular and lymphatic network with pulmonary edema, diuresis may improve the hypoxia. Digitalization has been of no therapeutic value in the absence of overt congestive heart failure. Because of the rapidly progressive nature of lymphangitic pulmonary carcinomatosis combination chemotherapy is generally the initial antitumor treatment of choice. Some authors have recommended the addition of prednisone in doses up to 70 mg daily to the other chemotherapeutic agents, although there has not been a randomized trial attesting to its efficacy.

Other Complications

Despite the high incidence of pituitary gland and adrenal gland metastases (25–50%) in various autopsy and surgical series the clinical appearance of adrenal or pituitary insufficiency has not been a major problem.

Intraocular metastasis is an uncommon clinical manifestation, although some studies report an incidence as high as 37% at autopsy. Retinal metastasis may be the first evidence of disseminated disease. Breast carcinoma and melanoma are the solid tumors with the greatest tendency to metastasize to the retina. Patients with breast carcinoma, especially those who develop visual symptoms, should have periodic, thorough funduscopic examinations. Local radiation therapy along with systemic treatment (either endocrine or chemotherapy) is the treatment of choice. Enucleation is generally not required.

INFLAMMATORY CANCER OF THE BREAST

Inflammatory carcinoma of the breast is an uncommon clinical presentation of breast malignancy occurring in 1–2% of patients with breast carcinoma (Robbins et al., 1974). It is seen most frequently in women with large, pendulous breasts and is often initially mistaken for a breast abscess. Yonemoto has established the following criteria for making a diagnosis of inflammatory breast carcinoma: (1) erythema and edema involving greater than one-third of the skin overlying the breast, (2) skin changes not due to direct extension of a growing breast mass; (3) skin thickening on mammography; and (4) presence of tumor cells in dermal lymphatic ducts (Yonemoto et al., 1970). Although some pathologists have attempted to define inflammatory breast carcinoma histologically (Ellis and Teitelbaum, 1974), it remains primarily a clinical diagnosis. The causative factors leading to this presentation are not well understood. Corall and Dao (1958) have demonstrated delayed hypersensitivity reactions in patients with inflammatory breast carcinoma to extracts of their own tumors.

The tumor has a poor prognosis with early distant metastases. Five-year survivals have been less than 5% in most series. Simple or radical mastectomy has not been effective in controlling the disease and for this reason many physicians consider inflammatory breast carcinoma a contraindication for mastectomy. Radiotherapy has caused transient tumor regression in approximately one half of the patients but 5-year survivals are less than 2% (Yonemoto et al., 1970). Oophorectomy combined with bilateral adrenalectomy appears to be the most effective palliative treatment available (Yonemoto et al., 1970). Responses have been seen with combination chemotherapy, but its ultimate therapeutic role has not been adequately assessed.

CYSTOSARCOMA PHYLLOIDES

Cystosarcoma phylloides is an uncommon tumor, comprising 0.5% of all breast tumors. Less than 20% of these tumors are malignant. Patients are younger than those with adenocarcinoma of the breast; the average age is 40 years. The tumor presents most commonly as a bulky mass (often larger than 10 cm in diameter) with prominent large veins on the overlying skin. Pain and ulceration are common and are usually secondary to avascular necrosis of the large tumor mass. Histologically the tumor consists of epithelial and stromal elements with the epithelial cells lining ductlike structures. Malignant changes, if present, occur only in the stromal components. There is a poor correlation between the initial histologic appearance and the subsequent course of the disease—some patients with apparently benign appearing tumors have subsequent metastatic involvement, and many with marked stromal atypia at diagnosis have a benign clinical course. Axillary metastases occur in only 5-15% of patients. Ipsilateral axillary adenopathy however, is not uncommon and is usually caused by inflammatory changes from adjacent tumor necrosis and infection.

Distant metastases are of stromal malignant components only and are seen most frequently in the lungs and skeletal system—although any part of the body can be involved (Treves and Sunderland, 1951; Kessinger et al., 1972).

The primary surgical therapy is simple mastectomy for lesions that are histologically benign. High incidences of local recurrence (up to 36%) have been reported when local excision alone has been utilized (Lawrence, 1972). For histologically malignant tumors removal of the breast and underlying pectoralis muscles have been recommended because of the tendency of cystosarcoma phylloides to invade locally. Since axillary lymph nodes are seldom involved with tumor routine axillary dissection is generally not performed. Most physicians have been discouraged with the results of radiotherapy in the treatment of primary, locally recurrent, or metastatic cystosarcoma phylloides (Kessinger et al., 1972). There have been no reported studies discussing the chemotherapy of metastatic disease.

BREAST SARCOMA

Pure breast sarcoma, i.e., sarcoma in which no epithelial cells are present, is uncommon, comprising between 0.3% and 1% of all breast tumors. As with cystosarcoma phylloides it occurs in a younger patient group than breast carcinoma (average age, 38 years) and presents as a breast mass with overlying dilated veins. Axillary lymph nodes are rarely involved although the tumor frequently extends locally to involve the pectoralis fascia and pectoralis major. Local pain is seen in one-third of the cases. The tumor may arise from a pre-existing benign fibroadenoma. Breast sarcoma may be rapidly growing and frequently presents as an accelerated growth of a previously stationary nodule. Fibrosarcoma is the most common histologic type (60-70% of all cases). The treatment of choice is local mastectomy with removal of the underlying pectoral fascia. Axillary lymph node dissection is not of value. Five-year disease free survival in most series occurs in 50-60% of all patients. Radiotherapy is of value in the treatment of recurrent anaplastic lesions, but its efficacy as an adjuvant to surgery as primary therapy has been largely unassessed. The value of chemotherapy in an adjuvant setting or for the treatment of metastatic disease has been essentially untested. At the current time metastatic disease should probably be treated with chemotherapy regimens effective for soft tissue sarcomas (see Chapter 26).

REFERENCES

Adair, F., Berg, J., Joubert, L., and Robbins, G. F. Long term follow-up of breast cancer patients; the 30-year report. Cancer, *33*: 1145–1150, 1974.

American Cancer Society. 1978 Cancer Facts and Figures. New York, 1978.

Anderson, D. E. Breast cancer in families. Cancer, *40*: 1855–1860, 1977.

Bloom, H. J. G. Survival of women with untreated breast cancer—past and present. In Prognostic Factors in Breast Cancer, edited by A. P. M. Forrest and P. B. Kunkler, pp. 3–19. E. & S. Livingstone, London, 1974.

Bonadonna, G., Valagussa, P., Rossi, A., Zucali, R., Tancini, G., Bajetta, E., Brambilla, C., De Lena, M., Di Fronzo, G., Banfi, A., Rilke, F., and Veronesi, U. Are surgical adjuvant trials altering the course of breast cancer? Semin. Oncol. *5:* 450–464, 1978.

Bond, W. H. The influence of various treatments on survival rates in cancer of the breast. In The Treatment of Carcinoma of the Breast: Proceedings of a Symposium held at Gonville & Caius College, Cambridge, 1967, edited by A. S. Jarrett, pp. 24–39. Excerpta Medica Foundation, London, 1968.

Broder, L., and Tormey, D. C. Combination chemotherapy of carcinoma of the breast—a review. Cancer Treat. Rev. *1:* 183–203, 1974.

Bruce, J., Carter, D. C., and Fraser, J. Patterns of recurrent disease in breast cancer. Lancet, *1:* 433–435, 1970.

Cooper, R. Combination chemotherapy in hormone resistant breast cancer (abstr.). Proc. Am. Assoc. Cancer Res., *10:* 15, 1969.

Corall, J. T., and Dao, T. L. The etiology of inflammatory relations in breast carcinoma. Surg. Forum, *9:* 611–614, 1958.

Culter, M. Tumors of the Breast, pp. 124–147. J. B. Lippincott, Philadelphia, 1962.

Dao, T., and Nemoto, T. An evaluation of adrenalectomy and androgen in disseminated mammary carcinoma. Surg. Gynecol. Obstet., *121:* 1257–1262, 1965.

Ellis, D. L., and Teitelbaum, S. L. Inflammatory carcinoma of the breast—a pathologic definition. Cancer, *33:* 1045–1047, 1974.

Fisher, B., Ravdin, R. G., Ausman, R. K., Slack, N. H., Moore, G. E., Noer, R. J., Cooperating Investigators. Surgical adjuvant chemotherapy in cancer of the breast; results of a decade of cooperative investigation. Ann. Surg., *168:* 337–356, 1968.

Fisher, B., Slack, N. H., Bross, I. D. J., and Cooperating Investigators. Cancer of the breast; size of neoplasm and prognosis. Cancer, *24:* 1071–1080, 1969.

Fisher, B. Cooperative clinical trials in primary breast cancer; a critical appraisal. Cancer, *31:* 1271–1286, 1973.

Fisher, B. Presented at the Breast Cancer Task Force Report to the Profession, Bethesda, Md., Sept. 30, 1974.

Greenspan, E. Response of advanced breast cancer to the combination of the antimetabolite, methotrexate, and the alkylating agent thio-TEPA. J. Mt. Sinai Hosp. N.Y., *30:* 246–267, 1963.

Greenspan, E. Combination cytotoxic chemotherapy in advanced disseminated breast cancer. J. Mt. Sinai Hosp. N.Y., *33:* 1, 1966.

Ingle, J. N., Tormey, D. C., Bull, J. M., and Simon, R. M. Bone marrow involvement in breast cancer; effect on response and tolerance to combination chemotherapy. Cancer, *39:* 104–111, 1977.

Ingle, J. N., Tormey, D. C., and Tan, H. K. The bone marrow examination in breast cancer; diagnostic considerations and clinical usefulness. Cancer, *41:* 670–674, 1978.

Kennedy, B. J. Systemic effects of androgenic and estrogenic hormones in advanced breast cancer. J. Am. Geriatr. Soc., *13:* 230–235, 1965.

Kessinger, A., Foley, J. F., Lemon, H. M., and Miller, D. M. Metastatic cystosarcoma phylloides; a case report and review of the literature. J. Surg. Oncol., *4:* 131–147, 1972.

Lawrence, G. A. Cystosarcoma phylloides. Indian J. Cancer *9:* 231–239, 1972.

Little, J. R., Dale, A. J. D., and Okazaki, H. Meningeal carcinomatosis; clinical manifestations. Arch. Neurol., *30:* 138–143, 1974.

Lynch, H. T., Guirgis, H., Brodkey, F., Maloney, K., Lynch, P. M., Rankin, L., and Lynch, J. Early age of onset in familial breast cancer. Arch. Surg., *111:* 126–131, 1976.

Manual for Staging of Cancer. American Joint Committee for Cancer Staging and End Results Reporting. Chicago, 1977.

McQuire, W. L., Carbone, P. P., Sears, M. E., and Escher, G. C. Estrogen receptors in human breast cancer; an overview. *In* Estrogen Receptors in Human Breast Cancer, edited by W. L. McQuire, P. P. Carbone, and E. P. Volmer, pp. 1–7. Raven Press, New York, 1975.

Olson, M. E., Chernik, N. L., and Posner, J. B. Infiltration of the leptomeninges by systemic cancer—a clinical and pathologic study. Arch. Neurol., *30:* 122–137, 1974.

Robbins, G. J., Shah, J., Rosen, P., Chu, F., and Taylor, J. Inflammatory carcinoma of the breast. Surg. Clin. N. Am., *54:* 801–807, 1974.

Seidman, K. Cancer of the Breast; Statistical and Epidemiological Data. American Cancer Society, New York, 1972.

Stjernsward, J. Decreased survival related to irradiation postoperatively in early operable breast cancer. Lancet, *2:* 1285–1286, 1974.

Strax, P., Venet, L., and Shapiro, S. Value of mammography in reduction of mortality from breast cancer in mass screening. A.J.R., *97:* 686–689, 1973.

Tormey, D. C. Combined chemotherapy and surgery in breast cancer—a review. Cancer, *36:* 881–892, 1975.

Tormey, D. C., and Neifeld, J. P. Chemotherapeutic approaches to disseminated breast cancer. *In* Breast Cancer Management—Early and Late, edited by B. A. Stoll, pp. 117–131. Year Book Medical Publishers, Chicago, 1977.

Treves, N., and Sunderland, D. A. Cystosarcoma phylloides of the breast. Cancer, *4:* 1286–1332, 1951.

Van Dyk, J. J., and Falkson, G. Extended survival and remission rates in metastatic breast cancer. Cancer *27:* 300–303, 1971.

Yonemoto, R. M., Keating, J. L., Byron, R. L., and Reihiwaki, D. M. Inflammatory carcinoma of the breast treated by bilateral adrenalectomy. Surgery, *68:* 461–467, 1970.

Chapter 21

Lung

HEINE H. HANSEN, M.D.

The treatment of lung cancer remains one of the major challenges in oncology. The disease is the most common lethal cancer among males and third among females with a rapidly rising incidence for both sexes within the last 20 years. The challenge is furthermore emphasized by the fact that the median survival from diagnosis has not changed appreciably during the period with the exception of small cell anaplastic carcinoma and continues to be close to 6 months. The 5-year survival for all patients with lung cancer is 10–12% with surgical resection being the main treatment modality offering any possibility of cure. Radiotherapy, chemotherapy and immunotherapy, which might be applied alone, combined or as adjunct to surgery currently constitute the other therapeutic alternatives.

The choice of treatment depends first of all on the histologic cell type and secondly on the stage of the disease. The most widely accepted histopathologic classification of lung cancer was proposed by the World Health Organization in 1967 (Table 21.1) (Kreyberg, 1967). Since then amended forms of this classification have been suggested (Yesner et al., 1965; Matthews, 1973). The most frequent cell types, which constitute more than 90% of all lung cancers, include the first four types of the WHO classification. Among those epidermoid carcinoma is twice as frequent as each of two anaplastic types and almost four times as frequent as adenocarcinoma of the lung.

Clinically a marked difference exists between the four cell types, a difference which also is reflected in the therapeutic results. In general, epidermoid carcinoma is characterized by its relatively slow growth rate. At the other end of the spectrum is the small cell carcinoma, which in addition to a higher growth rate also has a very high metastatic potential. Adenocarcinoma of the lung and large cell anaplastic carcinoma fall somewhere in between in these aspects (Strauss, 1977).

449

TABLE 21.1
World Health Organization (WHO) Classification of Lung Cancer by Histopathological Types[a]

I.   Epidermoid carcinoma
II. Small cell anaplastic carcinoma
     1. Fusiform cell type
     2. Polygonal cell type
     3. Lymphocyte-like ("oat-cell")
     4. Others
III. Adenocarcinomas
     1. Bronchogenic
        a. Acinar
        b. Papillary
     2. Bronchiolo-alveolar
IV. Large cell carcinomas
     1. Solid tumors with mucin-like content
     2. Solid tumors without mucin-like content
     3. Giant cell carcinomas
     4. "Clear" cell carcinomas
V.   Combined epidermoid and adenocarcinomas
VI. Carcinoid tumors
VII. Bronchial gland tumors
     1. Cylindromas
     2. Mucoepidermoid tumors
     3. Others
VIII. Papillary tumors of the surface epithelium
     1. Epidermoid
     2. Epidermoid with goblet cells
     3. Others
IX. "Mixed" tumors and carcinosarcomas
     1. "Mixed" tumors
     2. Carcinosarcomas of embryonal type ("blastomas")
     3. Other carcinosarcomas
X.   Sarcomas
XI. Unclassified
XII. Mesotheliomas
     1. Localized
     2. Diffuse
XIII. Melanomas

[a] From Kreyberg (1967).

The other major factor influencing the choice of treatment in addition to the cell type is the extent of the disease at the time of diagnosis. Careful clinical evaluation of intrathoracic and extrathoracic disease is indicated early, in order to avoid futile thoracotomy and local radiotherapy. Specifically the screening has to be emphasized for spread to mediastinal lymph nodes (mediastinoscopy) and for extrathoracic metastases in organs such as liver, brain, bones and adrenals. In addition to the utilization of biochemical parameters, radioisotopic scanning of the different organs combined with bone marrow examination and liver biopsy during peritoneoscopy have been of great value in the assessment of distant metastases (Hansen and Muggia, 1972; Margolis et al., 1975; Newman and Hansen, 1974).

For practical therapeutic purposes patients with lung cancer have been subdivided into three major groups with regard to the extent of the disease:

Stage A: "Regional disease," which includes patients, who technically can undergo a radical resection

Stage B: "Limited disease," including inoperable patients, in whom the disease is limited to one hemithorax with or without involvement of ipsilateral scalene lymphnodes

Stage C: "Extensive disease" including inoperable patients with intrathoracic or extrathoracic disease, which is not included in Stage B.

A more detailed staging classification of lung cancer according to the T (tumor) N (node) M (metastases) system and the correlation of the TNM classification to the above mentioned classification is described elsewhere (Dold, et al, 1972; Larsen, 1973; Selawry and Hansen, 1973; Mountain et al., 1974).

The choice of treatment for the different stages has until recently been surgery, radiotherapy and chemotherapy, respectively. However, increasing experience in staging has to a certain degree changed this approach by applying a combination of these modalities in appropriate circumstances.

REGIONAL DISEASE

For this group of patients, who constitute about 20% of all lung cancer patients, resection continues to be the treatment of choice. The results depend on the cell type, and 5-year postresection survival is according to a review of results from major series, 28% for epidermoid carcinoma, 17% for adenocarcinoma, 15% for patients with large cell anaplastic carcinoma and less than 5% for small cell anaplastic carcinoma (Selawry and Hansen 1973). The very poor prognosis for small cell carcinoma has recently been reemphasized by a randomized trial by the British Medical Research Council (Fox and Scadding, 1974). The 5-year survival for 144 patients with preoperative verified small cell anaplastic carcinoma, classified as having regional disease, was 3%. Furthermore, no difference was observed in the median survival for the two modalities of regional therapy, surgery and radiotherapy, respectively. Based on this trial and on similar experience from other centers (Jones et al., 1967; Lundar, 1970; Mountain,

1973) resection is not indicated in this cell type, unless it is combined with other modalities of therapy, as discussed below.

The use of adjuvant therapy to surgery has been evaluated in several prospective randomized trials. However, neither pre- nor postoperative irradiation have changed the median survival in patients undergoing resection. One exception might be the use of preoperative radiotherapy in patients with superior sulcus tumors, as described by Paulson (1966).

In contrast to radiotherapy adjuvant chemotherapy in connection with radical surgery has improved the survival of patients—however, only in small cell anaplastic carcinoma. By using cyclophosphamide the V.A. Adjuvant Surgical Group demonstrated an increase in 3-year survival from 8% to 22% in patients with this cell type. No beneficial effect of adjuvant chemotherapy was observed within the three other cell types (Higgins, 1972). The Swiss Cooperative Study Group has examined a similar group of patients with regional disease with the exception that the majority of the patients had epidermoid carcinoma. They demonstrated a significant shortening of survival in the adjuvant cyclophosphamide-treated group. Furthermore, the incidence of recurrences of the disease was significantly higher in the latter group, and they occurred earlier (Brunner et al., 1971). The explanation for this marked difference of adjuvant chemotherapy among the different cell types might not only be found in the selective sensitivity to the cytotoxic agents within the individual cell types, but might also be explained on the basis of interference with immunologic defense mechanisms. Of interest in that regard is the fact that a study using levamisole, a drug which possesses immunotropic properties, as an adjuvant to surgery, has indicated that the recurrence rate has decreased significantly after 1 year compared to placebo, particularly in patients with epidermoid carcinoma (Study Group for Bronchogenic Carcinoma, 1975).

More recently immunostimulation induced by instilling BCG in the pleural space has been demonstrated at least in one study to be of beneficial value when used at the time of surgery in patients with early disease (McKneally et al., 1976).

LIMITED DISEASE

For this group of patients (30% of all patients with bronchogenic carcinoma) radiotherapy has for years been the conventional mode of therapy. The symptomatic effect of irradiation has been well established in patients with atelectasis secondary to bronchial tumor obstruction, superior vena cava syndrome, Horner's syndrome with invasion of the ribs and brachial nerves, etc. However, the effect on survival has nonetheless been minimal. In controlled studies a statistically significant prolongation of survival has been documented only for epidermoid carcinoma from 3.5 months in the untreated groups as compared to 5.0 months for the treated group (Roswit et al., 1968). Several prospective randomized trials have combined radiotherapy with single agent chemo-therapy such as mechlorethamine, cyclophosphamide, 5-fluorouracil, ac-tinomycin D, and procarbazine, however, without significant changes in survival (Krant et al., 1963; Hall et al., 1967; Carr et al., 1971; Cohen et al., 1971; Durrant et al., 1971; Bergsagel et al., 1972; Landgren et al., 1973). One exception again is the use of cyclophosphamide in patients with small cell carcinoma, where three studies have demonstrated supe-riority of the combined treatment as compared to radiotherapy alone, using median survival as parameters (Bergsagel et al., 1972; Høst, 1973; Tucker et al., 1973). Similarly the administration of CCNU + hydroxyurea combined with radiotherapy was superior to radiotherapy alone (Petrov-ich et al., 1977). At present several ongoing studies by the cooperative groups are exploring the effect of combination chemotherapy and radio-therapy in small cell carcinoma and also adenocarcinoma based on encouraging results in some pilot studies (Hansen et al., 1972; Eagan et al., 1973).

Within the last 3–4 years more extensive radiotherapy including the use of "prophylactic" brain irradiation has been applied in some investi-gational trials for small cell carcinoma (Johnson et al., 1976; Livingstone et al., 1978).

The efficacy of this treatment remains still controversial, and many of the studies are inconclusive. At present, however, at least based on two prospective randomized trials (Tulloh et al., 1977; Hansen et al., 1977) no significant difference has been documented in median survival comparing "prophylactic" brain irradiation with none, and furthermore long term survivors (> 2 years) have been observed within both groups.

EXTENSIVE DISEASE

The effect of multiple chemotherapeutic compounds, applied either as single agents or in combinations, has been explored in multiple studies in this category of patients, who comprise almost half of all patients with lung cancer. Usually median survival and/or objective tumor regression have been utilized as parameters for the effectiveness of therapy.

SINGLE AGENT CHEMOTHERAPY

When using survival parameters as criteria the V.A. Lung Group has demonstrated superiority of mechlorethamine against an inert compound in epidermoid carcinoma and of cyclophosphamide against placebo in small cell anaplastic carcinoma. No significant prolongation of survival by the two agents as compared to placebo was observed in adenocarci-noma and large cell anaplastic carcinoma (Green et al., 1969). The same cooperative group has in a similar fashion evaluated 5-(3,3-dimethyl-1-triazeno)-imidazole-4-carboxamide (DTIC), BCNU (1,3-bis-(2-chloroethyl)-1-nitrosourea), hydroxyurea, vinblastine, methotrexate, streptozotocin, chlorambucil, dibromodulcitol and streptonigrin without any significant change in median survival (Green et al., 1969; Fink et al., 1970; Kaung et al., 1971; Mizgerd et al., 1971; Zelen, 1973). However, for the latter group of compounds no specific data are given by cell type. By using objective response rate instead of survival as parameters a number of different compounds have been demonstrated to have activity, including all cell types, but highest in small cell anaplastic carcinoma. Table 21.2 illustrates a review of the activity of the most commonly used compounds. A more detailed analysis has been published by Selawry and Hansen (1973) and Selawry (1977). It is noted in Table 21.2 that cyclophosphamide, mechlorethamine, 1,3-chloroethyl-1-cyclohexylnitrosourea (CCNU), hexamethylmelamine, methotrexate, 4'-demethylepipodophyllotoxin 9-(4,6-0-ethyliden-D-glucopyranoside (VP-16-213), procarbazine and Adriamycin are among the most active compounds. Other common agents such as thio-TEPA, busulfan, hydroxyurea, 5-fluorouracil, 6-mercaptopurine, cis-dichlorodiammine-platinum and streptonigrin have in published reports been tested only in a relatively few number of patients with lung cancer within each cell type. Therefore definitive statements on their value in the treatment of each cell type cannot be given.

COMBINATION CHEMOTHERAPY

Inspired by the progress in the treatment of acute childhood leukemia and lymphomas, combination chemotherapy of lung cancer has been

TABLE 21.2
Single Agent Chemotherapy in Lung Cancer Evaluated by Cell Type[a]

Drug	Epidermoid carcinoma	Small Cell Anaplastic Carcinoma	Adeno-carcinoma	Large Cell Anaplastic Carcinoma
Cyclophosphamide	+	++	+	+
Mechlorethamine	+	++	+	+
CCNU	+	+	+	+
Hexamethylmelamine	+	++	+	+
VP-16-213	+	++	+	0
Procarbazine	?	+	?	?
Methotrexate	+	+	+	+
Vinca alkaloids	+	++	+	?
Adriamycin	+	+	+	+
5-Fluorouracil	?	?	+	?
Bleomycin	0	0	?	0

[a] Based on reviews by Selawry and Hansen (1973), Selawry (1977), and unpublished data. ++ = 25–50% objective tumor response, + = 10–25% objective tumor response, 0 = < 10% objective tumor response, ? = drug not fully evaluated in cell type in question.

tested in the most recent years by several centers, and to a certain degree with some success. Tables 21.3–21.5 summarize the data on the effect of combination chemotherapy accumulated from controlled clinical trials. It is evident that the major progress has been achieved in small cell anaplastic carcinoma with an increase in median survival in patients presenting with advanced disease from 6 weeks without treatment to 36 weeks with intensive cytostatic therapy using a combination of vincristine, cyclophosphamide, CCNU and methotrexate, a combination which can easily be given on an outpatient basis. Similarly complete or partial objective response occurred in more than 75% of all patients using this combination or others including, e.g., Adriamycin (Livingstone at al.,

TABLE 21.3

Chemotherapy of Small Cell Anaplastic Carcinoma Controlled Clinical Trials Demonstrating Significant Differences

	Drugs	No. of Patients	Median Survival (Weeks)	Response Rate (%)	Reference
1.	Placebo	87	6	Not given	Green et al. 1969
	versus				
	CTX	57	16^a		
2.	CXT + MTX	27	23	38	Hansen et al. 1976
	versus				
	CTX + CCNU + MTX	26	32	56	
3.	CTX	118	17	22	Edmonson et al. (1976)
	versus				
	CTX + CCNU	110	20^b	43^a	
4.	CTX	25	—	17	Lowenbraun et al. (1975)
	versus				
	CTX + ADM + DTIC	25	—	77^a	
5.	CCNU + CTX + MTX	9	20	45	Cohen et al. (1977)
	low dose				
	versus				
	high dose (+prophylactic antibiotics)	23	43^a	96^a	
6.	CTX + CCNU + MTX	52	25	75	Hansen et al. 1978
	versus				
	CTX + CCNU + MTX + VCR	53	33^a	78	

^{a} $P < 0.05$.
^{b} $P = 0.07$.

CTX = cyclophosphamide, CCNU = 1,3-chloroethyl-1-cyclohexylnitrosourea, MTX = methotrexate, DTIC = dimethyl-triazeno-imidazole-carboxamide, VCR = vincristine.

TABLE 21.4

Chemotherapy of Adenocarcinoma Controlled Clinical Trials Demonstrating Significant Difference

Drugs	No. of Patients	Median Survival in Weeks	Response Rate (%)	Reference
1. a. CTX	79	16	12	Edmonson et al. (1976)
b. CTX + CCNU	83	26[a]	12	
2. a. CTX + MTX	21	17	6	Hansen et al. (1976)
b. CCNU + CTX + MTX	22	30[b]	38[c]	

[a] $P = 0.07$.
[b] $P = 0.007$.
[c] $P = 0.05$.
CTX = cyclophosphamide, MTX = methotrexate, CCNU = 1,3-chloroethyl-l-cyclohexylnitrosourea.

TABLE 21.5

Chemotherapy of Epidermoid Carcinoma Controlled Clinical Trials Demonstrating Significant Difference

Drugs	No. of Patients	Median Survival in Weeks	Reference
1. Placebo	229	15	Green et al. (1969)
Mechlorethamine	66	24[a]	
2. a. CTX	Total of 134[b]	10.7	Hyde et al. (1977)
b. CTX + CCNU		10	
c. CTX + ADM		24[d]	
d. CCNU + ADM		13.9	
e. CTX	Total of 82[c]	12.5	Hyde et al. (1977)
f. CTX + CCNU		24.4[e]	
g. CTX + ADM		23.3[e]	
h. CCNU + ADM		25.8[e]	

[a] $P = 0.005$.
[b] Well + moderately differentiated squamous cell cancer.
[c] Poorly differentiated squamous cell cancer.
[d] Superior to any of the three other regimens.
[e] All superior to single agent treatment with CTX.
The response rate (%) was not given. CTX, = cyclophosphamide, CCNU = 1,3-chloroethyl-1-cyclohexylnitrosourea, ADM = Adriamycin.

1978). In all recent studies a minor fraction of patients (5–15%) has been in remission for 1 year or more, with possible cure in a few patients. Present studies for small cell anaplastic carcinoma are focusing on the task of inducing remissions of longer durations either by, e.g., increasing the drug doses (Cohen et al., 1977), exploring combination chemotherapy in a cyclic fashion in an attempt to prevent or delay the development of resistant cell lines, or to incorporate new highly active compounds such as VP-16-213 in the initial therapy.

For adenocarcinoma and in particular for epidermoid carcinoma progress has been modest with regard to therapeutic improvement (Tables 21.4 and 21.5). For these cell types and also for large cell anaplastic carcinoma more optimal regimens are urgently needed.

Acknowlegment. Supported by a grant from Esper and Olga Boel's Foundation.

REFERENCES

Alberto, P., Brunner, K. W., Martz, G., Obrecht, J-P., and Sonntag, R. W. Treatment of bronchogenic carcinoma with simultaneous or sequential combination chemotherapy, including methotrexate, cyclophosphamide, procarbazine and vincristine. Cancer, *38:* 2208–2216, 1976.

Bergsagel, D. E., Jenkin, R. D. T., Pringle, J. D., White, D. M., Fetterly, J. C. M., Klaassen, D. J., and McDermot, R. S. R. Lung cancer; clinical trial of radiotherapy alone vs. radiotherapy plus cyclophosphamide. Cancer, *30:* 621–627, 1972.

Brunner, K. W., Marthaler, Th., and Müller, W. Unfavourable effects of long-term adjuvant chemotherapy with Endoxan, in radically operated bronchogenic carcinoma. Eur. J. Cancer, *7:* 285–294, 1971.

Carr, D. T., Childs, D. S., and Lee, R. E. Radiotherapy plus 5-FU compared to radiotherapy alone for inoperable and unresectable bronchogenic carcinoma. Cancer, *30:* 375–380, 1972.

Cohen, J. L., Krant, M. J., Shnider, B. I., Matias, P. I., Horton, J., and Baxter, I. Radiation plus 5-fluorouracil (NSC-19893); clinical demonstration of an additive effect in bronchogenic carcinoma. Cancer Chemother. Rep., *55:* 253–258, 1971.

Cohen, M. H., Creaven, P. J., Fossieck, B. J., Broder, L. E., Selawry, O. S., Johnston, A. V., Williams, C. L., and Minna, J. D. Intensive chemotherapy of small cell bronchogenic carcinoma. Cancer Treat. Rep., *61:* 349–354, 1972.

Dold, U., Schneider, V., and Krause, F. Applicability of the TNM-system on lung carcinoma, field trial, proposal of advanced TNM-classification including a category for diagnostic certainty degree. Z. Krebsforsch., *78:* 317–325, 1972.

Durrant, K. R., Berry, R. J., Ellis, F., Lidehalsch, F. R., Black, J. M., and Hamilton, W. S. Comparisons of treatment policies in inoperable bronchial carcinoma. Lancet, *1:* 715–719, 1971.

Eagan, R. T., Maurer, H., Forcier, R. J., and Tulloh, M. Combination chemotherapy and radiation therapy in small cell carcinoma of the lung. Cancer, *32:* 371–379, 1973.

Edmonson, J. H., Lagakos, S. W., Selawry, O. S., Perlia, C. P., Bennett, J. M., Muggia, F. M., Wampler, G., Brodovsky, H. S., Horton, J., Colsky, J., Mansour, E. G., Creech, R., Stolbach, L., Greenspan, E. M., Levitt, M., Israel, L., Ezdinly, E. Z., and Carbone, P. P. Cyclophosphamide and CCNU in the treatment of inoperable small cell carcinoma and adenocarcinoma of the lung. Cancer Treat. Rep., *60:* 925–932, 1976.

Einhorn, L. H., Fee, W. H., Farber, M. O., Livingston, R. B., and Gottlieb, J. A. Improved chemotherapy for small cell undifferentiated lung cancer. J.A.M.A., *235:* 1225–1229, 1976.

Fink, A., Finegold, S. M., Patno, M. E., Close, H. P., and Whittington, R. M. Vinblastine sulfate (NSC-49842) in the treatment of bronchogenic carcinoma. Cancer Chemother. Rep., *1:* 451–452, 1970.

Fox, W., and Scadding, J. G. Medical Research Council comparative trial of surgery and radiotherapy for primary treatment of small-celled or oat-celled carcinoma of bronchus (ten year follow-up). Lancet, *2:* 63–65, 1973.

Green, R. A., Humphrey, E., Close, H., and Patno, M. E. Alkylating agents in bronchogenic carcinoma. Am. J. Med., 46: 516–525, 1969.

Hall, T. C., Dederick, M. M., Chalmers, T. C., Krant, M. J., Shnider, B. I., Lynch, J. J., Holland, J. F., Ross, C., Koons, C. R., Owens, A. H., Frei, E., Brindley, C., Miller, S. P., Brenner, S., Hosley, H. F., and Olson, K. H. A clinical pharmacologic study of chemotherapy and x-ray therapy in lung cancer. Am. J. Med., 43: 186–193, 1967.

Hansen, H. H., Dombernowsky, P., Hirsch, F., and Rygård, J. Intensive combination chemotherapy plus localized or extensive radiotherapy in small cell anaplastic bronchogenic carcinoma (SMAC); randomized trial. Proc. Am. Soc. Clin. Oncol., 18: 350, 1977.

Hansen, H. H., Dombernowsky, P., Hansen, M., and Hirsch, F. Chemotherapy of advanced small cell anaplastic carcinoma; superiority in a randomized trial of a 4-drug combination to a 3-drug combination. Ann. Intern. Med., 89: 177–181, 1978.

Hansen, H. H., and Muggia, F. M. Staging of patients with unresectable bronchogenic carcinoma with special reference to bone marrow biopsy and peritoneoscopy. Cancer, 30: 1395–1401, 1972.

Hansen, H. H., Muggia, F. M., Andrews, R., and Selawry, O. S. Intensive combined chemotherapy and radiotherapy in patients with non-resectable bronchogenic carcinoma. Cancer, 30: 315–324, 1972.

Hansen, H. H., Selawry, O. S., Simon, R., Carr, D. T., van Wyk, C. E., Tucker, R. D., and Sealy, R. Combination chemotherapy of advanced lung cancer; a randomized trial. Cancer, 38: 2201–2207, 1976.

Higgins, G. A. The use of chemotherapy as an adjuvant to surgery for bronchogenic carcinoma. Cancer, 30: 1383–1387, 1972.

Hyde, L., Lowe, W. C., Phillips, R., and Wolf, J. Chemotherapy of squamous cell cancer of the lung. Proc. Am. Soc. Clin. Oncol., 18: 276, 1977.

Høst, H. Cyclophosphamide as adjuvant to radiotherapy in the treatment of unresectable bronchogenic carcinoma. Cancer Chemother. Rep., 4: 161–164, 1973.

Johnson, R. E., Brereton, H. D., and Kent, C. H. Small cell carcinoma of the lung; attempt to remedy causes of post therapeutic failure. Lancet, 2: 289–291, 1976.

Jones, J. C., Kern, W. H., Chapman, N. D., Meyer, B. W., and Lindesmith, G. G. Long-term survival after surgical resection for bronchogenic carcinoma. J. Thorac. Cardiovasc. Surg., 54: 383–393, 1967.

Kaung, D. T., Sbar, S., and Patno, M. E. Treatment of non-resectable cancer of the lung with hydroxyurea (NSC-32065) given intermittently. Cancer Chemother. Rep., 55: 87–89, 1971.

Krant, M. J., Chalmers, T. C., Dederick, M. M., Hall, T. C., Levene, M. B., Muench, H., Shnider, B. I., Gold, L., Hunter, C., Bersack, S. R., Owens, A. H., Leon, N., Dickson, R. J., Brindley, C., Brace, K. C., Frei, E., Gehan, E., and Salvin, L. Comparative trial of chemotherapy and radiotherapy in patients with non-resectable cancer of the lung. Am. J. Med., 35: 363–373, 1963.

Kreyberg, L. Histological Typing of Lung Tumours. World Health Organization, Geneva, 1967.

Landgren, R. C., Hussey, D. H., Samuels, M. L., and Leary, W. V. A randomized study comparing irradiation alone to irradiation plus procarbazine in inoperable bronchogenic carcinoma. Radiology, 108: 403–406, 1973.

Larsson, W. V. Pretreatment classification and staging of bronchogenic carcinoma. Scand. J. Thorac. Cardiovasc. Surg., Suppl. 10, 1973.

Livingstone, R. B., Moore, T. N., Heilbrun, L., Bottomley, R., Lehane, D., Rivkin, S. E., and Thigpen, T. Small cell bronchogenic carcinoma of the lung; combined chemotherapy and radiation. Ann. Intern. Med., 88: 194–199, 1978.

Lowenbraun, S., Krauss, S., Smalley, R., and Huguley, C. Randomized Study of cyclophosphamide (CTX) alone vs. CTX, Adriamycin (ADM) and Dimethyl triazeno imidazole carboxamide (DTIC) in small cell lung carcinoma. Proc. Am. Soc. Clin. Oncol., *16:* 246, 1975.

Lundar, J. Small-celled anaplastic lung carcinoma patients alive 5 years after operation. Scand. J. Respir. Dis., *72* (Suppl.): 139, 1970.

Margolis, R., Hansen, H. H., Muggia, F. M., and Kanhouwa, S. Diagnosis of liver metastases in bronchogenic carcinoma; a comparative study of liver scans, function tests and peritoneoscopy with liver biopsy in 111 patients. Cancer, *34:* 1825–1829, 1974.

Matthews, M. J. Morphologic classification of bronchogenic carcinoma. Cancer Chemother. Rep., *4:* 299–301, 1973.

McKneally, M. F., Maver, C., and Kausel, H. W. Regional immunotherapy of lung cancer with intrapleural BCG. Lancet, *1:* 377–379, 1976.

Mizgerd, J. B., Amick, R. M., Hilal, H. M., and Patno, M. E. Chemical study of 5-(3,3-dimethyl-1-triazeno) imidazole-4-carboxamide (NSC-45388) in carcinoma of the lung. Cancer Chemother. Rep., *55:* 83–86, 1971.

Mountain, C. F. The surgeon's viewpoint on collaborative research on lung cancer. Cancer Chemother. Rep., *4:* 307–309, 1973.

Mountain, C. F., Carr, D. T., and Anderson, W. A. D. A system for the clinical staging of lung cancer. A.J.R., *1:* 130, 1974.

Newman, S. J., and Hansen, H. H. Frequency, diagnosis and treatment of brain metastases in 247 consecutive patients with bronchogenic carcinoma. Cancer, *33:* 492–496, 1974.

Paulson, D. L. The survival rate in superior sulcus tumors treated by presurgical irradiation. J.A.M.A., *196:* 342–345, 1966.

Petrovitch, Z., Mietlowski, W., Ohanian, M., and Cox, J. Clinical report on the treatment of locally advanced lung cancer. Cancer, *40:* 72–77, 1977.

Roswitt, B., Patno, M. E., Rapp, R., Veinberg, A., Feder, B., Stuhlbars, J., and Reid, C. B. The survival of patients with inoperable lung cancer; a large-scale randomized study of radiation therapy versus placebo. Radiology, *90:* 688–697, 1968.

Selawry, O. S. Chemotherapy in lung cancer. *In* Lung Cancer, edited by M. J. Straus, pp. 199–222. Grune & Stratton, New York, 1977.

Selawry, O. S., and Hansen, H. H. 1973. Lung cancer. *In* Cancer Medicine, edited by J. F. Holland and E. Frei III, pp. 1473–1518. Lea & Febiger, Philadelphia, 1973.

Shields, T. W. Status report of adjuvant cancer chemotherapy trials in the treatment of bronchial carcinoma. Cancer Chemother. Rep., *4:* 119–124, 1973.

Straus, M. J. Growth characteristics of lung cancer. *In* Lung Cancer, edited by M. J. Straus, pp. 19–32. Grune & Stratton, New York, 1977.

Study Group for Bronchogenic Carcinoma. Immunopotentiation with levamisole in resectable bronchogenic carcinoma; a double-blind controlled trial. Br. Med. J., *3:* 461–464, 1975.

Tucker, R. P., Sealy, R., van Wyk, C., LeRoux, P. L. M., and Soskolne, C. L. A clinical trial of cyclophosphamide (NSC-26271) and radiation therapy for oat-cell carcinoma of the lung. Cancer Chemother. Rep., *4:* 159–161, 1973.

Tulloh, M. E., Maurer, L. H., and Forcier, R. J. A randomized trial of prophylactic whole brain irradiation in small cell carcinoma of lung. Proc. Am. Soc. Clin. Oncol., *18:* 268, 1977.

Yesner, R., Gerst, B., and Auerbach, L. Application of the World Health Organization classification of lung carcinoma to biopsy material. Ann. Thorac. Surg., *1:* 33–49, 1965.

Zelen, M. Keynote address on biostatistics and data retrieval. Cancer Chemother. Rep., *4:* 31–42, 1973.

Chapter 22

Head and Neck

PATRICK R. BERGEVIN, M.D.

The treatment of cancer of the head and neck requires the joint cooperative efforts of the pathologist, surgeon, radiotherapist, oral surgeon and medical oncologist. Tumors only centimeters apart are often approached quite differently. Sophisticated staging procedures help to determine the role of each therapist. The problem is complicated by the predisposition, by chronic irritation, or by poor oral hygiene, of an entire "field" to cancer, prompting attention to possible multifocal areas of malignancy. The histological appearance of the neoplasm is of less importance than the location, size and presence of metastases, but there is some correlation between the level of differentiation and aggressive behavior. Death frequently results from nodal or distant metastases rather than from the primary lesion, which is often controlled. Despite treatment with a maximally tolerable combination of radiotherapy and surgery, control of squamous cell carcinoma of the head and neck remains a vexing problem to the cancer specialist. Cure rates for Stage III and IV tumors are poor and generally do not exceed 35% (James, 1966), depending on the anatomic site, tumor differentiation, and presence or absence of metastatic disease.

ORAL CAVITY

In the United States well over 20,000 new cases of cancer of the oral cavity are diagnosed each year, and roughly half of this number will succumb to their disease. Epidermoid carcinomas of the oral mucosa tend to be well differentiated and less likely to have spread to regional nodes at the time of diagnosis than carcinomas further posteriorly.

Carcinoma of the lip is closely associated with chronic irritation, including prolonged exposure to sunlight and pipe smoking. The lower lip is most often involved and is usually curable in its early stages by either radiotherapy or surgery. Carcinomas of the upper lip pursue a more aggressive course with earlier nodal metastases.

Carcinoma of the buccal mucosa is related to local irritants such as tobacco and to leukoplakia and poor oral hygiene. If detected early they may be effectively treated by surgical excision or in some cases by radiation therapy. However, this tumor is prone to aggressiveness with a high recurrence rate, perhaps related to multicentric foci, and metastasizes to regional nodes in a high percentage of cases. A combination of radiotherapy and surgery may be required, and local control may be difficult.

Gingival tumors generally occur in premolar and molar regions, especially in the lower jaw, and may be superimposed on periodontal disease or leukoplakia. Although some superficial lesions can be effectively treated by surgery or radiotherapy, many lesions involve the adjacent bone and regional nodes and are best treated with extensive resection or a combination treatment with radiotherapy.

Cancer of the tongue is a frequent tumor of the oral cavity and is associated with leukoplakia, poor oral hygiene and the use of tobacco and alcohol. These tumors are usually located on the lateral border of the middle third of the tongue. Control of tumors in this region depends upon the size of the primary lesion and its histologic differentiation: these factors govern the risk of regional node involvement, which is present in over a third of patients at the time of diagnosis. Early cases can be effectively treated by surgery or radiotherapy, but extension into the floor of the mouth, mandible and posteriorly into the tonsillar area requires extensive surgical resection combined with radiotherapy. Carcinoma of the posterior third of the tongue tends to be clinically silent until extensive local spread and regional node metastases have already occurred, such that the prognosis for these tumors is exceedingly poor.

Floor of mouth tumors are usually quite advanced at the time of diagnosis with frequent involvement of adjacent structures, including tongue, gingiva, mandible and soft tissues with early regional node involvement. Combined treatment with preoperative radiotherapy and extensive surgical resection may help to salvage some advanced cases.

Tumors of the palate are generally of mucous or salivary gland origin. Certain superficial lesions are highly responsive to radiotherapy, but the more infiltrating types tend to involve adjacent sites, such as tonsils, tongue and buccal mucosa and must be managed by extensive surgical resection combined perhaps with pre- or postoperative radiotherapy.

PHARYNX

Oropharyngeal tumors are only slightly more than half as common as oral cancers. These are aggressive tumors with a high propensity to local spread and regional node and distant metastases. They tend to be undifferentiated or anaplastic and spread easily because of a rich lymphatic network. The principal mode of treatment is radiation therapy, although surgery is often employed for handling recurrent or residual disease.

The bulk of hypopharyngeal carcinomas arise in the piriform sinus. Most are poorly differentiated squamous cell tumors and have a poor prognosis because of extensive local invasion and regional node involvement. Radiotherapy has been used in combination with an extensive resection of the primary tumor, which may include laryngectomy and resection of the upper esophagus and mediastinal nodes.

The nasopharynx is one of the common "blind areas" in head and neck cancer. However, the primary tumor may grow so large as to obstruct the nasal fossa or eustachean tube or even extend into the orbit or cranial cavity and give rise to cranial nerve palsies, but cervical adenopathy is often the patient's first complaint. The frequent involvement of retropharyngeal and cervical nodes at the time of diagnosis calls for radiation therapy as primary treatment. It is gratifying that even patients with large cervical adenopathy may be radiocurable, but the overall 5-year survival is still only around 40%.

LARYNX

Cancer of the larynx tends to be a well differentiated squamous cell carcinoma and only rarely develops in nonsmokers. Carcinoma of the true vocal cord tends not to spread to regional nodes until it has extended into adjacent areas. Tumors arising from the supraglottic and subglottic areas tend to be less well differentiated with widespread mucosal spread and metastases to regional nodes. Pretherapeutic laryngographic studies are important to determine cord mobility and extent of disease. Carcinoma involving only the true vocal cord may be treated with radiotherapy or surgery with good long term control. Extension into adjacent muscle or arytenoid results in limitation of vocal cord mobility and is a serious prognostic finding. Advanced tumors are often approached with preoperative radiation therapy, followed by total laryngectomy and radical neck dissection.

NASAL FOSSA AND PARANASAL SINUSES

Primary carcinoma of the nasal fossa is uncommon and usually arises from the middle and inferior turbinates. Unilateral nasal obstruction and epistaxis are the most common presenting symptoms, although extension backward to involve the nasopharynx and base of the skull may occur. Radiotherapy and/or surgery have achieved good control, and survival for these tumors is better than for squamous cell carcinomas in the paranasal sinuses or nasopharynx.

Most paranasal sinus tumors are epidermoid carcinomas arising from the mucosa of the maxillary sinus. Bone involvement is common and extension into the nasal cavities or other sinuses may occur. Although surgery is the conventional mode of treatment, pre- or postoperative radiotherapy may be of benefit.

SALIVARY GLANDS

Roughly 80% of all salivary gland tumors are in the parotid, with the remaining tumors located in the submandibular and sublingual glands and in the small salivary glands of palate, tongue and buccal mucosa. Benign tumors are much more common than malignant ones and account for greater than 80% of parotid tumors but less than 50% of tumors of other salivary glands. Most parotid tumors present as a lump near the ear. Facial nerve paralysis, fixation of mass and ulceration of overlying skin point to a malignant process. Radical tumor resection is the treatment of choice. Lesser procedures usually result in recurrence of disease. Radiation therapy is employed for residual or recurrent disease.

CHEMOTHERAPY

The efficacy of single drug chemotherapy in carcinoma of the head and neck has been reviewed by Carter (1977). Methotrexate, an antimetabolite, with 40% overall response rates, has been studied the most. A comparison of various methotrexate regimens indicates that weekly or biweekly therapy may be superior to a monthly 5-day therapy (Leone et al., 1968; Papac et al., 1963, 1967; Lane et al., 1968; Huseby and Downing, 1962; Andrews and Wilson, 1967), although the median duration of response in most studies is less than 3 months. Leone et al. (1968) treated 35 patients with advanced head and neck cancer with methotrexate given intravenously (IV) at a dosage of 60 mg/m^2/week. Eleven patients achieved a complete response (CR) with median duration of response of 160 days. The overall response rate in this study was 57%. Response to methotrexate occurs with highest frequency in tumors of the oral cavity and oropharynx and with lowest frequency in tumors of the nasopharynx and hypopharynx.

Methotrexate has also been given as a prolonged infusion over 16–30 hours, with a response rate and duration of response equivalent to the conventional modes of administration. The use of drugs in large intermittent doses to kill maximum numbers of tumor cells has been emphasized by Skipper et al. (1964) in animal experiments. Skipper stressed that the proportion of cells killed at a given dose of drug is the same during each course of therapy. Thus, to kill the maximum number of cells in a large population, a high dose of antimetabolite should be given during the S phase and repeated often enough to prevent progressive disease. The length of infusion time necessary for maximal cell kill should theoretically depend upon the DNA synthesis time, which may be as long as 26 hours (Friedman et al., 1973). Levitt et al. (1972) reported the treatment of 16 patients with advanced head and neck cancer with a median maximal tolerated methotrexate dose of 1110 mg/m^2 as a twice weekly 30-hour infusion and achieved an overall response rate of 44%, but toxicity was unacceptable with four drug-related deaths. Reversal of systemic toxicity by leucovorin (citrovorum factor) allows high doses of methotrexate to be given over even longer periods of time (up to 42 hours (Levitt et al. (1972)). Leucovorin supplies tetrahydrofolic acid (THFA), which bypasses the methotrexate block. Methotrexate blocks the synthesis of thymidylic acid (and therefore of DNA) from deoxyuridylic acid by inhibiting dihydrofolate reductase, thus preventing formation of the essential coenzyme THFA. Leucovorin supplies THFA, which bypasses this block and, thereby, permits renewed DNA synthesis. Thus, leucovorin "rescues" normal cells whose synthesis of DNA had been inhibited by methotrexate, but were still viable. Mitchell et al. (1968) treated 19 patients with advanced head and neck cancer with three 24-hour infusions of methotrexate, spaced according to recovery from toxicity and each followed by leucovorin reversal. Maintenance treatment consisted of conventional weekly intravenous methotrexate. Nine out of 19 patients had > 50% tumor regression, and the median duration of response was 5 months. Similar results were obtained by Capizzi et al. (1970) utilizing the same mode of therapy.

In a few therapeutic trials, hydroxyurea seems to be another active agent. Papac and Fischer (1971) reported the use of cytosine arabinoside (ARA-C) in 20 patients, 8 of whom had received prior therapy with methotrexate and 1 with 5-fluorouracil. A partial response (> 50% tumor regression) was achieved in 4 patients, with the longest duration of response being 3 months. The value of ARA-C as a secondline agent to methotrexate is obvious; in addition, ARA-C infrequently causes mucositis or gastrointestinal side effects with conventional dosage schedules. Hexamethylmelamine (Wilson et al., 1970) and Adriamycin (Bonadonna et al., 1970) have shown activity against head and neck tumors, as well as BCNU (De Vita et al., 1965; Ramirez, 1972) high dose cyclophosphamide (Harrison et al., 1965), and bleomycin (Blum et al., 1973). cis-Diamminedichloroplatinum (II) (DDP) is an investigational agent which has moderate activity in head and neck cancer.

Responses to intra-arterial administration of single drugs in head and neck cancer are listed in Table 22.1. The best results (up to 75% response) are seen in patients not previously treated with surgery or radiotherapy. Better responses are also noted if the drug administration is prolonged in time. Theoretically, cell cycle specific drugs must be administered for the duration of the DNA synthesis time. Although intra-arterial chemother-

TABLE 22.1
Responses to Intra-arterial Administration of Single Agents in Head and Neck Cancer[a]

Drug	No. Evaluable	No. >50% Tumor Regression	Overall Percent Responses
Methotrexate	806	356	44
Cyclophosphamide	100	28	28
5-Fluorouracil	28	21	75
Vinblastine	24	6	25
Nitrogen mustard	20	10	50
Bleomycin	24	6	25

[a] Adapted from Bertino et al. (1973).

apy offers a maximal drug concentration to the tumor, it may be unsuccessful because a massive tumor may derive its blood supply from arteries which cannot all be included in the infused field. Regional and distant metastases are a major reason for the low cure rates seen. Complications inherent with intra-arterial chemotherapy are associated with catheter placement and function, especially catheter plugging, leakage, infection, hematoma, and other problems (Nervi et al., 1970).

There is little data regarding the efficacy of combination chemotherapy in head and neck cancer. Success with the MOPP schedule in Hodgkin's disease and the various drug combinations in the acute leukemias has prompted investigation into this area with regard to solid tumors. Hanham et al. (1971) applied the combination of cyclophosphamide-methotrexate-vincristine-5-fluorouracil to 10 patients with head and neck cancer and achieved 1 complete response and 7 partial responses, mainly in cases showing failure with or relapse following treatment with methotrexate, but the responses were short and the majority of these patients were dead within 9 months. The combination of Adriamycin and bleomycin allowed significant responses in two reports (Cortes et al., 1972; Tormey et al., 1973).

There is no clear clinical evidence that the susceptibility of neoplastic cells to radiation therapy is increased after exposure to methotrexate, although the action may be supplementary. Some drugs, notably hydroxyurea and dactinomycin, may cause reactivation of postirradiation erythema. Methotrexate or other antimetabolites may act by destroying relatively radioresistant cells in the S phase and by synchronizing other cells in a relatively radiosensitive phase (G_1), thus permitting more effective irradiation. The drug may also inhibit the repair process in those cells that receive potentially lethal irradiation. Clinical attempts to produce synchrony by chemotherapy have been numerous, but without much evidence of value. One of the major problems is that of the assessment of the optimal time at which to radiate. In any case, the chemotherapeutic agent frequently acts to reduce tumor size to allow radiotherapy a better chance in those large, poorly vascularized tumors with hypoxic and radioresistant cells.

Kramer (1971) gave 57 patients with advanced head and neck cancer methotrexate at a dosage of 2.5 mg 3 times daily, by mouth, followed in 5–7 days by radiotherapy. Combined therapy was continued to drug toxicity, whereupon the methotrexate was stopped and the radiation continued to full dose (6500 R in 6.5 weeks). Antitumor results with this combination were felt to be notably better than those obtained by irradiation alone in such patients with extensive tumors. Notably, at 3 years, 18 out of 57 patients were alive without disease. Enthusiasm for the combined use of methotrexate and radiotherapy has been voiced by others (Friedman et al., 1970; Kligerman et al., 1966; Condit et al., 1964).

The occurrence of prolonged remissions in patients with head and neck cancer after therapy with methotrexate and a less than curative course of radiotherapy suggests that methotrexate potentiates the therapeutic effects of radiation (Condit et al., 1964; Hardingham et al., 1972; Friedman and Daly, 1967). Hardingham et al. (1972) studied the effectiveness of a 16-hour methotrexate infusion followed by leucovorin and then a week later by a course of radiotherapy. Six patients got a short 8–12-day course of radiation; the other 5 patients received the conventional 4–6 week course. Five patients got a second methotrexate infusion postradiotherapy. In 8 patients, no sign of recurrent disease had been noted over periods ranging from 5 to 11 months. In this series, the short course radiation was as effective as the standard radiotherapy, when given with methotrexate; patient time in the hospital was reduced as a result.

Hydroxyurea has also been given in combination with radiotherapy in patients with head and neck cancer. Lipschultz and Lerner (1969) commented on the prompt primary tumor regression in their patients treated with a combination of hydroxyurea and radiotherapy, with 30 out of 60 patients clinically free of disease for periods of 4 months to over 3 years. Richards and Chambers (1969) felt that the most notable contribution of hydroxyurea in their patients was to increase the effectiveness of radiotherapy in eradication of tumor in nodes. Stefani et al. (1971, 1972), evaluated 154 patients in a double blind study comparing hydroxyurea with radiotherapy to placebo with radiotherapy. Hydroxyurea was given at a dosage of 80 mg/kg twice weekly by mouth during the period of radiotherapy only. All stages were accepted into the study except T₁ of the true vocal cord. Comparison of the two groups for primary tumor regression and length of tumor control, cervical node response and survival, failed to show statistically significant differences.

Ansfield et al. (1970) reported the use of 5-fluorouracil in combination with radiotherapy in patients with advanced head and neck cancer. In this randomized double blind study, 5-fluorouracil plus conventional radiotherapy was compared to radiotherapy alone. The 5-fluorouracil was given at a dosage of 10 mg/kg/day for 5 days every week intravenously through the period of radiotherapy only and then stopped. A prolonged survival was noted only for patients with intra-oral and tonsil tumors treated with 5-fluorouracil plus radiation (median survival 29 months) vs. radiation alone (13 months). Hall and Good (1961) and Foye et al. (1960) also noted good results with this combination.

REFERENCES

Andrews, N. C., and Wilson, W. L. Phase II study of methotrexate (NSC-740) in solid tumors. Cancer Chemother. Rep., *51*: 471–474, 1967.

Ansfield, F. J., Ramirez, G., Davis, H. L., Korbitz, B. C., Vermund, H., and Gollin, F. F. Treatment of advanced cancer of the head and neck. Cancer, *25*: 78–82, 1970.

Bertino, J. R., Mosher, M. B., and DeConti, R. C. Chemotherapy of cancer of the head and neck. Cancer, *31*: 1141–1149, 1973.

Blum, R. H., Carter, S. K., and Agre, K. A clinical review of bleomycin—a new antineoplastic agent. Cancer, *31*: 903–914, 1973.

Bonadonna, G., Monfardini, S., DeLena, M., Fossati-Bellani, F., and Beretta, G. Phase I and preliminary phase II evaluation of Adriamycin (NSC-123127). Cancer Res., *30*: 2572–2582, 1970.

Capizzi, R. L., DeConti, R. C., Marsh, J. C., and Bertino, J. R. Methotrexate therapy of head and neck cancer; improvement in therapeutic index by the use of leukovorin rescue. Cancer Res., *30*: 1782–1788, 1970.

Carter, S. K. The chemotherapy of head and neck cancer. Semin. Oncol., *4*: 413–424, 1977.

Condit, P., Ridingo, G., Coin, J., et al. Methotrexate and radiation in the treatment of patients with cancer. Cancer Res., *24*: 1524, 1964.

Cortes, E. P., Shedd, D., Albert, D. J., Ohnuma, T., and Hreshchyshyn, M. Adriamycin and bleomycin in advanced cancer. Proc. Am. Assoc. Cancer Res., *13*: 86, 1972.

DeVita, V. T., Carbone, P. P., Owens, A. H., Gold, G. L., Krant, M. J., and Edmonson, J. Clinical trials with 1,3-bis (2-chloroethyl)-1-nitrosourea (NSC-409962). Cancer Res., *25*: 1876–1881, 1965.

Foye, L. V., Willett, F. M., Hall, B. E., and Roth, M. The potentiation of radiation effects with 5-fluorouracil. Calif. Med., *93*: 288–290, 1960.

Friedman, M., DeNarvaes, F. N., and Daly, J. F. Treatment of squamous cell carcinoma of the head and neck with combined methotrexate and irradiation. Cancer, *26*: 711–721, 1970.

Friedman, M., Navi, C., Casole, C., Starace, G., Arcangeli, G., Page, G., and Ziparo, E. Significance of growth rates, cell kinetics, and histology in the irradiation and chemotherapy of the mouth. Cancer, *31*: 10–16, 1973.

Friedman, M., and Daly, J. F. The treatment of squamous cell carcinoma of the head and neck with methotrexate and irradiation. Am. J. R., *99*: 289–301, 1967.

Hall, B. E., and Good, J. W. Advanced neoplastic disease; treatment with 5-fluorouracil and irradiation. Calif. Med., *95*: 303–308, 1961.

Hanham, I. W. F., Newton, K. A., and Westbury, G. Seventy-five cases of solid tumors treated by a modified quadruple chemotherapy regime. Br. J. Cancer, *25*: 462–478, 1971.

Hardingham, M., Hulbert, M. H. E., and Walshwaring, G. P. Treatment of advanced carcinoma of the head and neck with a combination of high-dose infusions of methotrexate (NSC-740) and radiotherapy; a preliminary report on eleven cases. Cancer Chemother. Rep., *56*: 745–750, 1972.

Harrison, D., Espiner, H., and Glazebrook, G. Cyclophosphamide in head and neck cancer. *In* Cyclophosphamide, edited by G. Fanley and J. Simister, pp. 48–55. Williams & Wilkins, Baltimore, 1965.

Huseby, R., and Downing, V. The use of methotrexate orally in treatment of squamous cancers of the head and neck. Cancer Chemother. Rep., *16*: 511–514, 1962.

James, A. G. Cancer Prognosis Manual. American Cancer Society, New York, 1966.

Kligerman, M., Hellman, M., von Essen, C., and Bertino, J. Sequential chemotherapy and radiotherapy; preliminary results of clinical trial with methotrexate in head and neck cancer. Radiology, *86*: 247–250, 1966.

Kramer, S. Radiation therapy and chemotherapy combination. J.A.M.A., *217*: 946–947, 1971.

Lane, M., Moore, J. E., Levin, H., and Smith, F. E. Methotrexate therapy for squamous cell carcinoma of the head and neck. J.A.M.A., *204*: 561–564, 1968.

Leone, L. A., Albala, M. M., and Rege, V. B. Treatment of carcinoma of the head and neck with intravenous methotrexate. Cancer, *21*: 828–837, 1968.

Levitt, M., Mosher, M. B., DeConti, R. C., Farber, L. R., Marsh, J. C., Mitchell, M. S., Papac, R., Thomas, D., and Bertino, J. R. High-dose methotrexate (MTX) vs. methotrexate-leucovorin (N^5-formyltetrahydrofolate) in epidermoid carcinomas of the head and neck. Proc. Am. Assoc. Cancer Res., *13*: 20, 1972.

Lipschultz, H., and Lerner, H. Three-year observation of combined treatment for advanced cancer of the head and neck. Am. J. Surg., *118*: 698–700, 1969.

Mitchell, M. S., Wawro, N. W., DeConti, R. C., Kaplan, S. R., Papac, R., and Bertino, J. R. Effectiveness of high dose infusions of methotrexate followed by leukovorin in carcinoma of the head and neck. Cancer Res., *28*: 1088–1094, 1968.

Nervi, C., Arcangeli, G., Casale, C., Cortese, M., Guadagni, A., and LePera, V. A re-appraisal of intra-arterial chemotherapy. Cancer, *26*: 577–582, 1970.

Papac, R. J., and Fischer, J. J. Cytosine arabinoside (NSC-63878) in the treatment of epidermoid carcinoma of the head and neck. Cancer Chemother. Rep., *55*: 193–197, 1971.

Papac, R. J., Jacobs, E. M., Foye, L. V., and Donohue, D. M. Systemic therapy with amethopterin in squamous carcinoma of the head and neck. Cancer Chemother. Rep., *32*: 47–54, 1963.

Papac, R. J., Lefkowitz, E., and Bertino, J. R. Methotrexate in squamous cell carcinoma of the head and neck; II. Intermittent intravenous therapy. Cancer Chemother. Rep. *51*: 69–72, 1967.

Ramirez, G. Clinical trials with BCNU in solid tumors. Proc. Am. Assoc. Cancer Res., *13*: 83, 1972.

Richards, G. J., and Chambers, R. G. Hydroxyurea; a radiosensitizer in the treatment of neoplasm of the head and neck. A. J. R. *105*: 555–565, 1969.

Skipper, H. E., Schabel, F. M., and Wilcox, W. S. Experimental evaluation of potential anticancer agents; XIII. On the criteria and kinetics associated with "curability" of experimental leukemia. Cancer Chemother. Rep., *35*: 1–111, 1964.

Stefani, S., Eells, R. W., and Abbate, J. Hydroxyurea and radiotherapy in head and neck cancer. Radiology, *101*: 391–396, 1971.

Stefani, S., Eells, R. W., and Abbate, J. Treatment of advanced head and neck cancer by a combination of hydroxyurea and irradiation; a prospective controlled study in 154 patients. Proc. Am. Soc. Clin. Oncol., (abstract #59) 1972.

Tormey, D. C., Bergevin, P., Blom, J., and Petty, W. Preliminary trials with a combination of Adriamycin (NSC-123127) and bleomycin (NSC-125066) in adult malignancies. Cancer Chemother. Rep., *57*: 413–418, 1973.

Wilson, W. L., Bisel, J. F., Cole, D., Rocklin, D., Ramirez, G., and Madden, R. Prolonged low-dosage administration of hexamethylmelamine (NSC-13875). Cancer, *25*: 568, 1970.

Chapter 23

Odontogenic Tumors

ROGER E. FREILICH, D.M.D.

ODONTOGENESIS

Odontogenic cysts and tumors are developed from one or several types of tissues of the dental apparatus observed during embryogenesis. These tissues may appear in a lesion in either primitive or mature forms. A familiarity with dental development will therefore greatly enhance a comprehension of tumor formation. This information may be found in any standard oral pathology textbook and is beyond the scope of this chapter.

EPITHELIAL CYSTS OF ODONTOGENIC ORIGIN

Odontogenic cysts are tumors only in the loosest sense and have a common origin with true odontogenic tumors. Nevertheless, they may reach a formidable size and provide a nidus for further neoplastic development.

Odontogenic cysts develop because of an aberration in normal tooth formation, developing either before or after calcified tooth structures are formed. The dental epithelium associated with each cyst may be derived from one of the following sources: (1) tooth germ, (2) reduced enamel epithelium, (3) epithelial rests of Malassez, or (4) remnants of the dental lamina. Diagnosis is based on a correlation of clinical, microscopic and radiographic findings (Shafer et al., 1966; Bhaskar, 1969).

Two types of cysts, the primordial and the dentigerous, are both recognized as follicular cysts since they arise from the enamel organ or follicle. This is in contrast to the periodontal and gingival cysts, which are derived from the epithelial rests of Malassez (Shafer et al., 1966). Furthermore, on a histologic basis, all of the following cysts may be designated as odontogenic keratocysts if keratinization of the epithelial lining is observed (Robinson, 1975; Brannon, 1977).

Primordial Cyst

The primordial cyst is the least common, comprising less than 2% of odontogenic cysts. It develops in place of a tooth, being derived from dental embryonic tissues before calcification. The cyst is generally less than 1 cm in diameter. It may displace adjacent structures by pressure. It is painless and seldom clinically obvious. It occurs most frequently in the second and third decades of life with an equal sex distribution. Radiographically, a round, well defined radiolucent area may be seen situated near the apex of a tooth or, more often, in an edentulous space, particularly in the third molar area. Histologically, this is a true cystic lesion lined with stratified squamous epithelium. Treatment is by local curettage (Shafer et al., 1966; Bhaskar, 1969).

Dentigerous Cyst

This cyst develops through an alteration in the reduced enamel epithelium after the tooth crown has been completely formed. In one survey, 3.7% of impacted mandibular teeth and 1.5% of impacted maxillary teeth showed radiographic evidence sufficient to warrant the diagnosis of dentigerous cyst (Dachi and Howell, 1961). They comprise approximately 34% of all odontogenic cysts (Bhaskar, 1969). They are almost always associated with the coronal aspect of an unerupted permanent tooth, generally in the mandibular third molar and maxillary cuspid areas. These cysts have a tendency to be quite aggressive, causing pain, facial asymmetry, displacement or resorption of roots, and impingement on the maxillary sinus or mandibular nerve (Shafer et al., 1966).

One variant of this is the eruption cyst which is found coronal to erupting permanent or deciduous teeth. The mass is usually observed as a bluish compressible swelling of the alveolar ridge. It requires no treatment since it resolves upon tooth eruption.

Radiographically, the dentigerous cyst appears as a unilocular radiolucency surrounding a section of a tooth. A hyperostotic line may surround the cystic cavity. Histologically, this lesion is similar to other odontogenic cysts. Treatment is usually accomplished by extraction and a thorough curettage of the bony lumen. If the cyst is so large as to consider spontaneous fracture, a Partsch procedure (marsupialization) is recommended (Shafer et al., 1966).

It must be emphasized that the wall of primordial and especially dentigerous cysts contains small islands of odontogenic epithelium. In approximately 4% of these cases, the walls show signs of ameloblastic proliferation (Bhaskar, 1969). Also cases of intraosseous mucoepidermoid carcinoma arising in the walls of an odontogenic cyst have been reported, as well as other malignant transformations (Lapin et al., 1973; Marano and Hartman, 1974). This necessitates the submission for pathologic examination of all cystic material.

Periodontal Cysts

The apical periodontal cyst is the most common type. It originates from epithelial rests of Malassez secondary to an infected or traumatized dental pulp and is found associated with the apex of a tooth. These epithelial rests may remain after extraction, giving rise to a residual cyst (Shafer et al., 1966).

The lateral periodontal cyst however, arises from rests in the lateral periodontal membrane of an erupted tooth, although the specific mechanism is unknown (Standish and Shafer, 1958). This cyst is relatively rare but occurs in the mandibular bicuspid region most frequently. In contrast to the apical cyst, the lateral periodontal lesion is associated with a viable tooth (Shafer et al., 1966).

Radiographically both cysts may be seen as a small radiolucent area contiguous to the apical or lateral region of a tooth. Histologically, these cysts are like others except that the epithelial cells individually have a clear cytoplasm and small deeply staining nuclei. Treatment is directed toward curettage of the lesion and root canal therapy in an attempt to retain the tooth. There is little tendency for recurrence (Shafer et al., 1966).

Gingival Cyst

The gingival cyst may be found in the free or attached gingiva. Possible origins of this lesion are numerous but none have been fully substantiated (Ritchey and Orban, 1953). The cyst appears twice as frequently in the mandible, generally in the buccal gingiva in patients in the sixth decade of life. It is usually small, well circumscribed, and painless. In neonates this cyst appears as a large white swelling of the alveolar mucosa known as Epstein's pearls or Bohn's nodules. They resolve spontaneously a few weeks after their appearance (Bhaskar, 1969).

The gingival cyst is not generally observed on roentgenographic examination. Microscopically, the appearance is of a true cyst sometimes associated with evidence of calcification (Shafer et al., 1966). Treatment is by local surgical removal since these have no tendency to recur. Observation of the lesion in infants is indicated (Kreshover, 1957).

ODONTOGENIC TUMORS

Many attempts have been made to classify odontogenic tumors satisfactorily. Thoma and Goldman (1946) classified them according to origin, namely, ectodermal, mesodermal or mixed. This classification was adopted by the American Academy of Oral Pathology in 1950. In 1961, Gorlin et al. modified an existing classification based upon the embryonal inductive effect of one tissue on another.

Pindborg and Kramer's (1971) classification will be used in this chapter since former systematizations were indefinite (Table 23.1). Although

TABLE 23.1

World Health Organization (WHO) Classification by Histological Typing of Odontogenic Tumors, Jaw Cysts, and Allied Lesions[a]

I. Neoplasms and other tumors related to the odontogenic apparatus
  A. Benign
    1. Ameloblastoma
    2. Calcifying epithelial odontogenic tumor
    3. Ameloblastic fibroma
    4. Adenomatoid odontogenic tumor (adenoameloblastoma)
    5. Calcifying odontogenic cyst
    6. Dentinoma
    7. Ameloblastic fibro-odontoma
    8. Odontoameloblastoma
    9. Complex odontoma
    10. Compound odontoma
    11. Fibroma (odontogenic fibroma)
    12. Myxoma (myxofibroma)
    13. Cementomas
      a. Benign cementoblastoma (true cementoma)
      b. Cementifying fibroma
      c. Periapical cemental dysplasia (periapical fibrous dysplasia)
      d. Gigantiform cementoma (familial multiple cementomas)
    14. Melanotic neuroectodermal tumor of infancy
  B. Malignant
    1. Odontogenic carcinomas
      a. Malignant ameloblastoma
      b. Primary intraosseous carcinoma
      c. Other carcinomas arising from odontogenic epithelium including those arising from odontogenic cysts
    2. Odontogenic sarcomas
      a. Ameloblastic fibrosarcoma (ameloblastic sarcoma)
      b. Ameloblastic odontosarcoma
II. Neoplasms and other tumors related to bone
III. Epithelial cysts
  A. Developmental
    1. Odontogenic
      a. Primordial cyst (keratocyst)
      b. Gingival cyst
      c. Eruption cyst
      d. Dentigerous cyst
    2. Nonodontogenic
  B. Inflammatory: Radicular cyst (periodontal)

[a] From Pindborg and Kramer (1971).

imperfect, it attempts to define each lesion as specifically as possible and includes those tumors of uncertain status as well as clearly non-neoplastic ones. Benign and malignant types form the basis for this classification.

Odontogenic tumors comprise approximately 9% of all tumors of the oral cavity in the United States. However, this percentage may change geographically i.e. in Africa, an odontogenic tumor, the ameloblastoma, is responsible for more than 25% of all jaw tumors (Bhaskar, 1969). The rare types will not be discussed.

Odontogenic tumors are mostly neoplasms that arise from the dental lamina or any of its derivatives. They have in common the fact that most are benign and do not metastasize, although they may be quite deforming. Furthermore, most occur intraosseously and are slow growing (Shafer et al., 1966). The profile of these lesions is presented according to Gorlin's extensive review of the international literature and personal files (Table 23.2).

Other studies such as Bhaskar's collation of 429 cases must be used as a contrast since it reveals wide differences. The ameloblastoma accounts for only 18% of odontogenic tumors, whereas odontogenic fibroma, instead of being a rare lesion, is the most common (Bhaskar, 1969). Differences such as these further emphasize the need for a common denominator in defining such pathological entities.

BENIGN ODONTOGENIC TUMORS

Ameloblastoma (Adamantinoma)

The ameloblastoma, although the most common and aggressive of the odontogenic tumors of the jaw, comprises only 1% of all such tumors and

TABLE 23.2
Odontogenic Tumors[a]

Tumor	Cases		Male (%)	Female (%)	Average Age	Maxilla (%)	Mandible (%)
	No.	Percent					
Ameloblastoma	1258	57	52	48	39	19	81
Adenomatoid odontogenic tumor	100	4.5	47	53	16	61	39
Calcifying epithelial odontogenic tumor	50	2.2	48	52	42	27	73
Ameloblastic fibroma	43	1.9	49	51	16	21	79
Ameloblastic fibroma— granular cell	5	0.2	20	80	51	0	100
Ameloblastic fibrosarcoma	9	0.4	55	45	33	33	67
Immature dentinoma	9	0.4	55	45	17	22	78
Mature dentinoma	5	0.2	60	40	24	40	60
Ameloblastic odontoma	56	2.5	63	37	12	54	46
Complex odontoma	65	2.9	52	48	21	40	60
Compound odontoma	125	5.6	53	47	22	62	38
Myxoma or myxofibroma	116	5.2	52	48	31	43	57
Odontogenic fibroma	7	0.3	57	43	35	30	70
Cementoma (periapical cemental dysplasia)	375	16.8	11	89	39	20	80

[a] From Gorlin and Goldman (1970).

cysts (Small and Waldron, 1955; Gorlin and Goldman, 1970). Adamantinoma, which is sometimes used to designate this lesion, is misleading since no hard tissues are formed (Ivy and Churchill, 1930). These tumors also infrequently arise in soft tissue without bony involvement (Klinar and McManis, 1969; Wallen, 1972; Balfour et al., 1973).

The ameloblastoma is exclusively epithelial in composition, and formation from proliferation within dentigerous cyst walls is quite common (Quinn and Fournet, 1969; Taylor et al., 1971). Origin from a primordial, periodontal or radicular cyst is rare (Byrd et al., 1973). It is estimated that 25–33% of ameloblastomas are associated with follicular cysts (Bhaskar, 1969; Gorlin and Goldman, 1970). The ameloblastoma is slow growing, persistent, and generally painless (Small and Waldron, 1955). Because of its invasive properties and tendency to recur (approximately 33%), Gorlin considers this tumor locally malignant (Gorlin and Goldman, 1970), although this property seems to be dependent on the author's criteria of malignancy (Small and Waldron, 1955, Carr and Halperin, 1968). However, the ability to metastasize to the lung or lymph nodes, although minimal, has been documented (Tsukada et al., 1965; Keaton et al., 1974). The ameloblastoma may reach a massive size, eventually obstructing the airway, eroding major arteries or invading the middle cranial fossa (Hoffman et al., 1968; Kyriazis et al., 1971).

From a study of over 1000 cases of ameloblastoma, the average age at the time of discovery was 33, while the tumor was evenly divided between the sexes (Small and Waldron, 1955). Eighty percent originate in the mandible, generally in the posterior region. The site of occurrence may show normal or enlarged mucosa and bone with displacement of adjacent teeth (Bhaskar, 1969). Ameloblastomas occasionally have been reported in children (Dresser and Segal, 1967) and in the gingiva, where local excision is the treatment of choice (Bhaskar, 1969). On pathologic examination, the epithelium of the ameloblastoma may be in the form of sheets, islands or cords with the peripheral layer formed by ameloblast-like cells. The central mass of these islands resembles the stellate reticulum, while the connective tissue stroma is fibrous and usually dense. The tumor is not encapsulated, with tissue infiltrating the contiguous bone far beyond the extent of the lesion (Bhaskar, 1969).

Radiographically, the ameloblastoma shows a uni- or multilocular radiolucent area, giving a soap bubble effect. There may or may not be expansion or destruction of the bony cortex. Association with an impacted tooth is quite common (Bhaskar, 1969). Treatment of this tumor is directed toward wide resection since recurrence rates are high (Johnson and Topazian, 1968; Taylor, 1968; Keaton et al., 1974). Furthermore, reappearance of the lesion has been observed up to 30 years after primary removal (Small, 1956; Hayward, 1973). These facts plus the possibility of repeated surgery and ensuing malformations with possible local spread support the advisability of initial aggressive surgery (Emmings et al., 1971). In contrast, according to one author, a thorough curettage may be entirely satisfactory at selected times, depending on the operator's skill and the accessibility of the lesion (Kramer, 1963). Clinical features such as rate of growth, amount of invasion or dissemination, patient's age and health, and size and location of the tumor should be taken into account before deciding the proper course of action (Huffman and Thatcher, 1974). The use of radiation therapy is generally ineffective because of the tumor's radioresistance (Shafer et al., 1966), although Hair (1963) considers the ameloblastoma radiosensitive. Injection of a 5% solution of sodium psylliate to reduce the blood supply to the tumor has been utilized with success for an inoperable ameloblastoma (Schultz and Vazirani, 1960). Other contributors have advocated a conservative surgical approach for cystic lesions and a radical one for solid tumors (Gorlin and Goldman, 1970).

Calcifying Epithelial Odontogenic Tumor (Pindborg Tumor)

The calcifying epithelial odontogenic tumor is a locally invasive epithelial neoplasm whose origin is the reduced enamel epithelium of an unerupted tooth (Shafer et al., 1966). This tumor was first recognized as an entity in 1955, and subsequently over 113 cases have been published (Franklin and Pindborg, 1976). The Pindborg tumor is painless but slowly invasive and expands the contiguous bony structures causing noticeable swelling. The degree of aggressiveness, however, varies markedly. The lesion, which is generally found in the late fourth and early fifth decades, occurs most often in the posterior aspect of the mandible associated with an unerupted tooth (Chaudhry et al., 1972; Krolls and Pindborg, 1974). It may also be found extraosseously (Gorlin and Goldman, 1970). No sex predilection has been noted (Bhaskar, 1969). The histologic pattern is one of islands of closely packed, clear and polyhedral epithelial cells with well demarcated cell borders (Shafer et al., 1966). These islands are separated by a scanty connective tissue stroma (Gorlin and Goldman, 1970). Intercellular bridges are common. Within the cell masses are spherical acidophilic homogeneous foci which commonly calcify (Pindborg and Kramer, 1971). Radiographically, an impacted tooth with a radiolucent area around the crown is seen. Within this area are usually many variably sized radiopaque masses (Shafer et al., 1966). The tumor behaves somewhat like an ameloblastoma, having recurred up to 31 years following surgery (Gardner et al., 1968). Opinions vary as to definitive treatment from conservative therapy (Bhaskar, 1969) to wide resection (Shafer et al., 1966). Evidence exists that the extraosseous type is less active and therefore should be treated more conservatively (Gorlin and Goldman, 1970).

Ameloblastic Fibroma (Soft Mixed Odontoma)

The ameloblastic fibroma is a relatively uncommon neoplasm of odontogenic epithelium enclosed within cellular mesodermal tissue without the formation of true enamel or dentin (Pindborg and Kramer, 1971). It is probably derived from the epithelial root sheath of Hertwig (Spouge, 1967).

Clinically, this is a soft tumor which occurs routinely in patients under 25 years old, with a range between 6 months and 42 years. There is no sex preference. The lesion occurs most often in the posterior mandible, frequently associated with an unerupted tooth (Bhaskar, 1969). The tumor progresses as a slow growing, generally painless swelling of the affected site, causing bony expansion. However, on occasion pain, superimposed infection, and tooth migration are noted (Gorlin and Goldman, 1970). Although nonaggressive, the tumor does recur locally (Carr et al., 1970). In a study of 23 cases from the files of the Armed Forces Institute of Pathology, a recurrence rate of 43.5% was noted in a postoperative period of 10 months to 16.5 years (Trodahl, 1972).

Histologically, the tumor is formed by islands in many patterns composed of a peripheral layer of cuboidal to columnar ameloblast-like epithelial cells (Pindborg and Kramer, 1971). These thin islands are enclosed by numerous cells resembling the dental papilla. No hard tissues are present. Even though the tumor is not encapsulated, its peripheral tissue does not invade surrounding marrow (Bhaskar, 1969). However, at least one author considers the tumor encapsulated (Gorlin and Goldman, 1970). The likelihood that the ameloblastic fibroma is a stage in the eventual development of a complex odontoma (Cahn and Blum, 1952) is very much in doubt (Pindborg and Kramer, 1971).

The radiographic appearance is that of a solitary well defined radiolucent lesion which is rarely multilocular. Association with an unerupted tooth, expansion of cortical plates, and separation of roots are all occasionally seen (Bhaskar, 1969; Gorlin and Goldman, 1970). Treatment consists of curettage of the lesion which separates easily from its bony crypt. The small number of recurrences are probably secondary to incomplete removal (Gorlin and Goldman, 1970; Hager et al., 1978).

Adenomatoid Odontogenic Tumor (Adenoameloblastoma, Ameloblastic Adenomatoid Tumor)

This rare epithelial odontogenic tumor is commonly known as the adenoameloblastoma (Tchertkoff et al., 1969). However, this lesion should be differentiated from the more aggressive ameloblastoma, and thus the term adenomatoid odontogenic tumor is more appropriate (Philipsen and Birn, 1969). The tumor is probably derived from either the reduced enamel epithelium of the crown of a tooth or a cystic epithelial lining (Gorlin and Goldman, 1970). Its incidence is relatively rare, little more than 150 cases being reported in the literature (Courtney and Kerr, 1975; Tsaknis et al., 1977). From the more current analyses of this lesion, 75% of all adenomatoid odontogenic tumors occur in the second decade of life, with females predominating in a 2 to 1 ratio (Tchertkoff et al., 1969, Burzynski et al., 1970, Giansanti et al., 1970). While the maxilla is involved twice as often as the mandible, 90% of the cases involve the anterior teeth of either jaw (Bhaskar, 1969). Almost two-thirds of the tumors are associated with an impacted tooth (Gorlin and Goldman, 1970).

This tumor generally begins as an asymptomatic swelling, often arising in the wall of a dentigerous cyst (Khin et al., 1973). However, the adenomatoid odontogenic tumor may expand the cortical plates without invasion of approximating areas (Gorlin and Goldman, 1970). Recurrences are quite rare, the tumor being well circumscribed thus facilitating removal (Thoma and Goldman, 1960, Khin et al., 1973).

Microscopically the lesion is well encapsulated and is composed of epithelium in the form of strands, sheets or islands. Characteristic rings of ameloblast-like columnar cells resembling ducts are seen, but these may be scanty (Pindborg and Kramer, 1971). The connective tissue component includes a hyaline material which is probably dysplastic dentin. Interductile spaces are packed with loosely arranged epithelial cells. The lesion may be extensively calcified throughout the epithelial tissue and stroma (Gorlin and Goldman, 1970; Pindborg and Kramer, 1971). The surrounding marrow spaces are generally tumor free (Bhaskar, 1969).

Radiographically, the adenomatoid odontogenic tumor appears as a well circumscribed radiolucent area approximately 1 to 2 cm in diameter and frequently associated with an impacted tooth. The calcified tissue does not appear on x-rays (Gorlin and Goldman, 1970). Treatment of this lesion is removal by curettage or, less frequently, en bloc resection (Seymour et al., 1974). The lesion does not recur, being readily enucleated (Johnson and Topazian, 1968).

Calcifying Odontogenic Cyst (Keratinizing and Calcifying Odontogenic Cyst, Keratinizing and Calcifying Odontogenic Ameloblastoma)

The calcifying odontogenic cyst is a benign cystic lesion which has been described in the literature as "atypical ameloblastoma" (Boss, 1959). It may be found within bone in 75% of the cases but also in the overlying soft tissues. Infrequently, the lesion is found associated with a complex odontoma (Ulmansky et al., 1969; Altini and Farman, 1975). According to a survey of 70 cases, the lesion occurred at a mean age of 38.4 years with females comprising 54.2% of the patients. There was an equal distribution between the mandible and maxilla with 75% appearing anterior to the first molar. The calcifying odontogenic cyst generally presents itself as a firm noncompressible intraosseous swelling (Freedman et al., 1975).

Microscopically, the multicystic cavities are lined by islands of epithelium with a basal layer of columnar cells which resemble ameloblasts (Pindborg and Kramer, 1971). Overlying the basal layer are masses of swollen cells, pale individual cells, and sheets of large "ghost" epithelial cells (Gorlin and Goldman, 1970). Grossly the calcifying odontogenic cyst is tannish-brown to black in color and is usually cystic but may be in the form of solid tumor masses (Bhaskar, 1969, Freedman et al., 1975).

Radiographically, the tumor appears as a well circumscribed radiolucency containing varying amounts of radiopaque areas (Pindborg and Kramer, 1971). Treatment is by curettage of the lesion. Recurrences are rare, only one case being reported (Bhaskar, 1969; Pullman and Seldin, 1971).

Dentinoma

The dentinoma is a rare odontogenic tumor composed mainly or totally of dysplastic dentin and connective tissue. Odontogenic epithelium may be present (Bhaskar, 1969; Pindborg and Kramer, 1971). It occurs in two forms, the mature, and the rarer immature (ameloblastic fibrodentinoma) types. The dentinoma may be considered a further step in the maturation of the ameloblastic fibroma or as an odontoma, prior to enamel formation and thus may not be classified as a distinct pathologic entity (Gorlin and Goldman, 1970). This extremely rare and slow growing benign lesion may cause considerable destruction of bone as well as mucosal perforation (Shafer et al., 1966). Analysis of both types of dentinoma reveals a predilection for the mandibular molar area in association with the crown of an impacted tooth (Gorlin and Goldman, 1970). No sex pereference was noted but the lesion generally occurred in the third decade of life (Shafer et al., 1966). Occasionally an extraosseous lesion may be observed (Pindborg and Kramer, 1971). Microscopically, the immature dentinoma is frequently encapsulated, portions appearing identical with the ameloblastic fibroma. The epithelium occurs in the form of strands in intimate relationship to the dentin. Cells resembling odontoblasts are also present (Gorlin and Goldman, 1970). Dentinal tubules must be present to confirm the diagnosis of dentinoma. The unusual feature of this tumor is lack of enamel (Shafer et al., 1966). In the mature dentinoma, round or irregular areas of osteodentin are observed in a mesenchymal stroma. Cementum formation has also been reported. No epithelium is present (Gorlin and

Goldman, 1970). Radiographically, the lesion is a well demarcated radiolucency with one or several central radiopaque masses varying in size (Pindborg and Kramer, 1971). Treatment consists of a thorough curettage of the lesion, including removal of the connective tissue capsule which shells out easily (Gorlin and Goldman, 1970; Shafer et al., 1966).

Ameloblastic fibro-odontoma (Ameloblastic Odontoma)

The term ameloblastic fibro-odontoma may be used as a specific pathologic entity (Pindborg and Kramer, 1971) or to signify a transition state between the development of the complex or compound odontoma from an ameloblastic odontoma (Hooker, 1967; Sanders et al., 1974). Many authors also classify this lesion under the heading ameloblastic odontoma (Frissell and Shafer, 1953; Choukas and Toto, 1964). When used as a specific tumor classification, the ameloblastic fibro-odontoma refers to a neoplasm having the general features of an ameloblastic fibroma but containing dentin and enamel (Pindborg and Kramer, 1971). Clinically this tumor, although painless, enlarges by expansion and is frequently associated with impacted teeth, particularly in the area of the posterior dentition (Hooker, 1967; Hamner and Pizer, 1968). The mandible and maxilla as well as both sexes are affected equally. The average age of occurrence has varied from 6 months to 39 years with a mean age of 11.5 years (Sanders et al., 1974). Microscopically, the ameloblastic fibro-odontoma is quite similar to a developing complex odontoma as well as the ameloblastic fibroma. The epithelium does not resemble an ameloblastoma but appears as rests arranged as cords or nests resembling the enamel organ or the dental lamina. The calcified tissues are deposited in a stroma of embryonal-like connective tissues resembling the dental papilla (Sanders et al., 1974). Radiographically, the lesion appears as a well defined radiolucency, infrequently with calcified material intralumenally (Pindborg and Kramer, 1971). Treatment of the lesion is conservative since behavior is unlike the ameloblastoma (Sanders et al., 1974).

Odontoameloblastoma (Ameloblastic Odontoma)

Like the ameloblastic fibro-odontoma, the odontoameloblastoma is also frequently equated with the ameloblastic odontoma in the literature. Pindborg and Kramer (1971), however, do not regard the ameloblastic odontoma as a classifiable entity but as a developmental stage between the ameloblastic fibroma and an odontoma. The odontoameloblastoma is a rare benign odontogenic neoplasm containing tissues of both an ameloblastoma and a composite odontoma (Shafer et al., 1966; Gorlin and Goldman, 1970). Apparently, many reports of cases of an ameloblastoma or a complex odontoma have in reality been odontoameloblastomas

(Gorlin and Goldman, 1970). This tumor generally arises as an asymptomatic swelling of the alveolar process but may eventually deform the entire bony cortex (Worley and McKee, 1972). The lesion is not invasive (Gorlin and Goldman, 1970) but recurrences after removal have been reported (Thoma and Goldman, 1946; Frissel and Shafer, 1953). With few exceptions the tumor is found in children, 90% being under 15 years old. There is a slight propensity for occurrence in males and the maxilla (Gorlin and Goldman, 1970).

On histologic examination, ameloblastic epithelium, stellate reticulum, enamel, enamel matrix, dentin, dentinal matrix, and bone all may be observed, generally in a random arrangement. x-rays reveal a cystlike area, the lumen containing numerous radiopaque bodies of various sizes (Gorlin and Goldman, 1970; Pindborg and Kramer, 1971).

Since recurrences after curettage or enucleation of the lesion have been observed, a more radical approach is warranted. En bloc resection, preserving the inferior border of the jaw, will result in a permanent cure (Frissel and Shafer, 1953; Shafer et al., 1966).

Complex Odontoma (Complex Composite Odontoma)

An odontoma commonly denotes a malformation in which both mature enamel and dentin are formed, much like in a tooth. However, in a complex odontoma, these tissues are laid down in an abnormal pattern (Shafer et al., 1966). In contrast to the compound odontoma, morphodifferentiation is poor and therefore there is little resemblance to a normal tooth (Gorlin and Goldman, 1970).

Odontomas, in general, probably represent the most common odontogenic tumor, the compound type being seen more frequently than the complex odontoma. This latter benign, nonaggressive lesion is most often discovered in the second and third decades of life, showing a slight tendency for occurrence in males (Gorlin and Goldman, 1970). Although most are far smaller than a normal tooth, some may reach a formidable size. Approximately 70% are found in the third molar area. Dentigerous cyst development is also frequently associated with this lesion (Gorlin and Goldman, 1970). The complex odontoma, which is often found on routine x-ray examination, is usually self-limiting (Bhaskar, 1969). Local trauma or infection have been implicated as possible initiating factors (Shafer et al., 1966).

Microscopically, a random pattern of enamel, enamel matrix, dentin, dentinal matrix, cementum, and areas of pulp tissue are seen, sometimes associated with a cyst. The latter type of lesion is termed a cystic odontoma and must be excised (Hooker, 1967). A connective tissue capsule often surrounds the tumor (Gorlin and Goldman, 1970).

Radiographically, the pattern reveals disorganized, very dense, irregularly shaped radiopacities surrounded by a thin radiolucent ring (Gorlin and Goldman, 1970). The tumor should be removed thoroughly and carefully by enucleation during its early, predominantly soft tissue stage otherwise regrowth may occur (Pindborg and Kramer, 1971). With further maturation, the tumor is easily removed by separating the soft tissue capsule from the bone. After removal at this hard tissue phase, odontomas do not recur (Bhaskar, 1969).

Compound Odontoma (Compound Composite Odontoma)

Although the dividing line between compound and complex odontomas is indistinct, a compound odontoma refers to a tumor whose calcified structures are morphologically and structurally similar to a tooth. This lesion consists of many toothlike formations in which the enamel, dentin, cementum and pulp are normally interrelated. However, the tooth may have an abnormal shape (Pindborg and Kramer, 1971).

Clinically, this nonaggressive lesion usually occurs in the incisor-cuspid region of the maxilla. At least 60% occur in the second and third decades of life. Not uncommonly, these tumors arise in the mixed dentition stage and prevent permanent tooth eruption (Gorlin and Goldman, 1970).

Microscopically, the normal dental tissue relationship is seen in the form of teeth in a variety of sizes and shapes. Anywhere from 3 teeth to 2000 may be seen bound in a connective tissue capsule (Gorlin and Goldman, 1970). The compound odontoma may also be associated with a cyst in the form of a cystic odontoma or with complex odontomas (Hooker, 1967).

Radiographically, numerous small radiopaque toothlike structures surrounded by a narrow radiolucent band may be observed. They are usually located in interradicular spaces (Bhaskar, 1969). Treatment consists of enucleation of the tumor. Recurrences do not occur (Gorlin and Goldman, 1970).

Fibroma (Odontogenic Fibroma)

The odontogenic fibroma is a benign central neoplasm of the jaw which is variously described as being the most common odontogenic lesion (Bhaskar, 1969) or very rare or uncommon (Hamner et al., 1966; Hanley et al., 1971). This diversity of opinion is probably related to the author's definition of this lesion. The origin of the fibroma is the dental papilla or follicle (Shafer et al., 1966).

One extensive review of the English-language literature has produced only 13 verified cases, 5 being in a peripheral location (Farman, 1975). Bhaskar, on the other hand, cites this lesion as comprising 23% of all odontogenic tumors. It is a slow growing solid lesion which occurs in the second decade of life with an equal distribution between males and females. The third molar and cuspid area of the mandible are the most frequent sites of appearance. The lesion is generally asymptomatic and is ordinarily associated with an impacted tooth (Bhaskar, 1969). From Farman's 10 new reported cases of peripheral odontogenic fibromas and 5 previous cases, the mandible was the preferred site in 11 cases. The lesions appeared as firmly attached, sessile growths of the gingiva which simulate a fibrous epulis (Farman, 1975).

The odontogenic fibroma consists of odontogenic epithelium and loosely arranged fibrous tissue which is more mature and collagenous than the ameloblastic fibroma. The presence of epithelium is not constant and in such cases diagnosis is made if there is evidence that the tumor originates from odontogenic tissue. Peripheral lesions are similar except that epithelial proliferation may be quite prominent (Pindborg and Kramer, 1971). At times, the epithelium may be calcified, at which point the lesion is designated a calcifying odontogenic fibroma (Bhaskar, 1969).

Radiographic appearance is that of a variable-sized radiolucency associated with the coronal portion of a tooth (Bhaskar, 1969). The lesion resembles a dentigerous cyst or an ameloblastoma. The lesion "shells out" easily with curettage. Recurrences have not been reported (Gorlin and Goldman, 1970).

Myxoma (Myxofibroma)

The myxoma is a locally invasive, nonmetastasizing neoplasm, apparently of odontogenic origin, probably from the connective tissue of the dental papilla (Gorlin and Goldman, 1970; Pindborg and Kramer, 1971). Most if not all true osseous myxomas occur in the mandible and maxilla (Stout, 1948; Dahlin, 1969). Analysis of 116 reported cases revealed that 60% appear in the second and third decades of life. No pattern of sex distribution was apparent, the mandible being involved more frequently than the maxilla (Gorlin and Goldman, 1970). However, another report revealed the maxilla as the primary site of growth (Tiecke, 1965).

This usually slow growing and asymptomatic tumor is frequently associated with an impacted tooth (Bhaskar, 1969). However, bony expansion and tumor size may be marked causing sequellae such as facial deformity, severe pain, lip parasthesias, tooth displacement, and invasion of the maxillary sinus (Archer, 1960; Gorlin and Goldman, 1970; Gormley et al., 1975). Grossly, this soft tumor varies in color from grayish-white to amber. The surface is frequently bosselated (Gorlin and Goldman, 1970). Microscopically, the tissues contain rounded or angular cells with overabundant mucoid intercellular substance. The tumor shows little encapsulation, often invading bone and soft tissues (Pindborg and Kramer, 1971). Infrequently, odontogenic epithelium may be seen (Zimmerman and Dahlin, 1958).

Radiographically, the myxoma gives a multilocular radiolucent appearance, termed a "soap bubble" effect. The tumor is frequently poorly defined (Gorlin and Goldman, 1970; Pindborg and Kramer, 1971).

Because of its invasive characteristics and gelatinous consistency, proper removal is difficult and recurrences are common (Shafer et al., 1966). Enucleation followed by chemical or electric cautery may be used for smaller lesions, whereas en bloc resection is used for larger tumors (Large et al., 1960). Even though a 25% recurrence rate has been reported, the prognosis is good (Barros and Cabrini, 1969).

Cementoma

Cementomas consist of a group of lesions which contain cementumlike tissue (Pindborg and Kramer, 1971). This term has been traditionally used to describe a series of entities under a variety of names in the literature: ossifying fibroma, cementifying fibroma, cemento-ossifying fibroma, cementoma, cementoblastoma and fibro-osseous lesions. These tumors have been classified by each author's subjective evaluation of lesions containing a spectrum of histopathology with various amounts of cementum and bone. Furthermore, attempts to correlate the microscopic appearance with clinical and x-ray data have fared poorly. Pindborg and Kramer (1971) tried to simplify classification by dividing the cementoma into four groups to be specified here.

Collectively, cementomas show a striking tendency to occur in females (84%), in the mandible (86%), and during the third and fourth decades (75%), with approximately two-thirds appearing in Negroes. The clinical symptoms range from asymptomatic or slight pain and parasthesia to marked facial asymmetry. The vast majority of lesions are less than 4 cm in diameter (Waldron and Giansanti, 1973).

BENIGN CEMENTOBLASTOMA (TRUE CEMENTOMA)

The benign cementoblastoma is a neoplasm of cementum, arising from cementoblasts, and attached to the root of a tooth (Shafer et al., 1966). It is a slow growing and rare lesion, but may expand the bony cortical plates and cause pain (Curran and Collins, 1973; Abrams et al., 1974). Mandibular premolars or molars are most often involved (Kline et al., 1961; Gorlin and Goldman, 1970; Wiggins and Karian, 1975).

From the small number of reported cases, there seems to be no race predilection and the majority of patients were below 25 years old (Gorlin and Goldman, 1970; Cherrick et al., 1974). There is a tendency for occurrence in male patients (Pindborg and Kramer, 1971). The true cementoma may be differentiated from hypercementosis by its size, tendency for cortical expansion and its active histologic appearance (Shafer et al., 1966). Two reports suggest that the incidence of true cementomas may be more common than previously recognized and that it is not readily recognized by health care practitioners (Abrams et al., 1974; Cherrick et al., 1974).

Microscopic examination reveals numerous round bodies of cementum-like tissue with a small number of entrapped cells containing many reversal lines. The soft tissue aspect consists of vascular fibrous tissue containing osteoclasts (Pindborg and Kramer, 1971). The tumor appears to be encapsulated (Gorlin and Goldman, 1970). The cementoblastoma may simulate an osteoblastoma, atypical osteosarcoma, or Paget's disease (Pindborg and Kramer, 1971).

Radiographically, the tumor presents a well circumscribed dense radiopacity whose periphery is uniformly radiolucent (Wiggins and Karian, 1975). This appearance is pathognomonic (Cherrick et al., 1974). The suggested treatment is enucleation of the lesion since recurrence is rare (Abrams et al., 1974).

CEMENTIFYING FIBROMA

The cementifying fibroma is inconclusively classified as a true neoplastic growth (Hamner et al., 1968a). The probable origin of this lesion is mesenchymal "blast" cells possessing the capacity to form cementum, bone, and fibrous tissue (Hamner et al., 1968b). The lesion usually occurs in the posterior mandible of either men or women in their middle decades, not necessarily associated with the apices of teeth (Pindborg and Kramer, 1971). Although generally asymptomatic, the lesion may produce jaw enlargement and discomfort, sometimes attaining immense size (Champion et al., 1949). The possibility that this lesion represents a reparative reaction to trauma is dubious (Stafne, 1933).

The microscopic pattern varies according to the developmental stage. The lesion is generally composed of a cellular fibroblastic tissue and collagen bundles. Interspersed among this stroma are numerous accretions of rounded acellular cementum-like material (Hamner et al., 1968a; Bhaskar, 1969). In the early stages, the lesion is mainly fibroblastic and subsequently becomes almost a totally cementum-like lesion as the calcified masses fuse (Pindborg and Kramer, 1971). This cementum material may be easily confused with bone (Bhaskar, 1969).

On x-rays, initial formation of a radiolucent area secondary to bony destruction transforms in later stages to a similar picture with varying areas of radiopacity within the lesion (Hamner et al., 1968a). The tumor may eventually appear as a totally radiopaque area (Pindborg and Kramer, 1971). Since this lesion is generally self-limiting, no surgical intervention is indicated except possibly for diagnostic purposes (Hamner et al., 1968a).

PERIAPICAL CEMENTAL DYSPLASIA (PERIAPICAL FIBROUS DYSPLASIA)

Periapical cemental dysplasia is a relatively common lesion which is probably non-neoplastic (Shafer et al., 1966). However, some authors believe the lesion is neoplastic, being derived from the dental follicle (Gorlin and Goldman, 1970).

The incidence of periapical cemental dysplasia has been described as 2 or 3 per 1000 persons (Chaudhry et al., 1958). According to Bhaskar (1969), this periapical lesion represents 10% of all odontogenic tumors. The lesion has a predilection for females (91%), the third and fourth decades of life, and Negroes (83%) (Zegarelli and Ziskin, 1943; Zegarelli et al., 1964). The mandibular incisor area accounts for the location in a clear majority of cases. Trauma is apparently not a predisposing factor in formation (Chaudhry et al., 1958). The lesions grow quite slowly and occur in multiple numbers, each usually less than one centimeter in diameter (Zegarelli et al., 1964). The proximal teeth all remain viable (Bhaskar, 1969).

The microscopic picture is similar to cementifying fibroma, being principally fibroblastic initially, and subsequently composed of increasing amounts of cementum-like tissue with occasional trabeculae of woven bone (Pindborg and Kramer, 1971). The development of periapical cemental dysplasia has been divided into three stages: (1) osteolytic, (2) cementoblastic, and (3) mature reactive. The development time of the final stage is apparently 3–10 years (Scannell, 1949).

The radiographic appearance varies according to the developmental stage, simulating a cystlike radiolucency periapically at first. This is followed by areas of central calcification within the lesion. Finally, a discrete area of radiopacity surrounded by a thin radiolucent line separating the lesion from the tooth apex may be visualized (Bhaskar, 1969; Gorlin and Goldman, 1970). If this diagnosis has been confirmed, no treatment is indicated.

GIGANTIFORM CEMENTOMA (FAMILIAL MULTIPLE CEMENTOMA)

The gigantiform cementoma forms either as a result of a dysplastic process or a developmental anomaly (Pindborg and Kramer, 1971). The lesions are observed most frequently in middle aged Negro females and may reach a formidable size. Such enlargement may be observed in patients with Paget's disease (Gorlin and Goldman, 1970).

On histologic examination the lesion consists of a mass of dense avascular cementum (Bhaskar and Cutright, 1968). The tumor must be differentiated from hypercementosis in which secondary cementum is laid down in an orderly fashion on the root of a tooth (Pindborg and Kramer, 1971). Radiographically, the lesion is made up of large radiopaque masses without a radiolucent border (Bhaskar and Cutright, 1968). No surgical treatment is indicated.

Melanotic Neuroectodermal Tumor of Infancy (Melanotic Progonoma, Melano-ameloblastoma, Retinal Anlage Tumor)

The melanotic neuro-ectodermal tumor of infancy is quite rare and of dubious odontogenic origin, probably being derived from cells of the neural crest (Pindborg and Kramer, 1971). The tumor is benign and usually occurs in the anterior maxilla, almost exclusively in children under 1 year of age, although extraoral and extracephalic sites have been reported (Brekke and Gorlin, 1975). The maxilla is the favored site in 80% of the cases with 60% occurring in females (Lurie, 1961; Bhaskar, 1969). The lesion appears as a relatively rapid growing, firm, nonulcerating but aggressive swelling of the jaws which is darkly pigmented, much like an epulis (Shafer et al., 1966). In many cases it causes elevation of the upper lip, thus inhibiting breast or bottle feeding. The tumor does not metastasize (Bhaskar, 1969). Grossly, pigmentation varying from mottled gray patches to uniform black areas are seen in the specimen (Pindborg and Kramer, 1971). Microscopically, the lesion consists of two types of cells—cuboidal epithelial-like cells with abundant cytoplasm arranged in sheets, cords or ductlike structures, and lymphocyte-like cells in a fibrous stroma. Melanin granules are found in both cell types in varying proportions. At the periphery of the lesion are extensions into bone which may give an inaccurate invasive appearance (Pindborg and Kramer, 1971). The tumor is not encapsulated (Shafer et al., 1966).

Radiographs show a poorly circumscribed radiolucent area of varying sizes which gives the appearance of a possible malignant neoplasm (Shafer et al., 1966). Displacement of developing teeth is frequently seen (Bhaskar, 1969). Treatment is conservative, curettage being the management of choice. However, recurrences are common and many authors advocate more aggressive surgical modalities (Brekke and Gorlin, 1975).

MALIGNANT ODONTOGENIC TUMORS

Odontogenic Carcinomas

MALIGNANT AMELOBLASTOMA

This neoplasm is an ameloblastoma which shows evidence of metastasis. Furthermore, a squamous cell carcinoma may appear in association with an ameloblastoma. Whether this represents one or two separate tumors is controversial (Pindborg and Kramer, 1971).

PRIMARY INTRAOSSEOUS CARCINOMA

A squamous cell carcinoma may arise within the jaw, developing from odontogenic epithelium. The lesion is not related to the overlying mucosa, salivary gland tissue, or odontogenic cyst wall (Pindborg and Kramer, 1971).

OTHER CARCINOMAS ARISING FROM ODONTOGENIC EPITHELIUM, INCLUDING ODONTOGENIC CYSTS

The existence of malignant transformation of odontogenic epithelium is quite rare, only six well documented cases being reported in the literature until 1973 (Lapin et al., 1973; Hampl and Harrigan, 1973). Keratinizing odontogenic cysts are probably most likely to undergo this transformation (Pindborg and Kramer, 1971).

Odontogenic Sarcoma

AMELOBLASTIC FIBROSARCOMA (AMELOBLASTIC SARCOMA)

The ameloblastic fibrosarcoma represents a neoplasm, histologically similar to the ameloblastic fibroma, except for the presence of sarcomatous features in the mesenchymal portion with pleomorphism and mitoses (Pindborg and Kramer, 1971). Malignant transformation from ameloblastic fibromas, ameloblastic odontomas and ameloblastic fibro-odontomas has been suggested (Howell and Burkes, 1977). The lesion is extremely rare, rapid growing, and painful, causing loosening of teeth. No reported case of metastasis has been noted (Bhaskar, 1969). From a study of 17 cases, the average age of patients is 30, with occurrence most often in the mandible. No sex predilection was observed (Leider et al., 1972).

Radiographically, bony destruction and irregular margins of this unilocular lesion may be noted. Treatment is wide excision or radical resection of the area including hemimaxillectomy or hemimandibulectomy. In a follow-up of 5 of the 17 cases, 4 lesions recurred, although all patients were alive and well (Leider et al., 1972).

AMELOBLASTIC ODONTOSARCOMA

The ameloblastic odontosarcoma is another rare neoplasm which is similar to the ameloblastic fibrosarcoma but also contains small amounts of dysplastic dentin and enamel (Pindborg and Kramer, 1971). The stroma undergoes a malignant transformation from the ameloblastic odontoma (Villa, 1955).

REFERENCES

Abrams, A. M., Kirby, J. W., and Melrose, R. J. Cementoblastoma. Oral Surg., 38: 394–403, 1974.
Altini, M., and Farman, A. C. The calcifying ontogenic cyst. Oral Surg., 41: 751–759, 1975.
Archer, W. H. Myxoma of left maxilla. Oral Surg., 13: 139–141, 1960.
Balfour, R. S., Loscalzo, L. J., and Sulka, M. Multicentric peripheral ameloblastoma. J. Oral Surg., 31: 535, 1973.
Barros, P. E., and Cabrini, R. L. Myxoma of the jaws. Oral Surg., 27: 225–236, 1969.

Bhaskar, S. N. Oral pathology in the dental office; survey of 20,575 biopsy specimens. J. Am. Dent. Assoc., *76:* 761–766, 1968.

Bhaskar, S. N. 1969. Synopsis of Oral Pathology, Ed 3, pp. 204–257, 378–380, 505. C. V. Mosby, St. Louis, 1969.

Bhaskar, S. N., and Cutright, C. E. Multiple enostosis; report of 16 cases. J. Oral Surg., *26:* 321–326, 1968.

Boss, J. H. A rare variant of ameloblastoma. Arch. Pathol., *68:* 299–305, 1959.

Brannon, R. B. The odontogenic keratocyst. Oral Surg., *43:* 233–255, 1977.

Brekke, J. H., and Gorlin, R. J. Melanotic neuroectodermal tumor of infancy. J. Oral Surg., *33:* 858–865, 1975.

Burzynski, N. J., Rosenberg, C., Crider, R., and Martino, T. H. The ameloblastic adenomatoid tumor. Oral Surg., *29:* 880–882, 1970.

Byrd, D. L., Allen, J. W., and Dunsworth, A. R. Ameloblastoma originating in the wall of a primordial cyst; report of a case. J. Oral Surg., *31:* 301, 1973.

Cahn, L. H., and Blum, T. Ameloblastic odontoma; case report critically analyzed. J. Oral Surg., *10:* 169–170, 1952.

Carr, R. F., and Halperin, V. Malignant ameloblastomas from 1953 to 1966; review of the literature and report of a case. J. Oral Surg., *26:* 514, 1968.

Carr, R. F., Halperin, V., Wood, C., Krust, L., and Schoen, J. Recurrent ameloblastic fibroma. Oral Surg., *29:* 85–90, 1970.

Champion, A. H. R., Moule, A. W., and Wilkenson, F. C. Case report of an endosteal fibroma of the mandible. Br. Dent. J., *86:* 3–6, 1949.

Chaudhry, A. P., Hanks, C. T., Leifer, C., and Gargiulo, E. A. Calcifying epithelial odontogenic tumor. Cancer, *30:* 519–529, 1972.

Chaudhry, A. P., Spink, J. H., and Gorlin, P. J. Periapical fibrous dysplasia (cementoma). J. Oral Surg., *16:* 483–488, 1958.

Cherrick, H. M., King, O. H., Lucatorto, F. M., and Suggs, D. M. Benign cementoblastoma. Oral Surg., *37:* 54–63, 1974.

Choukas, N. C., and Toto, P. D. Ameloblastic odontoma. Oral Surg., *17:* 10–15, 1964.

Colby, R. A., Kerr, D. A., and Robinson, H. B. G. Color Atlas of Oral Pathology, Ed 2, pp. 1–14. J.B. Lippincott, Philadelphia, 1961.

Couch, R. D., Morris, E. E., and Vellios, F. Granular cell ameloblastic fibroma; report of two cases in adults with observations on its similarity to congenital epulis. Am. J. Clin. Pathol., *37:* 398–404, 1962.

Courtney, R. M., and Kerr, D. A. The odontogenic adenomatoid tumor. Oral Surg., *39:* 424–435, 1975.

Curran, J. B., and Collins, A. P. Benign (true) ameloblastoma of the mandible. Oral Surg., *35:* 168–172, 1973.

Dachi, S. F., and Howell, F. V. A survey of 3,874 routine fullmouth radiographs; II. A study of impacted teeth. Oral Surg., *14:* 1165, 1961.

Dahlin, D. C. Bone Tumors: General Aspects and Data on 3,987 Cases, Ed. 2. Charles C Thomas, Springfield, Ill., 1969.

Dresser, W. J., and Segal, E. Ameloblastoma associated with a dentigerous cyst in a six-year-old child. Oral Surg., *24:* 388–391, 1961.

Emmings, F. G., Gage, A. A., and Koepf, S. W. Combined curettage and cryotherapy for recurrent ameloblastoma of the mandible; report of a case. J. Oral Surg., *29:* 41, 1971.

Farman, A. G. The peripheral odontogenic fibroma. Oral Surg., *40:* 82–92, 1975.

Franklin, C. D., and Pindborg, J. J. The calcifying epithelial odontogenic tumor; a review and analysis of 113 cases. Oral Surg., *42:* 753–765, 1976.

Freedman, P. D., Lummerman, H., and Gee, J. K. Calcifying odontogenic cyst; a review and analysis of seventy cases. Oral Surg., *40:* 93–106, 1975.

Frissell, C. T., and Shafer, W. G. Ameloblastic odontoma; report of a case. Oral Surg., *6:* 1129, 1953.

Gardner, D. G., Michaels, L., and Liepa, E. Calcifying epithelial odontogenic tumor; an amyloid producing neoplasm. Oral Surg., *26:* 812–823, 1968.

Giansanti, J. S., Someren, A., and Waldron, C. A. Ontogenic adenomatoid tumor (adeno-Ameloblastoma); survey of 111 cases. Oral Surg., *30:* 69–86, 1970.

Gorlin, R. J., Chaudhry, A. P., and Pindborg, J. J. Odontogenic tumors. Cancer, *14:* 73–101, 1961.

Gorlin, R. J., and Goldman, H. M. (eds.). Thoma's Oral Pathology, Ed. 6, pp. 481–515. C.V. Mosby, St. Louis, 1970.

Gormley, M. B., Mallin, R. E., Solomon, M., Jarrett, W., and Bromberg, B. Odontogenic myxofibroma; report of two cases. J. Oral Surg., *33:* 356–359, 1975.

Hager, R. C., Taylor, C. G., and Allen, P. M. Ameloblastic fibroma; report of a case. J. Oral Surg., *36:* 66–69, 1978.

Hair, J. A. G. Radiosensitive adamantinoma. Br. Med. J., *1:* 105–106, 1963.

Hamner, J. E., and Pizer, M. E. Ameloblastic odontoma; report of two cases. Am. J. Dis. Child., *115:* 332–336, 1968.

Hamner, J. E., Gamble, J. W., and Gallegos, G. J. Odontogenic fibroma; report of two cases. Oral Surg., *21:* 113–118, 1966.

Hamner, J. E., Lightbody, D. M., Ketcham, A. S., and Swerdlow, H. Cemento-ossifying fibroma of the mandible. Oral Surg., *26:* 579–587, 1968a.

Hamner, J. E., Scofield, H. H., and Cornyn, J. Benign fibro-osseous jaw lesions of periodontal membrane origin. Cancer, *22:* 861–878, 1968b.

Hampl, P. F., and Harrigan, W. F. Squamous cell carcinoma possibly arising from an odontogenic cyst; report of a case. J. Oral Surg., *31:* 359, 1973.

Hanley, J. B., Looly, J. P., and Dincan, J. Odontogenic fibroma. J. Oral Surg., *29:* 52–54, 1971.

Hartman, K. S. Granular-cell ameloblastoma. Oral Surg., *38:* 241–253, 1974.

Hayward, J. R. Recurrent ameloblastoma 30 years after surgical treatment. J. Oral Surg., *31:* 368, 1973.

Hoffman, P. J., Baden, E., Rankow, R. M., and Potter, G. D. The fate of the uncontrolled ameloblastoma. Oral Surg., *26:* 419–426, 1968.

Hoke, H. F., and Harrelson, A. B. Granular cell ameloblastoma with metastasis to the cervical vertebrae. Cancer, *20:* 991–999, 1967.

Hooker, S. P. Ameloblastic odontoma; an analysis of twenty-six cases. Oral Surg., *24:* 375, 1967.

Howell, P. M., and Burkes, E. J. 1977. Malignant transformation of ameloblastic fibro-odontoma to ameloblastic fibrosarcoma. Oral Surg., *43:* 391–401, 1977.

Huffman, G. G., and Thatcher, J. W. Ameloblastoma—the conservative surgical approach to treatment; report of four cases. J. Oral Surg., *32:* 850–854, 1974.

Ivy, R. H., and Churchill, H. R. The need of a standardized surgical and pathological classification of the tumors and anomalies of dental origin. Am. Assoc. Dent. Sch. Trans., *7:* 240–245, 1930.

Johnson, R. H., and Topazian, R. G. The management of variants of ameloblastoma. Plast. Reconstr. Surg., *41:* 356, 1968.

Keaton, W. M., Kolodny, S. C., Roche, W. C., and Koutnik, A. W. Ameloblastoma; report of two cases. J. Oral Surg., *32:* 382–385, 1974.

Khin, U., Sanders, B., Kasper, E., and Adelman, H. Adenomatoid odontogenic tumor. J. Oral Surg., *31:* 607–612, 1973.

Klinar, K. L., and McManis, J. C. Soft tissue ameloblastoma. Oral Surg., *28:* 266–272, 1969.

Kline, S. N., Spatz, S. S., Zubrow, H. J., and Fader, M. Large cementoma of the mandible. Oral Surg., *14:* 1421–1426, 1961.

Kramer, I. R. Ameloblastoma; a clinicopathological appraisal. Br. J. Oral Surg., *1:* 13, 1963.

Kreshover, S. J. The Incidence and Pathogenesis of Gingival Cysts. Presented at 35th General Meeting, International Association for Dental Research, Zürich, 1957.

Krolls, S. O., and Pindborg, J. J. Calcifying epithelial odontogenic tumor; a survey of 23 cases and discussion of histomorphologic variations. Arch. Pathol., *98:* 206–210, 1974.

Kyriazis, A. P., Karkazis, G. C., and Kyriazis, A. A. Maxillary ameloblastoma with intracerebral extension. Oral Surg., *32:* 582, 1971.

Lapin, R., Garfinkel, A. V., Catania, A. F., and Kane, A. A. Squamous cell carcinoma arising in a dentigerous cyst. J. Oral Surg., *31:* 354–358, 1973.

Large, N. D., Nieble, H. H., and Fredricks, W. H. Myxoma of the jaws, report of two cases. Oral Surg., *13:* 1462–1468, 1960.

Leider, A. S., Nelson, J. F., and Trodahl, J. N. Ameloblastic fibrosarcoma of the jaws. Oral Surg., *33:* 559–569, 1972.

Lucas, R. B. Tumor of enamel organ epithelium. Oral Surg., *10:* 652–660, 1957.

Lurie, H. I. Congenital melanocarcinoma, melanotic adamantinoma, retinal anlage tumor, progonoma, and pigmented epulis of infancy. Cancer, *14:* 1090–1108, 1961.

Marano, P. D., and Hartman, K. S. Central mucoepidermoid carcinoma arising in a maxillary odontogenic cyst. J. Oral Surg., *32:* 915, 1974.

Philipsen, H. P., and Birn, H. The adenomatoid odontogenic tumor, ameloblastic adenomatoid tumor or adenoameloblastoma. Acta Pathol. Microbiol. Scand., *75:* 375–398, 1969.

Pindborg, J. J. Calcifying epithelial odontogenic tumor. Cancer, *11:* 838–843, 1958.

Pindborg, J. J., and Clausen, F. Classification of odontogenic tumors; suggestion. Acta Odont. Scand., *16:* 293–301, 1958.

Pindborg, J. J., and Kramer, I. R. H. Histological Typing of Odontogenic Tumours, Jaw Cysts, and Allied Lesions. World Health Organization, Geneva, 1971.

Pullman, S. F., and Seldin, R. The calcifying odontogenic cyst, report of a case. J. Oral Surg., *29:* 367–370, 1971.

Quinn, T. H., and Fournet, L. P. Dentigerous cyst with mural ameloblastoma; report of a case. J. Oral Surg., *27:* 662, 1969.

Ritchey, B., and Orban, B. Cysts of the gingiva. Oral Surg., *6:* 765, 1953.

Robinson, H. B. Primordial cyst versus keratocyst. Oral Surg., *40:* 362–364, 1975.

Sanders, D. W., Kolodny, S. C., and Jacoby, J. K. Ameloblastic fibro-odontoma; report of a case. J. Oral Surg., *32:* 281–285, 1974.

Scannell, J. M. Cementoma. Oral Surg., *2:* 1169–1180, 1949.

Schultz, L. W., and Vazirani, S. J. Use of sclerosing solution in treatment of ameloblastoma. Oral Surg., *13:* 150–156, 1960.

Seymour, R. L., Funke, F. W., and Irby, W. B. Adenomeloblastoma. Oral Surg., *38:* 860–865, 1974.

Shafer, W. G., Hine, M. K., and Levy, B. M. A Textbook of Oral Pathology, Ed. 2, pp. 200–236. W.B. Saunders, Philadelphia, 1966.

Sicher, H. (ed.). Orban's Oral Histology and Embryology. Ed. 6, pp. 18–38. C.V. Mosby, St. Louis, 1966.

Small, I. A. Recurrent ameloblastoma twenty-five years after hemimandibulectomy. Oral Surg., *9:* 699, 1956.

Small, I. A., and Waldron, C. A. Ameloblastoma of jaws. Oral Surg., *8:* 281–297, 1955.

Spouge, J. Odontogenic tumors. Oral Surg., *24:* 392–403, 1967.

Stafne, E. C. Cementoma; study of 35 cases. Dent. Surv., *9:* 27–31, 1933.

Standish, S. M., and Shafer, W. G. 1958. The lateral periodontal cyst. J. Periodontol., *29:* 27, 1958.

Stout, A. P. Myxoma; tumor of primitive mesenchyme. Ann. Surg., *127:* 706–719, 1948.

Taylor, B. G. Ameloblastoma of the mandible; a clinical study of 25 patients. Am. J. Surg., *34:* 57, 1968.

Taylor, R. N., Callins, J. F., Menell, H. B., and Williams, A. C. Dentigerous cyst with ameloblastomatous proliferation; report of a case. J. Oral Surg., *29:* 136–140, 1971.

Tchertkoff, V., Dalno, J. A., and Ehrenreich, T. Ameloblastic adenomatoid tumor. Oral Surg., *27:* 72–82, 1969.

Thoma, K. H., and Goldman, H. M. Odontogenic tumors; classification based on observation of epithelial, mesenchymal and mixed varieties. Am. J. Pathol., *22:* 433–471, 1946.

Thoma, K. H., and Goldman, H. M. Oral Pathology, Ed. 5. C.V. Mosby, St. Louis, 1960.

Tiecke, R. W. Oral Pathology, pp. 218–219, 276–277. McGraw-Hill, New York, 1965.

Trodahl, J. N. Ameloblastic fibroma. Oral Surg., *33:* 547–557, 1972.

Tsaknis, P. J., Carpenter, W. M., and Shade, N. L. Odontogenic adenomatoid tumor; report of case and review of the literature. J. Oral Surg., *35:* 146–149, 1977.

Tsukada, Y., de la Pava, S., and Pickren, J. W. Granular-cell ameloblastoma with metastasis to the lungs. Cancer, *18:* 916–925, 1965.

Ulmansky, M., Azaz, B., and Sela, J. Calcifying ondotogenic cyst. J. Oral Surg., *27:* 415–419, 1969.

Villa, V. G. Ameloblastic sarcoma in mandible; report of case. Oral Surg., *8:* 123–129, 1955.

Waldron, C. A., and Giansanti, J. S. Benign fibro-osseous lesions of the jaws; a clinical radiologic-histologic review of 65 cases. Oral Surg., *35:* 340–350, 1973.

Waldron, C. A., Thompson, C. W., and Conner, W. A. Granular-cell ameloblastic fibroma; report of two cases. Oral Surg., *16:* 1202–1213, 1963.

Wallen, N. G. Extraosseous ameloblastoma. Oral Surg., *34:* 95–97, 1972.

Wiggins, H. E., and Karian, B. K. Cementoblastoma of the maxilla; report of a case. J. Oral Surg., *33:* 302, 1975.

Worley, R. D., and McKee, P. E. Ameloblastic odontoma; report of a case. J. Oral Surg., *30:* 764–766, 1972.

Zegarelli, E. V., Kutscher, A. H., Napoli, N., and Iurono, F. The cementoma; a study of 230 patients with 435 cementomas. Oral Surg., *17:* 219–224, 1964.

Zegarelli, E. V., and Ziskin, D. E. Cementoma; report of 50 cases. Am. J. Orthod. (Oral Surg. Sect.), *29:* 285–292, 1943.

Zimmerman, D. C., and Dahlin, D. C. Myxomatous tumors of jaws. Oral Surg., *11:* 1069–1080, 1958.

Chapter 24

Brain

PATRICK R. BERGEVIN, M.D.

The gliomas comprise nearly half of all primary brain tumors and include mainly the astrocytoma and glioblastoma multiforme (astrocytoma Grade III-IV) with a lesser incidence of ependymoma, oligodendroglioma, medulloblastoma and miscellaneous types (Zimmerman, 1969). The astrocytoma is the commonest of the gliomas and occurs most often in the cerebral hemispheres in adults but subtentorially in children. Prognosis for the patient with an astrocytoma is clearly related to histologic grade (Zulch and Wechsler, 1968): Grade I may be cured or at least a long survival is expected; a 3-5-year survival is generally seen with Grade II; survival falls precipitously for Grade III-IV astrocytoma (glioblastoma multiforme), with median survival in the range of only 4-6 months and only 10% of patients alive at 18 months. Furthermore, the prognosis for glioblastoma multiforme has not been significantly improved in recent years by refinements in surgical and radiotherapeutic techniques. A review of the literature on glioblastoma multiforme would suggest that surgical debulking of tumor followed by whole brain irradiation at 5000-6000 R over 6-8 weeks will prolong life by 3-6 months (Frankel and German, 1958; Davis et al., 1949; Roth and Elridge, 1960; Jelsma and Bucy, 1976; Bouchard, 1966; Schultz et al., 1968).

Corticosteroids, particularly dexamethasone, have been employed to decrease cerebral edema and have led to a reduction in operative mortality (Jelsma and Bucy, 1967). It appears that corticosteroids act to stabilize cellular membranes and thus relieve edema, although in addition peritumoral blood flow is improved and more complex mechanisms may be operative (Weinstein et al., 1973). Renaudin et al. (1973) have emphasized the dose dependency of dexamethasone in patients with partially excised brain tumors: up to 96 mg/day were given to achieve additional antiedema effects without significant complications.

The obstacles to successful chemotherapy of the astrocytomas are as for other solid tumors with the addition of the so-called blood-brain barrier (BBB). In vivo cell kinetic studies of human gliomas (Hoshino et al., 1972) reveal the usual less than 10% labeling index seen with most other solid tumors, reflecting a decrease in growth fraction and thus a suboptimal response to chemotherapy. The BBB, located in the capillary endothelium, may effectively prevent most chemotherapeutic agents given systemically from entering the proliferating portion of the brain tumor (Tator, 1972). Long (1970), by ultrastructural studies, has demonstrated the virtual absence of the BBB within much of the tumor, although the peripherally situated, actively proliferating tumor cells are apparently confined within such a barrier (Wilson et al., 1972). Search for a substance which will pass the BBB (high lipid solubility, lack of ionization at physiologic pH and small molecular size (Rall and Zubrod, 1962) led to the use of nitrosoureas, which have become the best single agents in the treatment of advanced malignant astrocytomas.

Fewer et al. (1972) reported a 48% response rate in 81 patients with recurrent primary or metastatic brain tumors treated with 1,3-bis(2-chloroethyl)-1-nitrosourea (BCNU). In patients with glioblastoma multiforme the response rate was 53%. Most responsive in this series were the ependymomas and least responsive were metastatic brain tumors. A 33% response rate was noted in 38 patients with primary or metastatic brain tumors treated with 1-(2-chloroethyl)-3-cyclohexyl-1-nitrosourea (CCNU) (Fewer et al., 1972). No patients responded to CCNU who had previously shown progressive disease on BCNU. Equally promising results with the nitrosoureas have also been reported by Wilson et al. (1970) and Rosenblum et al. (1973). Walker (1973) studied 210 patients with glioblastoma multiforme randomized postoperatively to one of four treatment regimens and reported median survivals as follows:

1. Supportive therapy only   15 weeks
2. Chemotherapy with BCNU   21 weeks
3. Radiation therapy   30 weeks
4. Chemotherapy and radiotherapy   40 weeks

The survival of patients receiving radiotherapy or BCNU are little different after 1 year and by 18 months virtually all patients have died. In contrast, 25% of patients receiving both BCNU and radiotherapy were alive at 18 months.

Response rates seen with conventional administration of most of the standard chemotherapeutic agents are generally dismal (Broder and Rall, 1972; Shapiro and Ausman, 1969), with the exception of procarbazine, which crosses the BBB either directly or in metabolite form. Kumar et al. (1974) treated 29 patients with advanced primary or metastatic brain tumors with oral procarbazine and noted a definite clinical response in 12 patients, for a response rate of 41%. However, patients who had received previous chemotherapy either with CCNU or BCNU showed no response to procarbazine. The drug 4'-demethyl-epipodophylloxin-β-D-thenyli-dene-glucoside (PTG) is promising and may be of benefit in the patient with a primary brain tumor who has shown progressive disease while on one of the nitrosoureas (Sklansky et al., 1974). Both procarbazine and PTG are suitable agents for trials in combination regimens with nitrosoureas. One study indicates a slight superiority of procarbazine, CCNU and vincristine combination chemotherapy over procarbazine alone (Gutin et al., 1975).

Recognition that the BBB could be circumvented by giving the drug intrathecally led to the use of methotrexate in this manner. Responses to intrathecal methotrexate are occasionally seen but are usually of brief duration (Wilson and Norrell, 1969; Newton et al., 1968). The administration of methotrexate intraventricularly via the Ommaya reservoir is discussed by Rubin et al. (1966). Local application of various agents in the tumor cavity after partial resection has given no appreciable clinical benefit. Infusion and perfusion of chemotherapeutic drugs has generally not been beneficial (Shapiro and Ausman, 1969). Simultaneous administration of 5-fluorouracil with postoperative whole brain irradiation did not appear to alter survival (Edland et al., 1971).

The brain scan has proved to be the most useful means of following intracerebral tumor size, although it cannot distinguish active tumor from necrotic tumor or surrounding edema (Fewer et al., 1972). Computerized axial tomography (CAT) scans may help avert this problem. Differentiating the effects of corticosteroids from that of chemotherapy is a problem in the study of new drugs. The ability to discontinue corticosteroids following institution of chemotherapy is one means for evaluation. Survival from the time of institution of chemotherapy, however, remains the best indicator of drug activity. There are, however, certain patients with Grade III-IV astrocytomas who will have a considerably longer survival than most, even without treatment with chemotherapy. The longer a patient survives following surgery, the greater his chance of falling into this long term survival group. Patients therefore should be treated soon after their surgery for proper evaluation of the drug under study to be made.

Glioblastoma patients typically showed a decreased responsiveness to cutaneous antigens (Brooks et al., 1974). In one study (Young et al., 1977), autologous leukocytes were inoculated directly into recurrent glioblastomas with gratifying results in some patients.

Certain predominantly childhood central nervous system (CNS) tumors should be mentioned. The ependymoma is a slowly growing tumor derived from the ependymal-lining cells of the ventricles and central canal. It is very radiosensitive and long term survivors may be seen (Schultz et al., 1968). The medulloblastoma usually occurs subtentorially and is a highly malignant tumor of children and young adults. It frequently seeds throughout the cerebrospinal fluid and may metastasize outside the central nervous system. It is a highly radiosensitive tumor and often responds well to radiation therapy to the entire neuraxis, with approximately one third of patients surviving 10 years. Medulloblastomas will also often respond to intrathecal methotrexate, and its metastatic deposits may respond well to intravenous vincristine (Wilson, 1970).

REFERENCES

Bouchard, J. Radiation Therapy of Tumors and Diseases of the Nervous System, pp. 78–118. Lea & Febiger, Philadelphia, 1966.

Broder, L. E., and Rall, D. P. Chemotherapy of brain tumors. Progr. Exp. Tumor Res., *17:* 373–399, 1972.

Brooks, W. H., Cardwell, H. D., and Mortara, R. H. Immune responses in patients with gliomas. Surg. Neurol., *2:* 419–423, 1974.

Davis, L., Martin, J., Goldstein, S. L., and Ashkenazy, M. A study of 211 patients with verified glioblastoma multiforme. J. Neurosurg., *6:* 33–44, 1949.

Edland, R. W., Javrid, M., and Ansfield, F. J. Glioblastoma multiforme, an analysis of the result of postoperative radiotherapy alone vs. radiotherapy and concomitant 5-fluorouracil. A.J.R., *111:* 337–342, 1971.

Fewer, D., Wilson, C. B., Boldrey, E. B., Enot, K. J., and Powell, M. R. The chemotherapy of brain tumors; clinical experience with carmustine (BCNU) and vincristine. J.A.M.A., *222:* 549–552, 1972.

Fewer, D., Wilson, C. B., Boldrey, E. B., and Enot, J. K. Phase II study of 1-(2-chloroethyl)-3-cyclohexyl-1-nitrosourea (CCNU; NSC-79037) in the treatment of brain tumors. Cancer Chem. Rep., *56:* 421–427, 1972.

Frankel, S. A., and German, W. J. Glioblastoma multiforme; review of 219 cases with regard to natural history, pathology, diagnostic methods and treatment. J. Neurosurg., *15:* 489–503, 1958.

Gutin, P. H., Wilson, C. B., Kumar, A. R. V. et al. Phase II study of procarbazine, CCNU and vincristine combination chemotherapy in the treatment of malignant brain tumors. Cancer, *35:* 1398–1404, 1975.

Hoshino, T., Barker, M., Wilson, C. B., Boldrey, E. B., and Fewer, D. Cell kinetics of human gliomas. J. Neurosurg., *37:* 15–26, 1972.

Jelsma, R., and Bucy, P. C. The treatment of glioblastoma multiforme of the brain. J. Neurosurg., *27:* 388–400, 1967.

Kumar, A. R. V., Renaudin, J., Wilson, C. B., Boldrey, E. B., Enot, K. J., and Levin, V. A. Procarbazine hydrochloride in the treatment of brain tumors; phase II study. J. Neurosurg., *40:* 365–371, 1974.

Long, D. M. Capillary ultrastructure and the blood-brain barrier in human malignant brain tumors. J. Neurosurg., *32:* 127–144, 1970.

Newton, W. A., Sayers, M. P., and Samuels, D. L. Intrathecal methotrexate therapy for brain tumors in children. Cancer Chem. Rep., *52:* 257–261, 1968.

Rall, D. P., and Zubrod, C. G. Mechanisms of drug absorption and excretion. Passage of drugs in and out of the central nervous system. Ann. Rev. Pharmacol., *2:* 109–128, 1962.

Renaudin, J., Fewer, D., Wilson, C. B., Boldrey, E. B., Calogero, J., and Enot, K. J. Dose dependency of decadron in patients with partially excised brain tumors. J. Neurosurg., *34:* 302–305, 1973.

Rosenblum, M. L., Reynolds, A. F., Smith, K. A., Rumack, B. H., and Walker, M.D. Chloroethyl-cyclohexyl-nitrosourea (CCNU) in the treatment of malignant brain tumors. J. Neurosurg., *39:* 306–314, 1973.

Roth, J. G., and Elvidge, A. R. Glioblastoma multiforme; a clinical survey. J. Neurosurg., *17:* 736–750, 1960.

Rubin, R. C., Ommaya, A. K., Henderson, E. S., Bering, E. A., and Rall, D. P. Cerebrospinal fluid perfusion for central nervous system neoplasms. Neurology, *16:* 680–692, 1966.

Schultz, M. D., Wanc, C., Zimminger, G. F., and Tefft, M. Radiotherapy of intracranial neoplasms. *In* Progress in Neurological Surgery, edited by H. Krayenbuhl, P. E. Maspes, and W. H. Sweet, Vol. 2, pp. 318–370. Year Book Medical Publishers, Chicago, 1968.

Shapiro, W. R., and Ausman, J. I. The chemotherapy of brain tumors; a clinical experimental review. *In* Recent Advances in Neurology, edited by F. Plum, pp. 150–235. F. A. Davis, Philadelphia, 1969.

Sklansky, B. D., Mann-Kaplan, R. S., Reynolds, A. F., Rosenblum, M. L., and Walker, M. D. 4'-Demethyl-epipodophyllotoxin-β-D-thenylidene-glucoside (PTG) in the treatment of malignant intracranial neoplasms. Cancer, *33:* 460–467, 1974.

Tator, C. H. Chemotherapy of brain tumors; uptake of tritiated methotrexate by a transplantable intracerebral ependymoblastoma in mice. J. Neurosurg., *37:* 1–8, 1972.

Walker, M. D. Nitrosoureas in central nervous system tumors. Cancer Chem. Rep., *4:* 21–26, 1973.

Weinstein, J. D., Toy, F. J., Jaffe, M. E., and Goldberg, H. I. The effect of dexamethasone on brain edema in patients with metastatic brain tumors. Neurology *23:* 121–129, 1973.

Wilson, C. B., and Norrell, H. A. Brain tumor chemotherapy with intrathecal methotrexate. Cancer, *23:* 1038–1045, 1969.

Wilson, C. B. Medulloblastoma—current views regarding the tumor and its treatment. Oncology, *24:* 273–290, 1970.

Wilson, C. B., Boldrey, E. B., and Enot, K. J. 1-3-Bis(2-chloroethyl-1-nitrosourea) (NSC-409962) in the treatment of brain tumors. Cancer Chem. Rep., *54:* 273–281, 1970.

Wilson, C. B., Hoshino, T., Barker, M., and Downey, R. Kinetics of gliomas in rat and man. Progr. Exp. Tumor Res., *17:* 363–372, 1972.

Young, H., Kaplan, A., and Regelson, W. Immunotherapy with autologous white cell infusions ("lymphocytes") in the treatment of recurrent glioblastoma multiforme. Cancer, *40:* 1037–1044, 1977.

Zimmerman, H. M. Brain tumors; their incidence and classification in man and their experimental production. Ann. N.Y. Acad. Sci., *159:* 337–359, 1969.

Zulch, K. J., and Wecksler, W. Pathology and classification of gliomas. *In* Progress in Neurological Surgery, edited by H. Krayenbuhl, P. E. Maspes, and W. H. Sweet, Vol. 2, pp. 1–84. Year Book Medical Publishers, Chicago, 1968.

Chapter 25

Endocrine Tumors

JOHN S. MACDONALD, M.D., and PHILIP S. SCHEIN, M.D.

Major chemotherapeutic advances have been made in the treatment of malignancies of the endocrine glands. The most impressive results have been achieved in those tumors which have been recognized as being particularly drug sensitive: choriocarcinoma, testicular and ovarian carcinomas. However, a large variety of endocrine malignancies remain which oncologists are called upon to manage which may be treated by both cytotoxic and antihormonal chemotherapy. This chapter will be devoted to the medical management of several of these tumors including malignant islet cell tumors, adrenocortical carcinoma, thyroid carcinoma, malignant carcinoids and pheochromocytomas. Because of the potential of some of these tumors to secrete specific hormones, this group of malignancies possesses several unique clinical features. The hormones secreted by these neoplasms furnish readily measurable index materials that may be used not only in the diagnosis, but also in the assessment of the effectiveness of treatment of these diseases. These endocrine tumors are frequently characterized by slow growth, with the results of excessive hormone production frequently producing more morbidity than the actual tumor and its metastases. For this reason the management of this group of malignancies involves two distinct forms of drug treatment: cytotoxic and antihormonal chemotherapy. The former is directed against the primary tumor and its metastases, while the latter may offer significant palliation through the inhibition of synthesis, release, or direct cellular action of hormones produced in excess.

MALIGNANT ISLET CELL TUMORS

Insulinoma

The fundamental feature of insulinoma, of which approximately 10–25% are interpreted as malignant, is the development of hypoglycemia after a period of fasting (Laurent et al., 1971; Lundbaek et al., 1967;

Marks and Rose, 1965). Many patients will experience their initial symptoms during the morning hours prior to breakfast, or after exercise. The clinical features of this disease, representative of the recurrent episodes of lowered blood glucose, have been well described and, in many cases, will be misinterpreted as psychiatric or neurologic in origin (Marks and Rose, 1965). The diagnosis of benign or malignant insulinomas as the cause of hypoglycemia is dependent upon the concurrent measurement of plasma immunoreactive insulin (IRI) and blood glucose. The hallmark of the insulinoma is a state where the IRI is inappropriately high at a time when the blood glucose is low, which distinguishes this condition from other causes of fasting hypoglycemia, including extrapancreatic neoplasms, liver disease, adrenal and pituitary insufficiency, and glycogen storage diseases (Grunt et al., 1970). In investigations of patterns of insulin secretion in insulinoma, the proinsulin-like component (PLC), a presumed precursor protein of insulin (Steiner and Oyer, 1969), has been demonstrated to comprise a disproportionately high percentage of the total circulating basal IRI (Gorden et al., 1971a, 1971b; Gutman et al., 1971). While not specific for insulinoma, having also been found associated with hypokalemia (Gorden et al., 1972), assay of PLC may improve the future success in the diagnosis of this disease, and has already served as an important measure for assessing a patient's response to therapy (Blackard et al., 1970). Successful treatment should bring the percent PLC down to normal levels.

Based on the responsiveness of the neoplastic β cell to specific stimuli, a number of dynamic tests have been developed for diagnosis, which are also useful in following response to treatment in patients with insulinoma (Cunningham et al., 1971; Floyd et al., 1964). The tolbutamide test, with measurement of glucose and insulin, has proved the most efficient and will correctly identify approximately 80% of insulin secreting tumors.

False negatives with this test can be reduced by the simultaneous determination of percent PLC (Gutman et al., 1971). Also the use of additional provocative procedures such as L-leucine, glucose, or glucagon stimulation may decrease the likelihood of a false negative test.

The principal sites of metastatic spread are the liver and the regional lymph nodes. Preoperative hepatic scans and selective arteriography may not only demonstrate involvement of the liver, but the latter procedure will also facilitate both localization and determination of number and size of tumors (Basabe et al., 1970; Gray et al., 1970).

ANTIHORMONAL THERAPY

The recurrent attacks of hypoglycemia that characterize malignant insulinoma can often be palliated during the early stages of the disease with the use of diet and insulin antagonists. Frequent feedings between meals and at bedtime are administered with sufficient glucose to control symptoms. Adjustments in the carbohydrate content of the diet may be required depending upon the reactivity of the individual tumor, since the stimulus of a large glucose load may lead to an exaggerated release of insulin (Power, 1969). Parenteral glucose supplementation becomes an important adjunct in patients having frequent or sustained hypoglycemia attacks, and during emergencies, rapid intravenous injection of 50% glucose may be required and should always be available.

Corticosteroids, human growth hormone, and glucagon have been effective as palliative agents in individual patients (Laudau et al., 1958; Mahon et al., 1962; Marks and Rose, 1965; Roth et al., 1966), but, because of their overall limited effectiveness, they are best used in combination and with other antihormonal measures. Glucagon is a known stimulant of pancreatic insulin secretion, and it may produce a paradoxical exacerbation of a hypoglycemic episode.

A major advance in the palliation of malignant insulinoma came with the development of diazoxide, an antidiuretic benzothiadiazine. Its potent hyperglycemic properties, originally recognized during its initial use as an antihypertensive agent, have now been extended to the palliation of insulinoma and leucine-sensitive hypoglycemia of infancy (Dollery and Pentecost, 1962; Graber et al., 1966). The mechanisms by which diazoxide produces its hyperglycemic effects are twofold. First, the principal action is a direct inhibition of insulin release as has been well documented in perfused pancreas preparations (Basabe et al., 1970). There is no influence on insulin synthesis, leading to accumulation of the hormone within the β cell. A second or extrapancreatic mechanism involves a β-adrenergic stimulation of hepatic glucogenesis and a decrease in peripheral glucose utilization (Walfish et al., 1970). The compound is administered orally in divided doses, ranging from 100 to 1000 mg per day. While a patient's plasma insulin levels can, in many cases, be brought down to asymptomatic concentrations, the tumor will continue to grow and metastasize since diazoxide has no antitumor activity. Edema, on the basis of renal sodium retention, is an important toxicity. It may be corrected or prevented with the addition of a benzothiadiazine diuretic, such as chlorothiazide or chlormethiazide, which will also serve to synergize the hyperglycemic effects. Additional potential adverse drug reactions include gastric irritation, postural hypotension, supraventricular tachycardia, hyperuricemia, and hirsutism.

ANTITUMOR THERAPY

The conventional cancer chemotherapy agents have not been used extensively in the treatment of malignant insulinoma, but the literature does contain case reports describing the effectiveness of 5-fluorouracil and alkylating agents in the management of individual patients (Fonkalseud et al., 1964; Longmire et al., 1968; Thomas et al., 1968). The more systematic clinical trials in this disease have involved the use of compounds for which there has been some expectation for selective toxicity against the malignant islet cell tissue, based on toxicologic observations in normal animals. Historically, alloxan was the first agent with proven diabetogenic activity to be tested clinically (Lukens, 1948). While only rarely effective, it nevertheless demonstrated the potential efficacy of this approach to drug selection.

Tubercidin, 7-deazaadenosine, is an antibiotic isolated from the fermentation broth of *Streptomyces tubercidicus*. Biochemically, the drug has been shown to substitute effectively for the corresponding adenosine compound in a number of enzymatic reactions, and can be incorporated into DNA and RNA as a fraudulent purine with resultant inhibition of protein synthesis (Acs et al., 1964). Toxicologic studies carried out in dogs in preparation for clinical use of the compound demonstrated histologic lesions in the pancreatic islets of Langerhans with resulting glucose intolerance. At the present time, tubercidin has received only a limited clinical trial, but several cases of islet cell carcinoma, including one patient with the Zollinger-Ellison syndrome, have shown objective regression in tumor mass, lasting 6 months to over 1 year (Bisel et al., 1970; Grage et al., 1970; Longmire et al., 1968). Tubercidin's overall usefulness is limited by its severe toxicity to veins and local tissues which has necessitated the development of elaborate measures of administration (Bisel et al., 1970). A unit of whole blood is removed from the patient and is incubated with the prescribed dose of drug for 1 hour at 37°C. The blood is then retransfused, and the drug is slowly released from the red blood cells where it had been incorporated (Grage et al., 1970; Smith et al., 1970). Additional toxicities have included renal damage manifested by proteinuria and azotemia, nausea and vomiting, mild leukopenia and thrombocytopenia, and mild liver function abnormalities. The currently used dose schedule is 1500 μg/kg delivered on day 1 and 8 in red blood cells, followed by 750 μg/kg at monthly intervals as tolerated (Gray et al., 1970).

The chemotherapeutic agent most frequently used for the treatment of malignant insulinoma is streptozotocin, an antibiotic isolated from the fermentation cultures of *Streptomyces acromogenes*. Chemically, this drug is composed of the known anticancer agent, 1-methyl-1-nitrosourea, combined with glucose (Herr et al., 1967). The diabetogenic properties of streptozotocin were discovered during its initial preclinical toxicologic evaluation (Rakieten et al., 1969). It was demonstrated that a single intravenous dose could produce a permanent diabetic state in rodents, dogs, and monkeys, an action mediated through the selective destruction of the pancreatic β cell. Biochemically, this acute diabetogenic activity of streptozotocin has been related to an inhibition in the synthesis of pyridine nucleotides, and can be prevented in animals with the use of pharmacologic doses of nicotinamide (Schein et al., 1967, 1971). Because of the inherent diabetogenic properties of streptozotocin, an attempt has been made to exploit this "toxicity" in the treatment of malignant insulinomas.

In a series (Broder and Carter, 1972) of 29 cases of insulinoma where measurable disease was present, 48% of patients had an objective reduction in tumor mass, and 17% were considered to have obtained complete remission status with streptozotocin therapy. This therapeutic activity is not confined solely to the hormone-secreting tumors, since 5 of 8 patients with nonfunctioning islet cell carcinoma have also achieved some reduction in tumor size with treatment (Moertel et al., 1971). The average duration of these remissions has been approximately 1 year. With regard to hormonal response, 62% of patients had a lessening in severity of hypoglycemia or a lowering of an initially elevated insulin. In 26% of cases, there was a return of these hormonal paramf ' ers to normal levels. In these patients the median duration of hormon response is in excess of 1 year.

One of the noteworthy characteristics of the malignant insulinoma is the biologic capacity of some tumors to synthesize additional hormones, including gastrin, glucagon, ACTH, and serotonin. It is of interest that remissions with streptozotocin have not been limited to those tumors producing only insulin. In the original case report demonstrating the successful use of streptozotocin, Murray-Lyon et al. (1968, 1970) documented a concomitant reduction of initially elevated plasma insulin, gastrin, and glucagon values. In this connection in the series of 29 patients with insulinoma, all 3 cases treated with streptozotocin having documented secretion of both insulin and gastrin responded. The current data relating to the influence of streptozotocin treatment on survival in malignant insulinoma are preliminary. However, the median of 744 days for responders vs. 289 for nonresponders suggests that the drug will prove beneficial in prolonging life.

A weekly schedule of streptozotocin administration has been employed in the majority of successfully treated cases. The initial dose has been 1–2 g/m^2 and adjusted for subsequent courses based on signs of response or development of toxicity. There are, however, several cases in which remission has been obtained using a 5-day schedule at a dose of 500 mg/m^2/day (Moertel et al., 1971). At the present time, the optimal schedule of administration has not been determined. No controlled trials have been performed comparing the intra-arterial route of administration with the intravenous route. While there is one case reported in the literature documenting a response to celiac axis perfusion after failure with intravenous injection, it is impossible to determine what role the method of administration, vs. continued treatment, played in the production of this remission. It had been hoped that selective arteriographic injection might have avoided some of the renal complications of streptozotocin therapy, but this has not proven to be the case. In addition, a misplacement or slip of the catheter into the renal artery at the time of drug administration can be expected to have disastrous consequences (Sadoff, 1970).

The median time to response after streptozotocin therapy has been approximately 3 weeks (3 weekly injections), although with especially sensitive tumors, a functional remission can be documented almost immediately after the initial course. At the current time, there are no readily identifiable indices for prediction of an individual patient's response to treatment.

The toxicities associated with streptozotocin treatment have been well defined. Nausea and vomiting are experienced by almost all patients but with great variability as to severity. These symptoms are only partially prevented or controlled by phenothiazine antiemetics, but will usually diminish with each succeeding dose if the 5-day schedule is utilized. Renal tubular damage is the most common serious drug toxicity, and its occurrence severely limits the potential for further treatment (Sadoff, 1970). The earliest manifestation in our experience has been the development of proteinurea in the range of 400–1500 mg/24 hours. With more significant nephrotoxicity, excretion of up to 10 g of protein/24 hours has been documented. If unaccompanied by any other renal function abnormality, proteinuria is usually reversible in 2–4 weeks. However, with continued treatment pronounced signs of proximal tubular damage are produced including aminoaciduria, phosphaturia, uricosuria, glycosuria, and renal tubular acidosis, all of which are potentially reversible. Two investigators have reported development of nephrogenic diabetes insipidus after large doses of the drug, and varying degrees of azotemia have been observed (Murray-Lyon et al., 1970; Sadoff, 1970; Smith et al., 1971). Serious renal toxicity can be avoided by close monitoring of the urine for protein excretion and stopping treatment until full reversal of abnormal renal function has been demonstrated. In an attempt to determine the mechanism of nephrotoxicity, pharmacologic disposition studies (Schein, 1972) with streptozotocin have been carried out and have shown that 10–20% of each administered dose can be recovered in the urine with the N-nitroso group intact. It is possible that high concentrations of active drug in the renal tubule at physiologic pH could allow for local tubular damage by direct toxicity.

Mild abnormalities in liver function may occur after streptozotocin therapy. This is manifested by a transient elevation in serum transaminases observed at the end of each course of treatment in many patients. These biochemical abnormalities have had no apparent clinical significance (Moertel et al., 1971). While generally considered a nonmyelosuppressive antitumor agent, streptozotocin has produced mild degrees of leukopenia, which in almost all instances has not been dose limiting. There has, however, been one case (Schein et al., 1973) of profound bone marrow depression following a dose of 7.5 g/m^2 in a case of advanced malignant insulinoma previously treated with doses of 2.5 and 3.0 g/m^2. This degree of myelosuppression has never previously been reported, and the case must be considered unique.

Successful treatment with pulse doses of streptozotocin may cause destruction of large amounts of insulin-containing tissue. A sudden and profound rise in plasma insulin with accompanying hypoglycemia has been recorded in several cases, 4–7 hours after therapy, requiring that patients be monitored for this phenomenon with serial blood glucose determinations. Investigators working with streptozotocin in patients with a potential long life expectancy, as in the case of benign adenomas, must be aware that the compound contains a known carcinogen, 1-methyl-1-nitrosourea, and that streptozotocin itself has produced renal adenomas and hepatomas in rodents (Schein, 1972).

The Zollinger-Ellison Syndrome

The Zollinger-Ellison syndrome, which is characterized by recurrent gastric and small bowel ulceration with persistently elevated serum gastrin levels and gastric acid hypersecretion, is considered to be due to tumors of the δ cell of the islets of Langerhans. These tumors, even when metastatic to liver and/or bone, tend to be slow growing and the main morbidity and mortality of the syndrome is associated with the complication of recurrent gastrointestinal ulceration. The treatment of choice for symptomatic management is end organ removal, i.e., total gastrectomy (Schein, 1973). The operation must be a total gastrectomy as the parietal cell mass in patients with the Zollinger-Ellison syndrome may be hypertrophied as much as 6 times (Polack and Ellison, 1966) and attempts to leave small gastric remnants have lead to continued problems with gastrointestinal ulceration.

ANTIHORMONAL THERAPY

Until recently, there has been no antihormonal therapy to inhibit gastrin activity. However, within the last 5 years, two compounds that are able to pharmacologically inhibit the activity of gastrin have become available. Metiamide and cimetidine are analogs of histamine that have been shown to be inhibitors of the H_2 histamine receptor (Brimblecombe et al., 1978). It has previously been shown (Gibson et al., 1974) that there are two pharmacologically different histamine receptors. The H_1 receptor is inhibited by the commonly used antihistamines and is responsible for the contraction of gut and bronchial smooth muscle. The H_2 receptor is not inhibited by ordinary antihistamines but is inhibited by metiamide and cimetidine. The H_2 receptor mediates histamine induced inhibition of contraction of rat uterus, gastric acid secretion and increased auricular rate in rodents. Several workers (Kahn et al., 1978; Mainardi et al., 1974; Thjodleifsson and Wormsley, 1974) have shown in man, that metiamide is able to very significantly (>80%) inhibit gastric acid secretion in normals and in patients with peptic ulcer disease. The drug will inhibit acid production stimulated by histamine, pentagastrin and peptone meals. There was initially great clinical interest in the use of metiamide in the treatment of ulcer disease and the Zollinger-Ellison syndrome. However, reports (Mainardi et al., 1974) of transient agranulocytosis in patients receiving the drug on a chronic basis caused the cessation of clinical studies with metiamide.

Since metiamide is a thiourea analog of histamine and it was felt that the thiourea group might be an important determinant of the bone marrow toxicity of this drug (Brimblecombe et al., 1978) it was elected to study histamine analogs that did not bear the thiourea group. The prototype of this class of drug is cimetidine. This drug shows all of the H_2 receptor antagonist properties of metiamide and has been shown to be a potent inhibitor of histamine-mediated gastric acid secretion in man (Brimblecombe et al., 1978). Of note animal toxicology studies did not show evidence of acute or chronic myelosuppression after cimetidine administration (Brimblecombe et al., 1978). This is in direct contradiction to the findings in the toxicology studies of metiamide. Since the animal toxicology studies with metiamide were apparently predictive for myelosuppressive toxicity in man, it was felt highly unlikely that cimetidine would exhibit significant bone marrow toxicity in humans.

Cimetidine is now commercially available (Tagomet) and has gained widespread use as an inhibitor of gastric acid secretion. The drug has been found to be very safe with the only toxicities recorded in over 3000 patients being transient clinically insignificant increases in serum creatinine which disappeared when the drug was stopped. Gynecomastia also occurred in some patients on long term therapy.

There is now data to suggest that cimetidine therapy is a substitute for total gastrectomy in patients with the Zollinger-Ellison syndrome. McCarthy (1978) reviewed the clinical course of 61 patients with documented Zollinger-Ellison syndrome treated with cimetidine. When the drug was given in adequate doses, 56/61 (92%) patients had excellent clinical benefit with alleviation of pain and objective healing of gastric ulcers. One-half of the patients treated have remained on therapy for greater than 1 year with the only side effect being gynecomastia in 9% and transient liver dysfunction in 5%. McCarthy has pointed out that in patients with Zollinger-Ellison syndrome, it is critically important to maintain an adequate total dose of cimetidine and to administer the drug in divided doses every 6 hours. Only 40/61 (66%) patients initially responded to the standard dose of cimetidine (300 mg orally every 6 hours). Fourteen patients required doses as high as 600 mg every 6 hours before symptomatic improvement occurred. Attempts to decrease total dose or administer the drug less frequently than every 6 hours, almost invariably were followed by symptomatic relapse.

These results of cimetidine treatment in patients with the Zollinger-Ellison syndrome demonstrated that although this form of medical management does not affect the underlying tumor, it is a useful alternative to total gastrectomy as a palliative therapy.

CHEMOTHERAPY

There is little information available on the chemotherapy of metastatic islet cell carcinoma. Review of the older literature (Broder and Carter, 1973) shows uncertain results at best with alkylating agents and 5-fluorouracil. Streptozotocin has not been adequately assessed (Schein, 1972, 1973) in gastrin secreting islet carcinoma. We have had personal experience with a single patient with classic Zollinger-Ellison syndrome and hepatic metastases who responded to a single course of streptozotocin (1.5 mg/m^2 IV every 5 days repeated 5 times) with return of liver size to normal. This response lasted greater than 1 year. In a case report, as noted previously, tubercidin was reported to have produced an objective response in a patient with metastatic Zollinger-Ellison syndrome (Schein, 1973). Combination chemotherapy has not been adequately tested in metastatic islet cell carcinoma but a report by Moertel (1976) of 6 regressions in 8 patients treated with 5-fluorouracil and streptozotocin is encouraging.

Pancreatic Cholera Syndrome

There are over 50 cases in the literature of the pancreatic cholera syndrome. This clinical entity is characterized by diffuse watery diarrhea, hypokalemia, and metabolic acidosis in patients with non-β islet cell tumors (Sadoff, 1970). It has been distinguished from the Zollinger-Ellison syndrome in which diarrhea may be associated with gastric hypersecretion, by the absence of increased gastric acid, ulcer disease, and hypergastrinemia (Kraft et al., 1970). The hormones responsible for the clinical manifestations in the pancreatic cholera syndrome have not been clearly defined (Schein, 1973; Kahn et al., 1975). Secretin, glucagon, cholecystokinin, calcitonin, prostaglandins, gastric inhibitory peptide and vasoactive intestinal peptide have all been proposed as being the agents responsible, but there is no convincing proof to implicate any specific hormone. One half of the islet cell tumors associated with the pancreatic cholera syndrome are benign and the syndrome is surgically curable in these patients. Of the malignant tumors, 80% have metastases, usually to the liver, at the time of diagnosis (Schein, 1973).

ANTIHORMONAL THERAPY

Since the hormone or hormones responsible for the pancreatic cholera syndrome have not been clearly defined, no antihormonal therapy is currently feasible.

CHEMOTHERAPY

There are little data available on the chemotherapy of malignant pancreatic cholera syndrome. Glucocorticoids have been used and appear to be able to produce palliation in some patients (Kraft et al., 1970). Streptozotocin has been reported to have little effect in non-β islet cell carcinoma (Schein, 1973; Schein et al., 1973), so that the report of Kahn et al. (1978) reporting well documented tumor responses with streptozotocin in two patients with pancreatic cholera syndrome is of particular interest. Each patient was treated with from 3 to 5 doses of streptozotocin (1.5 g/m^2 every 5 days) infused into hepatic artery cathethers. After the first 2 doses of therapy, in both patients the stool volume began to decrease. In the first patient, after the total course of treatment, the stool volume decreased from 8000 to 600 ml each day. In the second patient, the stool volume decreased from 2000 to 200 ml per day. Serum potassium normalized, hepatic arteriography and liver scan showed marked decrease in liver metastasis in both patients. Neither patient developed any significant drug toxicity. The first patient required retreatment at 6 months when stool volume increased to 1.5 liters per day. After a course of streptozotocin, stool volume decreased 200 ml per day. The second patient was free of disease at 10 months after therapy and showed no evidence of metastatic disease on hepatic arteriography. Each of the patients had no significant treatment associated toxicity and in-dwelling hepatic artery catheterization for up to 1 year was tolerated well, except for asymptomatic celiac artery thrombosis in the first patient. This approach of direct hepatic artery infusion with streptozotocin deserves further trial both in metastatic pancreatic cholera syndrome and also in other islet cell neoplasms associated with significant liver metastases.

ADRENAL CORTICAL CARCINOMA

The clinical features of adrenal carcinoma at time of presentation include pain, abdominal mass, and a variety of symptoms and signs referable to one of a number of endocrine syndromes produced: Cushing's syndrome (essentially diagnostic in the pediatric age group), virilization, precocious puberty, and more rarely feminization or hyperglycemia. A functioning adrenal carcinoma typically produces large quantities of 17-ketosteroids (17-KS), documented in 67–91% of cases in different series (Hutter and Kayhoe, 1966a). An increase in the β fraction of the ketosteroids is suggestive of adrenal carcinoma, which in one series correlated with an augmented dehydroepiandrosterone (DHEA) excretion (Lipsett et al., 1963; Mason and Engstrom, 1950). Increased urinary 17-KS and 17-hydroxycorticoids (17-OHCS) occur in approximately 54% of patients, while only 5% of patients with functioning carcinomas will present with increased 17-OHCS alone (Hutter and Kayhoe, 1966a). Classically, the steroid secretion of adrenal carcinoma will not respond to ACTH stimulation, nor be suppressed with dexamethasone. However, there are several examples in the literature of patients with normal responses to these procedures (Lipsett et al., 1963). In addition, these tests do not distinguish between a carcinoma and an autonomously secreting benign adenoma.

In Lipsett's review of 184 cases of adrenal cortical carcinoma, 81 had no clinical manifestation of excessive hormone secretion, and 64% were males (Lipsett et al., 1963). This male predominance may lead to underestimation of the percentage of hormone-secreting tumors for several reasons. First, since the adult male is fully virilized, there is no clinical correlate of androgen excess in this group aside from polycythemia, and thus the tumor may appear to be nonfunctioning if the excessive hormone production is limited to the 17-KS. In addition, the total urinary 17-KS excretion does not necessarily correlate well with the degree of virilization in individual cases, since the 17-KS are derived from both androgenic and nonandrogenic precursors. Virilization will depend on the total contribution by androgens to the 17-KS, or transformation of a nonandrogenic steroid such as DHEA to an androgen. Conversely, virilization may occur with an entirely normal 17-KS if only a few milligrams of testosterone are produced (Lipsett et al., 1963).

Adrenal cortical carcinomas invade adjacent structures, such as kidney mesentery, retroperitoneal space, regional lymph nodes, and may enter local veins. With continued growth, the tumor tends to form a large intraabdominal mass which is palpable in approximately 40% of cases (Lipsett et al., 1963). The large size predisposes to central necrosis and hemorrhage, occasionally complicated by suppuration. The most common sites of distant metastases are the lung and liver, which are involved in approximately 50% of cases. Spread to bone, pleura, mediastinum, skin, and thyroid has been observed, but with a much lower incidence (Hutter and Kayhoe, 1966a).

Calcium deposition occurs in approximately one-third of cases of adrenal carcinoma and may be identified on a plain film of the abdomen

(Kahn, 1967). The presence of a soft tissue mass with displacement of the kidney may be recognized on an intravenous pyelogram with tomography. The tumors are usually moderately vascular, allowing determination of extent and metastases by an aortogram with selective adrenal and hepatic arteriography. Inferior vena cavography and selective renal venography has been advocated as a means of evaluating the size of the tumor and determining whether there is vein invasion (Bergenstal et al., 1960). Chest x-ray, liver function tests, hepatic scan, skeletal survey, and lymphangiography are useful in further delineating and following the extent of disease.

ANTIHORMONAL THERAPY

Metapyrone, an inhibitor of 11,β-hydroxylation in cortisol biosynthesis has been reported useful in the management of individual cases of Cushing's syndrome of adrenal carcinoma; however, it has largely proved ineffective in patients with advanced disease (Daniels et al., 1963). Chemical confirmation of effectiveness requires the direct measurement of plasma cortisol, since its immediate precursor, 11-deoxycortisol, will accumulate and increase its contribution to the Porter-Silber assay for 17-OHCS.

Aminoglutethimide (Elipten) had been used for several years as an anticonvulsant; however, with continued use, adrenal insufficiency and goitrous hypothyroidism have been observed. Further studies have demonstrated that the drug produces distinctive histologic changes in the adrenal gland and inhibition of the enzymatic conversion of cholesterol to Δ5-pregnenolone (Cash et al., 1967). Aminoglutethimide has been shown to be an effective, palliative treatment in Cushing's syndrome secondary to adrenocortical carcinoma, adenoma, and ectopic ACTH production by extra-adrenal carcinomas, with the potential for a rapid and sustained suppression of corticosteroid synthesis (Gorden et al., 1968; Schteingart et al., 1966). Because the drug has the capacity to alter the extra-adrenal metabolism of cortisol, measurement of urinary 17-OHCS excretion alone may overestimate the effectiveness of therapy; plasma cortisol concentrations are a more reliable index of drug effect for this hormone (Fishman et al., 1967). The usual clinical dose is in the range of 1 to 2 g/day, and the important toxicities include anorexia, dermatitis, somnolence, ataxia, and decreased thyroid function.

ANTITUMOR THERAPY

The use of o,p'-DDD in the treatment of adrenocortical carcinoma originated from the empirical observations of Nelson and Woodward in 1948, that the commercial insecticide DDD produced selective atrophy of the zona fasciculata and zona reticularis of the adrenal cortex of the dog (Nelson and Woodward, 1949). It was subsequently documented that the *ortho-para* isomer of the crude commercial preparation was the agent that both inhibited steroidogenesis and produced adrenal cortical necrosis (Cueto and Brown, 1958; Nichols and Hennigar, 1957; Vilar and Tullner, 1959). Biochemically, *o,p'*-DDD has been shown to inhibit dog adrenal glucose-6-phosphate dehydrogenase; this enzyme of the pentose pathway is responsible for the generation of NADPH, an essential cofactor in hydroxylation reactions for steroid synthesis, such as the conversion of cholesterol to Δ5-pregnenalone (Cazorla and Moncloa, 1962). It has also become apparent that, in addition to its direct effects on cortisol synthesis, *o,p'*-DDD can significantly alter the extra-adrenal metabolism of cortisol so as to invalidate its indirect measurement by 17-hydroxycorticosteroid excretion. As with the use of aminoglutethimide, direct measurement of plasma cortisol is required for an accurate estimate of the effect of *o,p'*-DDD on the secretion of this hormone (Bledsoe et al., 1964).

Based on the selective toxicity of *o,p'*-DDD for the dog adrenal gland, the compound underwent a clinical trial in man, and, in 1960, Bergenstal reported that the drug could both inhibit steroid secretion, and produce objective tumor regression in metastatic adrenocortical carcinoma (Bergenstal et al., 1960).

Between 1960 and 1965, 138 patients with adrenal cancer were treated with *o,p'*-DDD and the results of this series were reviewed by Hutter and Kayhoe (1966b). Eighty-two percent of patients studied had an initially increased excretion of 17-ketosteroids and/or 17-hydroxycorticosteroids. A 50% or greater decrease in hormone excretion was achieved in approximately 70% of cases. A minimum of 4 weeks of therapy was required to ensure an adequate therapeutic trial; of those patients who ultimately responded, only 37% did so by the 21 days, while, at 30 days of treatment, 87% of patients demonstrated a reduction in urinary 17-ketosteroid excretion. The average dose required for response was 8.5 g/day, and the median duration of steroid response was approximately 9 months.

Not all patients who had a hormonal response achieved a reduction in tumor mass. Of 59 patients with measurable disease 20, or 34%, demonstrated an objective response, which was accompanied by a decrease in steroid excretion in all cases. The median time to antitumor response from start of *o,p'*-DDD treatment was 6 weeks, with a mean duration of 10.2 months. Reinduction of remission after relapse is infrequent but has been reported.

In analyzing the clinical features of cases that demonstrated response to treatment, women had higher steroid and objective response rates (76% and 38%) than men (60% and 21%), but age, site of tumor, and location of metastases did not appear to influence the potential for benefit from *o,p'*-DDD. Prolongation of life was recorded for patients who obtained an objective tumor regression, compared to nonresponders; no difference in survival could be observed based on steroid response alone. The prognosis of female patients was better than that of males. Fifty-two percent of women and 38% of men lived 4 years after diagnosis, with median survivals of 56 and 19 months, respectively (Hutter and Kayhoe, 1966a; 1966b). There are no cases in which documented complete response of adrenocortical carcinoma has occurred as a result of o,p'-DDD treatment.

An additional 115 patients with adrenal carcinoma were treated with o,p'-DDD between 1965 and 1969, and the data have been reviewed by Lubitz et al. (1973). The measurable disease response in this series was 61% compared to the previous reported figure of 34%, and the steroid excretion response of 89% demonstrated an improvement over the 72% noted by Hutter and Kayhoe. It was estimated that 54% of patients derived overall benefit from treatment with favorable "clinical response" when the effects of drug toxicity were taken into consideration. The improved response rate is attributed to a shorter median time between diagnosis and treatment with o,p'-DDD. The majority of patients treated with o,p'-DDD have sustained some form of toxicity when dosage was brought up to the therapeutic range of 8–10 g/day. In general, it was mild, and commonly consisted of gastrointestinal symptoms consisting of anorexia, nausea, vomiting, or diarrhea. Neuromuscular toxicity has been recorded in 40–60% of cases and has usually taken the form of lethargy and somnolence. Dizziness or vertigo, and dermatologic toxicity are observed in 15% of cases, while leukopenia and liver function abnormalities are only rarely a problem (Hutter and Kayhoe, 1966b; Lubitz et al., 1978).

With successful treatment of a functioning tumor, a substantial proportion of patients will develop signs of adrenal insufficiency. This is probably mainly related to the suppressive effect of the longstanding massive steroid excretion of the tumor, to which o,p'-DDD may play an additive role. In patients demonstrating a hormonal response, the need for replacement glucocorticoid therapy should be anticipated.

THYROID CARCINOMA

Metastatic thyroid carcinoma has been considered resistant to chemotherapy (Gottlieb and Hill, 1974; Leeper, 1972). Advanced follicular and, to a lesser extent, papillary carcinomas that can be demonstrated to concentrate iodine-131, can be treated with thyroid stimulating hormone (TSH) stimulation and subsequent iodine-131 pulsing with good tumor response (Leeper, 1972). Medullary and giant or spindle cell carcinoma will not concentrate iodine and iodine-131 treatment is useless. The report of Gottlieb and Hill (1974) of a series of 30 patients with advanced thyroid carcinoma treated with Adriamycin supplies valuable information concerning the usefulness of chemotherapy in this disease. Of the 30 patients treated, 11 (37%) attained a partial remission with a median of 3 courses of therapy (Adriamycin given at 45–75 mg/m^2 IV every 3 weeks). Of particular interest were the 5 patients with medullary carcinoma and the 9 patients with spindle and giant cell carcinoma. Although advanced medullary carcinoma (Hill et al., 1973) has been felt to be resistant to medical management, Gottlieb demonstrated an objective response in 3 of 5 patients treated with Adriamycin. Of the 9 patients with spindle and giant cell carcinoma, which are particularly aggressive diseases the survival for responders was 11+ months (range 5+ to 40+) compared to 4 months (range 0.1 to 23+) for the nonresponders. These data indicate that Adriamycin is a useful single agent and may produce objective responses in approximately 30% of the patients with advanced thyroid carcinoma. Further studies with larger numbers of patients will be needed to confirm the effectiveness of Adriamycin in this disease.

MALIGNANT CARCINOID

Malignant carcinoid tumors are capable of secreting a number of biologically active materials including serotonin (5-hydroxytryptamine), 5-hydroxytryptophan, kallikrein, histamine, ACTH, insulin, and prostaglandins (Oates and Butler, 1967). The carcinoid syndrome, representing the clinical manifestation of this secretory capacity, has been most commonly associated with tumors of the jejunoileum where it has been described in 10% of patients and requires the presence of liver metastases (Wilson et al., 1978). However, in the cases of bronchial carcinoid and carcinoids arising from teratomas of the ovary, the syndrome may be present without evidence of metastatic disease, and will disappear with resection of the localized tumor. The probable explanation for this latter phenomenon is that in contrast to the gastrointestinal carcinoids, the venous drainage of the lung and ovary is systemic, and thus bypasses the liver where the excessive serotonin secretion would otherwise be metabolized by monoamine oxidase.

ANTIHORMONAL THERAPY

Based on their antagonism of the principal pharmacologic mediators of the carcinoid syndrome, serotonin, and bradykinin (Oates and Butler, 1967), the antiendocrine therapies for patients who exhibit humoral manifestations of this tumor can be divided into two categories. The serotonin-related symptoms of watery diarrhea, abdominal colic, and malabsorption have received the greatest attention and therapeutic investigation by clinical pharmacologists (Hill, 1971). When mild, these gastrointestinal manifestations may be successfully managed with simple measures, such as opiates and diphenoxylate hydrochloride with atropine (Lomotil), for long periods of time. With more severe symptoms, peripheral antagonists of serotonin, methysergide and cyproheptadine, have been effective in controlling diarrhea, and in some cases, malabsorption (Brown et al., 1960; Melmon et al., 1965b).

Another avenue of clinical investigation has been the use of agents that are known inhibitors of serotonin synthesis. One of the first to undergo clinical trial was α-methyldopa which partially inhibits the decarboxylation of 5-hydroxytryptophane (5-HTP) to serotonin. Results with this compound have been disappointing except for patients with the rare 5-HTP-secreting metastatic carcinoid of gastric origin (Mengel, 1965; Nelson and Woodward, 1949).

Parachlorophenylalanine (PCAC) is an inhibitor of the enzyme tryptophan 5-hydroxylase involved in the conversion of the amino acid to 5-HTP, the immediate precursor of serotonin. Engleman has demonstrated that PCAC at doses of 2–4 g/24 hours can reduce the urinary excretion of 5-hydroxyindoleacetic acid (an indirect measurement of 5-hydroxyindole synthesis) by 51–81% in patients with malignant carcinoid tumors (Engleman and Sjoerdsma, 1966; Sjoerdsma et al., 1970). This was accompanied by good-to-excellent control of diarrhea and other gastrointestinal symptoms. Several toxicities of PCAC have been defined. In addition to lethargy and light headaches, chronic administration may be accompanied by such mental aberrations as depression, anxiety, and confusional states. The development of an allergic eosinophilia appearing 2–9 weeks after initiation of treatment with PCAC has been observed in 50% of patients. This abnormality is rapidly reversible with withdrawal of the drug, reappears promptly with rechallenge, and is a definite sign for cessation of PCAC therapy. Continued treatment in the face of eosinophilia has lead to the development of urticaria, asthma, and pulmonary infiltrates (Loeffler's syndrome) (Sjoerdsma et al., 1970).

It is important to ensure that the patients with the carcinoid syndrome are not inadvertently placed on a monoamine oxidase inhibitor, such as iproniazid, which might block the degradation of serotonin to its inactive urinary excretion metabolites. It is recognized that carcinoid tumors may synthesize and release the proteolytic enzyme, kallikrein, which acts upon a specific α_2-globulin to generate bradykinin, the mediator of the flush (Oates and Sjoerdsma, 1962). Phenothiazines have been shown to antagonize the peripheral action of kinins and have been marginally effective in controlling flushing in some patients (Rocha e Silva and Garcia Lerne, 1963). Corticosteroids have been reported to significantly decrease or prevent the attacks of flushing, particularly in cases of bronchial carcinoid (Melmon et al., 1965a; Ureles et al., 1963). It is known that catecholamines can provoke an attack of flushing, and, on this basis, α-adrenergic blocking agents, such as phentolamine, have been proposed as therapeutic agents for patients with this syndrome (Adamson et al., 1969).

ANTITUMOR THERAPY

In contrast to the extensive work on the mechanisms and control of the carcinoid syndrome, drug treatment of the underlying malignancy has received remarkably little attention. In a significant proportion of patients, the disease may remain indolent, and active antitumor management may not necessarily be required (Moertel et al., 1961). However, there are patients with more aggressive tumor growth who will present in time with progressive liver metastases, signs of partial or impending complete intestinal obstruction, ascites, or severe and uncontrollable symptoms for whom anti-cancer therapy will be a consideration. Most of the information available on this subject is presently in the form of isolated case reports. This is, in part, related to the relative infrequency of this disease in any individual hospital center. Cyclophosphamide, thio-TEPA, and nitrogen mustard have all produced objective reductions in tumor mass accompanied by subjective improvement (Mengel, 1965; Vroom et al., 1962). 5-Fluorouracil has produced remissions when administered by either the intravenous or direct intra-arterial route (Reed et al., 1963). Most recently, streptozotocin has been reported to cause objective tumor regression in malignant carcinoid, but these remissions are usually short lived (Moertel et al., 1971). No response has been documented in 8 cases treated with a comparable route and schedule in National Cancer Institute (Schein et al., 1973, 1974) studies with streptozotocin. Recently case reports have suggested that Adriamycin and DTIC (Dacarbazine) may have single agent activity in this disease. Little information is available concerning combination chemotherapy in patients with malignant carcinoid tumors, but Moertel (1976) has reported response in 5 of 9 patients treated with the combination of 5-fluorouracil and streptozotocin. This regimen is being prospectively evaluated by the Eastern Cooperative Oncology Group and the results of that evaluation will be of great interest.

MALIGNANT PHEOCHROMOCYTOMA

Other than serving as a measure to maintain a patient for definitive surgery, medical management of pheochromocytoma is reserved for those cases where the tumor has metastasized, cannot be located at surgery, or when there are medical contraindications that preclude an exploratory laparotomy. Metastatic pheochromocytoma tends to be a slow growing tumor, and both the morbidity and mortality of this disease can be directly related to the cardiovascular complications produced by the prolonged elevation of catecholamine levels. A useful anticancer agent has not been identified, but long term symptomatic palliation can be obtained in some patients with the chronic oral administration of the α-adrenergic blocking agent, phenoxybenzamine (Engleman and Sjoerdsma, 1964). The drug is administered in divided doses, 30 to 100 mg/day, and the principal reported toxicity has been mild, transient sedation. Direct inhibition of catecholamine synthesis in patients with pheochromocytoma has been achieved with the experimental agent, α-methyl-p-L-tyrosine, which partially blocks the enzyme tyrosine hydroxylase (Engleman and Sjoerdsma, 1964).

REFERENCES

Acs, G., Reich, E., and Mori, M. Biological and biochemical properties of the analogue antibiotic tubercidin. Proc. Natl. Acad. Sci. U.S.A., 52: 493–501, 1964.

Adamson, A. R., Grahame-Smith, D. C., Peart, W. S., and Starr, M. Pharmacological blockade of carcinoid flushing provoked by catecholamines and alcohol. Lancet, 2: 293–296, 1969.

Basabe, J., Lopey, N., Viktora, J., and Wolff, F. Studies of insulin secretion in the perfused rat pancreas. Diabetes, 19: 271–281, 1970.

Bergenstal, D. M., Hertz, R., Lipsett, M. B., and Moy, R. H. Chemotherapy of adrenocortical cancer with o,p'-DDD. Ann. Intern. Med., 53: 672–682, 1960.

Bisel, H. F., Ansfield, F. J., Mason, J. H., and Wilson, W. L. Clinical studies with tubercidin administered by direct injection. Cancer Res., 30: 76–78, 1970.

Blackard, W. G., Garcia, A. R., and Brown, C. L., Jr. Effect of streptozotocin on qualitative aspects of plasma insulin in a patient with a malignant islet cell tumor. J. Clin. Endocrinol. Metab., 31: 215–219, 1970.

Bledsoe, T., Island, D. P., Ney, R. L., and Liddle, G. W. An effect of o,p'-DDD on the extra-adrenal metabolism of cortisol in man. J. Clin. Endocrinol. Metab., 24: 1301–1311, 1964.

Brimblecombe, R. W., Duncan, W. A. M., Durant, G. J., Emmett, C., Gandellin, C. R., Leslie, G. B., and Parsons, M. E. Characterization and development of cimetidine as a histamine H_2 receptor antagonist. Gastroenterology, 74: 339–347, 1978.

Broder, L., and Carter, S. Islet cell carcinoma (ICC); clinical features and results of therapy with streptozotocin (STR). Proc. Am. Assoc. Cancer Res., 13: 96, 1972.

Broder, L. E., and Carter, S. K. Results of therapy with streptozotocin in 52 patients. Ann. Intern. Med., 79: 108–118, 1973.

Brown, R. E., Hill, S. R., Jr., Berry, K. W., and Bing, R. J. Studies on several possible antiserotin compounds in the functioning carcinoid syndrome. Clin. Res., 8: 61, 1960.

Cash, R., Brough, A. J., Cohen, M. N. P., and Satoh, P. S. Aminoglutethimide (Elipten—Ciba) as an inhibitor of adrenal steriodogenesis; mechanism of action and therapeutic trial. J. Clin. Endocrinol. Metab., 27: 1239–1248, 1967.

Cazorla, A., and Moncloa, F.: Action of 1,1-dichloro-2-p-chlorophenyl-2-O-chlorophenyle-thane on dog adrenal cortex. Science, 136: 47, 1962.

Cueto, C., and Brown, J. H. Biological studies on an adrenocorticolytic agent and the isolation of the active components. Endocrinology, 62: 334–339, 1958.

Cunningham, G. R., Quickel, K. E., Jr., and Labovitz, H. E. The use of insulin dynamics in the evaluation of streptozotocin therapy of malignant insulinomas. J. Clin. Endocrinol. Metab., 33: 530–536, 1971.

Daniels, H., Van Amstel, W. J., Schopman, W., and Van Dommelen, C. Effect of metopirone in a patient with adrenocortical carcinoma. Acta Endocrinol., 44: 346–354, 1963.

Dollery, C. T., and Pentecost, B. L. Drug-induced diabetes. Lancet, 2: 735–737, 1962.

Engleman, K., and Sjoerdsma, A. Chronic medical therapy for pheochromocytoma. Ann. Intern. Med., 61: 230–241, 1964.

Engleman, K., and Sjoerdsma, A. Inhibition of catecholamine biosynthesis in man. Circ. Res. Suppl. *1:* 102–109, 1966.

Engleman, K., Lovenberg, W., and Sjoerdsma, A. Inhibition of serotonin synthesis by para-chloro-phenylalanine in patients with the carcinoid syndrome. N. Engl. J. Med., *277:* 1103–1108, 1967.

Feldman, J. M., Quickel, K. E., Jr., Marecek, R. L., and Lebovitz, H. E. Streptozotocin treatment of metastatic carcinoid tumors. South. Med. J., *65:* 1325–1327, 1972.

Fishman, L. M., Liddle, G. W., Island, D. P., Fleischer, N., and Kuchel, O. Effects of amino-glutethimide on adrenal function in man. J. Clin. Endocrinol. Metab., *27:* 481–490, 1967.

Floyd, J. C., Jr., Fajano, S. S., Kropf, R. F., and Conn, J. W. Plasma insulin in organic hyperinsulinism; comparative effects of tolbutamide, leucine, and glucose. J. Clin. Endocrinol. Metab., *24:* 747–760, 1964.

Fokalsrud, E. W., Dilley, R. B., and Longmire, W. P., Jr. Insulin secreting tumors of the pancreas. Ann. Surg., *159:* 730–741, 1964.

Gibson, R., Hirschowitz, B. I., and Hutchison, G. Action of metiamide, an H_2 histamine receptor antagonist, on gastric H+ and pepsin secretion in dogs. Gastroenterology, *67:* 93–99, 1974.

Gorden, P., Becker, C. E., Levey, G. S., and Roth, J. Efficacy of amino-glutethimide in the ectopic ACTH syndrome. J. Clin. Endocrinol. Metab., *28:* 921–923, 1968.

Gorden, P., Freychet, P., and Nankin, H. A unique form of circulating insulin in human islet cell carcinoma. J. Clin. Endocrinol. Metab., *33:* 983–987, 1971.

Gorden, P., Sherman, B., and Roth, J. Proinsulin-like component of circulating insulin in the basal state and in patients and hamsters with islet cell tumors. J. Clin. Invest., *50:* 2113–2122, 1971b.

Gorden, P., Sherman, B. M., and Simopoulos, A. P. Glucose intolerance with hypokalemia; an increased proportion of circulating proinsulin-like component. J. Clin. Endocrinol. Metab., *34:* 235–240, 1972.

Gottlieb, J. A., and Hill, C. S. Chemotherapy of thyroid cancer with Adriamycin. N. Engl. J. Med., *290:* 193–197, 1974.

Graber, A. L., Porte, E., Jr., and Williams, R. H. Clinical use of diazoxide and mechanism for its hyperglycemic effects. Diabetes, *15:* 143–148, 1966.

Grage, T. B., Rochlin, D. B., Weiss, A. J., and Wilson, W. L. Clinical studies with tubercidin administered after absorption into human erythrocytes. Cancer Res., *30:* 79–81, 1970.

Gray, R. K., Rosch, J., and Grollman, J. H. Arteriography in the diagnosis of islet cell tumors. Radiology, *97:* 39–44, 1970.

Grunt, J. A., Pallotta, J. A., and Soeldner, J. S. Blood sugar, serum insulin, and free fatty acid interrelationships during intravenous tolbutamide testing in normal young adults and in patients with insulinoma. Diabetes, *19:* 122–126, 1970.

Gutman, R. A., Lazarus, N. R., Penhas, J. C., Fajans, S., and Recant, L. Circulating proinsulin-like material in patients with functioning insulinomas. N. Engl. J. Med., *284:* 1003–1008, 1971.

Herr, R. R., Jahnke, H. K., and Argondelis, A. S. Structure of streptozotocin. J. Am. Chem. Soc., *89:* 4808–4809, 1967.

Hill, C. S., Ibanez, M. L., Samaan, N. A., Hearn, M. J., and Clark, R. L. Medullary (solid) carcinoma of the thyroid gland; an analysis of the M. D. Anderson Hospital experience with patients with the tumor, its special features, and its histogenesis. Medicine (Baltimore), *52:* 141–171, 1973.

Hill, G. J. Carcinoid tumors; pharmacological therapy. Oncology, *25:* 329–343, 1971.

Hutter, A. M., and Kayhoe, D. E. Adrenal cortical carcinoma, clinical features of 138 patients. Am. J. Med., *41:* 572–580, 1966a.

Hutter, A. M., and Kayhoe, D. E. Adrenal cortical carcinoma, results of treatment with o,p'-DDD in 138 patients. Am. J. Med., *41:* 581–592, 1966b.

Kahn, P. C. The radiologic identification of functioning adrenal tumors. Radiol. Clin. North Am., 5: 221–230, 1967.

Kahn, R., Levy, A., Gardner, J., Miller, J., Gorden, P., and Schein, P. Pancreatic cholera; beneficial effects of treatment with streptozotocin. N. Engl. J. Med. 292: 941–945, 1975.

Kanturek, S., Biernot, J., and Oleskay, J. Effect of metiamide, a histamine H_2 receptor antagonist, on gastric response to histamine pentagastrin, insulin and peptone meal in man. Am. J. Digest. Dis., 19: 609–616, 1974.

Kraft, A. R., Tompkins, R. K., and Zollinger, R. M. Recognition and management of the diarrheal syndrome caused by nonbeta islet cell tumors of the pancreas. Am. J. Surg., 119: 163–170, 1970.

Kruss, D. M., and Littman, A. Safety of cimetidine. Gastroenterology, 74: 478–483, 1978.

Landau, B. R., Levine, H. J., and Hertz, R. Prolonged glucagon administration in a case of hyperinsulinism due to disseminated islet cell carcinoma. N. Engl. J. Med., 259: 286–288, 1958.

Laurent, J., Debry, G., and Floquent, J. Hypoglycemic Tumours. Excerpta Medica, Amsterdam, 1971.

Leeper, R. D. Medical management of thyroid cancer. Sloan Kettering Clin. Bull., 2: 3–6, 1972.

Lipsett, M. B., Hertz, R., and Ross, G. T. Clinical and pathophysiologic aspects of adrenocortical carcinoma. Am. J. Med., 35: 374–383, 1963.

Longmire, W. P., Brown, J., Buckley, G. O., Cooke, A., Glober, G., Hanafee, W. N., Kantor, G., Matsumoto, K. K., Plested, W. G., Rochlin, D. B., and Wilkerson, J. A. Islet cell tumors of the pancreas. Ann. Intern. Med., 68: 203–221, 1968.

Lubitz, J. A., Freeman, L., and Okun, R. Mitotane in inoperable adrenal cortical carcinoma. J.A.M.A., 223: 1109–1111, 1973.

Lukens, F. D. W. Alloxan diabetes. Physiol. Rev., 28: 304–330, 1948.

Lundbaek, K., Lyngsoe, J., Madsen, B., Yde, H., and Orskov, H. The diagnosis of insulinoma. Acta Med. Scand., 181: 269–279, 1967.

Mahon, W. A., Mitchell, M. L., Steinke, J., and Raben, M. S. Effect of human growth hormone on hypoglycemic states. N. Engl. J. Med., 267: 1179–1183, 1962.

Mainardi, M., Maxwell, V., Sturdevant, R. A. L., and Isenberg, J. I. Metiamide, an H_2 receptor blocker, as inhibitor of basal and meal stimulated gastric acid secretion in patients with duodenal ulcer. N. Engl. J. Med., 291: 373–376, 1974.

Marks, V., and Rose, F. C. Hypoglycemia. Blackwell, Oxford, 1965.

Mason, H. L., and Engstrom, W. W. The 17-ketosteroids; their origin, determination and significance. Physiol. Rev., 30: 321, 1950.

McCarthy, D. M. Report on the United States experience with cimetidine in Zollinger-Ellison syndrome and other hypersecretory states. Gastroenterology, 74: 453–458, 1978.

Melmon, K. L., Sjoerdsma, A., and Mason, D. T. Distinctive clinical and therapeutic aspects of the syndrome associated with bronchial carcinoid tumors. Am. J. Med., 39: 568–581, 1965a.

Melmon, K. L., Sjoerdsma, A., Oates, J. A., and Laster, L. Treatment of malabsorption and diarrhea of the carcinoid syndrome with methysergide. Gastroenterology, 48: 18–24, 1965b.

Mengel, C. E. Therapy of the malignant carcinoid syndrome. Ann. Intern. Med., 62: 587–602, 1965.

Moertel, C. G., Reitemeier, R. J., Schutt, A. J., and Hahn, R. G. Phase II study of streptozotocin (NSC-85998) in the treatment of advanced gastrointestinal cancer. Cancer Chemother. Rep., 55: 303–307, 1971.

Moertel, C. G., Sauer, W. G., Dockerty, M. B., and Baggenstoss, A. H. Life history of the carcinoid tumor of the small intestine. Cancer, 14: 901–912, 1961.

Moertel, C. G. Chemotherapy of gastrointestinal cancer. Clin. Gastroenterol., 5: 777–793, 1976.

Murray-Lyon, I. M., Eddleston, A. C., Williams, R., Brown, M., Hogbin, B. M., Bennet, A., Edwards, J. C., and Taylor, K. W. Treatment of multiple-hormone-producing malignant islet cell tumor with streptozotocin. Lancet, 2: 895–898, 1968.

Murray-Lyon, I. M., Cassar, J., Coulson, R., Williams, R., Ganguli, P. C., Edwards, J. C., and Taylor, K. W. Further studies on streptozotocin therapy for a multiple-hormone-producing islet cell carcinoma. Gut, 12: 717–720, 1971.

Nelson, A. A., and Woodward, G. Severe adrenal cortical atrophy (cytotoxic) and hepatic damage produced in dogs by feeding 2,2-bis-(parachlorophenyl)-1,1-dichloroethane (DDD or TDE). Arch. Pathol., 48: 387–394, 1949.

Nichols, J., and Hennigar, G. Studies on DDD, 2,2-bis-(parachlorophenyl)-1,1-dichloroethane. Exp. Med. Surg., 15: 310–316, 1957.

Oates, J. A., and Butler, T. C. Pharmacologic and endocrine aspects of carcinoid syndrome. Adv. Pharmacol., 5: 109–128, 1967.

Oates, J. A., and Sjoerdsma, A. A unique syndrome associated with the secretion of 5-hydroxytryptophan by metastatic gastric carcinoids. Am. J. Med., 32: 333–342, 1962.

Polack, M. A., and Ellison, E. H. Parietal cell mass and gastric acid secretion in the Zollinger-Ellison syndrome. Surgery, 60: 606–614, 1966.

Power, L. A glucose-responsive insulinoma. J.A.M.A., 207: 893–896, 1969.

Rakieten, N., Rakieten, M. L., and Nadkarni, M. V. Studies on the diabetogenic action of streptozotocin (NSC-37917). Cancer Chemother. Rep., 29: 91–98, 1969.

Reed, M. L., Kuipers, F. M., Vaitkevicius, V. K., Clar, M. D., Drake, E. H., and Eyler, W. R. Treatment of disseminated carcinoid tumors including hepatic-artery catheterization. N. Engl. J. Med., 269: 1006–1010, 1963.

Rocha e Silva, M., and Garcia Lerne, J. Antagonists of bradykinin. Med. Exp., 8: 287–295, 1963.

Roth, H., Thier, S., and Segal, S. Zinc glucagon in the management of refractory hypoglycemia due to insulin-producing tumors. N. Engl. J. Med., 274: 493–497, 1966.

Sadoff, L. Nephrotoxicity of streptozotocin (NSC-85998). Cancer Chemother. Rep., 54: 457–459, 1970.

Schein, P. S. Chemotherapeutic management of the hormone-secreting endocrine malignancies. Cancer, 30: 1616–1626, 1972.

Schein, P. S., DeLillis, R. A., Kahn, C. R., Gorden, P., and Kraft, A. R. Islet cell tumors; current concepts and management. Ann. Intern. Med., 79: 239–257, 1973.

Schein, P. S., Alberti, K. G. M. M., and Williamson, D. H. Effects of streptozotocin on carbohydrate and lipid metabolism in the rat. Endocrinology, 89: 827–834, 1971.

Schein, P. S., Cooney, D. A., and Vernon, M. L. The use of nicotinamide to modify the toxicity of streptozotocin diabetes without loss of antitumor activity. Cancer Res., 27: 2324–2332, 1967.

Schein, P. S., Kahn, R., Jordan, P., Wells, S., and DeVita, V. T. Streptozotocin for malignant insulinoma and carcinoid tumor. Arch. Intern. Med., 132: 555–561, 1973.

Schein, P. S., O'Connell, M. J., Blom, J., Hubbard, S., MaGrath, I. T., Bergevin, P., Wiernik, P. H., Ziegler, J. L., and DeVita, V. T. Clinical antitumor activity and toxicity of streptozotocin (NSC-85998). Cancer, 34: 993–1000, 1974.

Schteingart, D. E., Cash, R., and Coon, J. W. Amino-glutethimide and metastatic adrenal cancer. J.A.M.A., 198: 1007–1010, 1966.

Sjoerdsma, A., Lovenberg, W., Engelman, K., Carpenter, W. T., Wyatt, R. J., and Gessa, G. L. Serotonin now; clinical implications of inhibiting its synthesis with para-chlorophenylalanine. Ann. Intern. Med., 73: 607–629, 1970.

Smith, C. G., Reineke, L. M., Burch, M. R., Shefner, A. M., and Muirhead, E. E. Studies on the uptake of tubercidin (7-deazaadenosine) by blood cells and its distribution in whole animals. Cancer Res., 30: 69–75, 1970.

Smith, C. K., Stoll, R. W., Vance, J., Ricketts, H., and Williams, R. H. Treatment of malignant insulinoma with streptozotocin. Diabetologia, 7: 118–124, 1971.

Steiner, D. F., and Oyer, P. E. The biosynthesis of insulin and a probable precursor of insulin by a human islet cell adenoma. Proc. Natl. Acad. Sci. U.S.A., *57:* 473–480, 1969.

Thjodleifsson, B., and Wormsley, K. G. Gastric response to metiamide. Br. Med. J., *2:* 304–306, 1974.

Thomas, R. L., Robinson, A. E., Johnsrude, I. S., Goodrich, J. K., and Lester, R. G. The demonstration of an insulin and gastrin producing pancreatic tumor by angiography and pancreatic scanning. A.J.R., *104:* 646–651, 1968.

Ureles, A. L., Murray, M., and Wolf, R. Results of pharmacologic treatment in the malignant carcinoid syndrome. N. Engl. J. Med., *267:* 435–438, 1963.

Vilar, O., and Tullner, W. W. Effects of *o,p'*-DDD on histology and 17 hydroxycorticosteroid output of the dog adrenal cortex. Endocrinology, *65:* 80–86, 1959.

Vroom, F. Q., Brown, R. E., Dempsey, J., and Hill, S. R., Jr. Studies on several possible antiserotonin compounds in a patient with the functioning carcinoid syndrome. Ann. Intern. Med., *56:* 941–945, 1962.

Walfish, P. G., Natale, R., and Chang, C. Beta-adrenergic receptor mechanisms in the metabolic effects of diazoxide in fasted rats. Diabetes, *19:* 228–233, 1970.

Wilson, H., Cheek, R. C., Sherman, R. T., and Storer, E. H. Carcinoid tumors. Curr. Probl. Surg. (in press), 1978.

Zimmer, F. E. Islet cell carcinoma treated with alloxan. Ann. Intern. Med., *61:* 543–548, 1964.

Chapter 26

Bone and Soft Tissue

PATRICK R. BERGEVIN, M.D., and STEPHEN C. COHEN, M.D.

BONE SARCOMAS

Primary bone tumors account for about 1.0% of all malignancies. Classification of primary bone tumors relates to the cell of origin. Tumors may originate from the osteoblast, chondroblast, fibroblast and from the endothelial, neural, vascular, hematopoietic or other supporting tissues of bone.

The evaluation of the patient with a suspected bone tumor requires the considerations of multiple medical specialists. Roentgenographic studies should include standard and tomographic films of the primary lesion as well as a good posteroanterior (PA) and lateral view of the chest and whole lung tomograms. A bone scan should also be performed. These studies are helpful in suggesting a probable diagnosis and to determine the extent of the lesion and its dissemination. An arteriogram is also useful to outline the extent of the primary lesion.

There are numerous lesions of the bone, both neoplastic and non-neoplastic, which are benign and must be clearly differentiated from malignant neoplasms, which require radical therapeutic approaches. Differentiation of such lesions can be most difficult and requires expertise by the pathologist.

Osteosarcoma is the most common primary malignant bone tumor with a peak age incidence at 10–25 years. The presentation is typically a mass at the involved bony site which may be accompanied by pain and redness of overlying skin. The lesion is more common in males and has a predilection for involvement of the lower extremity, particularly about the knee.

Radiographically these lesions show varying degrees of sclerosis, lucency, cortical destruction, periosteal new bone formation and an associated soft tissue mass. Histologically there is a sarcomatous stroma with osteoid formation.

The diagnosis of osteosarcoma has in the past implied an extremely poor prognosis with 5-year survival rates ranging up to only 20%. Pulmonary metastases occurred in the majority of patients within one year of surgical resection or amputation, followed by death within a few months. Surgical management is determined chiefly by location of the tumor: those bony sites not amenable to resection such as vertebrae or pelvis have a very poor prognosis following x-irradiation alone. Amputation of extremity lesions has been by disarticulation at the higher joint or by trans-medullary resection, although in the latter instance "skip" metastases along the medullary canal may be a factor in local recurrence and distant spread.

X-irradiation of the primary tumor up to 10,000 rads in the past has been used for control of the primary tumor in patients with pulmonary metastases. The same treatment schedule in patients without metastases given preoperatively with dismemberment planned 3–6 months later if no pulmonary metastases occur has served to select out those patients who will most benefit from surgery; a large number of patients would then be spared the functional and psychological sequelae of amputation (Allen and Stevens, 1973).

Response rates to the usual conventional chemotherapeutic agents was only in the range of about 20% with a negligible impact on survival. The demonstration of higher response rates to Adriamycin or high dose methotrexate with citrovorum factor rescue has prompted the use of these drugs in the adjuvant setting (Jaffe et al., 1974; Cortes et al., 1974). Current data suggest that 50–60% of patients so treated can expect an extended relapse free survival. Lowering the dose of Adriamycin to avoid leukopenia was associated with disease recurrence. More recently weekly high dose methotrexate was found to be superior to the original triweekly schedule in patients with metastatic disease (Jaffe et al., 1977). More aggressive adjuvant chemotherapy regimens have been used in studies designed to preserve a functional extremity. In one study (Rosen et al., 1976) a minimum of 2 months of preoperative chemotherapy with high dose methotrexate and citrovorum factor rescue and Adriamycin was given to patients with osteosarcoma of the distal femur or proximal tibia following which en bloc resection of the primary tumor with prosthetic replacement of involved bone was performed. Postoperative chemotherapy with high dose methotrexate and citrovorum factor rescue, Adriamycin and cyclophosphamide was given for 1 year. Another study (Morton et al., 1976) used intra-arterial Adriamycin and x-irradiation to the primary extremity tumor followed by radical local resection and cadaver allograft placement followed by postoperative chemotherapy with vincristine, high dose methotrexate with citrovorum factor rescue and Adriamycin. Beattie et al. (1975) have reported on the use of combined chemotherapy and thoracotomy for wedge resection of pulmonary tumor nodules. Such an approach has markedly contributed to a prolonged survival in these patients. Selecting out only those patients who respond to dinitrochlorobenzene and one of the recall skin test antigens and who have a metastatic tumor doubling time of greater than 40 days has allowed a 5-year survival of 63% after surgery (Holmes and Morton, 1977).

Certain variants of osteosarcoma deserve mention. Osteosarcoma arising within the mandible or facial bones are less aggressive than the classical osteosarcoma. Extraskeletal and multifocal osteosarcomas are very aggressive lesions and have a poor prognosis following surgery. Parosteal osteosarcoma occurs in a slightly older age group and is less aggressive locally and metastasizes late in its clinical course. En bloc resection may be performed if a good margin of normal tissue around the tumor can be obtained. Telangiectatic osteosarcoma presents in adolescents as a destructive osteolytic lesion and has a poor prognosis after surgery.

Ewing's sarcoma is the second commonest malignant bone tumor in children with a peak age incidence in the second decade of life. Males are predominantly affected, with presentation usually in the diaphysis of a long bone, signalled usually by pain and swelling in the affected area. Radiologically there is usually bone lysis with an overlying soft tissue component. Occasionally seen is lamellated new bone formation giving rise to an "onion skin" appearance on x-ray. Microscopically Ewing's sarcoma is a small cell tumor resembling certain other malignancies such as malignant lymphoma, neuroblastoma and rhabdomyosarcoma. PAS staining may reveal intracellular glycogen in the Ewing's sarcoma specimen which is absent in the other tumors. Urinary catecholamines should be determined in view of the frequency of neuroblastoma in this age group. Up to 30% of patients have obvious metastatic disease at the time of diagnosis, usually to lungs and bones.

Despite radical surgery and/or radiotherapy to the primary lesion, only about 10% of patients will survive 5 years. Single agent chemotherapy experience in patients with metastatic Ewing's sarcoma has yielded impressive response rates with cyclophosphamide, actinomycin D, Adriamycin and vincristine, prompting the use of these drugs in the adjuvant setting. Approximately 80% of patients with local disease treated by radiotherapy to the primary lesion followed by combined chemotherapy with vincristine, actinomycin D, and cyclophosphamide or the addition of Adriamycin to this regimen have been rendered disease free for periods varying from 2½ to 5½ years (Jaffe et al., 1976; Rosen et al., 1974). Of concern in some centers is the appearance of central nervous system disease upon relapse, prompting consideration of prophylactic whole brain irradiation with intrathecal chemotherapy (Marsa and Johnson, 1971; Mehta and Hendrickson, 1974).

Chondrosarcoma is a malignant tumor of cartilage arising de novo or from a benign cartilaginous lesion. This is generally a tumor of adults where long term survivals of up to 50% are seen after surgery, although in childhood chondrosarcoma pursues an aggressive course similar to osteosarcoma with development of pulmonary metastases in the majority within 8 months after treatment of the primary lesion. The tumor usually presents as swelling and pain in the proximal region of extremities. Roentgenographic findings include mottling, calcifications of the medulla and localized cortical destruction. The type of surgery employed depends upon the primary site of involvement: wide resection, amputation or hemipelvectomy may be required. Tumors not amenable to surgery are usually treated with x-irradiation, and a few patients so treated have enjoyed long term survivals. The use of adjuvant chemotherapy in chondrosarcoma is currently under study.

Giant cell tumor of bone is usually seen in patients in the third and fourth decades of life with a female predominance. Pain and swelling may be the presenting features. On x-ray the tumor is usually seen as a solitary area of radiolucency in the metaphyseal area of a long bone, frequently about the knee, with thinning of the adjacent cortex. Histologically the sarcomatous stroma consists of spindle or ovoid mononuclear cells with interspersed multinucleated or giant cells. This tumor may evolve from a benign giant cell tumor or from Paget's disease of bone.

The treatment of malignant giant cell tumor is usually surgical with the procedure of choice being wide local resection. Simple curettage is associated with a very high local recurrence rate. Amputation is usually reserved for recurrent disease after less radical surgery and for aggressive lesions which demonstrate perforation of adjacent cortex. Radiotherapy is generally ineffective and is reserved for lesions not amenable to surgery. The tumor uncommonly metastasizes to distant sites such as the lungs.

Fibrosarcoma of bone is usually seen in adults with pain and swelling about the involved site being the usual presenting features. The tumor originates in the medullary cavity of long bones, especially the femur and tibia and roentgenographically appears as an osteolytic lesion. Microscopically there is a fibroblastic proliferation in varying degrees of differentiation. Fibrosarcoma of bone may arise de novo or after radiation therapy to the involved bone, in giant cell tumors, Paget's disease of bone, fibrous dysplasia or long standing osteomyelitis. The treatment of choice for extremity lesions is usually amputation. Fibrosarcoma of bone is nearly as lethal as osteosarcoma, with early clinical development of pulmonary metastases and a five year survival of only about 25-30%. The use of adjuvant chemotherapy in this tumor is currently under study.

SOFT TISSUE SARCOMAS

Soft tissue sarcomas are malignant lesions originating from mesenchymal cells present in muscle, fibrous, adipose, vascular, connective, lymphatic, neural, fascial and synovial tissues. These tumors are infrequent, with an incidence of about 2/100,000 persons. The soft tissue sarcomas are more common in adults but rank sixth in frequency in the pediatric age group malignancies.

The etiology of most cases of soft tissue sarcomas is obscure. Some sarcomas seem clearly related to prior injury to tissues, e.g., radiation; occasional lesions, such as malignant schwannoma, may arise from a benign precursor. Prolonged edema of the upper extremity following mastectomy has been implicated as a cause of lymphangiosarcoma. Evidence for a viral agent as being causative for soft tissue sarcomas is mounting. Such evidence includes: isolation of type C viral particles in human sarcomas, demonstration of a common tumor specific antigen among multiple sarcomas and demonstration of antibodies to sarcoma specific antigens in patients with sarcomas and in their relatives and close associates (Morton et al., 1970).

Soft tissue sarcomas are usually discovered because of symptoms related to the encroachment of the tumor on surrounding tissues. The growth of the lesion is usually insidious and the mass is usually painless. Physical findings vary with the location of the tumor and the histological type. Efforts must be made to determine the tumor's relation to surrounding structures to identify, if possible, the tissue of origin and the possibility of surgical resection. Clues to the underlying primary can be gained by the knowledge that some tumors have a predilection for certain sites. For example, synovial sarcomas occur mainly in feet, hands and around the knee, while liposarcomas are common in the thighs.

Once the diagnosis is suspected, roentgenologic studies should be done to help define the extent of the tumor as well as its relationship to underlying bone and fascial planes. These studies can eliminate confusion with primary bone tumors and may help determine operability. Arteriography may help to determine the relationship of the tumor to surrounding structures and to estimate extent of disease. A bone scan and whole lung tomograms help to determine the presence of metastatic disease. Biopsy is the basis for diagnosis. The preferred procedure is an incisional biopsy, although a good needle biopsy may provide sufficient material for diagnosis. Multiple problems are encountered in seeking a histopathological diagnosis. Since all of these tumors have a common origin, the mesenchyma, there may be considerable histologic variation in different parts of the same tumor. Fibrotic proliferation is common in many sarcomas and can obscure the underlying primary tumor. In addition many tumors are too undifferentiated to determine the exact histogenesis.

Despite the great variety of soft tissue sarcomas and differences in their biologic activity, some generalizations can be made about management. The treatment of choice for a soft tissue sarcoma is surgical excision ensuring adequate margins. This may require extensive resection of surrounding muscles, nerves, vascular structures and regional lymphatics. Amputation may be necessary as the initial therapy in extensive lesions or in recurrent disease. Depending on the site of the primary, procedures such as hemipelvectomy or interscapulothoracic amputations may be necessary. Surgery has a definite role to play in some patients who develop pulmonary metastases after control of the primary seems relatively assured (Holmes and Morton, 1977). With proper selection long term survivals have been achieved with this technique.

In soft tissue sarcomas radiation therapy has a definite role in treating areas with known or suspected residual disease after surgery or for palliation. In cases where surgery is not possible or is rejected as a form of treatment, high dose radiotherapy in the range of 6000–7000 rads may allow long survivals (Scanlon, 1972). There is great variation in radiosensitivity among the sarcomas, and treatment must be individualized dependent upon cell type and location. It is apparent that in some tumors the combination of radiotherapy and surgery can yield better survivals than with surgery alone (McNeer et al., 1968). Suit and co-workers have demonstrated excellent local control and disease-free survival particularly in Stage I and II disease of the distal extremities with conservative surgery and high dose radiotherapy (Suit et al., 1973, 1975; Suit and Russell, 1975, 1977).

Several chemotherapeutic agents have been found to be effective in many soft tissue sarcomas. Some tumors, such as rhabdomyosarcoma, are very sensitive to combination therapy with vincristine, actinomycin D and cyclophosphamide. The combination of cyclophosphamide, vincristine, Adriamycin and DTIC (CYVADIC) appears to be one of the optimal regimens for treatment of patients with disseminated soft tissue sarcomas (Pinedo and Kenis, 1977). An overall response rate of 59% with 15% complete responses is seen. The median duration of a partial remission is about 6 months, but complete responses are durable, and over 70% of patients who enter complete response remain so at 30 months. A combined surgical, radiotherapeutic and chemotherapeutic approach is now being used in many sarcomas and will hopefully improve the survival of many patients (Jaffe et al., 1973).

The most recent modality to be used in treatment of soft tissue sarcomas is immunotherapy. Attempts are being made to enhance immunosurveillance by increasing levels of tumor specific antibodies by stimulation with BCG, irradiated tumor cells and cross transplantation of tumors (Krementz et al., 1974). While it is too early to draw conclusions about the efficacy of this therapy, it has been shown that it can increase titers of antibodies to tumor specific antigens (Morton et al., 1970).

Liposarcoma is the most frequent soft tissue sarcoma, making up about 15% of such lesions. The mean age of patients in most series is about 50 years with a slight male predominance; the tumor is rarely seen in patients under 30 years of age. The lesion has a predilection for deeper soft tissues with the extremities and retroperitoneum as favored sites of occurrence; however, the tumor may occur in any site where fat is present. Liposarcomas are almost always malignant from their inception and rarely arise from a pre-existing lipoma.

Liposarcoma usually presents as an inconspicuous swelling which progresses for up to 2–3 years before clinical detection. Large sizes may be attained particularly in the retroperitoneal space. On examination, liposarcomas are firm, deeply situated, nodular and fixed to surrounding tissues. Lipomas, on the other hand, are generally more superficial, soft and smooth. Microscopically, liposarcomas can be graded from a well differentiated type resembling embryonal fat with myxoid tissue to undifferentiated or round cell types with bizarre lipoblasts. Combinations of lesions may be seen. There is a strong relationship between histology and clinical behavior. The myxoid and well differentiated types are associated with as high as 80% 5-year survivals. The poorly differentiated types are subject to frequent local recurrences and distant metastases, usually pulmonary, in the majority of cases.

Treatment for localized disease is wide surgical excision and postoperative radiation therapy. With the use of postoperative radiation the local recurrence rate has been shown to decrease to as low as 20%. The well differentiated liposarcomas seem particularly susceptible to radiation therapy (Perry and Chu, 1962). Irradiation alone can in some cases lead to cure.

Fibrosarcoma is the second most common group of soft tissue sarcomas. These tumors usually arise de novo but may arise in areas of chronic draining infections, in scars or in previously irradiated benign lesions. Most patients are males between the ages of 40 and 70 years (Pritchard et al., 1974). Tumors are primarily located in the extremities or trunk. Patients often present with a firm mass after a delay of months to years. Pain, if present, is usually a late manifestation. Histologically, these tumors are composed of spindle-shaped cells in bands which are usually located in muscles. There is good correlation between the microscopic appearance of this tumor and the response to therapy (Pritchard et al., 1974). Many mesenchymal tumors cause fibrous proliferation and can be confused with fibrosarcoma.

The treatment of this tumor is wide local excision. Amputation is reserved for recurrent disease or extensive lesions. Long term survival rates as high as 70% can be obtained with surgical treatment alone (Castro et al., 1973). Radiation therapy has a limited role in the treatment of fibrosarcoma. There are cases, however, in which high dose radiation therapy was effective in controlling residual disease postsurgery, resulting in long term survivals (Scanlon, 1972). Metastatic disease is not uncommon, occurring in about 50% of cases (Castro et al., 1973; Pritchard et al., 1974).

Leiomyosarcoma is a rare tumor arising from smooth muscle and makes up about 5% of soft tissue sarcomas. The tumor occurs primarily in the viscera but can arise wherever there is smooth muscle. In adults the most common sites of involvement are the gastrointestinal tract, uterus and broad ligament. There is no sex predilection and no known etiologic association. Histologically, these lesions are composed of spindle cells arranged in intertwining bundles and whorls. Myofibrils can usually be seen. Differentiation from other tumors may be difficult because of an overlap of the various cellular types. Treatment is surgical excision. The tumors are generally considered radioresistant. Metastases occur in 50% of cases, primarily to lungs.

Synovial sarcomas comprise about 8% of soft tissue sarcomas. In most cases they arise from synovial membranes of joints, tendon sheaths and bursae. Most cases occur in the age group 20–40 years and are most common in males. The tumor is found almost exclusively in extremities, with tissues surrounding the knee being most frequently involved. Patients usually present with a painless swelling which may have been present for months to years. Histologically, the tumor reveals two cell types: spindle-shaped connective tissue cells and cuboid pseudoepithelial cells lining cleftlike spaces.

Treatment is radical surgical excision. Amputation leads to better survivals, since local recurrence rates with less radical surgery are extremely high (Cadman et al., 1965). Since lymph node metastases occur in 20% of cases nodal dissection has been recommended (Cadman et al., 1965). The 5-year survival in most studies is about 25%. Distant metastases, particularly to lungs and bones, are common.

Rhabdomyosarcomas are malignant tumors of skeletal muscles, making up the third largest group of soft tissue sarcomas. In children it is the most common soft tissue sarcoma and the third most frequent malignancy. The histopathologic patterns are varied.

Embryonal rhabdomyosarcoma—This type of tumor is seen primarily in infants and children. It is often located in the head and neck area and is particularly common in the orbit. Other common sites include the genitourinary tract, extremities, retroperitoneum and body wall. Because of the diverse locations of skeletal muscle, practically no site is immune. These patients generally present with a mass, with clinical manifestations related to the site of origin. Histologically these lesions are made up of spindle and round cells resembling primitive myoblasts, and cross striations are frequently absent.

Pleomorphic rhabdomyosarcoma—This variant occurs most commonly in adults over the age of 30 years with predilection for the lower extremities. It is rare in children. Patients usually present with a soft tissue mass with rapid growth. Histologically, this tumor is composed of spindle-shaped cells with little collagen. Myofibrils and cross striations are usually seen.

Alveolar rhabdomyosarcoma—The alveolar variant occurs mainly in young adults. It has a wide distribution but is seen mainly in the head and neck region and in the extremities. It is composed of round cells with a tendency to line connective tissue septa. Cross striations and giant cells are often found.

Botryoidal rhabdomyosarcoma—This tumor occurs in children with an average age of 7 years. It develops beneath a mucosal surface with predilection for the genital and urinary tracts, although many other sites may be involved. Grossly this tumor appears as a polypoid mass resembling grapes, and microscopically it resembles embryonal rhabdomyosarcoma.

Rhabdomyosarcomas are rapidly growing tumors with a variant symptomatology depending upon the sites of involvement. These tumors are infiltrative and subject to local recurrences. Frequently metastases are present at the time of diagnosis.

Treatment must be individualized for each patient with regard to type, site and extent of disease. In general, surgical excision is the primary approach. The treatment should be aggressive with wide excision. Extremely radical surgery should be avoided in embryonal rhabdomyosarcoma because of effective additional modalities of therapy. About one third of patients with pleomorphic rhabdomyosarcoma survive 5 years with surgical treatment (Keyhani and Bosher, 1968). Survival in alveolar rhabdomyosarcoma is extremely poor with a median survival of only about 9 months (Enzinger and Shiraki, 1969). Radiation therapy may be extremely effective in rhabdomyosarcoma of the embryonal type (McNeer et al., 1968). It is now used routinely in this tumor along with surgery and chemotherapy. Chemotherapy has been extensively utilized in rhabdomyosarcoma. It is especially effective in the embryonal types with other types being more resistant. The role of adjuvant chemotherapy with surgery and radiotherapy is being explored in the Intergroup Rhabdomyosarcoma Study. For further discussion the reader is referred to the chapter on pediatric tumors.

Malignant tumors of vascular origin are extremely rare. *Hemangiopericytomas* are derived from the capillary pericyte. They are usually locally invasive but may occasionally metastasize. Surgical excision is the treatment of choice and radiation treatment may be palliative. *Angiosarcomas* are rare tumors derived from endothelial cells and may arise in any tissue, occurring mainly in adults. These are aggressive tumors with 5–20% 5-year survivals after surgical excision.

Lymphangiosarcomas usually arise in swollen upper extremities as a complication of prolonged, massive postmastectomy lymphedema. Surgical excision is the treatment of choice with a radical interscapular thoracic amputation usually required.

Mesenchymomas are derived from primitive mesenchyme and made up of cells which have matured into several mesodermal cell types. They are widely distributed in the body. Treatment is by wide excision.

Kaposi's sarcoma is a common disease in Africa but uncommonly seen in the United States, making up about 2% of soft tissue sarcomas. In the United States it is most common in white males in the fourth to seventh decades and is more common in Jews and Italians (Brounstein et al., 1973). The tumor probably arises from blood vessels. Histologically it is composed of spindle cells and vascular channels with lymphocytic infiltrates. It is a systemic disease, usually beginning in the skin with subsequent visceral metastases. In most cases it pursues an indolent course but there are aggressive and infiltrating forms. Radiation therapy is the treatment of choice for skin disease and most lesions are cured with this treatment. With generalized involvement the prognosis is usually poor. Numerous chemotherapeutic agents have been shown to be effective, including DTIC, vinblastine, BCNU, actinomycin D, cyclophosphamide and bleomycin. The combination of actinomycin D plus vincristine allowed ten complete remissions and three partial responses in 14 patients with aggressive disease in the study of Vogel et al. (1973).

Malignant schwannomas arise from the neurilemma sheath. The tumor occurs mainly in the age group 20–40 years with more than half associated with neurofibromatosis. Peripheral nerve involvement can occur at any site but mainly occurs in the extremities and trunk. Patients usually present with an asymptomatic mass, but pain, muscle weakness and paresthesia may occur. The treatment is adequate wide excision since local recurrence is common with lesser surgical procedures. The 5-year survival is about 50%. The tumor is relatively radioresistant. An association with von Recklinghausen's disease signifies the tumor as more malignant with a poor prognosis (Ghosh et al., 1973).

The *malignant fibrous histiocytoma* is a tumor predominantly of middle-aged adults, presenting with an asymptomatic or slightly painful subcutaneous mass, most often on the extremities. The tumor is seen microscopically as a mixture of xanthomatous, histiocytic and giant cells and fibroblasts arranged in a storiform pattern. Malignant fibrous histiocytoma is often confused pathologically with other soft tissue sarcomas such as fibrosarcoma, liposarcoma or pleomorphic rhabdomyosarcoma. A wide local excision is required. Metastases may occur to regional nodes or lungs but long survival is possible, with median survivals of 1.5–8 years in three series (Leite et al., 1977).

REFERENCES

Allen, C. V., and Stevens, K. R. Preoperative irradiation for osteogenic sarcoma. Cancer, *31*: 1364–1366, 1973.

Beattie, E. J., Martini, N., and Rosen, G. The management of pulmonary metastases in children with osteogenic sarcoma with surgical resection combined with chemotherapy. Cancer, *35*: 618–621, 1975.

Brounstein, M. H., Shapiro, L., and Skolnick, P. Kaposi's sarcoma in community practice. Arch. Dermatol., *107*: 137–138, 1973.

Cadman, N. L., Soule, E. H., and Kelley, P. J. Synovial sarcoma; analysis of 134 tumors. Cancer, *18*: 613–627, 1965.

Castro, E. B., Hajdu, S. I., and Fortner, J. G. Surgical therapy of fibrosarcoma of extremities; a reappraisal. Arch. Surg., *107*: 284–286, 1973.

Cortes, E., Holland, J. F., Wang, J. J., Sinks, L. F., Blom, J., Senn, H., Bank, A., and Glidewell, O. Amputation and Adriamycin in primary osteosarcoma. N. Engl. J. Med. *291*: 998–1000, 1974.

Enzinger, F. M., and Shiraki, M. Alveolar rhabdomyosarcoma. Cancer, *24*: 18–31, 1969.

Ghosh, B. C., Ghosh, L., Huvos, A. G., and Fortner, J. G. Malignant schwannoma; a clinicopathologic study. Cancer, *31*: 184–190, 1973.

Holmes, E. C., and Morton, D. L. Pulmonary resection for sarcoma metastases. Orthop. Clin. North Am., *8*: 805–810, 1977.

Jaffe, N., Filler, R. M., Farber, S., Traggis, D. G., Vawter, G. F., Tefft, M., and Murray, J. E. Rhabdomyosarcoma in children; improved outlook with a multidisciplinary approach. Am. J. Surg., *125*: 482–487, 1973.

Jaffe, N., Frei, E., Traggis, D., and Bishop, Y. Adjuvant methotrexate and citrovorum factor treatment of osteogenic sarcoma. N. Engl. J. Med. *291*: 994–997, 1974.

Jaffe, N., Frei, E., Traggis, D., and Watts, H. Weekly high dose methotrexate-citrovorum factor in osteogenic sarcoma. Cancer, *39*: 45–50, 1977.

Jaffe, N., Traggis, D., Salian, S., and Cassady, J. R. Improved outlook for Ewing's sarcoma with combination chemotherapy (vincristine, actinomycin-D and cyclophosphamide) and radiation therapy. Cancer, *38*: 1925–1930, 1976.

Keyhani, A., and Booker, R. J. Pleomorphic rhabdomyosarcoma. Cancer, *22*: 956–967, 1968.

Krementz, E. T., Mansell, P. W. A., Hornung, M. O., Samuels, M. S., Sutherland, C. A., and Benes, E. N. Immunotherapy of malignant disease; the use of viable sensitized lymphocytes or transfer factor prepared from sensitized lymphocytes. Cancer, *33*: 394–401, 1974.

Leite, C., Goodwin, J. W., Sinkovics, J. G., Baker, L. H., and Benjamen, R. Chemotherapy of malignant fibrous histiocytoma. Cancer, *40*: 2010–2014, 1977.

Marsa, G. W., and Johnson, R. E. Altered pattern of metastasis following treatment of Ewing's sarcoma with radiotherapy and adjuvant chemotherapy. Cancer, *27*: 1051–1054, 1971.

McNeer, G. P., Cantin, J., Chu, F., and Nickson, J. J. Effectiveness of radiation therapy in the management of sarcoma of the soft somatic tissues. Cancer, *22*: 391–397, 1968.

Mehta, Y., and Hendrickson, F. R. Central nervous system involvement in Ewing's sarcoma. Cancer, *33*: 859–862, 1974.

Morton, D., Eilber, F. R., Joseph, W. L., Wood, W. C., Trahan, E., and Ketcham, A. S. Immunological factors in human sarcomas and melanomas; a rational basis for immunotherapy. Ann. Surg., *172*: 740–749, 1970.

Morton, D. L., Eilber, F. R., Townsend, C. M., Grant, T. T., Mirra, J., and Weisenburger, T. H. Limb salvage from a multidisciplinary treatment approach for skeletal and soft tissue sarcomas of the extremity. Ann. Surg., *184*: 268–278, 1976.

Perry, H., and Chu, F. Radiation therapy in the palliative management of soft tissue sarcomas. Cancer, *15*: 179–183, 1962.

Pinedo, H. M., and Kenis, Y. Chemotherapy of advanced soft tissue sarcomas in adults. Cancer Treat. Rev., *4*: 67–86, 1977.

Pritchard, D. J., Soule, E. H., Taylor, W. F., and Ivins, J. C. Fibrosarcoma—a clinicopathologic and statistical study of 199 tumors of the soft tissues of the extremities and trunk. Cancer, *33*: 888–897, 1974.

Rosen, G., Murphy, M. L., Huvos, A. G., Gutierrez, M., and Marcove, R. C. Chemotherapy, en bloc resection and prosthetic bone replacement in the treatment of osteogenic sarcoma. Cancer, *37*: 1–11, 1976.

Rosen, G., Wollner, N., Tan, C., Wu, S. J., Hajdu, S. I., Chan, W., D'Angio, G. J., and Murphy, M. L. Disease free survival in children with Ewing's sarcoma treated with radiation therapy and adjuvant four drug sequential chemotherapy. Cancer, *33*: 384–393, 1974.

Scanlon, P. W. Split dose radiotherapy for radioresistant bone and soft tissue sarcoma; ten years' experience. A.J.R., *114*: 544–552, 1972.

Suit, H. D., and Russell, W. O. Radiation therapy of soft tissue sarcomas. Cancer, *36*: 759–764, 1975.

Suit, H. D., and Russell, W. O. Soft part tumors. Cancer, *39*: 830–836, 1977.

Suit, H. D., Russell, W. O., and Martin, R. G. Management of patients with sarcoma of soft tissue in an extremity. Cancer, *31*: 1247–1255, 1973.

Suit, H. D., Russell, W. O., and Martin, R. G. Sarcoma of soft tissue clinical and histopathologic parameters and response to treatment. Cancer, *35*: 1478–1483, 1975.

Vogel, C. L., Primack, A., Dhru, D., Briers, P., Owor, R., and Kyalwazi, S. K. Treatment of Kaposi's sarcoma with a combination of actinomycin D and vincristine. Cancer, *31*: 1382–1389, 1973.

Chapter 27

Mycosis Fungoides

LOREN E. GOLITZ, M.D.

CLINICAL

Mycosis fungoides is a lymphoma that initially affects the skin with subsequent spread to lymph nodes and internal organs. Onset is predominantly in middle life, however, the disease may begin as early as the second or as late as the seventh decade. About two-thirds of those affected are men. Mycosis fungoides accounts for about 1% of deaths from lymphoma in the United States. The atypical cells which infiltrate the skin and viscera in mycosis fungoides represent a proliferation of abnormal thymus-derived lymphocytes (Edelson et al., 1974).

Clinically, three major types of mycosis fungoides have been described. The classic form which accounts for about 80% of all cases progresses through 3 overlapping stages that have a total duration of a few months to 40 years. The first stage which is called the erythematous or premycotic stage begins as localized patches of dermatitis which mimic eczema, psoriasis, contact dermatitis or neurodermatitis. Failure to respond to conventional topical medications is often the first clue that the rash is more than a nonspecific dermatitis. This initial phase of mycosis fungoides may persist for years with little effect on the patient's general health other than persistent pruritus. Spontaneous improvement may occur during the erythematous stage. Skin biopsies are often indistinguishable from chronic dermatitis during this stage, however, if mycosis fungoides is suspected biopsies should be repeated periodically.

The second, or plaque, stage is clinically and histologically the most characteristic and it is during this stage that the diagnosis is frequently made. Infiltrated plaques develop in areas of dermatitis or on normal appearing skin. The plaques enlarge peripherally, at times producing unusual annular lesions and areas of alopecia. Pruritus is prominent during this stage and skin biopsies commonly show atypical mononuclear cells in the dermis and characteristic microabscesses (so-called Pautrier's abscesses) within the epidermis.

531

During the third or tumor stage, cutaneous nodules and tumors appear and progress to ulcers which show little tendency to heal. Pruritus is typically decreased or absent during the tumor stage, however, painful ulcers and secondary pyodermas produce considerable discomfort. In about 50% of patients the definitive diagnosis of mycosis fungoides is not made until the tumor stage (Epstein et al., 1972).

The addition of a fourth stage of visceral involvement is helpful in understanding the current concept of mycosis fungoides as a single disease. For many years experts claimed that mycosis fungoides involved only the skin and that many patients subsequently developed visceral involvement with lymphocytic or histiocytic lymphoma or Hodgkin's disease. It is now clear that the visceral infiltrates in mycosis fungoides are the same as those in the skin and that extracutaneous involvement is present at autopsy in up to 75% of cases (Rappaport and Thomas, 1974; Long and Mihm, 1974).

Two other major forms of mycosis fungoides are recognized in addition to the classic form just described. About 10% of cases present with generalized erythroderma or exfoliative dermatitis. Patients with generalized erythroderma may progress to cutaneous tumors and visceral involvement. A variant of erythrodermic mycosis fungoides known as Sézary's syndrome has circulating atypical lymphocytes of thymic origin. Clendenning et al. (1964) have demonstrated that 20% of patients with classic mycosis fungoides have circulating abnormal cells indistinguishable from Sézary cells and Lutzner et al. (1971) were unable to distinguish the cells of Sézary's syndrome from those of mycosis fungoides by electron microscopy.

Mycosis fungoides d'emblee is the third major form of the disease. It accounts for slightly less than 10% of cases and is characterized by the onset of cutaneous tumors without preceding dermatitis or plaques (Epstein et al., 1972). Other forms of lymphoma have at times been confused with mycosis fungoides d'emblee.

While it is not always possible to predict which patient with an eczematous rash will develop mycosis fungoides, skin diseases such as poikiloderma atrophicans vasculare and parapsoriasis en plaque may evolve into mycosis fungoides after a number of years (Samman, 1964; Fleishmajer et al., 1965). Follicular mucinosis is associated with mycosis fungoides in a small percentage of cases (Ebling and Rook, 1968). This association is seen mainly in adults and histologically the deposits of hyaluronic acid within hair follicles are associated with a dermal infiltrate containing atypical mononuclear cells.

Lymphadenopathy can occur in any stage of mycosis fungoides, but is more common during the tumor stage or in those with generalized erythroderma. Biopsy of enlarged lymph nodes often reveals a nonspecific reactive process known as dermatopathic lymphadenitis. Late in the course of the disease, however, the lymph nodes may be invaded by atypical cells similar to those in the skin. The presence of palpable lymphadenopathy appears to be associated with a worse prognosis regardless of whether atypical infiltrates are found in the node histologically (Epstein et al., 1972).

LABORATORY

Routine laboratory tests are usually normal in mycosis fungoides. Anemia secondary to chronic disease may occur and mild eosinophilia is common. Patients with mycosis fungoides may have leukocytosis unrelated to obvious infection and about 20% have abnormal mononuclear cells in differential counts of their peripheral blood (Clendenning et al., 1964). Bone marrow examination is usually normal even in late stages of the disease. Lymphopenia is present in 45–76% of patients (Fuks et al., 1973; Cyr et al., 1966) and patients with less than 1000 lymphocytes per cubic millimeter unrelated to therapy appear to have a decreased survival rate (Fuks et al., 1973).

Pulmonary infiltrates and enlarged hilar nodes may be diagnosed by routine chest x-ray. In a study of patients who had staging laparotomies the intravenous pyelogram and inferior venacavogram were insensitive tests in identifying intra-abdominal lymphadenopathy and the lymphangiogram was frequently misleading (Griem et al., 1975). Three of 5 patients with abnormal spleen scans had myocosis fungoides of the spleen, however, abnormal liver scans did not correlate with liver involvement in 3 patients (Griem et al., 1975).

IMMUNOLOGY

A number of studies of immune function in mycosis fungoides have failed to identify any abnormality (Blaylock et al., 1966; Tan et al., 1974). Rostenberg and Bluefarb (1954), however, found decreased reactivity to a number of recall antigens and concluded there was a general depression of cell-mediated immunity. A depressed responsiveness to dinitrochlorobenzene has been reported (Vonderheid et al., 1977). Despite the relatively intact immune system in mycosis fungoides the incidence of infection, the types of microorganisms involved, the time of onset of infections, the number of infectious episodes per patient, and the incidence of septicemia are virtually identical to the infections seen in Hodgkin's disease (Casazza et al., 1966). Staphylococci and pseudomonas, the microorganisms most frequently involved, may produce a pyoderma and result in terminal pneumonia or septicemia. Recently it has been suggested that abnormal monocyte chemotaxis may be partly responsible for the high incidence of infection in mycosis fungoides (Seitz et al., 1977).

PATHOLOGY

In the erythematous stage of mycosis fungoides skin biopsies may show only nonspecific dermatitis. Characteristic changes which often appear during the plaque stage include a polymorphous dermal infiltrate of eosinophils, lymphocytes, histiocytes and atypical mononuclear cells, distribution of the infiltrate in a bandlike pattern in the upper dermis, and Pautrier's microabscesses, which contain atypical mononuclear cells, in the epidermis. During the tumor stage the epidermis may be ulcerated and the atypical infiltrate becomes more monomorphous. At the margins of the tumor, however, the characteristic mixture of cell types can often be seen.

Visceral involvement in mycosis fungoides is characterized by an atypical polymorphous infiltrate similar to that in the skin (Rappaport and Thomas, 1974; Long and Mihm, 1974). The infiltrate is arranged in a patchy distribution around blood vessels with little tendency to form tumors as seen in other lymphomas. Electron microscopy reveals that the atypical mononuclear cells in the skin and viscera have lobulated, cerebriform nuclei similar to the circulating atypical cells of Sézary's syndrome.

THERAPY

No form of therapy for mycosis fungoides has proved curative. A study by Epstein et al. (1972) failed to show improved survival of patients treated with new systemic drugs and treatment schedules when compared with those treated with earlier modes of therapy. Therapeutic responses are difficult to evaluate because the natural course of the disease may span many years with periods of spontaneous improvement and exacerbations. However, it appears that effective treatment depends on identifying patients early in their disease before widespread plaques and tumors develop. Several newer forms of therapy appear promising.

Topical nitrogen mustard has produced sustained complete remissions when applied at frequent intervals to the entire skin surface (Van Scott and Kalmanson, 1973). Most patients who experience complete remissions have erythematous or plaque stage disease. Delayed hypersensitivity reactions to nitrogen mustard characterized by contact dermatitis are frequent. While the reactions often enhance the clearing of cutaneous lesions in mycosis fungoides, they are not necessary for a therapeutic response.

Solutions of nitrogen mustard are prepared freshly on the day of use by dissolving 10 mg of drug in 60 ml of tap water. The patient should apply the mixture to the entire body surface by pouring small amounts into the palm and then applying it to the skin. Care must be taken to avoid the eyes and to wash the hands after use of the drug. Irritation may occur in intertriginous areas, and the drug should be used sparingly in the axilla, groin, and under the female breast. If nitrogen mustard solution is applied by medical personnel or spouses, protective gloves should be used to prevent contact sensitization. Initially the drug is applied daily but the frequency may be decreased after the patient has been completely clear of disease for 6–12 months. Topical applications of nitrogen mustard should be applied at a dose and frequency that will maintain a disease-free state for a minimum of 3 years (Vonderheid et al., 1977). Complete remissions of up to 7 years have been reported but further experience is needed to determine if these patients have been cured of their disease (Vonderheid et al., 1977). Long term topical therapy with nitrogen mustard appears to be safe, however, generalized hyperpigmentation occurs in almost all patients (Price, 1977).

Individuals that develop contact dermatitis to topically applied nitrogen mustard can generally be desensitized or hyposensitized by diluting 10 mg of the drug in 1 liter or more of water and gradually increasing the concentration as tolerated (Constantine et al., 1975). The concentration of the drug can be doubled weekly and most patients eventually tolerate a full dosage of 10 mg per 60 ml of water.

Nitrosourea compounds such as carmustine (BCNU) and lomustine (CCNU) may be an alternate form of topical therapy for patients who do not tolerate nitrogen mustard (Zackheim, 1972). Remissions with these drugs in patients with mycosis fungoides have been much shorter than with nitrogen mustard (Zackheim and Epstein, 1975).

Another therapeutic approach that shows promise in modifying the natural course of mycosis fungoides is the early and aggressive use of whole body electron beam radiation. Fuks et al. (1973) reported complete remissions in 58% of 132 patients treated with this modality. Fourteen patients were free of disease after 3–14 years. Response rates depend on the extent of cutaneous involvement. Patients with eczematous and limited plaque disease show complete remissions in 80%, while the results are 59% for generalized plaque disease and 30% for those with tumors. No patient who presented with tumors remained in remission for more than 1 year following electron beam therapy. All relapses occurred within 3 years after the first course of therapy. Electron beam therapy in this study consisted of total skin irradiation with 2.5 MeV electrons generated by a linear accelerator with doses varying from 800 rads in 10–15 days to 3000 rads in 50 days. Most centers are now utilizing total dosages of 4000–4500 rads of electron beam radiation. Whole body electron beam radiation followed by daily topical applications of nitrogen mustard may be more effective than either treatment alone. Acute side effects include erythema, pruritus, and loss of hair and nails while long term side effects are cutaneous atrophy, telangiectasia and xerosis. Patients should be evaluated periodically for actinic keratoses and skin cancer.

Photochemotherapy consisting of oral methoxsalen followed in 2 hours by longwave ultraviolet light was initially used for treating psoriasis but has been found to be effective in some cases of mycosis fungoides (Gilchrest et al., 1976). Erythematous lesions and plaques respond well to this therapy but cutaneous tumors are unresponsive (Roenigk, 1977). Longwave ultraviolet light penetrates deeper than shorter wavelength light and can produce clearing of deep dermal infiltrates.

When widespread cutaneous tumors or extracutaneous dissemination occurs in patients with mycosis fungoides systemic chemotherapy should be considered. The Mycosis Fungoides Cooperative Study Group Steering Committee (1975) uses a modification of the tumor-node-metastasis (TNM) system to stratify patients into numerous subgroups prior to randomization to topical nitrogen mustard, electron beam radiation or systemic chemotherapy. Levi and Wiernik (1975) have recently reviewed the chemotherapy of mycosis fungoides. While single agent chemotherapy may produce temporary remissions in a number of patients (Van Scott et al., 1962; Haynes and Van Scott, 1968) there is no evidence that it produces an improvement in the overall survival rate. Because of the improved outlook for patients with Hodgkin's disease and other lymphomas treated with combinations of chemotherapeutic agents, this form of therapy should be utilized for mycosis fungoides. Unfortunately no large controlled trials of multiple drug chemotherapy have been reported for mycosis fungoides. Conventional radiation therapy to individual cutaneous tumors may be used to supplement the treatment of patients who are not well controlled on systemic chemotherapy. General supportive care including wet compresses, topical steroids and systemic antibiotics is important in the management of mycosis fungoides.

REFERENCES

Blaylock, W. J., Clendenning. W. E., Carbone, P. P., and Van Scott, E. J. Normal immunologic reactivity in patients with the lymphoma mycosis fungoides. Cancer, *19:* 233–236, 1966.

Casazza, A. R., Duvall, C. P., and Carbone, P. P. Infection in lymphoma. J.A.M.A., *197:* 710–716, 1966.

Clendenning, W. E., Brecher, G., and Van Scott, E. J. Mycosis fungoides; relationship to malignant cutaneous reticulosis and the Sézary syndrome. Arch. Dermatol., *89:* 785–792, 1964.

Constantine, V. S., Fuks, Z. Y., and Farber, E. M. Mechlorethamine desensitization in therapy for mycosis fungoides: Topical desensitization to mechlorethamine (nitrogen mustard) contact hypersensitivity. Arch. Dermatol., *111:* 484–488, 1975.

Cyr, D. P., Geokas, M. C., and Worsley, G. H. Mycosis fungoides; hematologic findings and terminal course. Arch. Dermatol., *94:* 558–573, 1966.

Ebling, F. J. G., and Rook, A. Follicular mucinosis. *In Textbook of Dermatology*, edited by A. Rook, D. S. Wilkinson, and F. J. G. Ebling, pp. 1401–1403. F. A. Davis, Philadelphia, 1968.

Edelson, R. L., Kirkpatrick, C. H., Shevach E. M., Schein, P. S., Smith, R. W., Green, I., and Lutzner, M. Preferential cutaneous infiltration by neoplastic thymus-derived lymphocytes; morphologic and functional studies. Ann. Intern. Med., *80:* 685–692, 1974.

Epstein, E. H., Jr., Levin, D. L., Croft, J. D., Jr., and Lutzner, M. A. Mycosis fungoides; survival, prognostic features, response to therapy, and autopsy findings. Medicine, 15: 61-72, 1972.

Fleischmajer, R., Pascher, R., and Sims, C. F. Parapsoriasis en plaques and mycosis fungoides. Dermatologica, 131: 149-160, 1965.

Fuks, Z. Y., Bagshaw, M. A., and Farber, E. M. Prognostic signs and the management of the mycosis fungoides. Cancer, 32: 1385-1395, 1973.

Gilchrest, B. A., Parrish, J. A., Tannenbaum, E., Haynes, H. A., and Fitzpatrick, J. B. Oral methoxsalen photochemotherapy of mycosis fungoides. Cancer, 38: 683-689, 1976.

Griem, M. L., Moran, E. M., Ferguson, D. J., Mettler, F. A., and Griem, S. F. Staging procedures in mycosis fungoides. Br. J. Cancer, 31 (Suppl. 2): 362-367, 1975.

Haynes, H. A., and Van Scott, E. J. Therapy of mycosis fungoides. Progr. Dermatol., 3: 1-5, 1968.

Levi, J. A., and Wiernik, P. H. Management of mycosis fungoides—current status and future prospects. Medicine, 54: 73-88, 1975.

Long, J. C., and Mihm, M. C. Mycosis fungoides with extracutaneous dissemination; a distinct clinicopathologic entity. Cancer, 34: 1745-1755, 1974.

Lutzner, M. A., Hobbs, J. W., and Horvath, P. Ultrastructure of abnormal cells in Sézary syndrome, mycosis fungoides, and parapsoriasis en plaque. Arch. Dermatol., 103: 375-386, 1971.

Price, N. M. Topical mechlorethamine; cutaneous changes in patients with mycosis fungoides after its administration. Arch. Dermatol., 113: 1387-1389, 1977.

Rappaport, H., and Thomas, L. B. Mycosis fungoides; the pathology of extracutaneous involvement. Cancer, 34: 1198-1229, 1974.

Roenigk, H. H., Jr. Photochemotherapy for mycosis fungoides. Arch. Dermatol., 113: 1047-1051, 1977.

Rostenberg, A., and Bluefarb, S. M. Cutaneous reactions in the lymphoblastomas. Arch. Dermatol., 69: 195-205, 1954.

Samman, P. D. Survey of reticuloses and premycotic eruptions; A preliminary report. Br. J. Dermatol., 76: 1-9, 1964.

Seitz, L. E., Golitz, L. E., Weston, W. L., Aeling, J. E., and Dustin, R. D. Defective monocyte chemotaxis in mycosis fungoides. Arch. Dermatol., 113: 1055-1057, 1977.

Tan, R. S. H., Butterworth, C. M., McLaughlin, H., Malka, S., and Samman, P. D. Mycosis fungoides—A disease of antigen persistence. Br. J. Dermatol., 91: 607-616, 1974.

The Mycosis Fungoides Cooperative Study Group Steering Committee. Mycosis fungoides cooperative study. Arch. Dermatol., 111: 457-459, 1975.

Van Scott, E. J., Auerbach, R., and Clendenning, W. E. Treatment of mycosis fungoides with cyclophosphamide. Arch. Dermatol., 85: 499-501, 1962.

Van Scott, E. J., and Kalmanson, J. D. Complete remissions of mycosis fungoides lymphoma induced by topical nitrogen mustard (HN_2); control of delayed hypersensitivity to HN_2 by desensitization and by induction of specific immunologic tolerance. Cancer, 32: 18-30, 1973.

Vonderheid, E. C., Van Scott, E. J., Johnson, W. C., Grekin, D. A., and Asbell, S. O. Topical chemotherapy and immunotherapy of mycosis fungoides; intermediate-term results. Arch. Dermatol., 113: 454-462, 1977.

Zackheim, H. S. Treatment of mycosis fungoides with topical nitrosourea compounds. Arch. Dermatol., 106: 177-182, 1972.

Zackheim, H. S., and Epstein, E. H., Jr. Treatment of mycosis fungoides with topical nitrosourea compounds. Arch. Dermatol., 111: 1564-1570, 1975.

Chapter 28

Malignant Melanoma

LARRY NATHANSON, M.D., F.A.C.P.

Of tumors originating in the skin, only malignant melanoma appears to have predisposition to pursue an aggressive course with early dissemination either via lymphatic or hematogenous routes (Nathanson, 1967a, 1967b; DeVita and Fisher, 1976). This tumor is derived from the pigment cells in the basal layer of the epidermis which, during embryonic development, originate in the neural crest (Clark and Mihm, 1971). Although it has been considered a relatively uncommon tumor (representing approximately 2% of all human malignancies), its incidence is rising rapidly, and has doubled in the last decade in the United States. Thus, of the approximately 9600 cases diagnosed in 1978, approximately 4000 individuals will succumb to the disease (a 58% cure rate) (Silverberg and Holleb, 1978). In the United States, therefore, melanoma may be expected to account for more than twice as many deaths as is seen in Hodgkin's disease.

NATURAL HISTORY

Melanoma cells have a number of unique features which include the retention of the differentiated ability to synthesize melanin pigment (Fitzpatrick et al., 1971). This property is the basis of qualitative and quantitative tests, only partly successful for diagnosis or staging of the disease (Blois, 1976; Nathanson et al., 1971). The disease is also characterized by the well documented occurrence of spontaneous regression which is relatively common as a manifestation of the primary lesion, particularly in the skin, but which has only rarely been well documented in patients with metastatic disease (Nathanson, 1976): thus, the suggestion that host factors may play a role in determining the somewhat variable natural history of the disease. Studies of both in vitro and in vivo parameters have produced evidence of host mediated cellular and humoral immunity against tumor associated antigens (Mukherji and

Nathanson, 1973; Mukherji et al., 1975; Gutterman et al., 1975). Melanoma may arise in a number of sites including the mucous membranes and eye, but is predominantly a disease of the skin. Recent data has suggested that early recognition of characteristic symptoms including itching, bleeding, or ulceration, and signs including change in color and increased size of the lesion, together with the appearance of reddish, whitish, or bluish hues within the lesion, may contribute to early diagnosis and a higher cure rate of the disease (Mihm, 1973; Mihm et al., 1975). Whether better diagnosis is contributing to the increase in disease incidence, or whether this is due to some other environmental carcinogenic factor, such as actinic irradiation, is as yet unknown (Elwood and Lee, 1975). Melanoma families which are characterized by (1) frequent occurrence of multiple primary melanoma, (2) a tendency to have somewhat earlier age of onset (3rd and 4th decades of life), (3) similar age occurrence in the primary lesion in siblings suffering from the disease, and (4) a somewhat better prognosis than the sporadic variety, have been described (Anderson, 1971). These studies suggest the possibility of genetic factors in the etiology of the disease, although such factors are difficult to separate from indirect factors such as genetically determined pigmentation of the skin, which in turn accounts for superior protection from actinic irradiation.

TYPES OF PRIMARY MELANOMA

Four types of primary melanoma have been described (Clark et al., 1975; Seiji et al., 1977). These include, in the order of increasing aggressiveness: lentigo malignant melanoma (LMM), superficial spreading melanoma (SSM), nodular melanoma (NM), and palmar-plantar-mucosal melanoma (PPMM). LMM is a lesion primarily found in the elderly in exposed areas, especially the head and neck. It is usually a large (greater than 3 cm) lesion with highly irregular borders and heterogeneous distribution of pigmentation. SSM is the most common type of melanoma, accounting for 55% of all such lesions. It is somewhat smaller in size than LMM (usually less than 3 cm) and like LMM always has a radial component of tumor cells spreading horizontally through the superficial dermis prior to the development of an invasive component of melanoma cells. NM is the third type of primary melanoma and is characterized grossly by a relatively uniform deep-brown or blue-black colored nodule, which may be present as an elevated plaque or even in verrucous configuration. These lesions often measure less than 1 cm in size, always have an invasive component of tumor cells which frequently penetrate into the deeper layers of the dermis, and comprise about 30% of all melanomas. The fourth and rarest type of melanoma, PPMM, appears to be a histopathologic distinct entity (Seiji et al., 1977). It occurs in the

TABLE 28.1
Clinical Characteristics Mucocutaneous Malignant Melanoma

Type of Melanoma	Incidence (%)	Location	Median Age	Sex	"Latent" Period[a]	Mean Range Size (cm)	Margins	Color	Prognosis (5-Year) Survival[b]
Lentigo maligna	15	Exposed surfaces, especially head and neck	70	None	5–15 yr	3–5	Flat; highly irregular	Shades of brown, black; areas of hypopigmentation	55–80
Superficial spreading	50	All body surfaces	55	Lower extremity; predominantly female	1–5 yr	1–3	Palpable; somewhat irregular	Shades of brown, black, gray, pinkish; central or halo depigmentation	45–70
Nodular	30	All body surfaces	48	None	1–24 mo	1–2	Palpable nodule; regular	Regular bluish-black	25–50
Palmar-plantar mucosal	5	Palms, soles, mucous membrane	50	None	1–24 mo	1–2	Palpable nodule with irregular surrounding flat area	Black nodules irregularly colored macule	Mucosal < 10

[a] Period between first appearance of a nevus and clinical diagnosis of melanoma.
[b] Dependent on selection of invasive lesions.

mucous membranes, the palms and soles of the feet, is usually nodular with fairly sharply circumscribed margins and has only recently been defined. The declining prognosis in these four types of melanomas is described in Table 28.1.

LEVELS OF INVASION OF PRIMARY MELANOMA

All types of primary melanoma may be characterized by level of invasion into the dermis. An anatomic classification of such invasion includes 5 levels (Clark et al., 1975): Level I, an in situ and presumably premalignant lesion, contains tumor cells which are restricted to the dermoepidermal junction and do not penetrate the basement membrane of the epidermis; Level II contains neoplastic cells which have breeched the basement membrane and extended into the papillary dermis; Level III tumor extends to a somewhat ill defined interface between the papillary and reticular dermis; Level IV extends between the bundles of collagen fibers into the reticular dermis; and Level V shows invasion of subcutaneous tissues. As can be seen from Table 28.2, this leveling classification has significant prognostic implications. The same table shows a micrometric classification determined by measured extent of invasion from the basement membrane downward. Such thickness measurements (Breslow, 1970) probably are easier to relate to prognosis than anatomic leveling although racial, sex and anatomic differences may alter normal skin thickness to some extent.

STAGING

Staging of melanoma is critical for clinical therapy studies which hope to compare equivalent groups of patients treated in different ways. In Table 28.3, a four stage classification is indicated (Gutterman et al., 1978b; Nathanson, 1967a). It is most important to note the following points in this classification: (1) local disease must be distinguished prognostically from regional disease, (2) regional node involvement must be subdivided into clinical and histopathologic positive vs. clinically negative

TABLE 28.2
Melanoma: Levels of Invasion

Number	Depth (mm)	Incidence (%)	Approximate 5-Year Survival[a]	
			All primary sites	Extremity primary only
I	< 0.58	—	100	100
II	0.58	18	80	95
III	1.71	35	60	85
IV	3.31	38	35	65
V	7.02	9	15	?20

[a] With appropriate surgical excision.

TABLE 28.3
Staging and Prognosis of Malignant Melanoma

Stage	Primary Site[a]	
	Extremity	All other
0 "In situ"—corresponds to Level I melanoma	>95	>95
I Primary only (further staged by melanoma type and level)	25–95	15–70
A. Primary remaining	80	65
B. Primary excised		
C. Multiple primaries	85	70
II Local metastasis (<5 cm from primary site) (cutaneous and/or lymph node and/or subcutaneous)	50	35
III Regional metastases (≥5 cm from primary site)		
A. Intradermal (satellitosis)	25	15
B. Lymph nodes—clinical and pathologic	30	20
C. Lymph nodes—pathologic only		
IV Distant metastases		
A. Cutaneous	15	10
B. Lymph nodes	12	10
C. Soft tissue (subcutaneous, etc.)	8	8
D. Visceral	5	5

[a] In cases of multiple sites within a stage—use that with worst prognosis. Pathologic staging indicated by subscript "p".

and histopathologically positive categories, and (3) that patients with cutaneous, lymph node and soft tissue disease, at whatever stage, tend to have not only a superior survival, but also tend to be more responsive to chemotherapeutic treatment. Among visceral lesions, pulmonary lesions appear to be more responsive than lesions in liver, bone and brain, to chemotherapy. Melanoma may develop late recurrence, and although this occurs in a small minority of patients, one can demonstrate that patients who have survived 5 years with the disease have a decrement in survivorship from 5 to 10 years, which is approximately equal to that experienced in the first 5 years of the disease (Nathanson et al., 1967a). This clinical observation suggests the presence of host factors in the natural history of the disease, and emphasizes that restraint must be used in assuring patients, even though they may be disease-free for several years, that they are cured.

In order to stratify patients for chemotherapy studies into appropriate stages, a variety of techniques have been used to evaluate the extent of possible metastatic disease. The distribution of patients with recurrent disease is illustrated in Table 28.4 which estimates the percentage of patients in various stages of disease and how the natural history of the disease progresses. A routine workup in patients with early stage disease should include x-ray (posteroanterior (PA) and lateral) and possibly full

TABLE 28.4
Patterns of Development of Melanoma (All Numbers Are % Incidence)

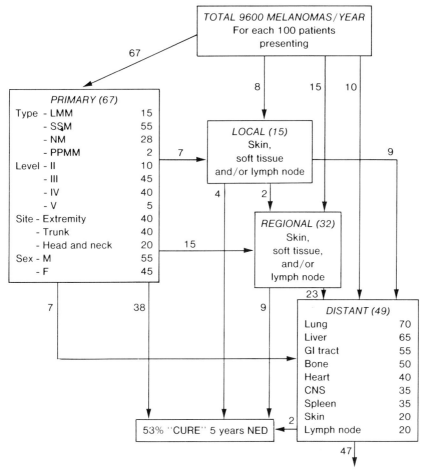

Note: All numbers on lines depicting natural history are in percentages of total patients presenting. Numbers in boxes labeled "Primary" or "Distant" are percentages of respective stages of disease only. "Primary" refers to patients who present with primary disease only. Note also that "5 years NED cure" rate is somewhat lower than the true value due to failure to exclude some non-melanoma deaths in melanoma patients.

lung tomography, as we have seen several patients in whom small lesions may be hidden behind the heart on the PA, adjacent to vertebral bodies on the lateral, etc. Thoracic computerized axial tomography (CAT) scanning may also be useful. Liver function tests are indicated, and although the yield is small in Stage I and II patients, liver-spleen scanning may be indicated in some patients. The presence of increased splenic uptake in some early stage patients appears to have an adverse prognostic significance (Nathanson et al., 1977). It may be related to splenic metastases, or to some remote effect of tumor presumably on the splenic reticuloendothelial system. In patients with lower extremity disease, especially those in whom positive lymph nodes are suspected, lower extremity lymphangiography (Musemeci et al., 1976) may be useful. Gastrointestinal (GI) films (which may demonstrate the characteristic bull's-eye lesion of melanoma metastatic to the bowel wall) are indicated in any patient with occult GI bleeding. Gallium scanning is of use in some patients for delineating unsuspected lesions anyplace in the body, as may be body CAT scanning. Bone marrow aspiration may also be helpful in any patient with suspected bone pain or positive bone scan. Urinary melanogens are positive in about 25% of patients with metastatic disease, but when negative are not helpful. This technique consists of adding a few drops of urine to a saturated solution of sodium ultroterrocyamide to glacial acetic acid and potassium hydroxide in that order. A blue-green color indicates positivity.

A variety of types of melanoma may require specialized therapeutic approaches. Prepubertal melanoma, melanoma seen in pregnancy (Shiu et al., 1976), melanoma spread by transplacental metastases (Trazak et al., 1975), ocular melanoma (uvula tract or ciliary body) (Davidorf and Lang, 1975), melanoma of the mucous membranes of mouth, anus or genitalia, and melanoma of the intestinal tract, upper respiratory tract, or brain may require specialized chemotherapeutic approaches. When relapse in these sites occurs following a long disease-free interval, the disease appears to pursue essentially as aggressive a course as it does in patients with rapid onset of metastatic disease.

SURGICAL THERAPY

It should be emphasized that the therapy of choice for all primary melanoma is surgical (Conrad, 1972; Davis, 1971). Following total excisional biopsy of the primary lesion, a histologic diagnosis of invasive melanoma (Levels III, IV, V) should indicate subsequent radical re-excision with 3–4 cm of free margin around the excised lesion, with grafting of the excision defect. A 1–2-cm free margin will suffice for Level II lesions (Balch et al., 1979). Publication of two major prospective randomized studies of regional node dissection in either extremity primary lesions, or other primary sites of melanoma, has failed to demonstrate any survival advantage resulting from early or prophylactic, regional lymph node dissection (Veronesi et al., 1977; Sim et al., 1978). In one study, there was a suggestion of benefit in patients with Level IV primary lesions (Veronesi et al., 1977). However, this benefit did not achieve statistical significance. If benefit is eventually demonstrated as a result of prophylactic regional node dissection in a subgroup of melanoma patients, it is likely that that degree of benefit will not be great. The use of regional node dissection to decrease the bulk of tumor in patients with clinically positive (or perhaps some high risk patients with clinically negative, e.g., Level V) lymph nodes, may well be justifiable, particularly where subsequent chemotherapy or chemoimmunotherapy is contemplated. Such surgery may also be indicated for staging purposes in selected patients. A very small group of Stage IV patients in whom (1) single distant metastases in lung (Cahan, 1973), brain and elsewhere have been identified; (2) who are young; (3) in whom the primary lesion is controlled; (4) in whom free interval is long (greater than 1 year); and (5) doubling time of the tumor appears to be slow (greater than 40 days), there may be a place for surgical removal of such distant disease (Holmes et al., 1977; Vidne et al., 1976). In general, however, such a procedure should be accompanied by some systemic form of therapy since cure will rarely be achieved by such a procedure.

RADIOTHERAPY

Conventional radiotherapy has proved to be relatively ineffective in controlling melanoma; several recent techniques have suggested that this approach may be more useful in the future. These techniques include high fraction doses of conventional gamma radiation radiotherapy (greater than 600 rads per dose) (Habermalz and Fischer, 1976); a combination of hyperthermia with radiotherapy; the use of high Let particle radiotherapy such as neutrons and pi mesons; or the use of radiosensitizing drugs. Although there are fragmentary data relative to all of these techniques, none has yet been proven to be clinically effective, and all will have to be studied further. Radiotherapy is predominantly used in melanoma with multiple CNS metastases, and there its effectiveness is marginal.

CHEMOTHERAPY

Methods of systemic therapy for disseminated melanoma may be categorized as follows:

1. Cytotoxic chemotherapy
2. Experimental chemotherapy
   a. Immunotherapy or chemoimmunotherapy
   b. Antipigmentary chemotherapy
   c. Hormonal therapy.

Of the above categories of treatment, cytotoxic chemotherapy and immunotherapy, although controversial, have fairly well defined data concerning efficacy. In antipigmentary chemotherapy and hormonal therapy, however, we have only experimental data to go on, and must look to the future for further definition of these techniques.

Cytotoxic Chemotherapy

In the discussion of chemotherapy only commercially available drugs will be mentioned in detail. Recent reviews should be consulted (Benjamin, 1975; Luce, 1975; Comis, 1974; Carter, 1976).

Principles of Chemotherapy. In order to evaluate the relative effectiveness of a large variety of chemotherapeutic regimens which have been employed to treat malignant melanoma, one must establish appropriate criteria for subjective or objective response in these patients. These criteria are somewhat variable in the studies to be reported, although the usual criteria for objective response is that of a 50% or greater reduction in surface area (profile of 3-dimensional lesions) of all measurable lesions for at least 1 month. Complete response indicates the disappearance of all clinically demonstrable disease. Duration of survival is obviously the most precise index of therapeutic efficacy, and both single and multiple drug programs described below have all been demonstrated to achieve superior survival in responding vs. nonresponding patients. Unfortunately, cross comparison of survival in total patient populations treated with specific single agents depends very much on the selection of patients and is frequently difficult. When such comparison is carried out, it is clear that single drug chemotherapy in this disease, at best, produces modest prolongation of mean survival (weeks or a few months) when compared to no treatment at all (Comis, 1976; Luce, 1975). Few if any single drug programs have been shown to produce median survival greater than 6 months in patients with disseminated disease. A number of general criteria of responsiveness have been suggested which include (Nathanson et al., 1971; Costanza et al., 1977): patients who are initially ambulatory (good performance status), female sex, have only soft tissue disease or a small number of visceral metastatic sites involved, are under 60 years of age, have not had prior chemotherapy or radiotherapy, have a normal hemogram, normal hepatic and renal function, and no central nervous system metastases. Thus, in weighing the chance of benefit against the risk of toxicity, all these factors should be kept in mind in selecting therapy for a given patient. There is no question that some patients who fall into several adverse prognostic categories may be more likely harmed than benefited by chemotherapy. Patients in whom such extensive disease exists that destruction of parenchymal organs is beyond the point of reversibility, clearly are not candidates for drug therapy. Nor, probably, are patients whose expected survival is less than 2–3 months. Histologic diagnosis of disease is a mandatory prerequisite for treatment.

A variety of cytokinetic studies have been carried out which may be helpful in selecting agents, or combinations of agents, with therapeutic value in melanoma. It has been suggested that humans can be classified according to the predominant pattern of DNA synthesis in the slowly proliferating cell fraction (Shackney, 1976). This classification scheme would group melanoma and carcinoma of the lung together in an intermediary classification between the slowest growing tumors such as breast and ovarian carcinoma and the most rapid ones such as acute myelogenous leukemia. Kinetic characteristics and drug response behavior may, under some circumstances, be related. Labeling index and/or cell labeling intensity may serve as useful guides to drug scheduling under some special circumstances (Shirakawa et al., 1970; Durie et al., 1977). By computer analysis techniques median duration G_2 phase of 5.3 hours and S phase of 21 hours have been obtained in human melanoma. Generation times (T_c) are highly variable with a median of 3 days. Growth fractions of 20–30% have been calculated and theoretical tumor generation time, as calculated from T_c and growth fracture, are found to be much shorter than the actual doubling time, indicating cell loss of approximately 70% in melanoma patients. Most doubling time (time for in vivo volume doubling) studies obtained from clinical analysis of growth of pulmonary and other metastatic lesions in patients, suggest 4–16 weeks doubling times with a median of approximately 8 weeks. DNA histograms on tissue obtained at biopsy have also been used as a source of predictive data for chemotherapeutic sensitivity (Schumann and Göhde, 1977). Recently the in vitro technique of stem cell cloning in soft agar (Salmon et al., 1978) has been utilized to predict in vivo tumor cell sensitivity in melanoma with preliminary success (unpublished data). A clear-cut relationship between the rate of generation of melanoma cells, rate of cell loss, growth fraction and the mechanism of cytotoxic drug effect or their antitumor efficacy has not been well demonstrated. However, the combination of single agents which are phase specific with those that are not has much influenced the design of combinations of cytotoxic agents (Comis and Carter, 1974). Animal models of melanoma including B-16, Fortner, Cloudman, S-91, and Harding Passay have also been of some value (Mabel et al., 1977) although overall such data have not been widely applied in practice.

Systemic Single Drug Therapy. A list of single cytotoxic chemotherapeutic agents currently available, which have antitumor activity in this disease, are noted in Table 28.5 with approximate expected objective response rates, and duration of response (Luce, 1975; Benjamin et al., 1975; Comis, 1976; Carter et al., 1976). Of these, the most commonly used are DTIC (Ahmann, 1976; Ahmann et al., 1974; Bellet et al., 1976; Burke et al., 1971; Costanza, 1976a, 1976b; Costanza et al., 1972; Johnson et al., 1976) and the nitrosoureas (Ahmann et al., 1974; Bellet et al., 1976; Falkson et al., 1972; Hoogstraten et al., 1973). Whereas DTIC must be

TABLE 28.5
Summary of Active Single Drug Studies in Malignant Melanoma

Chemical Name	Trivial or Trade Name	Objective Response (%)	Dose/Route
Cell cycle nonspecific:			
Phenylalanine mustard	PAM; melphalan	15	0.1–0.3 mg/kg/d PO to toxicity
Cyclophosphamide	Cytoxan	15	3 mg/kg/d PO 10–20 mg/kg/wk IV
Triethylenethiophosphoramide	Thio-TEPA; TSPA	15	0.5 mg/kg/wk IV
Actinomycin D	Dactinomycin	17	0.012–0.020 mg/kg/d for 5 days q 3 wk IV
Procarbazine	Matulane	15	50–100 mg/m²/d PO
Dimethyl-triazenoimidazole carboxamide	Dacarbazine; DTIC	20	200–250 mg/m²/d for 5 days q 3 wk IV *or* 650–950 mg/m² q 6 wk IV
Cyclohexylchloroethyl Nitrosourea	CeeNU; lomustine	20	100–130 mg/m² q 6 wk PO single dose
bis-Chloroethyl nitrosurea	BiCNU; carmustine	20	100–150 mg/m² q 3–6 wk IV single dose
S-Phase specific:			
Hydroxyurea	Hydrea	10	1000–1500 mg/m²/d PO
Mitotic inhibitors:			
Vincristine	Oncovin	15	0.015–0.03 mg/kg/wk IV
Vinblastine	Velban	20	0.1–0.3 mg/kg/wk IV

used intravenously, the nitrosoureas include both intravenous drugs such as BCNU and oral drugs such as CCNU or methyl-CCNU. DTIC is usually used in 3–5-day intravenous courses or in single doses every 3 weeks (Cowan and Bergsagel, 1971). The nitrosoureas are given in single doses approximately every 4–6 weeks because of delayed marrow suppression. Objective response rates for the alkylating agents (Nathanson et al., 1967a), vinca alkaloids (Ahmann et al., 1974; Bellet et al., 1976; Carter and Livingston, 1976; Chanes et al., 1971), actinomycin D (Chanes et al., 1971; Gerner et al., 1973) and procarbazine (Nordman and Mantyla, 1977), appear to be somewhat lower than those of DTIC or nitrosoureas.

Toxicity of these agents is variable. DTIC has predominantly GI toxicity, whereas the nitrosoureas are predominantly marrow suppressive. The vinca alkaloids, of course, are neurotoxic and other agents including actinomycin D and procarbazine exhibit both GI and marrow suppressive activity. Hydroxyurea is also mainly marrow suppressive.

The mechanisms of action of these drugs is variable and they are grouped according to the cytokinetic action in Table 28.5. This grouping is chosen to suggest the possibility that some of these agents may be combined in ways that make possible toxicities that are nonadditive and mechanisms of action which are diverse, so that either additive, or even possibly synergistic, actions may be obtained as a result of such combinations.

Systemic Drug Combinations. The best response rates and survival reported in the polychemotherapy (Comis and Carter, 1974; Beretta, 1976a, 1976b; Carmo-Pereira et al., 1976; Carter et al., 1976; Cohen et al., 1977; Coltman et al., 1971; Costanzi et al., 1975; Costanzi 1976a; DeWasch et al., 1976; Gardere et al., 1972; Gerner et al., 1973; McKelvey et al., 1977a, 1977b; Moon et al., 1975; Nordman and Mantyla, 1977; Wittes et al., 1978) trials in melanoma are those achieved by the combination of DTIC, BCNU (or methyl-CCNU or CCNU) and hydroxyurea ("BHD" or "MHD") (Table 28.6). This drug combination has been reported to produce a 27% objective response rate with a median survival of 5–6 months in patients, all of whom present with disseminated malignancy (Costanzi, 1976b). A similar drug combination "MHD" described below attempts to utilize the pharmacokinetic properties of these drugs by starting out with an S-phase specific agent, hydroxyurea. Eight hours following this drug dose, a significant increase in a cell population may result either at the G_1S interphase or in the G_2 phase. These cells then might be expected to be more sensitive to a nitrosourea, methyl-CCNU, as these are the sites of its predominant action in the cell cycle. Following the first dose of the nitrosourea, the remaining cells are then exposed to DTIC which is administered on the second to fifth days of the schedule. This drug has both an alkylating agent-like (phase nonspecific) as well as

TABLE 28.6
Combination Chemotherapy of Malignant Melanoma

I. BHD or MHD Regimen[a]

a)	Hydroxyurea	800–1400 mg/m²/d	d 1–5	q 3 wk	PO
b)	BCNC	100–150 mg/m²	d 1	q 6 wk	IV
	CCNU or Me-CCNU	100–150 mg/m²	d 1	q 6 wk	PO
c)	DTIC	100–150 mg/m²/d	d 1–5 or d 2–5	q 3 wk	IV

II. VAP Regimen[b]

a)	Vinblastine	5.0 mg/m²	d 1, 8	q 4 wk	IV
b)	Actinomycin D	0.5 mg/m²	d 1, 8	q 4 wk	IV
c)	Procarbazine	100 mg/m²	d 1–10	q 4 wk	PO

III. CVP Regimen[c]

a)	Cyclophosphamide	1000 mg/m²	d 1	q 3 wk	IV
b)	Vincristine	1.4 mg/m²	d 1	q 3 wk	IV
c)	Procarbazine	100 mg/m²	d 1–7	q 3 wk	PO

[a] Costanzi et al. (1975); Nathanson and Schoenfeld (1978).
[b] Perlin et al. (1975).
[c] Byrne (1976).

an antimetabolic (phase specific) activity as an inhibitor of purine biosynthesis. Whether this type of schedule makes optimal use of these three drugs is still not clear but a rather disappointing 20% objective response rate has been reported (Nathanson and Schoenfeld, 1978). The addition of vincristine to the three drugs, making it a four drug combination, might be logical because of its mechanism of activity as a mitotic inhibitor. Recent studies have suggested that vincristine, however, does not increase the response rate very much, although it may slightly increase median survival (Costanzi et al., 1975). Additional drug combinations for patients who have failed on the "MHD" combination include the combinations of either vinblastine, actinomycin D, and procarbazine (VAP), or Cytoxan, vincristine, procarbazine (CVP) with objective response rates of 20–30% (Table 28.6).

The importance of applying a constructively critical approach to this literature is emphasized by random choice of two examples. The premature prediction of an approximate 43-week median survival in melanoma with disseminated disease treated with "BHD" (Costanzi et al., 1975) was eventually followed by a reported median survival of about 21 weeks (Costanzi, 1976b, 1978) and the prediction of an objective response rate of 38% with a vinblastine, procarbazine and actinomycin D combination (Perlin et al., 1975) had a follow-up response rate of 22% (Kostinas et al., 1978).

Regional Chemotherapy. In patients with anatomically localized disease, the perfusion of an isolated arteriovenous circuit, with extracorporeal pump oxygenation, and recirculation of a chemotherapeutic agent, with or without hyperthermia (Stehlin et al., 1975) may be effective (Hersh et al., 1973). Drugs that have been traditionally used include the alkylating agents, such as phenylalanine mustard (L-PAM) or triethylenethiophosphoramide (thio-TEPA). However, more recently, DTIC (Costanzi, 1978) and the nitrosoureas have been used by an intra-arterial infusion system, and it is possible that these drugs may also be applied using the perfusion technique; DTIC being somewhat labile would require special care. Whether this technique is of benefit in patients in Stage I melanoma is still controversial (Sugarbaker and McBride, 1976). The intra-arterial infusion technique has been most often used for diseases in the liver (Costanzi, 1978) and in the lower extremities (Einhorn et al., 1973). The rate and duration of objective response appear to be somewhat better for infusion and perfusion than they are for conventional intravenous therapy. In patients with metastases in the central nervous system, the use of nitrosoureas, agents which are lipophilic, hence cross the blood-brain barrier, may be of some help (Costanza et al., 1972). However, CNS metastases rarely respond to any single agent chemotherapy.

Intracavitary (particularly intrapleural) chemotherapy has been employed in some patients using either triethylenethiophosphoramide (Dollinger, 1972) or sclerosing agents such as quinicrine (Dollinger, 1972) or tetracycline (Robinson and Bolooki, 1972). Introduction of a chest tube with total drainage of the pleural effusion prior to the use of such a chemotherapeutic approach is critical if good results are to be obtained. Furthermore, in most such patients repeated introduction of at least two to three doses of such chemotherapy at several days' intervals, clamping the tube approximately 24 hours after the introduction of each agent, yields a significantly high likelihood of prevention of subsequent recurrence of the effusion.

Adjuvant Chemotherapy. The use of DTIC (Hill et al., 1978) and polychemotherapy (Jacquillat et al., 1976) have both been evaluated in patients with surgical removal of all clinically demonstrable disease, with either deeply invasive primary melanoma or regional lymph node metastases, who are at high risk for recurrence. The largest trial of DTIC alone has failed to suggest that it either delays recurrence, or decreases rate of recurrence, in such patients (Hill et al., 1978). A polychemotherapy study, however, has been reported to decrease recurrence rate on a preliminary analysis (Jacquillat et al., 1976). Chemoimmunotherapy as an adjuvant has also been explored in a number of trials. The results of these trials are as yet inconclusive but, as will be discussed below, they show significant promise.

Experimental Chemotherapy

Immunotherapy. Immunotherapy so far tested in melanoma primarily consists of nonspecific active immunotherapy utilizing agents including BCG (Gutterman et al., 1975; Nathanson, 1972, 1974), *Corynebacterium parvum* (Presant et al., 1978; Gutterman et al., 1977), or levamisol (Spitler et al., 1978). A form of immunotherapy peculiarly appropriate to patients with intradermal satellitosis in melanoma is intralesional BCG (Nathanson, 1972, 1974). This therapy may, in fact, constitute specific active immunotherapy because it introduces a nonspecific adjuvant directly in contact with tumor cells. It produces complete regression (including noninjected lesions) in 20% and clinically useful regression in another 60% of such patients.

No large studies with specific active immunotherapeutic reagents have been carried out, and in small studies the results have been highly controversial (McIllmurray et al., 1977; Simmons et al., 1978). Randomized, prospective studies of patients with high risk (Level III, IV, V) Stage I melanoma have included both positive (Beretta, 1978; Kaufman et al., 1978) and negative (Cunningham et al., 1978) results. Among the prospective nonrandomized studies in node positive patients (Stage III) one has suggested that BCG appears to delay onset of recurrence (Eilber et al., 1976) but in a subsequent randomized verson (Morton et al., 1978) the addition of a specific tumor cell preparation, together with BCG, did not further increase the effectiveness. In the Eastern Cooperative Oncology Group (ECOG) study (Cunningham et al., 1978), the largest carried out to date in a prospective and randomized format, little difference in recurrence rate has been demonstrated between BCG and BCG plus DTIC in poor risk Stages I, II, or III (regional node positive) patients. This data, however, is incompletely analyzed at the time of this review.

Studies of chemoimmunotherapy have either been in the adjuvant role following surgical excision of all clinically demonstrable disease, or in patients with disseminated metastases trying to optimize the immunosuppressive and augmentative effects (Cheema and Hersh, 1971). Two prospective randomized studies have compared BCG with or without DTIC in Stages I and III patients and have suggested optimal benefit of chemoimmunotherapy (Kaufman et al., 1978; Beretta, 1978). Use of chemoimmunotherapy in advanced disease has undergone several trials which have been suggested by their authors to demonstrate the additive effects of BCG when given with single or multiple drug chemotherapy (Gutterman et al., 1973, 1976, 1978a). These trials, although large, were not randomized. Randomized trials have, in general, failed to demonstrate that BCG increases objective response rates achieved by chemotherapy alone. However, a distinct suggestion of increased survival in BCG treated patients has been reported in these same studies (Nathanson and Schoenfeld, 1978; Costanza, 1976b). Other prospective randomized trials are underway at this time but have failed to suggest any additional benefit when an immunoadjuvant is added to chemotherapy (Kostinas et al., 1978; Costanzi, 1978; Mastrangelo, 1978a, 1978b). Toxicity of BCG is generally tolerable but may on occasion be serious or life threatening (Norton et al., 1978).

One might make the following generalizations about the significance of data currently available:

1. The use of active adjuvant immunotherapy or chemoimmunotherapy in early melanoma has shown evidence of benefit in well designed studies, but further data is needed to confirm this observation;
2. The degree of benefit exhibited is of a low order of magnitude making it difficult to separate out statistically significant effects;
3. The addition of chemotherapy to immunotherapy may be a technique which has significant advantages over the use of either modality alone, especially in the adjuvant setting; and
4. The use of chemoimmunotherapy in patients with advanced disease is controversial, although it may produce modest benefit when properly used.

The use of passive immunotherapy, that is, the transfusion of preformed humeral antibody or immunocompetent lymphocytes, or a factor derived from it, has also been tested in melanoma. For example, transfer factor (Greco, 1976), Thymosin and serum from black patients, which has been stated to be high in "unblocking factor" in vitro (Wright et al., 1978), have been clinically used in the disease. Whether these materials confer cellular or humeral immunity to melanoma associated antigens upon patients in whom they are transfused, or whether they in fact clinically benefit melanoma patients at any stage in the disease is still uncertain.

Antipigmentary Chemotherapy. This approach has been based upon the premise that certain compounds which interfere with pigment cell metabolism in the melanocyte may also interfere with respiration and/or growth of malignant pigmented cells. Initially, several methods were used to inhibit tyrosinase, the key enzyme in pigment biosynthesis. These methods included (1) depletion of the normal substrates for melanin pigment (tyrosine and phenylalanine) (Demopoulos, 1966); (2) the use of competitive inhibitors of tyrosinase such as α-methyltyrosine or phenyllactate (Demopoulos, 1965); (3) chelators of copper, a component of tyrosinase, with penicillamine or triethylene tetramine dihydrochloride; (4) the use of phosphodiesterase inhibitors, such as caffeine or aminophylline (Wick, 1977); (5) the use of various compounds such as 6-hydroxy-DOPA (Wick and Byers, 1977) or isopropyl catechol (Bleehan, 1976) which may be oxidized by tyrosinase to free radicals; or (6) the coupling of compounds which may have specific target affinity for melanocytes such as melanocyte-stimulating hormone coupled to daunomycin (Varga et al., 1977). Several of these approaches have been shown to have significant inhibitory properties for cell growth or replication in vitro or even inhibition of DNA synthesis (Wick and Ratliff, 1978). Others, including α-methyltyrosine (Voorhees, 1971), mimosine (Nathanson et al., 1977), or α-methyl-DOPA (Wick and Ratliff, 1978) may also have antitumor activity in vivo in B-16 melanoma or other animal tumors. None have, as yet, undergone clinical trials.

Hormonal Therapy. Clinical features of melanoma including the rarity of the disease in pre-pubertal children, the occasional regression of tumor following term pregnancy, the superior survival of premenopausal women, and the normal sensitivity of melanocytes to MSH, have all suggested that endocrine influences may affect growth of malignant melanocytes (Nathanson et al., 1967a). This effort has received some recent encouragement from the observation that tumors from some melanoma patients may contain estrogen binding protein receptors (Fisher et al., 1976). The proportion of melanoma patients in whom such receptors are present is still debated, but the use of estrogen (Fisher et al., 1978) and estracyt (Didolkar et al., 1978) have both been employed in the treatment of melanoma patients. One study has shown objective responses in 2 of 18 patients with melanoma on diethylstilbesterol but both were patients with soft tissue or nodal disease, and neither had estrogen binding protein receptors (Fisher et al., 1978). In another study estramustine phosphate responses were observed in 4 of 20 patients (Didolkar et al., 1978). These responses were primarily in females and, of course, because this drug is a complex of estradiol and nitrogen mustard, the nitrogen mustard alone could have accounted for the observed responses. Antitumor hormones need further study, particularly with reference to the use of such compounds in a polychemotherapy program.

SUMMARY

In summary, melanoma is a disease which has a high potential for cure when early diagnosis is possible. When dissemination occurs, it may take place through lymph node, hematogenous or combined routes of dissemination. The clinical characteristics of patients with disseminated disease who are likely to respond to chemotherapy may give important clues concerning indications, and contraindications for the use of such systemic therapy. Single agent chemotherapy in general produces low response rates with relatively short durations of response. Polychemotherapy has increased response rates up to the 35–40% range but median survival in such patients still remains in the 8–12 month range. The addition of immunotherapy, antipigmentary chemotherapy, hormone therapy, or new radiotherapy programs, is still being evaluated. Occasionally, localized manifestations of disseminated tumor may be treated with surgery, radiotherapy, infusion or perfusion chemotherapy, intracavitary chemotherapy, or steroids. Although a number of new research leads look promising, available therapy for disseminated malignant melanoma is still largely unsatisfactory.

REFERENCES

Ahmann, D. L. Nitrosoureas in the management of disseminated malignant melanoma. Cancer Treat. Rep., 60: 747–751, 1976.

Ahmann, D. L., Hahn, R. G., and Bisel, H. F. Evaluation of MeCCNU versus combined DTIC and vincristine in palliation of disseminated malignant melanoma. Cancer, 33: 615–618, 1974.

Anderson, D. E. Clinical characteristics of the genetic variety of cutaneous melanoma in man. Cancer, 28: 721–725, 1971.

Balch, C. K., Murad, T. M., Soong, S., Griffin, A. L., Richards, P. C., and Maddox, W. A. Tumor thickness as a guide to surgical management of clinical stage I melanoma patients. Cancer 43: 883–888, 1979.

Bellet, R. E., Mastrangelo, M. J., Laucius, J. F., and Bodurtha, A. J. Randomized prospective trials of DTIC (NSC-45388) alone versus BCNU (NSC-409962) plus vincristine (NSC-67574) in the treatment of metastatic malignant melanoma. Cancer Treat. Rep., 70; 595–601, 1976.

Benjamin, R. S., Gutterman, J. Y., McKelvey, E. M., Einhorn, L. M., Livingston, R. B., and Gottlieb, J. A. Systemic chemotherapy for melanoma. In Neoplasms of the Skin and Malignant Melanoma, pp. 460–471. Year Book Medical Publishers, Chicago, 1975.

Beretta, G., Bonadonna, G., Bajetta, E., Tancini, G., DeLena, M., Azzarelli, A., and Veronesi, U. Combination chemotherapy with DTIC (NSC-45388) in advanced malignant melanoma, soft tissue sarcomas, and Hodgkin's disease. Cancer Treat. Rep., 60: 205–211, 1976a.

Beretta, G., Bonadonna, G., Cascinelli, N., Morabito, A., and Veronesi, U. Comparative evaluation of three combination regimens for advanced malignant melanoma; results of an international cooperative study. Cancer Treat. Rep., 60: 33–40, 1976b.

Beretta, G. Controlled study for prolonged chemotherapy, immunotherapy, and chemotherapy plus immunotherapy as an adjuvant to surgery in stage I–II malignant melanoma: Preliminary report. In Immunotherapy of Cancer: Present Status of Trials in Man, edited by W. D. Terry and D. Windhorst, p. 65. Raven Press, New York, 1978.

Bleehen, S. S. Selective lethal effect of substituted phenols in cell cultures of malignant melanocytes. In Pigment Cell Melanomas: Basic Properties and Clinical Behavior. Proceedings of the 9th International Pigment Cell Conference, edited by B. Riley. Karger, Basel, 1976.

Blois, M. S. Urinary melanogens—correlations of multiple metabolites with clinical disease. Cancer Res., 36: 3317–3322, 1976.

Breslow, A. Thickness, cross sectional areas and depth of invasion in the prognosis of melanoma. Ann. Surg., 172: 902–908, 1970.

Burke, P. J., McCarthy, W. H., and Milton, G. W. Imidazole carboxamide therapy in advanced malignant melanoma. Cancer, *27:* 744–750, 1971.

Byrne, M. J. Cyclophosphamide, vincristine, and procarbazine in the treatment of malignant melanoma. Cancer, *38:* 1922–1924, 1976.

Cahan, W. G. Excision of melanoma metastases to lung. Ann. Surg., *178:* 703–709, 1973.

Carmo-Pereira, J., Costa, F. O., and Pimentel, P. Combination cytotoxic chemotherapy for metastatic cutaneous malignant melanoma with DTIC, BCNU, and vincristine. Cancer Treat. Rep., *60:* 1381–1384, 1976.

Carter, R. D., Krements, E. T., Hill, G. J. II, Metter, G. E., Fletcher, W. S., Golomb, F. M., Grage, T. B., Minton, J. P., and Sparks, F. C. DTIC (NSC-45388) and combination therapy for melanoma. I. Studies with DTIC, BCNU (NSC-409962), CCNU (NSC-79037), vincristine (NSC-67574), and hydroxyurea (MSC-32065). Cancer Treat. Rep., *60:* 601–610, 1976a.

Carter, S. K., and Livingston, R. B. Plant products in cancer chemotherapy. Cancer Treat. Rep., *60:* 1141–1156, 1976b.

Chanes, R. E., Condit, P. T., Bottomley, R. H., and Misimblat, W. Combined actinomycin D and vincristine in the treatment of patients with cancer. Cancer, *27:* 613–617, 1971.

Cheema, A. R., and Hersh, E. M. Patient survival after chemotherapy and its relationship to in vivo lymphocyte blastogenesis. Cancer, *28:* 851–855, 1971.

Clark, W. H., and Mihm, M. C. Moles and malignant melanoma. *In* Dermatology in General Medicine, Chap. 2, edited by T. B. Fitzpatrick, K. A. Arndt, W. H. Clark, et al. McGraw Hill, New York, 1971.

Clark, W. H., Ainsworth, A. M., Bernardino, E. A., Yang, C. H., Mihm, M. C., and Reed, R. J. Developmental biology of primary human malignant melanoma. Semin. Oncol., *2:* 83–104, 1975.

Cohen, S. M., Greenspan, E. M., Ratner, L. H., and Weiner, M. J. Combination chemotherapy of malignant melanoma with imidazole carboxamide, BCNU and vincristine. Cancer, *39:* 41–44, 1977.

Coltman, E. A., Jr., Costanzi, J. J., Dudley, G. M., Haut, A., Lane, M., and Gehan, E. A. Further clinical studies of combination chemotherapy using cyclophosphamide, vincristine, methotrexate and 5-flourouracil in solid tumors. Am. J. Med. Sci., *261:* 73–78, 1971.

Comis, R. L. DTIC (NSC-45388) in malignant melanoma; a perspective. Cancer Treat. Rep., *60:* 165–172, 1976.

Comis, R. L., and Carter, S. K. Integration of chemotherapy into combined modality of solid tumors; IV. Malignant melanoma. Cancer Treat. Rep., *1:* 285–304, 1974.

Conrad, F. G. Treatment of malignant melanoma, wide excision alone vs. lymphadenectomy. Arch. Surg., *104:* 587–593, 1972.

Costanzi, J. J. DTIC (NSC-45388) studies in the Southwest Oncology Group. Cancer Treat. Rep., *60:* 189–192, 1976a.

Costanzi, J. J. Combination chemoimmunotherapy for disseminated malignant melanoma (DMM). Proc. Am. Soc. Clin. Oncol., *17:* 241, 1976b.

Costanzi, J. J. Chemotherapy and BCG in the treatment of disseminated malignant melanoma. *In* Chemotherapy and BCG in the Treatment of Disseminated Malignant Melanoma, edited by W. D. Terry and D. Windhorst, p. 87. Raven Press, New York, 1978.

Costanzi, J. J., Vaitkevicius, V. K., Quagliana, J. M., Hoogstraten, B., Coltman, C. A., and Delaney, F. C. Combination chemotherapy for disseminated malignant melanoma. Cancer, *35:* 342–346, 1975.

Costanza, M. E., Nathanson, L., Wolter, J., Lenhard, R., Taylor, S., Colsky, J., Oberfield, R. A., and Schilling, A. Therapy of malignant melanoma with an imidazole carboxamine and bis-chloroethyl-1-nitrosourea. Cancer, *30:* 1457–1461, 1972.

Costanza, M. E., Nathanson, L., Costello, W. G., Wolter, J., Brunk, S. F., Colsky, J., Hall,

T., Oberfield, R. A. and Regelson, W. Results of a randomized study comparing DTIC with TIC mustard in malignant melanoma. Cancer, *37:* 1654–1659, 1976.

Costanza, M. E., Nathanson, L., Schoenfeld, D., Wolter, J., Colsky, J., Regelson, W., Cunningham, R., and Sedransk, N. Results with methyl-CCNU and DTIC in metastatic melanoma. Cancer *40:* 1010–1015, 1977.

Cowan, D. H., and Bergsagel, D. E. Intermittent treatment of metastatic malignant melanoma with high dose 5-(3,3-dimethyl-l-triazeno) imidazole-4-carboxamide (NSC-45388). Cancer Chemother. Rep., *55:* 175–181, 1971.

Cunningham, T. J., Schoenfeld, E., Nathanson, L., Wolter, J., Patterson, W. B., and Cohen, M. H. A controlled study of adjuvant therapy in patients with stage I and II malignant melanoma. *In* Immunotherapy of Cancer: Present Status of Trials in Man, edited by W. D. Terry and D. Windhorst, p. 19. Raven Press, New York, 1978.

Demopoulos, H. B. Effects of reducing the phenylalanine-tyrosine intake of patients with advanced malignant melanoma. Cancer, *19:* 657–664, 1966.

Demopoulos, H. B., Gerving, M. A., and Bagdoyan, H. Selective inhibition of growth and respiration of melanomas by tyrosinase inhibitors. J. Natl. Cancer Inst., *35:* 823–827, 1965.

Davidorf, F. H., and Lang, J. R. Natural history of malignant melanoma of the carotid; small vs. large tumors. Trans. Am. Acad. Ophthalmol. Otolaryngol., *79:* op310–op320, 1975.

Davis, N. C. Elective lymph node dissection for melanoma. Br. J. Surg., *58:* 820–823, 1971.

DeVita, V. T., Jr., and Fisher, R. I. Natural history of malignant melanoma as related to therapy. Cancer Treat. Rep., *60:* 153–157, 1976.

DeWasch, G., Bernheim, J., Michel, J., Lejeune, F., and Kenis, Y. Combination chemotherapy with three marginally effective agents, CCNU, vincristine, and bleomycin, in the treatment of stage III melanoma. Cancer Treat. Rep., *60:* 1273–1276, 1976.

Didolkar, M. S., Catane, R., Lopex, R., and Holyoke, E. D. Estramustine phosphate (estracyt) in advanced malignant melanoma resistant to DTIC treatment. Proc. Am. Soc. Clin. Oncol., *19:* 381, 1978.

Dollinger, M. R. Management of recurrent malignant effusions. CA *22:* 138–147, 1972.

Durie, B. G. M., Vaught, L., and Salmon, S. E. Prognostic significance of tritiated thymidine labeling index (L.I.) in multiple myeloma and acute myeloid leukemia. Proc. Am. Assoc. Cancer Res., *18:* 80, 1977.

Eilber, F. T., Morton, D. L., Holmes, E. M., Sparks, F. C., and Ramming, K. P. Adjuvant immunotherapy with BCG in treatment of regional lymph-node metastases from melanoma. N. Engl. J. Med., *294:* 237–240, 1976.

Einhorn, L. H., McBride, C. M., Luce, J. K., Caoli, E., and Gottlieb, J. A. Intra-arterial infusion therapy with DTIC for malignant melanoma. Cancer, *32:* 749–755, 1973.

Elwood, J. M., and Lee, J. A. H. Recent data on the epidemiology of malignant melanoma. Semin. Oncol., *2:* 149–154, 1975.

Falkson, G., van der Merwe, A. M., and Falkson, H. C. Clinical experience with BCNU in the treatment of metastatic malignant melanoma. Cancer Chemother. Rep., *56:* 671, 1972.

Fisher, R. I., Neifeld, J. P., and Lippman, M. E. Estrogen receptors in human malignant melanoma. Lancet, *2:* 337, 1976.

Fisher, R. I., Young, R. C., and Lippman, M. E. Diethylstilbesterol therapy of surgically non-resectable malignant melanoma. Proc. Am. Soc. Clin. Oncol., *19:* 339, 1978.

Fitzpatrick, T. B., Quevedo, W. C., Szabo, G., and Seiji, M. The melanocyte system. *In* Dermatology in General Medicine, edited by T. B. Fitzpatrick, K. A. Arndt, W. H. Clark, et al., Chap. 18. McGraw-Hill, New York, 1971.

Gardere, S., Hussain, S., and Cowan, D. H. Treatment of malignant melanoma with the combination of DTIC, cyclophosphamide and vincristine. Cancer Chemother. Rep., *56:* 357–362, 1972.

Gerner, R. E., Moore, G. E., and Didolkar, M. S. Chemotherapy of disseminated malignant melanoma with DTIC and dactinomycin. Cancer, *32:* 756–760, 1973.

Greco, R. S. Application of transfer factor to clinical immunotherapy. Surg. Gynecol. Obstet., *142:* 765–778, 1976.

Gutterman, J. U., McBride, C., Freireich, E. J. Active immunotherapy with BCG for recurrent melanoma. Lancet, *1:* 1208–1212, 1973.

Gutterman, J. U., Mavligit, G. M., Reed, R. C., Gottlieb, J. A., Burgess, M. A., McBride, C. M., Einhorn, L., Freireich, E. J., and Hersh, E. M. Chemoimmunotherapy for regional and disseminated malignant melanoma. *In* Cancer Chemotherapy—Fundamental Concepts and Recent Advances, p. 455. Year Book Medical Publishers, Chicago, 1974.

Gutterman, J. U., Mavligit, G., Reed, R., Rechman, S., McBride, C. E., and Hersh, E. M. Immunology and immunotherapy of human malignant melanoma; historic review and perspectives for the future. Semin. Oncol., *2:* 155–174, 1975.

Gutterman, J. U., Mavligit, G. M., Reed, R., Burgess, M. A., Gottlieb, J., and Hersh, E. M. Bacillus Calmette-Guerin immunotherapy in combination with DTIC (NSC-45388) for the treatment of malignant melanoma. Cancer Treat. Rep., *60:* 177–182, 1976.

Gutterman, J., Hersh, E., Benjamin, R., Mavligit, G., Burgess, M., and Bodey, G. An effective new chemoimmunotherapy regimen for disseminated malignant melanoma. Proc. Am. Soc. Clin. Oncol., *18:* 300, 1977.

Gutterman, J. U., Hersh, E. M., Mavligit, G. M., Burgess, M. A., Richman, S. P., Schwarz, M., Rodriquez, and Valdivieso, M. Chemoimmunotherapy of disseminated malignant melanoma with BCG: Follow-up report. *In* Immunotherapy of Cancer: Present Status of Trials in Man, edited by W. D. Terry and D. Windhorst, p. 103. Raven Press, New York, 1978a.

Gutterman, J. U., Mavligit, G. M., McBride, C. M., Richman, S. P., Burgess, M. A., and Hersh, E. M. Postoperative immunotherapy for recurrent malignant melanoma: An updated report. *In* Immunotherapy of Cancer: Present Status of Trials in Man, edited by W. D. Terry and D. Windhorst, p. 35. Raven Press, New York, 1978b.

Habermalz, H. J., and Fischer, J. J. Radiation therapy of malignant melanoma—experience with high individual treatment doses. Cancer, *38:* 2258–2262, 1976.

Hersh, E. M., McBride, C. M., and Geschwind, C. Local and systemic efforts of perfusion therapy for malignant melanoma. Surg. Gynecol. Obstet., *137:* 461–464, 1973.

Hill, G. J., Moss, S., Fletcher, W., Golomb, T., and Grage, T. DTIC melanoma adjuvant study: Final report. Proc. Am. Soc. Clin. Oncol., *19:* 309, 1978.

Holmes, E. C., Ramming, K. P., Eilber, F. R., and Morton, D. L. The surgical management of pulmonary metastases. Semin. Oncol., *4:* 65–69, 1977.

Hoogstraten, B., Gottlieb, J. A., Caoili, E., Turner, W. G., Talley, R. W., and Haut, A. CCNU in the treatment of cancer. Cancer, *32:* 38–43, 1973.

Jacquillat, C., Banzet, P., Civatz, J., Puissant, A., and Chastang, C. Chemotherapy as an adjunct to the surgical resection of naevocarcinoma. Proc. Am. Assoc. Cancer Res., *17:* 42, 1976.

Johnson, R. O., Metter, G., Wilson, W., Hill, G., and Krementz, E. Phase I evaluation of DTIC (NSC-45388) and other studies in malignant melanoma in the Central Oncology Group. Cancer Treat. Rep., *60:* 183–187, 1976.

Kostinas, J. E., Leone, L. A., and Rege, V. B. Procarbazine, vinblastine and dactinomycin in stage III and IV melanoma with or without MER. Proc. Am. Soc. Clin. Oncol., *19:* 355, 1978.

Kaufman, S. D., Carey, R. W., Cosimi, A. B., and Wood, W. C. Randomized trial of adjuvant therapy for "high risk" primary malignant melanoma. Proc. Am. Soc. Clin. Oncol., *19:* 374, 1978.

Luce, J. K. Chemotherapy of malignant melanoma. Semin. Oncol., *2:* 279–285, 1975.

Mabel, J. A., et al. Combination chemotherapy against B16 melanoma bleomycin/vinblastine, bleomycin/cisdiamminedichloroplatinum, 5-fluorouracil/CCNU and 5-fluorouracil/

methylCCNU. Cancer 42: 1711-1719, 1978.

Mastrangelo, M. J., Bellet, R. E., Berd, D., and Lustbader, E. A randomized prospective trial comparing methylCCNU + vincristine to methylCCNU + vincristine + BCG + allogeneic tumor cells in patients with metastatic malignant melanoma. In Immunotherapy of Cancer: Present Status of Trials in Man, edited by W. D. Terry and D. Windhorst, p. 95. Raven Press, New York, 1978a.

Mastrangelo, M. J., Bellet, R. E., and Berd, D. A randomized prospective trial comparing methylCCNU + vincristine with methylCCNU + vincristine + BCG + allogeneic tumor cells in patients with metastatic malignant melanoma. Proc. Am. Soc. Clin. Oncol., 19: 319, 1978b.

McIllmurray, M. B., Embleton, M. J., Reeves, W. G., Langman, M. J. S., and Deane, M. Controlled trial of active immunotherapy in management of stage IIB malignant melanoma. Br. Med. J., 1: 540-542, 1977.

McKelvey, E. M., Luce, J. K., Talley, R. W., Hersh, E. M., Hewlett, J. S., and Moon, T. E. Combination chemotherapy with bis-chloroethyl-nitrosourea (BCNU), vincristine and dimethyl triazenoimidazole carboxamide (DTIC) in disseminated malignant melanoma. Cancer, 39: 1-4, 1977a.

McKelvey, E. M., Luce, J. K., Vaitkevicius, V. K., Talley, R. W., Bodey, G. P., Lane, M., and Moon, T. E. Bis-chloroethyl-nitrosourea, vincristine, dimethyl triazenoimidazole carboxamide and chlorpromazine combination chemotherapy in disseminated malignant melanoma. Cancer, 39: 5-10, 1977b.

Mihm, M. C. Early detection of primary cutaneous malignant melanoma: a color atlas. N. Engl. J. Med., 289: 989-996, 1973.

Mihm, M. C., Clark, W. H., and Reed, R. J. Clinical diagnosis of malignant melanoma. Semin. Oncol., 2: 108-115, 1975.

Moon, J. H., Gailani, S., Cooper, M. R., et al. Comparison of the combination of BCNU and vincristine with two dose schedules of DTIC in the treatment of disseminated malignant melanoma. Cancer, 35: 368-371, 1975.

Morton, D. L., Holmes, E. C., Eilber, F. R., Sparks, F. C., and Ramming, K. P. Adjuvant immunotherapy of malignant melanoma: Preliminary results of a randomized trial in patients with lymph node metastases. In Immunotherapy of Cancer: Present Status of Trials in Man, edtied by W. D. Terry and D. Windhorst, pp. 57-64. Raven Press, New York, 1978.

Mukherji, B., and Nathanson, L. Studies of humoral and cell mediated immunity in human melanoma. Yale J. Biol. Med., 46: 681-692, 1973.

Mukherji, B., Vassos, D., Flowers, A., Binder, S. C., and Nathanson, L. Variables and specificity of in vitro lymphocyte-mediated cytotoxicity in human melanoma. Cancer Res., 35: 3721-3730, 1975.

Musemeci, R., LaMonica, G., Orefice, S., et al. Lymphangiographic evaluation of 250 patients with malignant melanoma. Cancer, 38: 1568-1573, 1976.

Nathanson, L. Regression of intradermal malignant melanoma after intralesional injection of mycobacterium bovis strain BCG. Cancer Chemother. Rep., 56: 659-665, 1972.

Nathanson, L. Use of BCG in treatment of human tumors. Semin. Oncol., 1: 337-350, 1974.

Nathanson, L. Spontaneous regression of malignant melanoma; a review of the literature of incidence, clinical features, and possible mechanisms. Natl. Cancer Inst. Monogr., 44: 67-76, 1976.

Nathanson, L., and Kahn, P. Splenic uptake of Tc^{99m} sulfur colloid in malignant melanoma. J. Nucl. Med., 18: 1040, 1977b.

Nathanson, L. and Schoenfeld, D. Report on ECOG 1675. Minutes of ECOG meeting, Madison, Wisc., June 1, 1978.

Nathanson, L., Hall, T. C., Vawter, G., and Farber, S. Melanoma as a medical problem. Arch. Intern. Med., 119: 479-492, 1967a.

Nathanson, L., Hall, T. C., and Farber, S. Biological aspects of human malignant melanoma. Cancer, 20: 650–655, 1967b.

Nathanson, L., Horton, J., Wolter, J., Colsky, J., and Schilling, A. Characteristics of prognosis and response to imidiazole carboxamide in malignant melanoma. Clin. Pharm. Ther., 12: 955–962, 1971.

Nathanson, L., Khwaja, T. A., and Hall, T. C. Selective cytotoxicity of α-N-(3-hydroxy-4 pyridone)-β-aminopropionic acid (L-mimosine) for malignant pigment cells. Int. Pigment Cell Conf., 10: 87 (abstr.), 1977.

Nordman, E. M., and Mantyla, M. Treatment of metastatic melanoma with combined 5-fluorouracil and procarbazine. Cancer Treat. Rep., 61: 1709–1710, 1977.

Norton, J. A., Shulman, N. R., Corash, L., Smith, R. L., Au, F., and Rosenberg, S. A. Severe thrombocytopenia following intralesional BCG therapy. Cancer, 41: 820–826, 1978.

Perlin, E., Engeler, J., Reid, J. W., Lokey, J. L., and Kostinas, J. Treatment of malignant melanoma with vinblastine (NSC-49842), procarbazine (NSC-77213), and actinomycin D (NSC-3053). Cancer Chemother. Rep., 59: 767–768, 1975.

Pinsky, C. M., Hirshaut, Y., Wanebo, H. J., Hilal, E. Y., Fortner, J. G., Miké, V., Schottenfeld, D., and Oettgen, H. F. Surgical adjuvant immunotherapy with BCG in patients with malignant melanoma: Results of a prospective randomized trial. In Immunotherapy of Cancer: Present Status of Trials in Man, edited by W. D. Terry and D. Windhorst, p. 27. Raven Press, New York, 1978.

Presant, C. A., Bartolucci, A. A., Smalley, R. V., and Vogler, W. R. Effect of corynebacterium parvum on combination chemotherapy of disseminated malignant melanoma. In Immunotherapy of Cancer: Present Status of Trials in Man, edited by W. D. Terry and D. Windhorst, p. 113. Raven Press, New York, 1978.

Rubinson, R. M. and Bolooki, H. Intrapleural tetracycline for control of malignant pleural effusion; a preliminary report. South. Med. J., 65: 847–849, 1972.

Salmon, S. E., Hamburger, A. W., Soehnlen, B., Durie, B. G. M., Alberts, D. S., and Moon, T. E. Quantitation of differential sensitivity of human tumor stem cells to anticancer drugs. N. Engl. J. Med., 298: 1321–1327, 1978.

Schumann, J., and Göhde, W. Short term test of the effects of cytostatic agents on human malignant melanoma in vivo. Proc. Am. Assoc. Cancer Res., 18: 146, 1977.

Seiji, M., Mihm, M. C., Sober, A. J., et al. Malignant melanoma of the palmar-plantar-mucosal type; clinical and histopathologic features. Int. Pigment Cell Conf., 10: 124 (abstr.), 1977.

Shackney, S. E. Role of radioautographic studies in clinical investigative oncology and chemotherapy. Cancer Treat. Rep., 60: 1873–1886, 1976.

Shirakawa, S., Iver, J. K., Tannock, I., and Frei, E. Cell proliferation in human melanoma. J. Clin. Invest., 49: 1188–1199, 1970.

Shiu, M. H., Schottenfeld, D., MacLean, B., and Fortner, J. G. Adverse effect of pregnancy on melanoma. Cancer, 37: 181–187, 1976.

Silverberg, E., and Holleb, A. I. Cancer Statistics. Ca, 28: 25, 1978.

Sim, F. H., Taylor, W. F., Ivins, J. C., Pritchard, D. J., and Soule, E. H. A prospective randomized study of the efficacy of routine elective lymphadenectomy in management of malignant melanoma. Cancer, 41: 948–956, 1978.

Simmons, R. L., Aranha, G. V., Gunnarsson, A., Grage, T. B. and McKhann, C. F. Active specific immunotherapy for advanced melanoma utilizing neuraminidase-treated autochthonous tumor cells. In Immunotherapy of Cancer: Present Status of Trials in Man, edited by W. D. Terry and D. Windhorst, p. 123. Raven Press, New York, 1978.

Spitler, L. E., Sagebiel, R. W., Glogau, R. G., Wong, P. P., Malm, T. M., Chase, R. H., and Gonzalez, R. L. A randomized double-blind trial of adjuvant therapy with levamisole versus placebo in patients with malignant melanoma. In Immunotherapy of Cancer: Present Status of Trials in Man, edited by W. D. Terry and D. Windhorst, p. 73. Raven Press, New York, 1978.

Stehlin, J. S., Giovanella, B. C., Ipoly, P. D., Muenz, R. R., and Anderson, R. F. Results of hyperthermic perfusion for melanoma of the extremities. Surg. Gynecol. Obstet., *140:* 339–348, 1975.

Sugarbaker, E. V., and McBride, C. M. Survival and regional disease control after isolation-perfusion for invasive stage I melanoma of the extremities. Cancer, *37:* 188–198, 1976.

Trazak, D. J., Rowland, W. D., and Hu, F. Metastatic malignant melanoma in prepubertal children. Pediatrics, *55:* 191–204, 1975.

Varga, J. M., Asato, N., Lande, S., and Lerner, A. B. Hormone-receptor mediated selective destruction of cultivated murine melanoma cells by a melanotropin-daunomycin conjugate. Clin. Res., *25:* 533A, 1977.

Vidne, B. A., Richter, S., and Levy, M. J. Surgical treatment of solitary pulmonary metastasis. Cancer, *38:* 2561–2563, 1976.

Veronesi, U., Adamus, J., Bandiera, D. C., et al. Inefficacy of immediate node dissection in stage I melanoma of the limbs. N. Engl. J. Med., *297:* 627–630, 1977.

Wanebo, H. J., Woodruff, J., and Fortner, J. G. Malignant melanoma of the extremities; a clinicopathologic study using levels of invasion (microstage). Cancer, *35:* 666–676, 1976.

Voorhees, M. E. α-Methyl DOPA in BCG experimental melanoma. Cancer, Res., *31:* 1450-1455, 1971.

Wick, M. M. Synergistic inhibition of growth of melanoma cells by α-melanocyte stimulating hormone and theophylline. Clin. Res., *25:* 533A, 1977.

Wick, M. M., and Byers, L. Selective toxicity of 6-hydroxydopa (6-HDA) for S-91 Cloudman melanoma in vitro. Proc. Am. Assoc. Cancer Res., *18:* 37, 1977.

Wick, M. M., and Ratliff, J. M. L-DOPA methyl ester—a new antitumor agent. Proc. Am. Assoc. Cancer Res., *19:* 160, 1978

Wittes, R. E., Wittes, J., and Golbey, R. B. Combination chemotherapy in metastatic malignant melanoma. A randomized study of three DTIC-containing combinations. Cancer, *41:* 415–421, 1978.

Wright, P. W., Hellström, K. E., Hellström, I., Warner, G., Prentice, R., and Jones, R. F. Serotherapy of malignant melanoma. *In* Immunotherapy of Cancer: Present Status of Trials in Man, edited by W. D. Terry and D. Windhorst, p. 135. Raven Press, New York, 1978.

Chapter 29

Skin Cancer and Precancerous Dermatoses

LOREN E. GOLITZ, M.D.

Skin cancer is by far the most common form of human malignancy. Excluding malignant melanomas which account for only 1% of all human cancer, basal cell and squamous cell carcinomas of skin are the malignancies seen most often in clinical practice. A number of observations lend support to the theory relating the high incidence of cutaneous malignancy to chronic sunlight exposure. Skin cancers occur predominantly on exposed parts of the body with over 90% involving the face, ears, neck and dorsa of the hands. Individuals who work outdoors and those with a fair complexion have a higher incidence of skin cancer and actinic keratoses. The incidence of actinically induced skin cancer is high in persons with albinism but low in blacks who are protected from ultraviolet radiation by abundant melanin pigment. Finally, southern areas of the United States where sunlight is most intense have the highest incidence of cutaneous malignancy.

PRECANCEROUS DERMATOSES

Actinic Keratosis (Solar Keratosis, Senile Keratosis)

Actinic keratoses are the most common of the precancerous dermatoses, a term which has also been applied to Bowen's disease, arsenical keratoses and chronic radiation dermatitis. While most actinic keratoses remain only a cosmetic problem, a small percentage of untreated lesions will subsequently develop into squamous cell carcinoma.

Actinic keratoses occur mainly after middle age in fair-skinned individuals and are the result of the cumulative effect of years of exposure to sunlight. Clinically they are erythematous and slightly elevated with an adherent yellow to brown scale. The edges are well defined without significant induration. Actinic keratoses usually occur as multiple lesions of the face and upper extremities and are commonly associated with solar elastosis which gives the skin a course, yellow, wrinkled appearance.

THERAPY

The individual with a history of actinic keratoses or skin cancer should be cautioned to wear protective clothing or sunscreens when outdoors and to avoid sunbathing. Sunscreens containing 5% p-aminobenzoic acid in 55–70% ethanol are effective in protecting the skin against those wavelengths of ultraviolet radiation which cause sunburn (Poh-Fitzpatrick, 1977).

A simple method for treating patients with a small number of actinic keratoses is to freeze each area briefly with liquid nitrogen applied with a cotton-tipped applicator. The applicator should be touched to the keratoses for a few seconds until a superficial freezing is seen. A similar method utilizes a carbon dioxide slush which is prepared just prior to use by mixing crushed dry ice with a small amount of acetone. Following superficial freezing with liquid nitrogen or carbon dioxide, the keratoses peel off within a few days and the skin heals without significant scarring. Curettage with a surgical curette followed by gentle electrodesiccation is a simple and effective means of treatment if only a few lesions are present, however, it is less convenient than freezing since a local anesthetic is required.

Topically applied 5-fluorouracil is the therapy of choice for patients with widespread superficial actinic keratoses. The topical use of this drug followed the observation of Falkson and Schultz (1962) that patients treated for cancer with systemic 5-fluorouracil experienced the resolution of actinic keratoses.

When applied topically, 5-fluorouracil has little or no effect on normal skin but produces marked inflammation of actinic keratoses followed by desquamation and complete clearing of the lesions. The drug which is available for topical use in 1, 2, and 5% concentrations is applied with the fingertips to the skin of the entire affected area. Frequently actinic keratoses which are clinically inapparent will become inflamed. The inflammatory response becomes apparent within 4–6 days and is usually maximum in about 2 weeks. One treatment course should take about 2–3 weeks and, once completed, the inflammation can be quickly controlled with a steroid cream such as triamcinolone acetonide. A recent study (Breza et al., 1976) demonstrated that topical applications of 5-fluorouracil followed immediately by potent (0.4–0.5%) triamcinolone cream was as effective as 5-fluorouracil alone in treating actinic keratoses but avoided the inflammatory reaction. These findings indicate that the effectiveness of 5-fluorouracil does not depend on nonspecific inflammation and suggest that the resolution of actinic keratoses is related to chemotherapeutic properties of the drug.

Bowen's Disease (Squamous Cell Carcinoma in Situ)

Bowen's disease is an uncommon but not rare precancerous dermatosis which occurs both on sun-exposed and covered parts of the body. Most of those affected are over 40 years of age and about 35% have multiple lesions (Graham and Helwig, 1959). The incidence in men and women is approximately equal.

Microscopically, Bowen's disease is an intraepidermal squamous cell carcinoma with dysplasia of the entire thickness of the epidermis. In about 5% of individuals Bowen's disease progresses to locally invasive squamous cell carcinoma, while 2% of all patients with Bowen's disease eventually develop metastatic squamous cell carcinoma (Graham and Helwig, 1972).

About 25% of individuals with Bowen's disease have associated primary internal cancer (Graham and Helwig, 1972). Some studies suggest that the association with internal malignancy is seen predominantly with Bowen's disease of nonsun-exposed skin (Peterka et al., 1961) while other investigators feel there is no correlation between the anatomic location of the dermatosis and the presence or absence of visceral cancer (Graham and Helwig, 1972). The association with internal malignancy may be related to arsenic ingestion, although a history of arsenic exposure is present in only about 5% of those with Bowen's disease.

Clinically, Bowen's disease is a sharply marginated tan to brown plaque one to several centimeters in diameter. The slightly elevated lesion may be scaly, keratotic, nodular or ulcerated.

THERAPY

Surgical excision is the treatment of choice for Bowen's disease. The pathologist should be asked to check surgical margins to be sure they are free of residual tumor. While shave biopsy followed by electrodesiccation and curettage has been associated with frequent recurrences in some series (Graham and Helwig, 1972), others have reported cure rates of 98% in patients followed a minimum of 4 years (Honeycutt and Hansen, 1973). When performed by experienced physicians, electrodesiccation and curettage appears to be an effective form of treatment for Bowen's disease. Radiotherapy may be the preferred treatment for Bowen's disease in a small percentage of patients. It should be considered in elderly patients, in lesions which have recurred following surgery or electrodesiccation and curettage, and in lesions which are located on areas such as the nose, ear or eyelid where surgery would result in a significant cosmetic defect. If radiotherapy is utilized, a full tumor dosage should be administered as described in the section on squamous cell carcinoma. While 5-fluorouracil applied topically with polyethelene film occlusion may be effective in some cases (Fulton et al., 1968) it is associated with a high recurrence rate and should not be used in Bowen's disease.

SKIN CANCER

Squamous Cell Carcinoma (Epidermoid Carcinoma)

Squamous cell carcinoma of the skin occurs predominantly in individuals over 40 years of age with a history of chronic exposure to sunlight. The incidence is increased in fair-skinned individuals living in the southern United States and is approximately twice as common in men as in women. Squamous cell carcinoma has also been reported to occur in thermal burn scars, chronic sinuses, chronic radiodermatitis, and following exposure to inorganic arsenic or hydrocarbons. Renal transplant patients and other individuals on immunosuppressive therapy have an increased incidence of squamous cell carcinoma of skin and malignant lymphoma. In one survey of renal transplant recipients the risk of skin cancer was over 7 times that expected (Hoxtell et al., 1977).

The reported incidence of metastases from squamous cell carcinoma of the skin is 0.5-2% (Lund, 1965; Epstein et al., 1968). Squamous cell carcinomas that arise in actinic keratoses may be less prone to metastasize (Graham et al., 1969). However, in a study of 142 squamous cell carcinomas with metastases, over two-thirds of the presumed primary lesions occurred on sun-exposed areas of the body (Epstein et al., 1968). Squamous cell carcinomas which arise from mucous membranes or which occur in chronic sinuses or areas of radiation dermatitis are biologically more aggressive than those that develop on sun-exposed skin.

Clinically, squamous cell carcinoma begins as an indurated, firm papule or plaque. The lesion may be scaly or verrucous and frequently is ulcerated. The margins of the carcinoma may have a yellowish-red color with hyperemia of the surrounding skin.

THERAPY

Squamous cell carcinomas of the skin less than 2 cm in diameter can be effectively treated by electrodesiccation and curettage. Five-year cure rates of over 96% have been reported in large series of cases treated with this modality (Freeman et al., 1964; Honeycutt and Jansen, 1973). Squamous cell carcinomas larger than 2 or 3 cm in diameter are best treated by surgical excision or radiation therapy. It has been demonstrated that a surgical margin of 1 cm beyond the gross tumor removes microscopic areas of invasion in 99% of squamous cell carcinoma of the skin (Beirne and Beirne, 1959). In cases which are felt by the pathologist to be inadequately excised the actual recurrence rate is about 50% (Glass et al., 1966). Radiation therapy is effective in many squamous cell carcinomas that are not amenable to surgery. It is of particular value for lesions of the nose or eyelid where surgery may produce excessive deformity and for lesions of the nasolabial fold which often invade deeply. The radiotherapy dosage schedule should be tailored to the specific case, but one schedule that has proven effective is 4500 rads fractionated in 9–15 treatments with a half-value layer of aluminum of 0.68–1.64 mm depending on the size and depth of the tumor (Honeycutt and Jansen, 1973). Mohs' chemosurgery may be required for difficult cases. This technique is described fully in the section on basal cell carcinoma. Topical chemotherapy has little or no place in the management of squamous cell carcinoma of the skin.

Basal Cell Carcinoma (Basal Cell Epithelioma)

Basal cell carcinomas account for 65–75% of all skin cancer (Wermuth and Fajardo, 1970) and have been reported to be 2–9 times more common than squamous cell carcinomas of the skin. A close relationship to chronic sunlight exposure accounts for the relatively high incidence of this cancer on sun-exposed parts of the body. Like actinic keratoses and squamous cell carcinomas, basal cell carcinomas occur more frequently in fair-skinned individuals living in the southern United States.

Patients with a history of skin cancer should have yearly follow-up examinations since at least 20% will develop additional skin cancers (Epstein, 1973; Bergstresser and Halprin, 1975). The occurrence of multiple basal cell carcinomas during the first 2 decades of life suggests the diagnosis of the nevoid basal cell carcinoma syndrome. This syndrome is characterized by autosomal dominant inheritance, distinctive pits in the keratin of the palms and soles, jaw cysts, calcification of the falx cerebri, boney abnormalities such as bifid ribs and multiple basal cell carcinomas which develop early in life. Ingestion of inorganic arsenic in the form of medication, insecticides, or contaminated well water is associated with an increased incidence of Bowen's disease, squamous cell carcinomas and basal cell carcinomas which may be multiple. If arsenic exposure is suspected the patient should also be evaluated for internal malignancy.

Metastases from basal cell carcinomas are rare, having been reported in less than 100 cases (Mikhail et al., 1977). In a hospital study of over 9000 basal cell carcinomas, the incidence of metastases was about 0.1% (Cotran, 1961). The incidence in a less selected population of patients has been reported to be as as low as 0.0028% (Paver et al., 1973). Lesions which metastasized did not differ histologically from other tumors but were characterized clinically by a prolonged course, failure to respond to repeated surgery and x-ray, and by extensive local invasion. Metastases usually spread to regional lymph nodes and rarely to the lung. The average survival time after metastasis to the lungs, bone, and internal organs is about 10 months (Mikhail et al., 1977).

Clinically, basal cell carcinomas usually appear as papules or nodules 0.5–2 cm in diameter. The margins tend to be elevated, smooth, and translucent with a pearly appearance. Telangiectatic vessels commonly overlie the tumor margins and central ulceration may produce the so-called rodent ulcer. Basal cell carcinomas are generally skin colored but may contain abundant melanin pigment and mimic the clinical appearance of malignant melanoma. Morphea-like basal cell carcinomas are relatively flat with a sclerotic appearance and little or no pigmentation.

THERAPY

Electrodesiccation and curettage is the treatment of choice for most basal cell carcinomas. This modality produces a cure rate of about 95% in the hands of experienced physicians (Kopf et al., 1977). After local anesthesia, the tumor is scraped away from the underlying tissue with a surgical curette. The base of the tumor is then treated by electrodesiccation which destroys any remaining tumor with heat and desiccation produced by the passage of a high frequency electrical current. This procedure is repeated serially a total of 3 times after which the lesion heals leaving a flat slightly depigmented scar. Hypertrophic scars are an occasional complication. Recurrences after this form of therapy are most common for basal cell carcinomas located on the nose, forehead or nasolabial folds.

Surgical excision is an effective treatment for basal cell carcinoma and has the advantage of producing a linear scar which may be cosmetically more acceptable in some instances than the flat scar produced by electrodesiccation. An elliptically shaped incision is performed with a margin of 3–4 mm. Sutures should generally be removed in 4–7 days. In lesions with histologic extension of the basal cell carcinoma to the surgical margin only about one-third recur and these can usually be managed successfully by re-excision or radiation therapy (Gooding et al., 1965).

Radiation therapy is a useful form of treatment for basal cell carcinomas, particularly those occurring on the nose or eyelid and those involving the nasolabial fold. A common treatment schedule for small lesions consists of 4000–5000 rads of 80–120 kV radiation with a half-value layer of 0.6–1.0 mm of aluminum. This may be administered at 500 rads daily for 8–10 days. Fractionation of x-ray therapy over 10 days reduces the incidence of complications such as acute radiation dermatitis and chondritis. Tumors over 10 cm in diameter do not respond well to radiation therapy. X-ray treatment should also be avoided on acral parts of the body where postradiation sequelae may be severe. The cure rates with radiation therapy are comparable to those for electrodesiccation and curettage. At times radiation therapy is the preferred treatment for far-advanced skin cancer (Farina et al., 1977).

Basal cell carcinomas can be treated by cryosurgery (Zacarian, 1968). A thermocouple needle is placed beneath the tumor mass to measure the temperature during the application of liquid nitrogen spray. Special equipment is required to administer the liquid nitrogen to assure a temperature of at least −20°C at the base of the tumor. Liquid nitrogen applied with a cotton-tipped applicator is inadequate for treating most skin cancers as it freezes only to a depth of 1.0–1.5 mm. A new cryotherapy technique utilizing standardized 30-sec freeze-thaw cycles produced a 97.7% cure rate of basal cell carcinomas without the use of thermocouple needles (McLean et al., 1978).

Topical therapy with cytotoxic drugs has not found wide acceptance in the treatment of basal cell carcinomas because of the high degree of effectiveness of electrodesiccation and curettage. Belisario (1970) has reported on 10 years' experience with various skin cancers treated with topical cytotoxic agents. In general, the cure rates for topically applied drugs such as colcemid, methotrexate and 5-fluorouracil are less than that for electrodesiccation and curettage.

Basal cell carcinomas which have repeatedly recurred, which are large, or which cannot be safely treated by the above methods, may be treated by Mohs' chemosurgery. This technique employs in situ fixation of the tumor followed by removal in multiple histologically controlled stages. Mohs' chemosurgery has been effective in over 90% of basal cell carcinomas that appeared too difficult to treat by conventional therapy (Mohs and Ghosh, 1969).

After estimation of the extent of the lesion dichloroacetic acid is applied until the skin turns white. This allows for penetration of the keratin layer by the zinc chloride fixative paste which fixes the tissue in situ and allows for preservation of histologic detail. An occlusive dressing is applied and after 4–24 hours the area is mapped and numbered so that specific areas can be identified. The fixed tissue is excised in a horizontal plane and frozen sections are prepared for microscopic examination. There is no bleeding from the fixed tissue and anesthesia is not required although the zinc chloride may produce some pain. Deeper fixation and excision is carried out as indicated by the results of the microscopic evaluation. The area heals producing a flat white scar.

Because of the discomfort produced by standard Mohs' chemosurgery and the time required for fixation, some surgeons have now changed to a fresh tissue modification of the Mohs' technique (Tromovitch and Stegman, 1974). This modality allows microscopically controlled excision of skin cancer, saves time for the physician, and has better patient acceptance, while producing a cure rate of over 95% in patients followed 3–8 years.

REFERENCES

Belisario, M. C. Ten years' experience with topical cytotoxic therapy for cutaneous cancer and precancer; type and number of cases and lesions treated (Part 1 and Part 2). Cutis, 6: 293–306 and 401–412, 1970.

SKIN CANCER AND PRECANCEROUS DERMATOSES 569

Beirne, G. A., and Beirne, C. G. Observations on the critical margin for the complete excision of carcinoma of the skin. Arch. Dermatol., 80: 344-345, 1959.

Bergstresser, P. R., and Halprin, K. M. Multiple sequential skin cancers; the risk of skin cancer in patients with previous skin cancer. Arch. Dermatol., 111: 995-996, 1975.

Breza, T., Taylor, R., and Eaglestein, W. H. Non-inflammatory destruction of actinic keratoses by fluorouracil. Arch. Dermatol., 112: 1256-1258, 1976.

Cotron, R. S. Metastasizing basal cell carcinomas. Cancer, 14: 1036-1040, 1961.

Epstein, E., Epstein, N. N., Bragg, K., and Linden, G. Metastases from squamous cell carcinomas of the skin. Arch. Dermatol., 97: 245-251, 1968.

Epstein, E. Value of follow-up after treatment of basal cell carcinoma. Arch. Dermatol., 108: 798-800, 1973.

Falkson, G., and Schulz, E. J. Skin changes in patients treated with 5-fluorouracil. Br. J. Dermatol., 74: 229-236, 1962.

Farina, A. T., Leider, M., Newall, J., and Carella, R. J. Modern radiotherapy for malignant epitheliomas; a measure of last resort. Arch. Dermatol., 113: 650-654, 1977.

Freeman, R. G., Knox, J. M., and Heaton, C. L. The treatment of skin cancer. Cancer, 17: 535-538, 1964.

Fulton, J. E., Carter, D. M., and Hurley, H. J. Treatment of Bowen's disease with topical 5-fluorouracil under occlusion. Arch. Dermatol., 97: 178-180, 1968.

Glass, R. L., Spratt, J. S., and Perez-Mesa, C. The fate of inadequately excised epidermoid carcinoma of the skin. Surg. Gynecol. Obstet., 122: 245-248, 1966.

Gooding, C. A., White, F., and Yatsuhashi, M. Significance of marginal extension in excised basal-cell carcinoma. N. Engl. J. Med., 273: 923-924, 1965.

Graham, J. H., Bendl, B. J., and Johnson, W. C. Solar keratosis with squamous cell carcinoma; a new biologic concept. Am. J. Pathol., 55: 26a, 1969.

Graham, J. H., and Helwig, E. B. Bowen's disease and its relationship to systemic cancer. Arch. Dermatol., 80: 133-159, 1959.

Graham, J. H., and Helwig, E. B. Premalignant cutaneous and mucocutaneous diseases. In Dermal Pathology, edited by J. H. Graham, W. C. Johnson, and E. B. Helwig, pp. 561-624. Harper & Row, Hagerstown, Md., 1972.

Honeycutt, W. M., and Jansen, G. T. Treatment of squamous cell carcinoma of the skin. Arch. Dermatol., 108: 670-672, 1973.

Hoxtell, E. O., Mandel, J. S., Murray, S. S., Schuman, L. M., and Goltz, R. W. Incidence of skin carcinoma after renal transplantation. Arch. Dermatol., 113: 436-438, 1977.

Kopf, A. W., Bart, R. S., Schrager, D., Lazar, M., and Popkin, G. L. Curettage-electrodesiccation treatment of basal cell carcinomas. Arch. Dermatol., 113: 439-443, 1977.

Lund, H. A. How often does squamous cell carcinoma of the skin metastasize? Arch. Dermatol., 92: 635-637, 1965.

McLean, D. I., Haynes, H. A., McCarthy, P. L., and Baden, H. P. Cryotherapy of basal-cell carcinoma by a simple method of standardized freeze-thaw cycles. J. Dermatol. Surg. Oncol., 4: 175-177, 1978.

Mikhail, G. R., Nims, L. P., Kelly, A. P., Jr., Ditmars, D. M., and Eyler, W. R. Metastatic basal cell carcinoma: Review, pathogenesis and report of two cases. Arch. Dermatol., 113: 1261-1269, 1977.

Mohs, J. B., and Ghosh, B. C. Chemosurgery for basal cell carcinoma. J.A.M.A., 210: 1759-1761, 1969.

Paver, K., Poyzen, K., Burry, N., and Deikin, M. The incidence of basal cell carcinomas and their metastases in Australia and New Zealand. Aust. J. Dermatol., 14: 53, 1973.

Peterka, E. S., Lynch, F. W., and Goltz, R. W. An association between Bowen's disease and internal cancer. Arch. Dermatol., 84: 623-629, 1961.

Poh-Fitzpatrick, M. B. The biologic actions of solar radiation on skin with a note on sunscreens. J. Dermatol. Surg. Oncol., 3: 199-204, 1977.

Tromovitch, T. A., and Stegman, S. J. Microscopically controlled excision of skin tumors.

Chemosurgery (Mohs): Fresh tissue technique. Arch. Dermatol., *110:* 231–232, 1974.

Wermuth, B. M., and Fajardo, L. F. Metastatic basal cell carcinoma; a review. Arch. Pathol., *90:* 458–462, 1970.

Zacarian, S. A. Cryosurgery in dermatologic disorders and in the treatment of skin cancer. J. Cryosurg., *1:* 70–75, 1968.

Chapter 30

Childhood Malignancies

FREDERICK B. RUYMANN, M.D.

Malignancy ranks second only to accidents as a killer of children. This fact continues to impress the young house officer as he progresses in his pediatric training. In somewhat converse fashion the attending staff, if not directly involved in the practice of oncology, may think infrequently of malignancy in childhood. Leukemia accounts for half of the annual mortality due to malignancy (Miller, 1969; Table 30.1). The treatment of Wilms' tumor, neuroblastoma, rhabdomyosarcoma, retinoblastoma, hepatoblastoma, and teratoma will be discussed in this chapter; other chapters in this text are devoted to malignancies of the lymphoreticular system, central nervous system, and bone. An early awareness of malignancy in the differential diagnosis of masses in children is prerequisite to proper diagnosis and treatment. This point is emphasized by Farber's statement:

> Every solid, semi-solid, or semi-cystic mass in an infant or child should be regarded as a malignant tumor until its exact nature is determined by histologic examination of the removed tumor (Farber, 1969).

An excisional biopsy remains the preferred diagnostic procedure for any tumor arising in childhood. Unnecessary delay in biopsy is the major factor contributing to the morbidity and mortality of childhood malignancy.

WILMS' TUMOR

Nephroblastoma or Wilms' tumor is an embryonal renal malignancy having its original description in the 19th century. It is one of the more common, primary abdominal tumors of early childhood with about 500 new cases reported annually in the United States (D'Angio, 1972) and accounts for 5.4% of the mortality due to childhood malignancy (Miller,

TABLE 30.1
Death Rate and Distribution of Malignancy from 0 to 15 years, 1960–1966[a]

Diagnosis or Site	Death Rate (Million/Year)	Distribution (%)
Leukemia	34.55	48.4
CNS	11.36	15.8
Lymphoma	5.41	7.6
Neuroblastoma	5.08	7.2
Wilms' tumor	3.85	5.4
Bone	2.87	4.0
Rhabdomyosarcoma	1.56	2.2
Liver	0.87	1.2
Retinoblastoma	0.59	0.8
Teratomata	0.57	0.8
Other	4.77	6.6
Total	71.48	100.0

[a] Adapted from Miller (1969).

1969). The typical presentation of Wilms' tumor is by accidental discovery of an abdominal mass; fever, and gross hematuria are the next most common symptoms (Kinzel et al., 1960). Such a presentation is in sharp contrast to the symptoms of renal tumors in adults where the order is reversed. Hypertension has been found in as many as 50% of children with Wilms' tumor (Silva-Sosa and Gonzalez-Cerna, 1966). With increasing size the tumor may press on adjacent structures causing obstruction of the inferior vena cava with subsequent ascites or edema; similarly pressure on the intestines can cause intestinal obstruction. Occasionally the initial symptoms of the tumor may be with cough due to pulmonary metastases. An intravenous pyelogram is prerequisite in evaluating a child with an abdominal mass. In Wilms' tumor the calyceal system usually shows distortion with inferior and medial displacement; there is, however, no diagnostic radiographic picture. Presumptive diagnosis of Wilms' tumor by intravenous pyelogram is incorrect in 6% of cases (D'Angio et al., 1974). Calcification commonly attributed to neuroblastoma may be present in as many as 15% of children with Wilms' tumor (Marsden and Steward, 1968). An enlarged hydronephrotic kidney is the most common cause of an abdominal mass in childhood. Xanthogranulomatosis pyelonephritis, a chronic suppurative renal infection, may appear very similar to Wilms' tumor or neuroblastoma on intravenous pyelogram (Graivier and Vargos, 1972). Renal angiography is useful in placing the lesion within or outside the kidney and may suggest the type of malignancy within the kidney. In Wilms' tumor abnormal vessels are demonstrated on the angiogram, while the less common hypernephroma or renal adenocarcinoma shows arteriovenous shunting (Shanberg et al., 1970). Differentiation of an enlarged spleen from an abdominal tumor may be difficult. Usually the edge of the spleen is sharp and lateral but when the edge is rounded or difficult to feel an intravenous pyelogram should resolve the question.

Early detection of Wilms' tumor by biochemical studies has shown some progress with reports of elevated serum and urine mucopolysaccharide (Morse and Nussbaum, 1967). The similarity of these mucopolysaccharides to those obtained from Wilms' tumor extracts has raised the hope of easily available diagnostic screening (Allerton et al., 1970). Polycythemia has been shown to occur in Wilms' tumor in response to increased levels of erythropoietin. Anemia may be due to urinary blood loss secondary to pelvic ureteral invasion. Although uncommon, metastatic Wilms' tumor cells, similar in appearance to cells of rhabdomyosarcoma, have been found in the bone marrow and may be the cause of anemia (O'Neil and Pinkel, 1968).

Routine liver function studies should be performed prior to surgery. Abnormalities in the serum alkaline phosphatase, lactic acid dehydrogenase, and glutamic oxaloacetic transaminase may suggest liver, bone or lung metastases. Radioisotopic scanning of these organs is of great help in evaluating hematogenous spread. As with any tumor disseminated intravascular coagulation may be present; preoperative screening with fibrinogen, partial thromboplastin time, platelet count, and fibrin split product assays are of value. Genitourinary anomalies, sporadic aniridia, hemihypertrophy, and multiple hamartomas have all been reported in association with Wilms' tumor (Miller, 1968). Children presenting with any of these physical findings, although showing no abnormalities of their intravenous pyelogram, deserve careful follow-up by physical and radiographic examinations. Preliminary information suggests an increased incidence of brain tumors among relatives of children with Wilms' tumor (D'Angio et al., 1974).

Local metastases by direct extension of the tumor from the kidney occur in a majority of cases with involvement of the perirenal tissue, lymph nodes, liver, diaphragm, and abdominal muscle. Distant metastases are most common to the lung and the result of embolization following renal vein invasion. Involvement of the liver and contralateral kidney is not uncommon. The congenital Wilms' tumor or benign congenital mesoblastic nephroma presenting in infancy is a pathologically more differentiated tumor of improved prognosis, in comparison to Wilms' tumor presenting at an older age (Bolande et al., 1967). Nephrectomy alone is the treatment of choice thus avoiding the hazards of other therapeutic modalities (Bachman and Kroll, 1969; Pochedly et al., 1971).

Treatment

The presently high cure rate in Wilms' tumor has evolved over 35 years of cooperative study. A review of the literature from 1940 to 1958 showed a survival rate of 21% using nephrectomy alone (Klapproth, 1959). Individual series have been reported with cure rates up to 30% (Ladd, 1938; Lattimer and Conway, 1968). Postoperative radiation to the tumor bed increased survival in some series to 50% (Gross and Neuhauser, 1950). In other reviews radiotherapy and nephrectomy resulted in only a 26% cure rate (Klapproth, 1959).

CHEMOTHERAPY

A breakthrough was clearly made by Farber and co-workers in 1960 when actinomycin D was given in combination with radiotherapy to 29 children with metastatic Wilms' tumor (Farber et al., 1960). Ten of these children showed no evidence of disease at 4–33 months follow-up. A single dose versus multiple dose actinomycin D program indicated an increased number of pulmonary metastastes with single dose therapy (Wolff et al., 1968). Because of the aggressive, multidisciplinary pursuit of pulmonary metastases in the single dose actinomycin D treatment group, long term evaluation of the two treatment groups showed no significant differences in survival. Long term follow-up showed 49 of 73 patients living with a 67% survival rate (Wolff et al., 1974). The demonstration of vincristine activity in Wilms' tumor (Sutow et al., 1963) was subjected to randomized analysis by the National Wilms' Tumor Study in patients with Group II and III disease (Table 30.2). Group I patients treated with vincristine and actinomycin D have a projected disease free survival of 90%. A multivariate statistical analysis in National Wilms' Tumor Study—I has identified anaplastic or sarcomatous histology, specimen weight over 250 g, positive regional lymph nodes, treatment with only a single drug and age over 2 years as the most important predictors of relapse (Breslow et al., 1978). The first three factors predict mortality as well as relapse. Twenty-eight of 49 patients with either anaplasia or sarcomatous lesions died of tumor (Beckwith and Palmer, 1978). This mortality of 57.1% for patients with unfavorable histology is contrasted with a 6.9% mortality in 378 patients with favorable histology.

Adriamycin has definite activity in Wilms' tumor (Tan et al., 1973) and is undergoing randomized study in National Wilms' Tumor Study—II. In a recent bulletin (D'Angio et al., 1978) a significantly lower relapse rate has been demonstrated in Group II and III patients receiving triple agent

TABLE 30.2
Clinical Grouping National Wilms' Tumor Study

Group I	Tumor limited to kidney and completely resected
Group II	Tumor extends beyond the kidney but is completely resected
Group III	Residual nonhematogenous tumor confined to abdomen
Group IV	Hematogenous metastases
Group V	Bilateral renal involvement either initially or subsequently

chemotherapy. For this reason Group II, III, and IV patients, regardless of histology, have been recommended to receive triple therapy with vincristine, actinomycin D, and Adriamycin. In addition Group I patients with unfavorable histology would also receive triple agent chemotherapy. The addition of Adriamycin late in the course of maintenance chemotherapy is felt by the National Wilms' Tumor Study—II committee to be of dubious value and balanced by the unknown potential for late cardiac damage. The cumulative toxicity of Adriamycin in a patient previously exposed to actinomycin D and radiotherapy must be respected; an Adriamycin cumulative dose limit of 550 mg/m^2 has been found safe in patients with osteosarcoma.

SURGERY

Surgery is the critical first step in the diagnosis and treatment of Wilms' tumor. A wide transperitoneal incision will facilitate nephrectomy and minimize spillage of the tumor. Clamping of the renal pedicle prior to mobilization of the involved kidney will limit hematogenous spread. The liver, periaortic nodes, and perihilar nodes are inspected and any suspicious areas biopsied. The bilaterality of Wilms' tumor demands a careful inspection of the contralateral kidney. Metal clips are used to demarcate the tumor bed and any area of residual disease. When initial, complete resection is not possible chemotherapy and/or radiotherapy should be followed by a second look to remove residual tumor.

RADIOTHERAPY

Age adjusted radiation to the tumor bed in a dose of 2000–4000 rads is routinely recommended for patients in Groups II, III, and IV. The low incidence of flank recurrence in Group I patients, 5% or less, has promoted the elimination of local radiation in Group I patients. The National Wilms' Tumor Study Group is also undertaking a randomized comparison of 6 months versus 15 months combination vincristine and actinomycin D therapy for Group I patients. Accurate clinical grouping at the time of surgery then becomes a critical point for all members of the treatment team. Besides the standard tumor dose Group III patients receive therapy to the entire peritoneal cavity with exclusion of the femoral heads; the remaining kidney is limited to 1500 rads. A rupture of the tumor in the superior pole of the right kidney necessitates a liver dose of up to 3000 rads. With pulmonary metastases both lungs are treated to 1400 rads regardless of the number or location of visible metastases. Liver metastases should be evaluated for resectability before resorting to radiotherapy. Doses of 3000 rads are given to the involved portions of the liver. Metastases to brain, bone and lymph nodes would generally receive doses comparable to that given the liver. Cerebral metastases although rare represent some of the most difficult to treat. Lesions may arise originally in the interdiploic space with direct extension through the inner table into the brain. Brain scans are useful in delineating the size of the metastases if the cerebral hemispheres are involved. Initial treatment of the whole brain is preferred; combination treatment with vincristine, actinomycin D and/or Adriamycin should be continued for 1 year following radiation. With the initial presentation of pulmonary metastases a 2-month course of chemotherapy along with bilateral pulmonary radiotherapy should precede attempts at surgical resection. This allows for control of microscopic disease not visible on lung scan or lung tomograms; if the lesions show a complete remission a thoracotomy may be avoided. Continued chemotherapy for at least a year is indicated regardless of whether pulmonary resection is performed. Cooperative management of pulmonary metastases may be expected to show a 50% long term survival rate as shown by Table 30.3. Several resections may be necessary in the case of multiple or recurrent lesions.

BILATERAL WILMS' TUMOR

A bilateral Wilms' tumor occurred in 4.9% of 307 patients on the National Wilms' Tumor Study and must be considered as an immediate or potential threat (D'Angio et al., 1974). Whether this represents a multicentric process or the extension of a single tumor remains unresolved. Usually the kidney most grossly involved is removed and the remaining kidney is irradiated (Leen and Williams, 1971). In some instances the remaining kidney can be partially resected and spared from radiation; in 12 cases the median number of months from initial diagnosis to contralateral involvement of the other kidney was nine months with a range of 6–15 months (Jagasia et al., 1964). Bilateral Wilms' is not a hopeless situation; aggressive multimodal therapy should improve the survival of these children (Ragab et al., 1972).

NEUROBLASTOMA

Neuroblastoma is one of the most common solid tumors in infancy and childhood and arises from immature undifferentiated neuroblasts of

TABLE 30.3
Survival with Multidisciplinary Treatment of Pulmonary Metastases in Wilms' Tumor

Reference	Patients Presenting	Patients Surviving	Survival Time from Pulmonary Resection
Howard (1965)	7	3	$4^1/_2$ to 5 yr
Kilman et al. (1969)[a]	8	6	4 mo to 3 yr
Kilman et al. (1969)[b]	22	16	20 mo to 7 yr
Martin and Rickham (1970)	16	7	19 mo to 21 yr
Total	54	32	

[a] Personal series.
[b] Cases included in review.

neural crest ectoderm. Neuroblastomas are found wherever there is sympathetic nervous tissue. On Wright's stain neuroblasts resemble lymphoblasts. The tumor may be arranged in sheets or palisades; neuroblasts in the marrow form rosettes or pseudorosettes. With hemorrhage or necrosis the tumor may appear cystic. About one-third of neuroblastomas occur under 1 year of age; the male/female distribution is equal. Of 212 cases reviewed in one series, 63% arose from the retroperitoneal space (DeLorimier et al., 1969).

The mediastium is the second most common site of origin. Almost three quarters of children presenting beyond the age of 2 years will have distant metastases at the time of diagnosis. The most common metastases are to the liver, lymph nodes, marrow, skeleton and brain. Increased urinary catecholamine excretion with neural crest tumors has been known for several years (Voorhess and Gardner, 1960). A simple qualitative spot test developed by LaBrosse has been found to be of practical value in the diagnosis and management of children with neuroblastoma (LaBrosse, 1968; Evans et al., 1971a). In one study the spot test was positive in 32 of 35 patients with known neuroblastoma giving a 91% accuracy; 34 of 35 patients showed abnormal quantitative studies in 3 of 4 catecholamine metabolites in the urine (Gitlow et al., 1970). In Stage IV patients a low urinary vanillylmandelic acid (VMA)/ homovanillic acid (HVA) ratio and increased amounts of cystathionine (CTH) correlated with a poor prognosis (Laug et al., 1978). The presence of increased catecholamines is not specific for malignancy; increased excretion has been noted in the entire spectrum of neural crest tumors (Greenfield and Shelley, 1965). Norepinephrine in the unbound state accounts for symptoms of tachycardia, increased perspiration, flushing, diarrhea, and hypertension. All these symptoms may be noted in children with neural crest tumors. After the tumor is removed catecholamine excretion will return to normal and the symptoms of diarrhea will subside (Hamilton et al., 1968). In congenital neuroblastoma symptoms of sweating, headache, paroxysmal hypertension, palpitation, and tingling in the fingertips and toes may occur in the mother due to fetal catecholamine entering the maternal circulation. Any gravidas showing the symptoms of pheochromocytoma or eclampsia should have analysis of urinary catecholamines performed (Voûte et al., 1970). Several descriptions of infantile polymyoclonia and opsoclonus have been reported in association with neural crest tumors (Soloman and Chutorian, 1968; Moe and Nellhaus 1970; Voûte et al., 1970). Another presentation of neuroblastomas has been as an acute cerebellar ataxia (Bray et al., 1969; Korobkin et al., 1972). These symptoms have resolved gradually after removal of the tumor; the neurological signs appear not directly attributable to the fall in urinary catecholamine and may in fact represent an immune state which is somewhat misdirected at the host's nervous system. There is extensive interest in the complex immune response known to be present in patients with neuroblastoma (Hellstrom et al., 1968, 1970). Both humoral cytotoxic antibody and cellular immune mechanisms are operative in the host defense of neuroblastoma. Progression of the tumor is associated with the appearance of a blocking antibody which inhibits the tumor directed, cytotoxic lymphocytes and humoral antibody. The microscopic pattern of the tumor is a critical prognostic guide; the slightest sign of differentiation such as increased nuclear size, presence of visible cytoplasm or cytoplasmic processes offer a favorable prognosis (Mäkinen, 1972). A proposed staging for children with neuroblastoma by the Children's Cancer Study Group A emphasizes the favorable prognosis of children under one year of age with a specialized Stage IV-S (Table 30.4) (Evans et al., 1971b). In a recent review of 109 cases of IV-S neuroblastoma, Stephenson et al. (1979) have shown that children under 6 weeks of age without skin metastases have a poorer prognosis relative to other IV-S patients. Reported instances of neuroblastoma in situ is 1 in 200 live births (Beckwith and Perrin, 1963). Several reports of familial neuroblastoma underline the need for further investigation of such kindreds (Hardy and Nesbit, 1972). Certainly this data suggests that neuroblastomas are very common and that immunologic integrity is critical to the regression of this exceedingly common tumor. Persistently elevated carcinoembryonic antigen levels have been associated with recurrent neuroblastoma (Frens et al., 1976). Factors reported to influence the prognosis of neuroblastoma are summarized in Table 30.5.

Treatment

Comparative studies between 1956 and 1968 have failed to show that chemotherapy has had a significant effect on survival; this is in sharp contrast to the improved survival shown in Wilms' tumor during the same period of time (Sutow, et al., 1970a). More recent reviews of

TABLE 30.4
Neuroblastoma Staging

Stage I	Tumors confined to organ or structure of origin
Stage II	Tumors extending in continuity beyond the organ or structure of origin but not crossing the midline; regional lymph nodes may be involved bilaterally[a]
Stage III	Tumors extending in continuity beyond the midline; regional lymph nodes may be involved bilaterally
Stage IV	Remote disease involving skeleton, organs, soft tissues or distant lymph node groups, etc.
Stage IV–S	Patients who otherwise would be Stage I or II but who have remote disease confined to one or more of the following sites: liver, skin or bone marrow (without radiographic evidence of metastases on complete skeletal survey)

[a] For tumors arising in midline structures (e.g., the organs of Zuckerkandl), penetration beyond the capsule and involvement of lymph nodes on the same side shall be considered Stage II. Bilateral extension of any type shall be considered Stage III.

TABLE 30.5
Factors Influencing Prognosis of Neuroblastoma

Factors	Favorable	Unfavorable
Age of diagnosis	Under 2 years	Over 2 years
	Over 6 weeks in IV-S	Under 6 weeks in IV-S
Stage of disease	I, IV-S, or II	III or IV
Location	Mediastinal or cervical	Abdominal
Metastatic spread	Skin in IV-S	Skeletal lesions or bone marrow invasion as in IV
Maturation to ganglion cells	Present	Absent
Lymphocytic and plasma cell infiltration	Present	Absent
Secretory granules on E/M	Present	Absent
Peripheral and marrow lymphocytosis	Present	Absent
Initial catecholamine excretion	Increased VMA/HVA ratio and decreased CTH in stage IV	Decreased VMA/HVA ratio and increased CTH in stage IV
Carcinoembryonic antigen	Return to normal	Persistently elevated
Cell mediated cytotoxicity and cytotoxic antibodies	Present	Absent
Blocking factors	Absent	Present

chemotherapy in advanced neuroblastoma have come to the same negative conclusion (Breslow and McCann, 1971; Leikin et al., 1974).

SURGERY

Complete surgical resection is recommended whenever possible and is usually practical in children with Stage I and II disease. Technical problems become greater with advancing stages; tumors arising from the celiac axis may not yield to complete resection (Koop, 1968). Aggressive surgery in Stage IV patients with retroperitoneal primaries must be evaluated individually and weighed against the complications of pancreatitis or bleeding. Although an aggressive surgical approach has been advocated in Stage IV disease by Fortner et al. (1968), such an approach would not be advisable in a Stage IV-S patient who stands an excellent prognosis with only minimal chemotherapy. A second look procedure for nonresectable primaries is desirable, as in Wilms' tumor, this may be accomplished after the tumor has shown regression with radiotherapy and chemotherapy. Children with mediastinal neuroblastomas have a distinctly improved prognosis over those presenting with neuroblastoma at other locations. Although the primary tumor was completely excised in only 8 of 27 mediastinal neuroblastomas there was an 85% survival rate (Filler et al., 1972). Neuroblastomas in the posterior mediastinum or in the retroperitoneal space may extend via the intervertebral foramina to the extradural space in a dumbbell or hourglass configuration causing compression of the spinal cord. Although this condition has occurred more commonly in the older child it has also been reported in the newborn (Rothner, 1971). A laminectomy should be performed to prevent further destruction of nervous tissue.

RADIOTHERAPY

Even though neuroblastoma is a relatively radiosensitive tumor, radiotherapy has not been routinely advised in the Stage I or Stage IV patient. Radiation therapy in the range of 1200–2500 rads was found to be effective in prolonging the survival of patients with Stage III disease (Koop and Johnson, 1971). Increased application of radiotherapy with combination chemotherapy has been advocated in Stage IV patients (Perez et al., 1967). This may improve the response of patients with advanced disease.

CHEMOTHERAPY

Combination chemotherapy with vincristine and cyclophosphamide has been found effective in prolonging the disease free survival of neuroblastoma (James et al., 1965; Evans et al., 1969). Although not as striking as the former two agents in combination, daunorubicin also has shown activity against the tumor (Tan et al., 1967; Sutow et al., 1970b; Samuels et al., 1971). Adriamycin, a compound very similar to daunorubicin, has also shown some activity in neuroblastoma (Bonadonna et al., 1970; Wang et al., 1971a; Tan et al., 1973). A 60% response rate has been reported in 20 patients with a combination of vincristine, cyclophosphamide and daunorubicin (Helson et al., 1972). In responders the median response duration was 17 months with a median survival time of 18 months in patients over 2 years of age. On the hypothesis that a non-cell cycle specific drug would be effective in neuroblastoma, combination chemotherapy with cyclophosphamide, vincristine, and imidazole carboxamide was applied to children with Stage IV disease; 19 of 26 children evaluable showed a complete or partial response (Finklestein, et al., 1974). This response rate of 73% represents the best so far reported in Stage IV neuroblastoma. Using a basic triple drug regimen of vincristine, cyclophosphamide and Adriamycin, Necheles et al., (1978) have increased the median remission time of patients with Stage III and IV neuroblastoma by adding intradermal MER, the methanol-extracted residue of BCG. In this nonrandom study, patients receiving the triple drug regimen had a median duration of complete remission less than one year while those receiving additional MER had remissions in excess of 24 months.

RHABDOMYOSARCOMA

The most common soft tissue sarcoma occurring in childhood is the rhadomyosarcoma; these tumors arise from mesenchymal cells located in striated muscle. Seven of 43 children autopsied with rhabdomyosarcoma had associated congenital anomalies (Ruymann et al., 1977). Four of these 7 cases involved malformations of the central nervous system including 1 case each of lumbosacral meningomyelocele with hydrocephalus, hemiatrophy of the left cerebral hemisphere and right cerebellar hemisphere, localized microgyria of the left operculum and diffuse cerebral microgyria. The embryonal rhabdomyosarcoma is more common in the younger age group; when arising from under a mucosal surface it will present as a grapelike tumor, sarcoma botryoides. The alveolar rhabdomyosarcoma is more common in adolescents while pleomorphic rhabdomyosarcomas occur only rarely in childhood; undifferentiated sarcomas may be treated as embryonal rhabdomyosarcomas. The presentation of sarcomas in childhood is very deceptive since they can arise from any site on the body. The most common location for embryonal rhabdomyosarcoma is the head and neck area. In one series of 78 children with a mean age of 5 years and 7 months, 48 of the rhabdomyosarcomas occurred in that area (Sutow et al., 1970c). The prognosis in childhood has been related to the age at diagnosis, location of primary, extent of disease, histologic variety, and treatment (Sutow et al., 1970a). Survival has been shown to be affected mainly by the extent of disease at the time of diagnosis (Ehrlich et al., 1971; Pratt et al., 1972). The high incidence of hematogenous and lymphatic spread account for the early, distant metastases to bone marrow, liver, lungs, bones and lymph nodes. Bone marrow metastases at diagnosis are more common with alveolar histology and have a high incidence of concomitant metastases to bone, lymph node and lung (Ruymann et al., 1979). The outcome in earlier series with irregular application of surgery, radiotherapy and chemotherapy was largely fatal. In one study from 1946 to 1966 there were no long term survivors with inoperable or metastatic disease (Sutow et al., 1970a). The Intergroup Rhabdomyosarcoma Study grouping is shown in Table 30.6. This working classification is primarily dependent on the surgeon; several

TABLE 30.6
Intergroup Rhabdomyosarcoma Study Staging

Group I	Localized disease, completely resected with regional nodes not involved
	a. Confined to muscle or organ of origin
	b. Contiguous involvement with infiltration outside the muscle or organ of origin, as through fascial planes
Group II	a. Grossly resected tumor with microscopic residual disease and negative nodes
	b. Regional disease, completely resected with nodes either positive or negative
	c. Regional disease with involved nodes, grossly resected but with evidence of microscopic disease
Group III	Incomplete resection or biopsy with gross residual disease
Group IV	Metastatic disease present at onset

diagnostic studies, however, are desirable. In all cases the chest roentgenogram, complete skeletal survey and bone marrow aspiration with biopsy
are indicated. Radioisotopic scans of the liver, brain, and bones are of
great value in evaluating the patient preoperatively. Early extension of
nasopharyngeal, paranasal sinus, and middle ear rhabdomyosarcomas
through the dura make cytological examination of the spinal fluid necessary. Angiography is useful in the differentiation of abdominal rhabdomyosarcoma, from Wilms' tumor or neuroblastoma.

Treatment

SURGERY

A wide local excision of the primary tumor to achieve Group I or II is
desirable if not excessively destructive. The false capsule commonly
found with these tumors may be very misleading with the growing edge
of tumor well beyond the assumed margins. In superficial tumors of the
head and neck, where extension into bone has been demonstrated from
the onset needle biopsy may be used to establish a histological diagnosis.
The current trend in surgical management is away from routine exenteration of orbital and pelvic primaries (Maurer et al., 1977). A more limited
surgery for pelvic primaries is being proposed in Intergroup Rhabdomyosarcoma Study II. Tumors arising in the nasopharyngeal space or in the
middle ear cannot be easily resected and the surgical role is primarily
one of diagnostic biopsy. A review of 40 cases of rhabdomyosarcoma of
the middle ear showed no survivors (Jaffe et al., 1971). More recently
several cases with long term survival have been reported (Conte and
Sagerman, 1971; Edland, 1972; Fish et al., 1972; Cunningham and Kung,
1972; Webb and McFarland, 1973). Combination chemotherapy with
radiotherapy was applied in all 5 of the surviving individuals; only 2
patients had radical mastoidectomy. The common extension of paratesticular and spermatic rhabdomyosarcomas to the retroperitoneal nodes
makes node dissection desirable (Burrington, 1969; Malek et al., 1972).
Testicular tumors in childhood have recently been reviewed and the
question of bilateral versus unilateral retroperitoneal node dissection in
paratesticular rhabdomyosarcomas remains unanswered (Giebink and
Ruymann, 1974). In the Intergroup Rhabdomyosarcoma Study a high
incidence of lymphatic spread has been documented in both genitourinary
and extremity primaries. Whereas, the incidence of lymphatic spread is
only 5% in other sites, genitourinary and extremity sites have been 19%
and 17%, respectively (Lawrence et al., 1977; Raney et al., 1978). As in
earlier studies, patients subjected to amputation for extremity primaries
in Intergroup Rhabdomyosarcoma Study I have done poorly (Hays et al.,
1977).

RADIOTHERAPY

Rhabdomyosarcoma is a tumor of moderate radiosensitivity (Nelson, 1968; Sagerman et al., 1972). Following an excisional biopsy with a wide margin, supravoltage radiation in the range of 5000–6000 rads will usually achieve complete local control. The Intergroup Rhabdomyosarcoma Study is currently randomizing patients in Group I to receive or not receive local irradiation. A preliminary report of Intergroup Rhabdomyosarcoma Study I (Maurer et al., 1977) suggests that no advantage is gained by irradiating the primary site in Group I patients. At last report, 92% of both the irradiated and nonirradiated groups of patients enjoy a disease free status with a median follow-up of 72 weeks. Special attention has been called to sites at high risk for direct meningeal extension (Tefft et al., 1978). In 20 of 57 rhabdomyosarcomas arising in the nasopharynx, paranasal sinuses, and middle ear, meningeal involvement presented at diagnosis or shortly thereafter. Special radiotherapy guidelines have been established in Intergroup Rhabdomyosarcoma Study I and Study II to prevent this usually fatal complication (Maurer et al., 1977).

CHEMOTHERAPY

Tumor regression with actinomycin D occurred in 26% of patients with rhabdomyosarcoma as summarized by Pratt (1969). Cyclophosphamide resulted in tumor regression in 57% of 37 patients with rhabdomyosarcoma (Haddy et al., 1967; Pratt et al., 1968). Vincristine used as a single agent resulted in tumor regression in 50% of patients treated (Sutow et al., 1966; Pratt et al., 1968). The use of these three chemotherapeutic agents in combination was applied to 7 patients with advanced rhabdomyosarcoma; all patients responded with a median response time of 4 months (Pratt, 1969). A prolonged tumor-free survival in 7 of 20 patients was also reported using these same agents (Pratt et al., 1972). Patients with localized tumors were treated for 6 months while those with generalized tumors were treated 12 months. Wilbur and co-workers at the M. D. Anderson Hospital initially reported on a group of patients with rhabdomyosarcoma in which two-thirds of the patients were doing well without evidence of disease (Wilbur et al., 1971). Subsequent follow-up on these patients showed that of 32 patients with embryonal rhabdomyosarcoma or undifferentiated sarcoma who had not received previous chemotherapy or radiotherapy, 22 were alive with no evidence of disease (Wilbur and Etcubanas, 1974). This report is all the more remarkable since 75% of these 32 patients had inoperable or metastatic disease. Several series have reported the use of adriamycin in rhabdomyosarcoma; the average response rate in these series is 58% (Bonadonna et al., 1970; O'Bryan et al., 1973; Tan et al., 1973).

Preliminary results of the Intergroup Rhabdomyosarcoma Study I in 278 evaluable patients reveal a 92% disease free survival for Group I patients receiving vincristine, dactinomycin and cyclophosphamide (VAC) in combination for 2 years. Postoperative radiotherapy to the tumor bed did not enhance disease control in Group I patients. In Group II 85% of the patients exhibited no evidence of disease with either 2 years of VAC or 1 year of vincristine and dactinomycin. All Group II patients received radiotherapy. Patients with Group III and Group IV rhabdomyosarcoma were randomized on Intergroup Rhabdomyosarcoma Study I to treatment regimens which included either "pulse" VAC or "pulse" VAC plus Adriamycin. Early results suggest that no significantly increased response or survival is achieved by the addition of Adriamycin at 60 mg/m^2 (Maurer et al., 1977). In Group III patients, 69% remain in continuous response with a median follow-up time of 41–44 weeks. With similar median follow-up 50% of Group IV patients are alive. A more extensive "pulse"-VAC regimen with or without adriamycin has been planned for trial in clinical Group III and IV patients in the Intergroup Rhabdomyosarcoma Study II. Imidazole carboxamide in combination with adriamycin has shown activity in a variety of soft tissue sarcomas (Gottlieb et al., 1972).

RETINOBLASTOMA

Retinoblastoma is a malignancy of retinal neuroepithelium occurring almost exclusively in young children with an incidence of 1/14,000 births (Francois and Matton-VanLeuven, 1964). The improved survival of patients with retinoblastoma and other genetic factors may account for the increasing frequency of this tumor. The distribution of hereditary and sporadic cases is 40% and 60%, respectively. A two-step mutational model best satisfies the occurrence of hereditary and sporadic retinoblastoma (Knudson, 1971). In this model all bilateral cases are considered hereditary while only 15% of unilateral cases are hereditary. A slight predominance of males has been noted in bilateral retinoblastoma by Leelawongs and Regan (1968), despite the generally accepted autosomal inheritance of this malignancy. A patient with the inherited germ cell mutation is more likely to develop retinoblastomas which are multiple and occur at a younger age.

The average age of diagnosis is 18 months; two-thirds of children present with a white pupillary or cat's eye reflex. It is not uncommon for the white pupillary reflex to be seen in early childhood photographs taken with a flash bulb. Macular involvement causes strabismus as a presenting sign in 20% of the patients. About 10% of the presentations are atypical and include glaucoma, chemosis, pain, irritability, conjunctival hemorrhage, corneal cloudiness, and ocular wasting (Andrew and Smith, 1965;

Schuster and Ferguson, 1970). Initial misdiagnosis in 14.9% of patients in a review of 825 cases and delay in treatment of correctly diagnosed patients resulted in increased mortality (Stafford et al., 1969). Since 25–30% of retinoblastomas are bilateral, meticulous examination of the retina in both eyes by indirect ophthalmoscopy is necessary for accurate diagnosis and staging. A useful staging system (Table 30.7) has been developed, based on the extent of intraocular disease (Reese, 1955; Ellsworth, 1969). The number, size, description and location of ocular lesions must be accurately recorded under general anesthesia with the pupils fully dilated. Other diagnostic studies include chest x-ray and a skull series with special views of the orbital and optic foramina. Brain scan, bone scan, bone marrow aspiration, and spinal fluid examination are indicated in most instances. With active disease urinary catecholamine catabolite values have been reported elevated by Brown (1966). Both neuroblastoma and retinoblastoma are of neural crest origin and may form rosettes.

The major published experience with retinoblastoma is from the Columbia-Presbyterian Medical Center where 900 patients have been examined from 1938 through 1968 (Ellsworth, 1969; Tapley and Tretter, 1973). The team approach emphasized by these publications and those of others is essential to proper management (Leelawongs and Regan, 1968).

Treatment

A small tumor of Group I, II, or III in a child with a family history of retinoblastoma may be treated by irradiation without a tissue diagnosis in some cases. Early suspicious lesions occurring in the absence of a

TABLE 30.7
Retinoblastoma Staging

Group I	Prognosis very favorable
	a. Solitary tumor, less than 4 disc diameters in size, at or behind the equator
	b. Multiple tumors, none over 4 disc diameters in size, all at or behind the equator
Group II	Prognosis favorable
	a. Solitary tumor, 4–10 disc diameters in size, at or behind the equator
	b. Multiple tumors, 4–10 disc diameters in size, all behind the equator
Group III	Prognosis doubtful
	a. Any lesion anterior to the equator
	b. Solitary tumors larger than 10 disc diameters behind the equator
Group IV	Prognosis unfavorable
	a. Multiple tumors, some larger than 10 disc diameters
	b. Any lesion extending anteriorly to the ora serrata
Group V	Prognosis very unfavorable
	a. Massive tumors involving over half the retina
	b. Vitreous seeding

hereditary precedent will require serial ophthalmoscopy. Occasionally in such a patient enucleation will be necessary. Trials of radiation therapy to establish diagnosis are not recommended. With bilateral retinoblastoma the dilemma of preserving vision versus removing the tumor comes into sharper focus. Even if the least involved eye is a Group V effort should be made to salvage vision. When there is no hope for achieving useful vision, the more extensively diseased eye should be removed.

Removal of the eye with a long segment of optic nerve is desirable. If tumor cells have invaded the optic nerve proximal to the major retinal vessels entrance and exit, then spread to the subarachoid space is a certainty and orbital exenteration would be unnecessary.

Radiotherapy with an 18–22 meV Betatron in a dose of 3500 rads over 3 weeks is standard for Groups I, II and III. Details regarding size, angle of the beam and shielding must be adhered to so as to preserve vision in the contralateral eye, minimize cataract formation in the treated eye, and maximize cure (Tapley and Tretter, 1973). Light coagulation may be adjunctive to radiotherapy in the treatment of lesions anterior to the equator. The more advanced tumors in Groups IV and V are treated through an anterior portal with 1000–1500 rads and a posterior retinal port with 4500 rads in 4 weeks. Choroidal extension, larger, recurrent tumors and small solitary tumors on the nasal side are suitable for surface applicators (Stallard, 1962). Several patterns of regression have been observed; generally control is probable if the tumor remains smaller than the original lesion. Recurrent retinoblastoma represents a major problem and may require a second course of irradiation. Blindness may complicate treatment after a second course of irradiation (Ellsworth, 1969). Complications of active residual tumor and hemorrhage with secondary glaucoma is distributed equally in eyes removed after tumor regrowth and retreatment. Shukovsky and Fletcher (1972) reported that retinal doses in excess of 6800 rads over 6 weeks will result in blindness within 2–5 years. In 11.6% of the patients secondary tumors of osteosarcoma and rhabdomyosarcoma occur within the field of irradiation (Sagermann et al., 1969). The majority of these secondary malignancies occur at tumor doses in excess of 8000 rads with latent periods of 4–30 years. Besides light coagulation, cryotherapy to isolated tumor masses has merit (Rubin, 1968). Since 1953 triethylene melamine (TEM) has been used by the Columbia-Presbyterian group with questionable success. A nonrandom experience reported by Krementz et al. (1966) showed improved survival and vision in the TEM treated group. However, a randomized experience using TEM intramuscularly in Groups I and II failed to show any improvement (Tapley, 1964). Expectations remain that in advanced disease, Groups IV and V, TEM may be of value. Injection of TEM at 0.08–0.1 mg/kg into the internal carotid artery under direct exposure 24 hours prior to beginning irradiation has been used in patients with extensive retinal involvement (Tapley and Tretter, 1973). The response of metastatic disease to cyclophosphamide, chlorambucil, actinomycin D, vincristine, and methotrexate by Sitarz et al. (1965) has prompted investigators at St. Jude's Medical Center to use these drugs in newly diagnosed advanced group patients (C. B. Pratt, unpublished data). The prognosis for patients with demonstrated subarachnoid spread at the time of diagnosis remains extremely poor but prolonged survival with metastatic disease in the central nervous system has been observed (Wilbur and Etcubanus, 1974).

Extensive combination therapy with whole brain irradiation, systemic CCNU and the use of intrathecal methotrexate, cytosine arabinoside, and hydrocortisone may be required in such instances. As yet there is no statistical support for the use of chemotherapy in early disease. The overall mortality of 15% is attributable primarily to good surgical judgments and improved radiotherapeutic techniques (Tapley and Tretter, 1973). Randomized studies of combination chemotherapy now in progress may show further improvements in advanced groups. Perhaps more than in any other childhood malignancy, experienced team management is essential for good results in retinoblastoma.

HEPATOBLASTOMA

The treatment of primary tumors of the liver has recently been reviewed by Remichovsky et al. (1974). The two major hepatic malignancies are hepatoblastoma, usually presenting under 3 years of age and hepatoma which is more common in children over 5 years. Ishak and Glunz (1967) have reviewed a series of 47 cases from the Armed Forces Institute of Pathology. Both hepatoblastoma and hepatoma occur predominantly in male caucasians. Hepatoblastomas comprise 75% of Izhak and Glunz's series and arise solely in the left lobe in only 4 of 35 patients. The relatively less common hepatomas of children are histologically identical to those of adults.

Although chronic active hepatitis, cirrhosis, Australian antigen positivity, androgen therapy, and aflatoxin have been associated with the pathogenesis of hepatomas no such relationships have been found for hepatoblastoma.

Elevated α-fetoprotein levels are found commonly in both malignancies (McIntire et al., 1972). As with Wilms' tumor and adrenal carcinoma, hepatoblastoma has been associated with hemihypertrophy (Geiser et al., 1970). We have recently treated a child with hepatoblastoma who in the course of his illness exhibited pathological fractures, osteoporosis and virilization. Both in vivo and in vitro production of human chorionic gonadotropin and α-fetoprotein were demonstrated (Braunstein et al.,

1972). Additional associations of hepatoblastomas with Fanconi's syndrome, cystathionuria, hypercholesterolemia, and hypercalcemia emphasize the varied metabolic interactions of this malignancy.

Progressive abdominal enlargement, weight loss, anorexia and vomiting are the most common presenting symptoms. An abdominal mass is palpable in 75% of the children with additional findings being pallor, emaciation, splenomegaly, and abdominal venous distention. Mild to moderate abnormalities in liver function studies are common. Since neuroblastoma is the most common metastatic tumor found in the liver a screening study for urinary VMA is desirable (LaBrosse, 1968). Intravenous pyelography is helpful in delineating primary malignancies of the retroperitoneal space; however, a hepatoblastoma arising in the right lobe of the liver will commonly cause inferior and posterior displacement of the right kidney. A radioisotopic liver-spleen scan and arteriography are more definitive and will provide the surgeons with essential preoperative data (Wang et al., 1971b).

The benign hemangioendothelioma may be confused with a malignant hepatoma (McSweeney et al., 1973). Intractable, high output heart failure from arteriovenous shunting is suggested by progressive respiratory distress in an infant with an enlarged liver and hepatic bruit. Arteriography is prerequisite to the proper diagnosis and surgical management of this benign vascular tumor (Leonidas et al., 1973). In one series benign hamartomas accounted for 7 of 39 liver tumors presenting under three years of age (Keeling, 1971).

Treatment

The published survival of primary malignancies of the liver in children is 30–40% (Kasai and Watanabe, 1970). Younger children with hepatoblastoma may be expected to do better than the older child with hepatoma. Complete, aggressive, surgical resection of the malignant hepatic tumor, whether hepatoblastoma or hepatoma, remains the primary goal in management. Survival will depend directly on the degree to which initial resection is achieved (Foster, 1970). An estimated 20% of remaining liver tissue is thought sufficient for survival (Remischovsky et al., 1974). The surgical anatomy of liver resection has been carefully described by Nixon (1965) and Raffucci and Ramirez-Schon (1970). Postoperative support may require infusions of glucose and albumin as well as intravenous hyperalimentation. The remarkable regenerative and functional capacity of the child's liver permits an aggressive, surgical approach to hepatic malignancy.

Although not curative in primary hepatic malignancies, radiotherapy has a distinct role in reducing tumor size to improve palliation or achieve resectability. If half of the liver is irradiated a dose up to 4500 rads may be given; whole liver exposure should be limited to 2500 rads. Caution is required in the simultaneous administration of actinomycin D and whole liver irradiation (Tefft et al., 1971). Enhancement of radiation induced hepatitis by actinomycin D is attributable to is radiomimetic effect on biological tissues and to the delayed excretion of actinomycin D by a compromised liver.

Although tumor regression has been reported with a variety of single agents no consistent treatment has emerged. Preliminary studies by Children's Cancer Study Group A with combination actinomycin D, vincristine and cyclophosphamide have not been encouraging (Remischovsky et al., 1974). Patients with recurrence or metastases are placed on weekly 5-fluouracil. Limited responses have been achieved in a small series of adult hepatomas using adriamycin 75 mg/m^2 every 3 weeks (Olweny et al., 1975).

TERATOMA

Teratomas are tumors of germ cell origin and contain tissue arising from all three embryonic layers, ectoderm, mesoderm and endoderm. The site of these tumors is predominantly midline or gonadal. In order of frequency the location of teratomas in children is as follows: ovarian, sacrococcygeal, testicular, intrathoracic, retroperitoneal, intracranial and cervical (Partlow and Taybi, 1971).

The incidence of sacrococcygeal teratomas has been reported as 1 in 40,000 live births (Gelb et al., 1964). Careful physical examination and radiographic studies of skin-covered sacrococcygeal masses in infants and children are prerequisite to their evaluation. Presacral components are best demonstrated by anterior displacement of the rectum on a lateral radiograph. A positive rectal examination is a consistent finding with presacral extension (Lemire et al., 1971). Calcification within the mass is commonly seen in sacrococcygeal and gonadal teratomas (Lemire et al., 1971; Wooley et al., 1967).

Congenital anomalies of the lower gastrointestinal and urinary tracts are higher than expected in patients with sacrococcygeal teratomas (Berry et al., 1970). The female to male ratio is 4.5 to 1 in the 111 cases reviewed by Waldhausen et al. (1963). The earlier report by Gross et al. (1951) of a family history of twins in over half the patients has not been confirmed.

Pathological classification of teratomas is confusing at best which makes comparison of treatments doubly confounding. A recent review of embryonal adenocarcinoma arising in the sacrococcygeal region emphasizes the basic teratomatous quality of this malignancy (Chretien et al., 1970).

Similarly, in testicular tumors of childhood embryonal carcinoma, choriocarcinoma, and teratoma are closely related and may be classified respectively as immature, intermediate, and mature teratomas (Melicow, 1955). A recent review of 609 testicular tumors in childhood by Giebink and Ruymann (1974) emphasizes the relative decreased incidence of germinal tumors, 69% in children compared to 98% in adult males (Dixon and Moore, 1952).

Mature, well differentiated teratomata are treated by simple surgical excision. For embryonal carcinomas of the testis bilateral retroperitoneal node dissection with combination chemotherapy and radiotherapy has been recommended (Duckett et al., 1974). Firm recommendations for teratocarcinoma, of lower grade malignancy are less clear. A series of 21 patients with embryonal adenocarcinoma, an anaplastic sacrococcygeal teratoma, showed universal recurrence despite resection and irradiation (Chretien et al., 1970). Extensive hematogenous spread was indicated by pulmonary metastases in 19 patients. Early surgical removal with normal margins and postoperative chemotherapy has been recommended by the authors. The surgical approach to sacrococcygeal tumors utilizes a combined abdominal and sacrococcygeal approach if there is a presacral component (Waldhausen et al., 1963). Experiences with the chemotherapy of teratomas in children are extremely limited as noted by Smith and Rutledge (1973). The largest experience has been at M. D. Anderson Hospital where several basic regimens have had success (Table 30.8). The VAC regimen evolved primarily out of success with rhabdomyosarcoma at the same institution. Obviously, the treatment of malignant teratomas is unsettled but there is a definite move toward earlier, definitive surgery with node dissection, radiotherapy, and combination chemotherapy.

TABLE 30.8
Commonly Used Treatment Regimens in Childhood Solid Tumors[a]

VAC	
Vincristine:	2 mg/m² IV weekly for 12 weeks (maximum 2 mg)
Actinomycin D:	0.075 mg/kg/course IV over 5 days (maximum 0.5 mg/day) every 3 months for 5 courses
Cyclophosphamide:	2.5 mg/kg/day PO for 2 years
PULSE-VAC	
Vincristine:	2 mg/m² IV weekly for 12 weeks (maximum 2 mg)
Actinomycin D:	0.075 mg/kg/course IV over 5 days (maximum 0.5 mg/day) every 3 months for 5 courses
Cyclophosphamide:	10 mg/kg/day for 7 days IV or PO every 6 weeks
ACT-FU-CY	(course repeated every 3 weeks)
Actinomycin D:	0.075 mg/kg/course IV over 5 days
5-Fluorouracil:	40–50 mg/kg/course IV over 5 days
Cyclophosphamide:	30–40 mg/kg/course IV over 5 days

[a] Wilbur and Etcubanas (1974); Smith and Rutledge (1973).

REFERENCES

Allerton, S. E., Beierle, J. W., Powars, D. R., and Bavetta, L. A. Abnormal extracellular components in Wilms' tumor. Cancer Res., *30:* 679–688, 1970.

Andrew, J. M., and Smith, D. R. Unsuspected retinoblastoma. Am. J. Ophthalmol., *60:* 536–540, 1965.

Bachmann, K. D., and Kröll, W. Wilms' tumor in the first year of life. Dtsch. Med. Wochenschr., *94:* 2598–2602, 1969.

Beckwith, J. B., and Palmer, N. F. Histopathology and prognosis of Wilms' tumor; results from the First National Wilms' Tumor Study. Cancer, *41:* 1937–1948, 1978.

Beckwith, J. B., and Perrin, E. V. In situ neuroblastomas; a contribution to the natural history of neural crest tumors. Am. J. Pathol., *43:* 1089–1104, 1963.

Berry, C. L., Keeling, J. and Hilton, C. Coincidence of congenital malformation and embryonic tumours of childhood. Arch. Dis. Child., *45:* 229–231, 1970.

Blom, J., and Brodovsky, H. S. Comparison of the treatment of metastatic testicular tumors with actinomycin D or actinomycin D, bleomycin, and vincristine (abstr.). Am. Soc. Clin. Oncol., *16:* 247, 1975.

Bolande, R. P., Brough, A.J., and Izant, R. J., Jr. Congenital mesoblastic nephroma of infancy. Pediatrics, *40:* 272–278, 1967.

Bonadonna, G., Monfardini, S., Delang, M., Fossati-Bellani, F., and Beretta, G. Phase I and preliminary phase II evaluation of Adriamycin (NSC-123127). Cancer Res., *30:* 2572–2582, 1970.

Braunstein, G. D., Bridson, W. E., Glass, A., Hall, E. W., and McIntire, K. R. In vivo and in vitro production of human chorionic gonadotropin and alpha-fetoprotein by a virilizing hepatoblastoma. J. Clin. Endocrinol. Metab., *35:* 857–862, 1972.

Bray, P. F., Ziter, F. A., Lahey, M. E., and Myers, G. G. The coincidence of neuroblastoma and acute cerebellar encephalopathy. J. Pediatr., *75:* 983–990, 1969.

Breslow, N., and McCann, B. Statistical estimation of prognosis for children with neuroblastoma. Cancer Res., *31:* 2098–2103, 1971.

Breslow, N. E., Palmer, N. F., Hill, L. R., Buring, J., and D'Angio, G. J. Wilms' tumor; prognostic factors for patients without metastases at diagnosis; results of the National Wilms' Tumor Study. Cancer, *41:* 1577–1589, 1978.

Brown, D. H. The urinary excretion of vanillyl mandelic acid (VMA) and homovanillic acid (HVA) in children with retinoblastoma. Am. J. Ophthalmol., *62:* 239–243, 1966.

Burrington, J. D. Rhabdomyosarcoma of the paratesticular tissues in children; report of eight cases. J. Pediatr. Surg., *4:* 503–509, 1969.

Chretien, P. B., Milan, J. D., Foote, F. W., and Miller, T. R. Embryonal adenocarcinomas (a type of malignant teratoma) of the sacrococcygeal region. Cancer, *26:* 522–535, 1970.

Conte, P. J., and Sagerman, R. H. Embryonal rhabdomyosarcoma of the middle ear with long term survival. N. Engl. J. Med., *284:* 92–93, 1971.

Cortes, E. P., Holland, J. F., Wang, J. J., Sinks, L. F., Blom, J., Senn, H., and Glidewell, Amputation and Adriamycin in primary osteosarcoma. N. Engl. J. Med., *291:* 998–1000, 1974.

Cunningham, M. D., and Kung, F. H. Combined therapy for middle ear rhabdomyosarcoma. Am. J. Dis. Child., *124:* 401–402, 1972.

D'Angio, G. J. Management of children with Wilms' tumor. Cancer, *30:* 1528–1533, 1972.

D'Angio, G. J., Beckwith, J. B., Bishop, H. C., Breslow, N., Evans, A. E., Goodwin, W. E., King, L. R., Pickett, L. K., Sinks, L. F., Sutow, W. W., and Wolff, J. A. Childhood cancer; the National Wilms' Tumor Study; a progress report. Urology, *3:* 798–806, 1974.

D'Angio, G. J., et al. National Wilms' Tumor Study-2; Informational Bull. No. 8, 1978.

DeLorimier, A. A., Bragg, K. U., and Linden, G. Neuroblastoma in childhood. Am. J. Dis. Child., *118:* 441–450, 1969.

Dixon, F. J., and Moore, R. A. Tumors of the male sex organs. *In* Atlas of Tumor Pathology, Sec. VIII, Fasc. 31b and 32. Armed Forces Institute of Pathology, Washington, D.C., 1952.

Duckett, J. W., Jr., Cromie, W. B., and Bongiovanni, A. M. Genitourinary tumors in children. Semin. Oncol., 1: 71–75, 1974.

Edland, R. W. Embryonal rhabdomyosarcoma of the middle ear. Cancer, 29: 784–788, 1972.

Ehrlich, F. E., Haas, J. E., and Kiesewetter, W. B. Rhabdomyosarcoma in infants and children; factors affecting long-term survival. J. Pediatr. Surg., 6: 571–577, 1971.

Ellsworth, R. M. The practical management of retinoblastoma. Trans. Am. Opthalmol. Soc., 67: 462–534, 1969.

Evans, A. E., Heyn, R. M., Newton, W. A., Jr., and Leikin, S. L. Vincristine sulfate and cyclophosphamide for children with metastatic neuroblastoma. J.A.M.A., 207: 1325–1327, 1969.

Evans, A. E., Blore, J., Hadley R., and Tanindi, S. The LaBrosse spot test; a practical aid in the diagnosis and management of children with neuroblastoma. Pediatrics, 47: 913–915, 1971a.

Evans, A. E., D'Angio, G. J., and Randolph, J. A proposed staging for children with neuroblastoma. Cancer, 27: 374–378, 1971b.

Farber, S. The control of cancer in children; The Guy H. Heath and Dan C. C. Heath Memorial Lecture. In the University of Texas M. D. Anderson Hospital and Tumor Institute; Neoplasia in Childhood, p. 323. Year Book Medical Publishers, Chicago, 1969.

Farber, S., D'Angio, G. J., Evans, A., and Mitus, A. Clinical studies on actinomycin D., with special reference to Wilms' tumors in children. Ann. N.Y. Acad. Sci., 89: 421–425, 1960.

Filler, R. M., Traggis, D. G., Jaffe, N., and Vawter, G. F. Favorable outlook for children with mediastinal neuroblastoma. J. Pediatr. Surg., 7: 136–143, 1972.

Finklestein, J. Z., Leikin, S., Evans, A., Klemperer, M., Bernstein, I., Hittle, R., and Hammond, G. D. Combination chemotherapy for metastatic neuroblastoma (abstr.). Proc. Am. Assoc. Cancer Res., 15: 44, 1974.

Fish, C. A., Koch, H. F., and Canales, L. Survival in rhabdomyosarcoma. Am. J. Dis. Child., 124: 408–409, 1972.

Fortner, J., Nicastri, A., and Murphy, M. L. Neuroblastoma; natural history and results of treating 133 cases. Ann. Surg., 167: 132–142, 1968.

Foster, J. H. Survival after liver resection for cancer. Cancer, 26: 493–502, 1970.

Francois, J., and Matton-VanLeuven, M. T. Recent data on the heredity of retinoblastoma. In Ocular and Adnexal Tumors, edited by M. Boniuk, pp. 123–141. C. V. Mosby, St. Louis, 1964.

Frens, D. B., Bray, P. F., Wu, J. T., and Lahey, M. E. The carcinoembryonic antigen assay; prognostic value in neural crest tumors. J. Pediatr., 88: 591–594, 1976.

Geiser, C. F., Baez, A., Schindler, A. M. and Shih, V. E. Epithelial hepatoblastoma associated with congenital hemihypertrophy and cystathionuria; presentation of a case. Pediatrics, 46: 66–73, 1970.

Gelb, A., Rosenblum, H., Jaurigue, V. G., Liboro, C., and Francisco, P. Sacrococcygeal teratoma. Del. Med. J., 36: 119–123, 1964.

Giebink, G. S., and Ruymann, F. B. Testicular tumors in childhood; review and report of three cases. Am. J. Dis. Child., 127: 433–438, 1974.

Gitlow, S. E., Bertani, L. M., Rausen, A., Gribetz, D., and Dziedzic, S. W. Diagnosis of neuroblastoma by qualitative and quantitative determination of catecholamine metabolites in urine. Cancer, 25: 1377–1383, 1970.

Gottlieb, J., Baker, L. H., Ouayliana, J. M., Luce, J. K., Whitecar, J. P., Sinkovics, J. G., Rivkin, S. E., Brownlee, R., and Frei, E. Chemotherapy of sarcomas with a combination of Adriamycin and dimethyltriazeno-imidazole carboxamide. Cancer, 30: 1632–1638, 1972.

Graivier, L., and Vargas, M. A. 1972. Xanthogranulomatous pyelonephritis in childhood. Am. J. Dis. Child., 123: 156–158, 1972.

Greenfield, L. J., and Shelley, W. M. The spectrum of neurogenic tumors of the sympathetic nervous system; maturation and adrenergic function. J. Natl. Cancer Inst., 35: 215–226, 1965.

Gross, R. E., and Neuhauser, E. B. D. Treatment of mixed tumors of the kidneys in childhood. Pediatrics, *6:* 843–852, 1950.

Gross, R. E., Clatworthy, H. W., and Meeker, I. A., Jr. Sacrococcygeal teratomas in infants and children. Surg. Gynecol. Obstet., *92:* 341–354, 1951.

Haddy, T. B., Nora, A. H., Sutow, W. W., and Vietti, J. J. Cyclophosphamide treatment for metastatic soft tissue sarcoma; intermittent large doses in the treatment of children. Am. J. Dis. Child., *114:* 301–308, 1967.

Hamilton, J. R., Radde, I. C., and Johnson, G. Diarrhea associated with adrenal ganglio-neuroma. Am. J. Med., *44:* 453–463, 1968.

Hardy, P. C., and Nesbit, M. E. Familial neuroblastoma; report of a kindred with a high incidence of infantile tumors. J. Pediatr., *80:* 74–77, 1972.

Hays, D. M., Sutow, W. W., Lawrence, W., Moon, T. E., and Tefft, M. Rhabdomyosarcoma; surgical therapy in extremity lesions in children. Orthop. Clin. North Am., *8:* 883–902, 1977.

Hellstrom, I. E., Hellstrom, K. E., Pierce, G. E., and Bill, A. H. Demonstration of cell-bound and humoral immunity against neuroblastoma cells. Proc. Natl. Acad. Sci. U.S.A., *60:* 1231–1238, 1968.

Hellstrom, I. E., Hellstrom, K. E., Bill, A. H., and Pierce, G. E. Studies on cellular immunity to human neuroblastoma cells. Int. J. Cancer, *6:* 172–188, 1970.

Helson, L., Vanichayangkul, P., Tan, C. C., Wollner, N., and Murphy, M. L. Combination intermittent chemotherapy for patients with disseminated neuroblastoma. Cancer Chemother. Rep., *56:* 499–503, 1972.

Howard, R. Actinomycin D in Wilms' tumour; treatment of lung metastases. Arch. Dis. Child., *40:* 200–202, 1965.

Ishak, K. G., and Glunz, P. R. Hepatoblastoma and hepatocarcinoma in infancy and childhood. Cancer, *20:* 396–422, 1967.

Jaffe, B. F., Fox, J. E., and Batsakis, J. G. Rhabdomyosarcoma of the middle ear and mastoid. Cancer, *27:* 29–37, 1971.

Jagasia, K. H., Thurman, W. G., Pickett, E., and Grabstaldt, H. Bilateral Wilms' tumors in children. J. Pediatr., *65:* 371–376, 1964.

James, D. H., Jr., Hustu, O., Wrenn, E. L., Jr., and Pinkel, D. Combination chemotherapy of childhood neuroblastoma. J.A.M.A., *194:* 123–126, 1965.

Kasai, M., and Watanabe, I. Histologic classification of liver-cell carcinoma in infancy and childhood and its clinical evaluation. Cancer, *25:* 551–563, 1970.

Keeling, J. W. Liver tumors in infancy and childhood. J. Pathol., *103:* 69–85, 1971.

Kilman, J. W., Kronenberg, M. W., O'Neill, J. A., Jr., and Klassen, K. P. Surgical resection for pulmonary metastases in children. Arch. Surg., *99:* 158–165, 1969.

Kinzel, R. C., Mills, S. D., Childs, D. S., Jr., and DeWeerd, J. H. Wilms' tumor; a review of 47 cases. J.A.M.A., *174:* 1925–1929, 1960.

Kithier, K., Jusher, J., Brought, J., and Poulik, M. D. Effect of therapy on the serum level of alpha$_1$-fetoprotein in embryonal cell carcinoma. J. Pediatr. *81:* 71–75, 1972.

Klapproth, H. J. Wilms' tumor; a report of 45 cases and an analysis of 1,351 cases reported in the world literature from 1940 to 1958. J. Urol. *81:* 633–647, 1959.

Knudson, A. G. Mutation and cancer; statistical study of retinoblastoma. Proc. Natl. Acad. Sci. U.S.A., *68:* 820–823, 1971.

Koop, C. E. The role of surgery in resectable, nonresectable and metastatic neuroblastoma. J.A.M.A., *205:* 157–158, 1968.

Koop, C. E., and Johnson, D. G. Neuroblastoma; an assessment of therapy in reference to staging. J. Pediatr. Surg., *6:* 595–600, 1971.

Korobkin, M., Clark, R. E., and Palubinskas, A. J. Occult neuroblastoma and acute cerebellar ataxia in childhood. Radiology, *102:* 151–152, 1972.

Krementz, E. T., Schlosser, J. V., and Rumage, J. P. Combined radiation and regional chemotherapy in the treatment of retinoblastoma. A.J.R., *96:* 141–146, 1966.

LaBrosse, E. H. Biochemical diagnosis of neuroblastoma; use of a urine spot test (abstr.). Proc. Am. Assoc. Cancer Res., *9:* 39, 1968.

Ladd, W. E. Embryoma of the kidney; Wilms' tumor. Ann. Surg., *108:* 885–902, 1938.

Lattimer, J. K., and Conway, G. F. The place of surgery in Wilms' tumors. J.A.M.A., *204:* 985–986, 1968.

Laug, W. E., Siegel, S. E., Shaw, K. N. F., Landing, R., Baptistri, J., and Guttenheim, M. Initial catecholamine metabolite concentrations and prognosis in neuroblastoma. Pediatrics, *62:* 77–83, 1978.

Lawrence, W., Hays, D., and Moon, T. Lymphatic metastases with childhood rhabdomyosarcoma. Cancer, *39:* 556–559, 1977.

Leelawongs, N., and Regan, D. D. J. Retinoblastoma; a review of ten years. Am. J. Ophthalmol., *66:* 1050–1060, 1968.

Leen, R. L. S., and Williams, I. G. Bilateral Wilms' tumor. Cancer, *28:* 802–806, 1971.

Leikin, S., Evans, A., Heyn, R., and Newton, W. The impact of chemotherapy on advanced neuroblastoma; survival of patients diagnosed in 1956, 1962, and 1966–1968 in Children's Cancer Study Group A. J. Pediatr., *84:* 131–134, 1974.

Lemire, R. J., Graham, C. B., and Beckwith, J. B. Skin-covered sacrococcygeal masses in infants and children. J. Pediatr., *79:* 948–954, 1971.

Leonidas, J. C., Strauss, L., and Beck, A. R. Vascular tumors of the liver in newborns. Am. J. Dis. Child., *125:* 507–510, 1973.

Mäkinen, J. Microscopic patterns as a guide to prognosis of neuroblastoma in childhood. Cancer, *29:* 1637–1646, 1972.

Malek, R. S., Utz, D. C., and Farrow, G. M. Malignant tumors of the spermatic cord. Cancer, *29:* 1108–1113, 1972.

Marsden, H., and Steward, J. Wilms' tumor, *In* Tumors in children, edited by H. Marsden and J. Steward, p. 225. Springer-Verlag, New York, 1968.

Martin, J., and Rickham, P. P. Pulmonary metastases in Wilms' tumor; treatment and prognosis. Arch. Dis. Child., *45:* 805–807, 1970.

Maurer, H. M., Moon, T., Donaldson, M., Fernandez, C., Gehan, E. A. Hammond, D., Hays, D., Lawrence, W., Newton, W., Ragab, A., Raney, B., Soule, E. H., Sutow, W. W. and Tefft, M. The intergroup rhabdomyosarcoma study; A preliminary report. Cancer, *40:* 2015–2026, 1977.

McIntire, K. R., Vogel, C. L., Princler, G. L., and Patel, I. R. 1972. Serum alpha-fetoprotein as biochemical marker for hepatocellular carcinoma. Cancer Res., *32:* 1941–1946, 1972.

McSweeney, W. J., Bove, K. E., and McAdams, A. J. Spontaneous regression of a putative childhood hepatoma. Am. J. Dis. Child., *125:* 596–598, 1973.

Melicow, M. M. Classification of tumors of testis; clinical and pathological study based on 105 primary and 13 secondary cases in adults and 3 primary and 4 secondary cases in children. J. Urol., *73:* 547–574, 1955.

Miller, R. W. Relation between cancer and congenital defects; an epidemiologic evaluation. J. Natl. Cancer Inst., *40:* 1079–1085, 1968.

Miller, R. W. Fifty-two forms of childhood cancer; United States mortality experience, 1960–1966. J. Pediatr., *75:* 685–689, 1969.

Moe, P. G., and Nellhaus, G. Infantile polymyoclonia-opsoclonus syndrome and neural crest tumors. Neurology, *20:* 756–764, 1970.

Morse, B. S., and Nussbaum, M. The detection of hyaluronic acid in the serum and urine of a patient with nephroblastoma. Am. J. Med., *42:* 996–1002, 1967.

Necheles, T. F., Rausen, A. R., Kung, F. H., and Pochedly, C. Immunochemotherapy in advanced neuroblastoma. Cancer, *41:* 1282–1288, 1978.

Nelson, A. J., III. Embryonal rhabdomyosarcoma; report of twenty-four cases and study of the effectiveness of radiation therapy upon the primary tumor. Cancer, *22:* 64–68, 1968.

Nixon, H. H. Hepatic tumours in childhood and their treatment by major hepatic resection. Arch. Dis. Child., *40:* 169–172, 1965.

O'Bryan, R. M., Luce, J. K., Talley, R. W., Gottlieb, J. A., Baker, L. H., and G. Bonadonna, G. Phase II evaluation of Adriamycin human neoplasia. Cancer, *32:* 1–8, 1973.

Olweny, C. L. M., Toya, T., McBidde, E. K., Mugerma, J., Kyalwaji, S. K., and Cohen, M. 1975. Treatment of hepatocellular carcinoma with Adriamycin; preliminary communication. Cancer, *36:* 1250–1257, 1975.

O'Neill, P., and Pinkel, D. Wilms' tumor in bone marrow aspirate. J. Pediatr., *72:* 396–398, 1968.

Partlow, W. F., and Taybi, H. Teratomas in infants and children. A.J.R., *112:* 155–166, 1971.

Perez, C. A., Vietti, T., Ackerman, L. V., Eagleton, M. D., and Powers, W. E. Tumors of the sympathetic nervous system in childhood; An appraisal of treatment and results. Radiology, *88:* 750–760, 1967.

Pochedly, C., Colucci, J. A., Kenigsberg, K., and Loesevitz, A. Hazards of chemotherapy in congenital Wilms' tumor. J. Pediatr., *79:* 708–709, 1971.

Pratt, C. B. Response of childhood rhabdomyosarcoma to combination chemotherapy. J. Pediatr., *74:* 791–794, 1969.

Pratt, C. B., James, D. H., Jr., Holton, C. P., and Pinkel, D. Combination therapy including vincristine (NSC-67574) for malignant solid tumors in children. Cancer Chemother. Rep., *52:* 489–495, 1968.

Pratt, C. B., Hustu, O., Fleming, I. D., and Pinkel, D. Co-ordinated treatment of childhood rhabdomyosarcoma with surgery, radiotherapy, and combination chemotherapy. Cancer Res., *32:* 606–610, 1972.

Raffucci, F. L., and Ramirez-Schon, G. Management of tumors of the liver. Surg. Gynecol. Obstet., *130:* 371–385, 1970.

Ragab, A. H., Vietti, T. J., Crist, W., Perez, C., and McAllister, W. Bilateral Wilms' tumor. Cancer, *30:* 983–988, 1972.

Raney, R. B., Hays, D., Lawrence, W., Soule, E., Tefft, M., and Donaldson, M. Paratesticular rhabdomyosarcomas in childhood. Cancer, *42:* 729–736, 1978.

Reese, A. B., Hyman, G. A., Merriam, G. R., Jr., Forrest, A. W., and Kligerman, M. M. Treatment of retinoblastoma by radiation and triethylenemelamine. Arch. Ophthalmol., *53:* 505–513, 1955.

Remischovsky, J., Schnaufer, L., and Gloebl, H. Treatment of primary liver tumors. Semin. Oncol., *1:* 65–69, 1974.

Rothner, A. D. Congenital "dumbbell" neuroblastoma with paraplegia. Clin. Pediatr., *10:* 235–236, 1971.

Rubin, M. L. Cryopexy treatment for retinoblastoma. Am. J. Ophthalmol., *66:* 870–871, 1968.

Ruymann, F. B., Newton, R. W., Rajab, A., and Gehan, E. A. Bone marrow metastases at diagnosis in childhood rhabdomyosarcoma. Am. Assoc. Cancer Res. Proc., *20:* 194, 1979.

Ruymann, F. B., Gaiger, A. M., and Newton, W., Jr. Congenital anomalies in rhabdomyosarcoma (abstr.). Birth Defects Conference, June 8–10, Memphis, Tenn., 1977.

Sagerman, R. H., Cassady, J. R., Tretter, P., and Ellsworth, R. M. Radiation induced neoplasia following external beam therapy for children with retinoblastoma. A.J.R. *105:* 529–535, 1969.

Sagerman, R. H., Tretter, P., and Ellsworth, R. M. The treatment of orbital rhabdomyosarcoma of children with primary radiation therapy. A.J.R., *114:* 31–34, 1972.

Samuels, L. D., Newton, W. A., and Heyn, R. Daunorubicin therapy in advanced neuroblastoma. Cancer, *28:* 831–834, 1971.

Schuster, S. A. D., and Ferguson, E. C., III. Unusual presentations of retinoblastoma. South. M. J., *63:* 4–8, 1970.

Shanberg, A. M., Srouji, M., and Leberman, P. R. Hypernephroma in the pediatric age group. J. Urol., *104:* 189–192, 1970.

Shukovsky, L. J., and Fletcher, G. H. Retinal and optic nerve complications in a high dose technique of ethmoid sinus and nasal cavity irradiation. Radiology, *104:* 629–634, 1972.

Silva-Sosa, M., and Gonzalez-Cerna, J. L. Wilms' tumor in children. *In* Progress in Clinical Cancer, edited by I. M. Ariel, Vol. 2, pp. 323–337. Grune & Stratton, New York, 1966.

Sitarz, A. L., Heyn, R., Murphy, M. L., Origenes, M. L., Jr., and Severo, N. O. Triple drug therapy with actinomycin D, chlorambucil, and methorexate in metastatic solid tumors in children. Cancer Chemother. Rep., *45:* 45–51, 1965.

Smith, J. P., and Rutledge, F. Malignant gynecologic tumors. *In* Clinical Pediatric Oncology, edited by W. W. Sutow, T. J. Vietti, and D. J. Fernbach, pp. 515–524. C. V. Mosby, St. Louis, 1973.

Solomon, G. E., and Chutorian, A. M. Opsoclonus and occult neuroblastoma. N. Engl. J. Med., *279:* 475–477, 1968.

Stafford, W. R., Yanoff, M., and Parnell, B. L. Retinoblastomas initially misdiagnosed as primary ocular inflammations. Arch. Ophthalmol., *82:* 771–773, 1969.

Stallard, H. B. The conservative treatment of retinoblastoma; Doyle Memorial Lecture. Trans. Ophthalmol. Soc. U.K., *82:* 473–534, 1962.

Stephenson, S. R., Mease, A. D., and Ruymann, F. B. The prognostic significance of metastases in stage IV-S neuroblastoma. Am. Soc. Clin. Oncol. Proc., *20:* 433, 1979.

Sullivan, M. P., Nora, A. H., Kulapongs, P., Lane, D. M., Windmiller, J., and Thurman, W. G. Evaluation of vincristine sulfate and cyclophosphamide chemotherapy for metastatic neuroblastoma. Pediatrics, *44:* 685–694, 1969.

Sutow, W., Thurman, W., and Windmiller, J. Vincristine (Leucoristine) sulfate in the treatment of children with metastatic Wilms' tumor. Pediatrics, *32:* 880–887, 1963.

Sutow, W. W., Berry, D. H., Haddy, T. B., Sullivan, M. P., Watkins, W. L., Windmiller, J. Vincristine sulfate therapy in children with metastatic soft tissue sarcoma. Pediatrics, *38:* 465–472, 1966.

Sutow, W. W., Gehan, E. A., Heyn, R. M., Kung, F. H., Miller, R. W., Murphy, M. L., and Traggis, D. G. Comparison of survival curves: 1956 versus 1962, in children with Wilms' tumor and neuroblastoma. Pediatrics, *45:* 800–811, 1970a.

Sutow, W. W., Fernbach, D. J., Thurman, W. G., Holton, C. P., and Watkins, W. L. Daunomycin (NSC-82151) in the treatment of metastatic neuroblastoma. Cancer Chemother. Rep., *54:* 283–289, 1970b.

Sutow, W. W., Sullivan, M. P., Reid, H. L., Taylor, H. G., and Griffith, K. M. Prognosis in childhood rhabdomyosarcoma. Cancer, *25:* 1384–1390, 1970c.

Tan, C., Tasaka, H., Yu, K. P., Murphy, M. L., and Karnofsky, D. A. Daunomycin, an antitumor antibiotic; in the treatment of neoplastic disease. Cancer, *20:* 333–353, 1967.

Tan, C., Etcubanas, E., Wollner, N., Rosen, G., Gilladoga, A., Showel, J., Murphy, M. L., and Krakoff, I. H. Adriamycin; an antitumor antibiotic in the treatment of neoplastic diseases. Cancer, *32:* 9–17, 1973.

Tapley, N. 1964. Treatment of retinoblastoma with radiation and chemotherapy. *In* Ocular and Adnexal Tumors, edited by M. Boniuk, pp. 158–170. C. V. Mosby, St. Louis, 1964.

Tapley, N., and Tretter, P. Retinoblastoma. *In* Clinical Pediatric Oncology, edited by N. Tapley and P. Tretter, pp. 411–430. C. V. Mosby, St. Louis, 1973.

Tefft, M., Mitus, A., and Jaffe, N. 1971. Irradiation of the liver in children; acute effects enhanced by concomitant chemotherapeutic administration. A.J.R., *111:* 165–173, 1971.

Tefft, M., Fernandez, C., Donaldson, M., Newton, W., and Moon, T. E. Incidence of meningeal involvement by rhabdomyosarcoma of the head and neck in children. Cancer *42:* 253–258, 1978.

Voorhess, M. L., and Gardner, L. I. Catecholamine metabolism in neuroblastoma. Lancet, *2:* 651–652, 1960.

Voûte, P. A., Jr., Wadman, S. K., and VanPutten, W. L. Congenital neuroblastoma; symptoms in the mother during pregnancy. Clin. Pediatr., *9:* 206–207, 1970.

Waldhausen, J. A., Kilman, J. W., Vellios, F., and Battersby, J. S. Sacococcygeal teratoma. Pediatr. Surg., *54:* 933–949, 1963.

Wang, J. J., Cortes, E. P., Sinks, L. F., and Holland, J. F. Therapeutic effect and toxicity of adriamycin in patients with neoplastic disease. Cancer, 28: 847–843, 1971a.

Wang, I., Wood, D. E., Colapinto, R. F., and Langer, B. Scintigraphy and arteriography in the diagnosis of diseases of the liver. Can. Med. Assoc. J., 104: 989–993, 1971b.

Wilbur, J. R., and Etcubanas, E. Solid tumors in children. In Advances in Pediatrics, edited by I. Schulman, pp. 281–313. Year book Medical Publishers, Chicago, 1974.

Wilbur, J. R., Sutow, W. W., Sullivan, M. P., Castro, J. R., Kaizer, H., and Taylor, H. G. Successful treatment of inoperable embryonal rhabdomyosarcoma (abstr.). The American Pediatric Society and the Society for Pediatric Research, Atlantic City, N.J., 1971.

Webb, B. M., and McFarland, J. J., Jr. Rhabdomyosarcoma of the ear rejmia long-term survival. Laryngoscope, 83: 778–782, 1973.

Wolff, J. A., Krivit, W., Newton, W. A., Jr., and D'Angio, G. J. Single versus multiple dose dactinomycin therapy of Wilms' tumor. N. Engl. J. Med., 279: 290–294, 1968.

Wolff, J. A., D'Angio, G., Hartmann, J. R., Krivit, W. and Newton, W. A. Long term evaluation of single versus multiple courses of antinomycin D therapy of Wilms' tumor. N. Engl. J. Med., 290: 84–86, 1974.

Wooley, M. M., Ginsburg, S., DiCenso, S., Snyder, W. H., Jr., Mirabal, V. Q., and Landing, B. H. Teratomas in infancy and childhood; a review of the clinical experience at the Children's Hospital of Los Angeles. Z. Kinderchir., 4: 289–303, 1967.

IV.
Additional
Topics
on
Cancer

Chapter 31

Design of Clinical Trials

ROBERT L. COMIS, M.D.

The intention of this chapter is to present a general introduction to the principles and problems involved in designing clinical research studies in cancer chemotherapy. Well designed clinical trials in medical oncology represent the efforts of both clinicians and biomedical statisticians, who together attempt to design studies which will answer precise, pertinent questions of clinical importance. The ultimate goal of clinical research studies in oncology is to explore and define better methods of treatment for the cancer patient.

Before embarking on a clinical investigation, the clinician should have completed an explicit written statement of the question posed and the precise method of executing the study to answer it—a self-contained document known as a protocol. It must be written so that everyone involved in the care of the patient, from the research nurse to the principal investigator, completely understands its rationale and requirements. The essential elements of a protocol are presented in Table 31.1. Guidelines for protocol writing have been presented by Gehan and Schneiderman (1973).

The catalog of effective anticancer drugs has increased dramatically since the discovery of the antitumor effects of nitrogen mustard and aminopterin in the 1940s (Farber et al., 1948; Gilman, 1963). The armamentarium of the medical oncologist now includes at least 40 drugs, exclusive of hormones, which have documented effectiveness against a variety of malignancies. Most of these compounds have been obtained through an orderly series of steps: (1) acquisition and purification, (2) antitumor screening in animals, (3) drug formulation, (4) large animal toxicology, and (5) clinical evaluation. Before the last step is taken, the animal systems must have revealed not only that the drug has experimental antitumor activity, but also the toxicities which should be ex-

TABLE 31.1
Elements of a Protocol

1. Introduction and scientific background for the study
2. Study objectives
3. Patient selection
4. Study design (including schematic diagram)
5. Treatment programs
6. Procedures in event of response, no response, or toxicity
7. Required clinical and laboratory data
8. Criteria for evaluating the effect of treatment
9. Statistical considerations
10. Informed consent
11. Record forms
12. References
13. Study coordinator and telephone number

pected in man and what would be a safe dose for initiating human trials.

ANIMAL TUMOR SYSTEMS IN THE PREDICTION OF TOXICITY IN MAN

Any new drug considered for human use must undergo adequate toxicologic evaluations in animals before being employed in man. The answers sought in animal toxicology studies are qualitative, i.e., what general organ system toxicities should be expected in man; and semi-quantitative, i.e., what would be an appropriate starting dose in man. The relationship of the qualitative and quantitative aspects of animal toxicology to human toxicity have been extensively analyzed.

Qualitative Predictability

Both Owens (1962) and Schein et al. (1973) have retrospectively compared toxicities observed in several animal species to those observed in man for several classes of anticancer compounds. These studies have shown that human toxicity observed in the hematopoietic, gastrointestinal, renal, and hepatic systems, are generally predicted by animal toxicology studies. However, for each of these organ systems, the two most commonly used large animal species (dog and monkey) tend to overpredict toxicity, i.e., a toxic effect observed in the animal is not seen in man. Overprediction of toxicity has been particularly striking in the renal and hepatic systems. Specific parameters of toxicity (i.e., anemia or leukopenia in the hematopoietic system or vomiting and diarrhea in the gastrointestinal system) are less accurately predicted than the broader major organ toxicities. In other words, although anemia may be the most significant hematopoietic toxicity in animals, another manifestation of hematologic toxicity may predominate in man. In animals many of the reported organ system toxicities are produced after the administration of severely toxic, often lethal, drug doses. This may account for some of the overprediction since in man the drugs are not purposefully administered at such high levels.

Skin, cardiac, pulmonary and nervous system toxicities have generally not been well predicted. But, as active drugs with specific organ toxicities become available, animal toxicity screening systems are often designed in an attempt to predict these toxicities. This has been the case for Adriamycin and bleomycin, both of which have demonstrated significant antitumor activity, and have specific dose-limiting organ system toxicities. The dose-limiting toxicity of Adriamycin is a cardiomyopathy, while the limiting toxicity of bleomycin is pulmonary fibrosis. Currently several laboratories are employing various animal screening systems to test analogs of these drugs in an attempt to establish systems which will predict agents with comparable antitumor effects but less toxicity.

"Quantitative" Predictability

The second concern in animal toxicology is of a more quantitative nature. Is there any relationship between the dose administered and the observed toxic or therapeutic effects among different species? If such a relationship exists, it might offer a guide both for establishing a safe initial dose for human trials and for indicating the dose expected to produce toxicity.

Several studies (Pinkel, 1958; Freireich et al., 1966; Homan, 1972) have shown that a better correlation exists between toxic doses among various animal species and man when the dose is expressed in terms of body surface area (mg/m^2) rather than body weight (mg/kg). This correlation also exists when toxic doses are expressed in mg/m^2 within species, e.g., adults versus children. As a result, doses of chemotherapeutic agents are now commonly administered on the mg/m^2 basis.

Certain investigators have attempted to define a potentially safe starting dose for man by correlating toxicologic data among a variety of animal species and man. Freireich et al. (1966) suggested that one-third the "maximum tolerated dose" defined by the weighted estimate of 5 animal species, expressed in mg/m^2, would be a safe clinical dose for most chemotherapeutic agents. In a similar analysis, Homan (1972) has shown that, when one-third "the dose which produced only minimal reversible toxicity" of the most sensitive large animal species is employed, there is a 6% probability of finding toxicity in man.

Another analysis of this type has been performed by Goldsmith et al. (1975). One-third of the "toxic dose low" (TDL) for the dog and one-third the LD_{10} in normal mice were compared to the "commonly used clinical dose" in man. The TDL is defined as the "lowest dose to produce pathologic alterations in hematologic, chemical, clinical, or morphologic parameters; doubling this dose produces no lethality." The mouse LD_{10}

is the dose that kills 10% of the animals. Although the "commonly used clinical dose" in man may not represent the human maximally tolerated dose, it is the dose that generally produces toxicity and may yield therapeutic effects. The analysis of Goldsmith et al. was performed to establish how often the commonly used clinical dose would have been exceeded if the starting dose in man had been based upon the doses predicted by animal studies.

Because of the retrospective nature of the analysis, identical doses and schedules of administration were not always available for both animals and man. In fact, only 4 of the 30 drugs in the analysis had identical schedules in all animal species and man. For this reason, the cumulative doses from the animal schedules were converted to those used in humans by a method described by Freireich et al. (1966) based on the work of Griswold et al. (1963). For example, the total dose in man might have been given as a daily injection for 10 days, while data were available only for single dose administration in animals. In this situation the total single dose administered to the animal was divided by 10 to obtain a schedule comparable to the one used in man. This simple conversion is based on the assumption that the toxic effects of drugs are related to the cumulative effect of the total dose regardless of schedule. The validity of this assumption, and therefore the conversion, is not completely established.

The starting dose used in initial clinical trials sponsored by the National Cancer Institute is ⅓ the TDL of the most sensitive large animal species. In this connection, Goldsmith et al. showed that complete reliance on ⅓ the TDL for every drug would have exceeded the commonly used clinical dose for 5 (17%) of the drugs available. Thus, strict adherence to the ⅓ TDL "guideline" may not be appropriate for all drugs. Interestingly, the Goldsmith et al. study found that the use of ⅓ the LD_{10} (mg/m²) in normal mice would have exceeded the human dose in only 2 of 19 instances (10.5%).

Other investigators are currently reanalyzing the relative predictive value of large animal versus small animal toxicology screens. Small animal toxicology can be performed more quickly and less expensively than large animal studies. If the data indicate that rodent toxicology screens are equivalent to large animal systems, toxicology screening would become much more efficient, inexpensive and less time consuming.

In summary, studies of animal toxicology provide a reasonable, but not wholly precise, guide to qualitative and quantitative drug toxicity in man.

DESIGN OF CLINICAL STUDIES

Phase I Study

The Phase I study is the first clinical evaluation of a new anticancer drug in man. The purposes of a Phase I study are:

1. To establish the maximum tolerated dose (MTD) on a given schedule and route of administration.

2. To establish the patterns of toxicity and to determine whether the toxicities encountered are predictable, tolerable and reversible.

3. To establish the pharmacology of the drug in man.

Although the primary purposes of the initial human trial are toxicologic and pharmacologic, the study, as with all other investigations, is therapeutic in intent. The drugs being tested have shown promising antitumor activity in animal screening systems, and may prove effective in the treatment of human malignancies.

Patients are candidates for Phase I studies if they have been unsuccessfully treated on appropriate standard therapy, including surgery, radiotherapy, and chemotherapy, or if there is no currently available treatment of known benefit for their disease type and stage. However, they must not be so ill as to preclude adequate follow-up or toxicity evaluation.

Concerning the ethics of Phase I study, it must be remembered that the patients entered into the study have a disease state for which there is no established therapy of benefit, and the drugs being investigated have shown promising antitumor activity in animal systems. In addition, the patients are meticulously monitored by expert clinical investigators to prevent or treat any untoward drug effects.

As mentioned previously, the first dose level employed in patients entered onto Phase I studies is ⅓ of the TDL in the most sensitive large animal species. The choice of the route and schedule of administration is based upon several factors. The choice of the route of administration in humans generally results from preclinical investigations into the physiochemical, pharmacologic and therapeutic characteristics of the compound such as its lipid solubility, the pharmacology of oral versus parenterally administered drug in animals and the relative therapeutic effects of different routes of administration. The schedule to be used is sometimes based upon the results of differential therapeutic effects of various schedules noted in animal tumor systems. In addition, the schedules employed in Phase I studies must have been evaluated in large animal toxicology studies. As the pharmacologic data generated in initial human studies become established, other variations in scheduling may be based upon this information. Several different schedules of administration are investigated by separate institutions in concurrent Phase I studies throughout the country.

After the appropriate initial dose and schedule are decided upon, the next problem is to reach the maximum tolerated dose in a safe and efficient fashion. With the heterogeneity of anticancer drugs, it is not surprising that a variety of approaches have been tested. Gold (1962) proposed a geometric progression of dose escalations starting with $\frac{1}{100}$ the LD_{50} in rodents but, with its progressively increasing doses per escalation, the method would probably result in excessive toxicity. Another method, used in the Eastern Cooperative Oncology Group Phase I study of BCNU (DeVita et al., 1965), has been randomization of patients to one of three starting doses and schedules using fixed, predetermined dose escalations. Gottlieb (1975) has described a method currently used in the Developmental Therapeutics Department at M. D. Anderson Hospital. Starting at $\frac{1}{3}$ TDL, the dose is increased by 50% increments until toxicity is encountered and then decreased to 25% increments until the maximally tolerated dose is reached. Recently, interest has been renewed in a dose escalation schema based on a numerical series described by the famed 13th century Italian mathematician Leonardo Pisano, alias Fibonacci (Schneiderman, 1966). The modified Fibonacci search scheme, used by Hansen et al. (1971), employs a series of predetermined decreasing dose escalations. When mild, but reproducible, toxicity is observed at any dose, 30–35% escalations are employed until the MTD is established. It has been suggested that this method would require 5 ($\pm$ 3) dose escalations for most drugs. Goldsmith et al. (1975) estimated the number of escalations necessary to reach the commonly used clinical dose for 30 compounds, using $\frac{1}{3}$ the TDL in dogs as the starting dose. Three agents (10%), including 2 antimetabolites and 1 alkylating agent, would have required more than 8 steps if the modified Fibonacci search had been rigidly employed.

Practically, no statistical model for dose escalation is inherently safe and efficient for every compound. Most investigators generally start with large increments (rarely exceeding $2n$) when no toxicity is observed and decrease the escalations when minimal toxicity is encountered. Three patients are placed on the initial dose and adequate time($\sim$2–4 weeks) is allowed to evaluate the possibility of delayed toxicity before entering patients on the subsequent dose. As toxicity is encountered, more patients ($\sim$6) are entered at each dose until the MTD is reached. Doses are generally not escalated in individual patients because it would be difficult to know whether a toxic effect is the result of the cumulative dose administered or the current dose level being given to the patient.

The theoretical goal of a Phase I study is to reach a single MTD for a particular schedule. In practice, the MTD reached is often a function of the degree of prior therapy to which patients have been exposed. For example, patients with extensive prior chemotherapy or radiotherapy tolerate less amounts of drug, particularly those which are bone marrow suppressive, than patients without extensive prior treatment. In the Phase I study of MeCCNU (Gottlieb et al., 1972), significant thrombocytopenia was more frequent and more severe in previously treated patients compared to those without prior therapy. As a result of this trial the doses recommended for Phase II study were 200 mg/m^2 for previously untreated patients and 150 mg/m^2 for previously treated patients. In addition, the maximally tolerated dose and the dose limiting toxicity may vary greatly depending upon the disease being treated. This variation is most striking when comparing the MTD of a specific drug in the treatment of acute leukemia versus the solid tumors. Bone marrow aplasia is a therapeutic goal in the treatment of leukemia, while it may be considered a severe toxic side effect in a solid tumor patient. Therefore, the MTD may be severalfold higher in a Phase I study in solid tumor patients, and the dose limiting organ system toxicity may be different. When analyzing the results of a Phase I study it is imperative to be cognizant of these selection factors before deciding the dose for further clinical investigation.

The Phase I study design tends to preclude a judgment of true therapeutic potential. The patients treated have far advanced, generally refractory, disease and many of them receive low and probably ineffective doses of chemotherapy. Also, the study population encompasses a broad range of malignancies and the number of patients with any single tumor type is not sufficient to signal specific antitumor activity. Unfortunately, in spite of these very real limitations in design, enthusiasm for pursuing further studies with a drug often wanes if the Phase I trial gives no hint of antitumor activity.

Once the Phase I study has been completed, the next step is to attempt to define the antitumor activity of the agent in a variety of malignancies.

Phase II Study

The Phase II study is designed to establish whether the drug has antitumor activity in a variety of different cancers. The doses and schedules of drugs employed in the Phase II study are those which have been defined in the previous Phase I study.

Since the Phase II study is a screen for antitumor activity there must be a clear, objective, and measurable end point for judging response. In clinical cancer studies, the size of the lesion and patient survival from a fixed time point are the major disease parameters that meet this need.

Currently, the end point used in most Phase II studies is a measurable and reproducible decrease in the size of a lesion for a specified period of time. Some of the commonly used criteria for objective response and disease progression are defined in Table 31.2. In general, the duration of a partial or complete response must be at least 1 month. Moertel and Hanley (1976) have shown that a 50% change in the products of the longest perpendicular diameters of a measurable lesion is a reasonably accurate and reproducible measurement. Hopefully, research on immu-

TABLE 31.2
Commonly Used Criteria for Objective Response and Disease Progression in Solid Tumors

Complete response:	Complete disappearance of all demonstrable disease
Partial response:	≥50% reduction in the sum of the products of the longest perpendicular diameters of discrete measurable disease, with no demonstrable disease progression elsewhere
No response:	No change in the size of any measurable lesion or <50% reduction of measurable disease as defined above
Progression:	>50% increase in the sum of the products of the largest perpendicular diameter of any measurable lesion

nological and biochemical markers will, in time, allow more precise definitions of response in solid tumors.

The second method of evaluating response, which is less commonly employed and somewhat more problematic, is measurement of survival. The problems of using this end point have been extensively reviewed by both Carter (1972) and Feinstein et al. (1969). Briefly, this approach is of limited value because patients may die from diseases not directly related to their malignancy or from causes induced by the therapy (Byar, 1972). Such an end point also suffers from the shortcoming that patients are "locked in" until death on a specific therapy in order to properly assess the impact of therapy on survival.

There are two predominant approaches to Phase II studies. The first is the *drug-oriented study* in which a large number of patients with a variety of diseases are treated with a particular drug. This has been the classical Phase II investigation through which drugs, such as 5-fluorouracil (Moore, et al., 1968), cyclophosphamide (Rundles et al., 1962), methotrexate (Condit et al., 1962), and Adriamycin (O'Bryan et al., 1973), have been detected. Although the total patient numbers are sometimes quite large, there are often relatively few patients in each disease category. In addition, little attention is generally given to disease states and patient characteristics which might affect the ability of the drug to induce a response.

There are many diseases and patient characteristics which alter the ability of a drug to induce objective response or to favorably affect survival. For example, the performance status of the patient has a marked effect upon survival in lung cancer (Zelen, 1973) and on the objective response rate in colon cancer (Moertel et al., 1974). Prior chemotherapy affects the objective response rate in solid tumors (Moertel et al., 1974) as well as in the hematologic malignancies (Frei et al., 1973). Various metastatic sites respond differently within the same disease category, such as soft tissue versus visceral disease in breast cancer (Broder and Tormey, 1974) and malignant melanoma (Carter and Friedman, 1972).

Since the list of variables which affect response and survival are unique for each disease, it is not surprising that selection factors can significantly alter the results of small uncontrolled drug oriented trials. The greatest danger of drug oriented studies is not the overestimation of antitumor activity, since an agent showing significant activity in a broad Phase II study will probably undergo further trials. The real pitfall lies in a spurious judgment that the drug has no activity and does not merit further study.

These considerations have led to the second major type of Phase II trial, *the disease oriented study.* The essence of this approach is that the study is directed to specific types of patients with a specific disease entity and/or stage. The prognostic variables which are known to affect response are accounted for prospectively in the study design. When possible, studies include patients with host and disease parameters that may make them likely to respond to a reasonably active agent.

Restrictions on patient entry may be imposed to limit the study to groups with specific prognostic variables or, in large studies, specific prognostic groups may be analyzed separately after completion of the study. For example, instead of evaluating the activity of a particular drug in the treatment of all types of cancer, the study may be designed particularly for gastric cancer. The performance status of patients acceptable for investigational treatment is defined in the protocol. The disease categories are decided upon prospectively, e.g., patients with metastatic disease will be included and not patients with locally advanced disease. The study may be limited to previously untreated patients only or might be written to include patients with prior chemotherapy.

In the last several years, the *disease oriented* approach to Phase II studies has appropriately become more prevalent. Currently, *disease oriented* Phase II studies are being performed in nonrandomized, consecutive series of patients, as well as in series of patients randomized to various Phase II treatment options. The necessity for randomized Phase II studies versus nonrandomized Phase II studies is currently under debate. As long as the study is precisely written and executed, the screening nature of the study can be effectively accomplished in either a nonrandomized, consecutive series of patients or in patients randomized to different treatments.

The priorities for the disease oriented, Phase II testing of new drugs vary for different diseases. For instance, there are certain malignancies against which most of the standard chemotherapeutic agents have been evaluated and a few drugs have been reported to have some antitumor activity. Examples of such situations include the use of cyclophosphamide in non-oat cell lung cancer (Selawry, 1973), 5-fluorouracil in colon cancer (Moertel, 1973) and imidazole carboxamide in malignant melanoma

(Carter and Friedman, 1972). These drugs have marginal activity and the majority of patients do not respond favorably. It would be important to evaluate new agents in these diseases in an attempt to uncover drugs with significant antitumor activity which could be used as first line therapy.

There are other malignancies (e.g., bladder, prostate and cervix cancer) against which most standard and investigational agents have never been adequately evaluated (Carter and Soper, 1974). Priorities in these diseases would lie in evaluating untested standard drugs which have shown activity in other tumors, as well as in evaluating new agents.

In the examples cited above, new chemotherapeutic agents or conventional ones that have not been adequately evaluated could be tested in relatively good risk, previously untreated patients. A different situation exists with the malignancies in which a number of active drugs, used singly or in combination, have significantly increased response rates or survival, e.g., acute lymphoblastic leukemia in children, Hodgkin's disease, and non-Hodgkin's lymphomas. New drug evaluation is needed but it must be subordinated to an exhaustive list of effective primary and secondary combination chemotherapy regimens, as well as tertiary single agents. The patients available for new drug testing are far advanced cases and probably only highly active drugs will be detected. In this setting, the activity of Adriamycin (O'Bryan et al., 1973) and bleomycin (Yagoda et al., 1972) has been determined for Hodgkin's and non-Hodgkin's lymphomas. An analogous situation exists in breast cancer where combination chemotherapy has increased the response rate and duration of response over that achieved by single agent therapy (Taylor et al., 1974). Top priority now is being given to establishing new and potentially more effective combinations of currently available drugs for patients with metastatic disease. In addition, chemotherapy is now being employed as an effective adjuvant to primary surgery (Bonadonna et al., 1976); therefore, new agents will again be tested in heavily treated patients.

Other factors affecting the priorities in Phase II studies include drug related characteristics such as cell cycle and phase specificity, the mechanisms of action of a compound, and the relative immunosuppressive and myelotoxic properties of the drug.

The Phase II study attempts to detect clinical activity rapidly, efficiently, and in a reasonably accurate fashion with a relatively small number of patients. The actual number needed to accept or reject an agent for further study depends upon the level of activity sought, the design of the study, and the relative heterogeneity of the patient groups. An approach to estimating the minimum number of patients for Phase II studies has been devised by Gehan (1961).

Although the primary goal of the Phase II study is detection of clinical activity, valuable information concerning drug toxicity is obtained as more patients are exposed to the doses and schedules employed in previous Phase I studies. A better understanding of the therapeutic index of a drug may be an important factor in its development. For example, an agent having activity comparable to the more standard approach, but at the expense of more severe toxicity, may be less desirable than a drug yielding a response rate similar to the conventional agent with less quantitative or different qualitative toxicity.

Once potential therapeutic activity has been uncovered the next step is to focus upon the role of the new treatment in a particular disease. Depending upon the disease entity, the drug may be definitively compared to standard therapy as a single agent or it may be integrated into a new combination chemotherapy regimen. In the latter instance it would essentially be "recycled" to a Phase I setting, where the appropriate dose ratios, schedules, and sequences of administration, as well as parameters of toxicity, can be established for the new combination. The myriad theories and problems in dealing with these factors are beyond the scope of this chapter but they have been excellently detailed by Carter (1974) and others.

Phase III Study

The Phase III study is a clinical trial designed to establish the relative value of different treatment programs. It must be a comparative trial. In general, a new treatment is compared to the currently available standard treatment, termed a control group. The *sine qua non* of this study is that the patients treated with the various therapeutic options are comparable with regard to important factors which predispose for, or against, a response. This requirement must be met to be confident that observed differences in response to a particular therapy are directly attributable to the treatment program, rather than being a function of differences in the patient populations treated. In addition, this end also requires that patients are managed in a comparable fashion as they are entered into the study, managed while on study and as the data are analyzed after the study is completed.

Various techniques are employed in an attempt to establish comparability of patient groups. One is called randomization, in which patients are randomly allocated to treatment programs. Unfortunately, randomization does not ensure that important variables within treatment groups are balanced unless there are large numbers of patients included in the study. Therefore, when analyzing a randomized trial it is imperative that a detailed analysis of the important patient and disease characteristics for each treatment has been presented by the author and scrutinized by the reader. It is incorrect to assume that because a study has randomized patients to treatment options, it has ensured comparability of patient groups.

Another method employed to accomplish comparability of treated groups is to use a prerandomization "stratification" of patients. "Stratification" is employed before the patients are randomly allocated to two or more therapeutic regimens. Patients entering the study are categorized by sets of known important prognostic factors and the individuals falling within each set form a group or "stratum." Then the patients within each "stratum" are separately randomized to the treatment programs (Zelen, 1974). This procedure attempts to ensure a balance of important prognostic variables among the treatments being compared, so that no single treatment group is inordinately weighted with poor or good risk factors.

Randomization does control for the conscious or unconscious bias of the investigator in selecting a treatment program. The importance of this concept is illustrated in the analysis of a study by the Eastern Cooperative Oncology Group (Schneiderman, 1967) as shown graphically in Figure 31.1. This study compared three alkylating agents in the treatment of malignant lymphoma prior to the advent of combination chemotherapy and analyzed the survival data according to the initial prognostic risk category ascribed to the patient by the physician. There was a significant correlation between the physician's initial judgment and survival for all

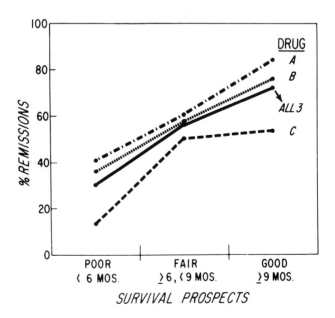

Fig. 6.1. Response to chemotherapy and survival prospects in malignant lymphoma.

treatments. Although treatment A appears superior to C for each risk category, it is not inconceivable that an investigator could bias such a study by treating only those patients with "good" survival prospects with drug C and "poor" survival prospects with drug A. If this were done the response rate could conceivably be higher for drug C than drug A, and an erroneous judgment of drug activity would result from investigator selection rather than a true therapeutic difference.

Currently, most Phase III studies in cancer research employ a randomization, but not all investigators ascribe to this concept. Arguments for or against randomization can be found in the literature (Chalmers et al., 1972; Schneiderman, 1975; Mathé, 1973; Gehan and Freireich, 1974).

There are two basic types of control groups, i.e., patients treated concurrently and those selected from past records, termed "historical controls." Most Phase III cancer chemotherapy trials now employ randomized, concurrent, control groups where patients are prospectively and randomly assigned to a treatment program. The patient selection factors, therapy, supportive care, follow-up, and definitions of response remain essentially constant throughout the trial, as long as the protocol is precisely written and executed, and the study does not take an inordinately long time for completion.

The necessity for a concurrent, randomized control group is not accepted by all investigators. It has been suggested that careful selection of controls from the literature, matched controls from a particular group or institution, or controls from sequential studies may provide an adequate group for comparison with a new therapy (Mathé, 1973; Gehan and Freireich, 1974). However, none of these methods accounts for the vagaries of changing institutional personnel, advances in supportive and diagnostic capabilities, or the pressure of an increasingly aware public, both lay and medical, seeking earlier medical care for cancer. Another major criticism of this method voiced by Dr. Marvin Schneiderman (1975) is that it "almost assumes that you know all you will ever need to know about what makes for response in patients."

Newly discovered and important prognostic variables may arise for which data do not exist among historical controls. For instance, with the recent interest in immunologic evaluation and "immunotherapy," the battery of sophisticated tests for immune function is increasing. There is some indication that immunocompetent patients are more likely to respond to treatment than others who have depressed immune systems (Takita and Brugorolas, 1973; Gutterman and Maglivit, 1974). Comparable immunological function data may not be available in the historical control group. Research on immunological and biological markers may uncover new prognostic categories that are not available in the retrospective control group. Using concurrent control groups, similar parameters may be followed in all patients and all treatment groups can be equally evaluated as a new, important, characteristic develops during a study.

The common denominator in the debate surrounding "historical" versus concurrent, randomized control groups is the need for comparability of patients in the different treatment programs being tested.

Another factor important in analyzing any controlled study is whether the patients considered "evaluable" for analysis are comparable to patients considered "nonevaluable" for each treatment. Most protocols involve specific patient selection factors. Thus, the outcome of the study is related to the particular patients treated in a specific manner. Every study involves the following sequential flow of patient numbers:

1. Number *evaluated* for entrance into the study, i.e., all patients with the disease type and stage for which the protocol has been written.
2. Number *eligible* for entrance into the study, i.e., those patients who fit the specific criteria for admission into the study within the disease type and stage.
3. Number *entered.*
4. Number *evaluable,* i.e., those patients for whom the protocol has been precisely followed and there is the required data for analysis.
5. Number *"adequately" treated,* i.e., those patients who have received a certain number of treatment courses specified by the protocol.

If the denominator used in determining response rate becomes progressively smaller, from those considered for entrance to those "adequately treated," the selection phenomenon inherent in the protocol may be markedly compounded. There must be a careful presentation and analysis of patients considered "nonevaluable." In any study, patients may move away, some (hopefully few) investigators may not abide by the protocol, or patients may die from causes unrelated to the disease or treatment. These patients might be justifiably considered "nonevaluable." On the other hand, it would be misleading to eliminate patients who satisfy the protocol eligibility requirements, but suffer severe drug-related toxicity or "early" death after treatment begins. The treatment in the first instance may be evaluable from the standpoint that it is too toxic for certain patients, whereas in the second case the treatment may be incapable of arresting rapidly advancing disease or disease in drug-resistant sites. In either case, valid information concerning the treatment and its effect on the disease in the patient group defined by the protocol should not be lost or disregarded.

Combined Modality Studies

A combined modality study employs more than one type of treatment modality in a certain disease category and/or stage. It may include a combination of the modalities most effective in treating clinically localized disease (i.e., *surgery* and *radiotherapy*), where the risk for local recurrence is high. More importantly, combinations of effective local and systemic therapy may be used against certain tumors in an attempt to eradicate both clinically localized and disseminated subclinical disease. *Chemotherapy,* including cytotoxic as well as hormonal drugs, is presently the only firmly established method of controlling disseminated disease. *Immunotherapy* is undergoing intensive clinical evaluation and may have a significant role in future combined modality approaches.

Until recently, chemotherapy has been almost exclusively relegated to treating patients with advanced and widely disseminated disease. In view of the massive tumor cell burden in these patients, it is remarkable that the cell kill potential of chemotherapy is significant enough to induce objective measurable regression. Data from animal hematologic and solid tumor systems indicate not only that the curative ability of chemotherapy is inversely related to tumor cell burden, but also that combined surgery and effective chemotherapy has greater curative potential than either modality used alone (Skipper and Schabel; 1973; Mayo et al., 1972).

Recently, combined modalities of therapy have made significant strides in controlling some of the rapidly proliferating childhood malignancies, e.g., acute lymphoblastic leukemia (Simone et al., 1972), Wilm's tumor (Wolff et al., 1974), and Ewing's sarcoma (Hustu et al., 1972). Surgical adjuvant chemotherapy studies in adult solid tumors have been performed in the past, most of them employing short courses of chemotherapy of minimal intensity (VA Cooperative Surgical Adjuvant Group, 1965). The expressed purpose of these studies was to eradicate circulating tumor cells dislodged at the time of surgery but they have yielded largely negative or, at best, equivocal results.

Most adult solid tumors are thought to have low growth fractions and long doubling times; in addition, most chemotherapeutic agents are thought to kill cells by first order kinetics (Skipper and Schabel, 1973). Killing by first order kinetics means that the same proportion of cells is killed with the same effective dose of a drug regardless of the tumor cell burden, i.e., it would require as much chemotherapy to lower the tumor cell burden from 10^{12} to 10^{9} as from 10^{4} to 10^{1}. Therefore, prolonged, intensive chemotherapy will probably be needed to eradicate even small micrometastases. Recently, the use of intensive surgical adjuvant chemotherapy has been shown to be effective in preventing relapse in premenopausal patients with breast cancer at high risk for recurrence (Bonadonna et al., 1976).

A prerequisite to embarking on any combined modality study of a specific disease or disease stage is a thorough knowledge of the therapeutic potential and limitations of each modality. The first step is a comprehensive review of the available current and past data to define the patient groups, either clinically, pathologically, and/or immunologically, that have a high risk of recurrence after "curative" primary therapy. The review should also provide information on the systemic treatment of advanced disease which might be of potentially greater benefit in less advanced disease. One report has described this step, as well as the rationale and strategy for integrating chemotherapy into the combined modality approach to 16 major solid tumors (Carter and Soper, 1974).

Each modality has its own potential range of toxic effects, and combination of these modalities may significantly increase overall toxicity. Therefore, a prime concern must be the means of combining the modalities to avoid development of toxicity. Before proceeding with a large study, trials with relatively few patients can be used to determine appropriate dosages, sequences and schedules of administration.

The principles and problems of the design of combined modality studies are similar to those detailed for Phase III, including the need for a concurrently randomized control group. The potential for benefit is great, but the long term risks of intensive chemotherapy in patients with minimal disease is unknown. Therefore, it is imperative that a control group be used to precisely define the benefits and potential liabilities of this approach.

REFERENCES

Bonadonna, G., Brusamolino, E., Valagusa, F., et al. Combination chemotherapy as an adjuvant treatment in operable breast cancer. N. Engl. J. Med., 294: 405–411, 1976.

Broder, L., and Tormey, D. Combination chemotherapy of carcinoma of the breast. Cancer Treat. Rev., 1: 183–204, 1974.

Byar, D. P. Treatment of prostatic cancer by the Veterans Administration Cooperative Urological Group. Bull. N.Y. Acad. Med., 48: 751–766, 1972.

Carter, S. K. Study design principles for the clinical evaluation of new drugs as developed by the chemotherapy program of the National Cancer Institute. In The Design of Clinical Trials in Cancer Therapy, edited by M. Staquet, pp. 242–289. Editions Scientifiques Europeenes, Brussels, 1972.

Carter, S. K. Planning combined therapy—the interaction of experimental and clinical studies. Cancer Chemother. Rep. 4(Part 2): 3–12, 1974.

Carter, S. K., and Friedman, M. A. 5-(3,3-Dimethyl-1-triazeno)-imidazole-4-carboxamide (DTIC, DIC, NSC 45388)—a new antitumor agent with activity against malignant melanoma. Eur. J. Cancer, 8: 85–92, 1972.

Carter, S. K., and Soper, W. T. Integration of chemotherapy into combined modality treatment of solid tumors; I. The overall strategy. Cancer Treat. Rev., 1: 1–13, 1974.

Chalmers, T. C., Block, J. B., and Lee, S. Controlled studies in clinical cancer research. N. Engl. J. Med., 287: 75–78, 1972.

Condit, P., Shnider, B., and Owens, A. H. Studies on the folic acid vitamins; VII. The effect of large doses of aminopterin in patients with cancer. Cancer Res., 22: 706–710, 1962.

DeVita, V. T., Carbone, P. P., Owens, A. H., Gold, C. L., Krant, M. J., and Edmonson, J. Clinical trials with 1,3-bis-(2-chloroethyl)-1-nitrosourea, NSC 409962. Cancer Res. 25: 1876–1882, 1965.

Farber, S., Diamond, L. K., Mercer, R. D., Sylvester, R. F., and Wolff, J. A. Temporary remissions in acute leukemia in children produced by folic acid antagonist 4-aminopteroylglutamic acid (aminopterin). N. Engl. J. Med., 238: 787–791, 1948.

Frei, E., III, Luce, J. K., and Gamble, J. F. Combination chemotherapy in advanced Hodgkin's disease; induction and maintenance of remission. Ann. Intern. Med., *79:* 376–382, 1973.

Feinstein, A. R., Pritchett, J. A., and Schimpff, C. R. The epidemiology of cancer therapy; II. The clinical course: Data, decision and temporal demarcations. Arch. Intern. Med., *123:* 323–343, 1969.

Freireich, E. J., Gehan, E. A., Rall, D. A., Schmidt, L. H., and Skipper, H. A. Quantitative comparison of toxicity of anti-cancer agents in mouse, rat, hamster, dog, monkey and man. Cancer Chemother. Rep., *50:* 219–244, 1966.

Gehan, E. A. The determination of the number of patients required in a preliminary and follow up trial of a new chemotherapeutic agent. J. Chronic Dis., *13:* 346–353, 1961.

Gehan, E. A. and Freireich, E. J. Non-randomized controls in cancer clinical trials. N. Engl. J. Med., *290:* 198–203, 1974.

Gehan, E. A., and Schneiderman, M. A. Experimental design of clinical trials. *In* Cancer Medicine, edited by J. F. Holland and E. Frei III, pp. 499–524. Lea & Fibiger, Philadelphia, 1973.

Gilman, A. The initial clinical trial of nitrogen mustard. Am. J. Surg., *105:* 574–578, 1963.

Gold, L. Coordinated Phase I studies for cooperative chemotherapy groups. Cancer Chemother. Rep., *16:* 99–105, 1962.

Goldsmith, M. A., Slavik, M., and Carter, S. K. Quantitative prediction of drug toxicity in humans from toxicology in small and large animals. Cancer Res., *35:* 1354–1364, 1975.

Gottlieb, J. A. New drugs introduced into clinical trials. *In* Cancer Chemotherapy, pp. 79–98. Yearbook Medical Publishers, Chicago, 1975.

Gottlieb, J. A., McCredie, K. B., and Frei, E., III. Initial clinical studies with 1,2-(chloroethyl)-3-(4-methylcyclohexyl)-1-nitrosourea (methyl CCNU) (abstr.). Proc. Am. Assoc. Cancer Res., *13:* 79, 1972.

Griswold, D. P., Laster, W. R., Snow, M.Y., Schabel, F. M., Jr., and Skipper, H. E. Experimental evaluation of potential anticancer agents; XII. Quantitative drug response of Sa 180, Ca 755, and leukemia L1210 systems to a "standard list" of "active" and "inactive" agents. Cancer Res. (Suppl.), *23* (No. 4, Part 2): 271–520, 1963.

Gutterman, J. U., and Maglivit, G. M. Chemoimmunotherapy (CI) of disseminated malignant melanoma (DMM) with imidazole carboxamide (DTIC) and BCG (abstr.). Am. Soc. Clin. Oncol., *15:* 182, 1974.

Hansen, H., Selawry, O. S., Muggia, F. M., and Walker, M. D. Clinical studies with 1-(2-chloroethyl)-3-cyclohexyl-1-nitrosourea (NSC 79037). Cancer Res., *31:* 223–227, 1971.

Homan, E. R. Quantitative relationships between toxic doses of antitumor chemotherapeutic agents in animals and man. Cancer Chemother. Rep. (Part 3), *3:* 13–19, 1972.

Hustu, H. O., Pinkel, D., and Pratt, C. B. Treatment of clinically localized Ewing's sarcoma with radiotherapy and combination chemotherapy. Cancer, *30:* 1522–1527, 1972.

Mathé, G. 1973. Clinical examination of drugs, a scientific and ethical challenge. Biomedicine, *18:* 169–172, 1973.

Mayo, J. G., Laster, W. R., Andrews, C. M., and Schabel, F. M., Jr. Success and failure in the treatment of solid tumors; III. "Cure" of metastatic Lewis lung carcinoma with MeCCNU (NSC 95441) and surgery. Cancer Chemother. Rep., *56:* 183–195, 1972.

Moertel, C. G. Clinical management of advanced gastrointestinal cancer. Semin. Drug Treat., *3:* 55–68, 1973.

Moertel, C. G., and Hanley, J. A. The effect of measuring error on the results of therapeutic trials in advanced cancer. Cancer, *38:* 387–394, 1976.

Moertel, C. G., Schutt, A. J., Hahn, R. G., and Reitemeier, R. S. Effects of patient selection on results of Phase II chemotherapy trials in gastrointentinal cancer. Cancer Chemother. Rep., *58:* 257–260, 1974.

Moore, G. E., Bross, I., and Ausman, R. Effects of 5-fluorouracil (NSC 19893) in 389 patients with cancer. Cancer Chemother. Rep., *52:* 641–650, 1968.

O'Bryan, R. M., Luce, J. K., Talley, R. W., Gotlieb, J. A., Baker, L. H., and Bonadonna, G. Phase II evaluation of adriamycin in human neoplasia. Cancer, *32:* 1–8, 1973.

Owens, A. H. Predicting anti-cancer drug effects in man from animal laboratory studies. J. Chronic Dis., *15:* 223–228, 1962.

Pinkel, D. The use of body surface area as a criterion of drug dosage in cancer chemotherapy. Cancer Res., *18:* 853–856, 1958.

Rundles, W. R., Laszlo, J., and Garrison, F. The antitumor spectrum of cyclophosphamide. Cancer Chemother. Rep., *16:* 407–412, 1962.

Schein, P. S., Davis, R. D., and Cooney, D. A. Qualitative aspects of drug toxicity in prediction from laboratory animals to man. *In* Pharmacology and the Future of Man. Proceedings of the 5th International Congress on Pharmacology, Vol. 3, pp. 304–314, Albert J. Phiebig, White Plains, N.Y., 1973.

Schneiderman, M. A. Mouse to man; statistical problems in bringing a drug to clinical trial. *In* Proceedings of the Fifth Berkeley Symposium on Mathematical Statistics and Probability, pp. 855–866. University of California Press, Berkeley, Calif., 1966.

Schneiderman, M. A. Non-objective art and objective evaluation in cancer chemotherapy. *In* Cancer Chemotherapy, edited by I. Brodsky and S. B. Kahn, pp. 67–76. Grune & Stratton, New York, 1967.

Schneiderman, M. A. How do you know you've done any better? Cancer *35:* 64–69, 1975.

Selawry, O. S. The monochemotherapy of bronchogenic carcinoma with special reference to cell type. Cancer Chemother. Rep., *4:* 177–188, 1973.

Simone, J., Rhomes, J. A., Aur, J. A., Hutsu, H. O., and Pinkel, D. "Total therapy" studies of acute lymphocytic leukemia in children. Cancer, *30:* 1488–1494, 1972.

Skipper, H. E. and Schabel, F. Quantitative and cytokinetic studies in experimental models. *In* Cancer Medicine, edited by J. F. Holland and E. Frei III, pp. 629–650. Lea & Febiger, Philadelphia, 1973.

Takita, H., and Brugorolas, A. Effect of CCNU (NSC 79037) on bronchogenic carcinoma. J. Natl. Cancer Inst., *50:* 49–53, 1973.

Taylor, S. G., III, Canellos, G. P., Band, P., and Pocock, S. Combination chemotherpay for advanced breast cancer; randomized comparison with single drug therapy (abstr.). Am. Soc. Clin. Oncol., *15:* 175, 1974.

Veterans Administration Cooperative Surgical Adjuvant Group Study. Use of thiotepa as an adjuvant to the surgical treatment of carcinoma of the stomach. Cancer, *18:* 291–297, 1965.

Wolff, J. A., D'Angio, G. D., Hartmann, J., Krivit, W., and Newton, W. A., Jr. Single versus multiple course actinomycin D therapy in Wilm's tumor. N. Engl. J. Med., *290:* 84–86, 1974.

Yagoda, A., Mukherji, B., Young, C., Etcubanas, E., Lamonte, C., Smith, J. R., Tan, C. T. C., and Krakoff, I. H. Bleomycin, an antitumor antibiotic; clinical experience in 274 patients. Ann. Intern. Med., *77:* 861–870, 1972.

Zelen, M. Keynote address on biostatistics and data retrieval. Cancer Chemother. Rep., *4*(Part 3): 31–42, 1973.

Zelen, M. The randomization and stratification of patients to clinical trials. J. Chronic Dis., *27:* 365–375, 1974.

Chapter 32

Hemostatic Disorders in Neoplastic Diseases

SALVATORE J. SCIALLA, M.D., AND DANIEL B. KIMBALL, JR., M.D.

The hemostatic mechanism is a delicately balanced system that requires interaction between vascular tissue components, platelets, and plasma factors. In response to vascular injury a series of physical-biological events take place which eventually lead to the arrest of hemorrhage and maintenance of vascular integrity. Malignancy is associated with abnormalities of hemostasis as listed in Table 32.1.

VASCULAR DEFECTS

A feature common to these conditions is the inability of the vessel to maintain its integrity. The hemorrhagic tendency in Kaposi's hemorrhagic sarcoma results from a neoplastic proliferation of vascular elements. Abnormal proteins of high viscosity, such as cryoglobulins and macroglobulins, may block flow in small veins producing vascular rupture as demonstrated in the fundi of patients with macroglobulinemia. Patients with acute leukemia and very high white blood cell counts are at risk of bleeding. Severe leukostasis probably causes toxic changes and degeneration of small blood vessels (Al-Mondhiry, 1975a; Lisiewicz, 1978). When this occurs in association with thrombocytopenia, bleeding results. The chemotherapeutic agent, mithramycin, causes vascular injury demonstrating endothelial and perivascular leukocytic infiltration (Monto et al., 1969).

PLATELET DEFECTS

Platelet disorders causing a hemostatic defect are related to altered platelet number and/or platelet function. Decreased platelet concentrations in plasma are usually secondary to an absolute decrease in production (zero to decreased megakaryocytes in the bone marrow), but ineffective production (normal to increased megakaryocytes in the bone mar-

619

TABLE 32.1

Classification of Hemostatic Disorders in Neoplastic Diseases

I. Vascular defects
    A. Kaposi's hemorrhagic sarcoma
    B. Malignant dysproteinemic states
    C. Leukostasis
    D. Chemotherapy-induced
II. Platelet defects
    A. Quantitative
    B. Qualitative
       1. Intrinsic
          a. Myeloproliferative disorders
          b. Drug-induced
       2. Extrinsic
          a. Dysproteinemic states
          b. Fibrinolysis
          c. Liver disease
          d. Uremia
III. Disorders of blood coagulation
    A. Deficient synthesis of plasma factors
    B. Circulating anticoagulants
    C. Defibrination syndromes
    D. Dysfibrinogens

row), or increased utilization (increased megakaryocytes in the bone marrow and large platelets in the peripheral blood) may also play a role (Slichter and Harker, 1974). Defective and ineffective platelet production may be secondary to neoplastic involvement of the bone marrow, widespread metastases, or secondary to chemotherapy. Increased utilization can be seen in enhanced platelet destruction secondary to infection, disseminated intravascular consumption, and sequestration secondary to hypersplenism. There is a significant correlation between decreased platelet survival and decreased fibrinogen survival, both of which correlate with tumor load (Slichter and Harker, 1974), and both of which improve following objective response to therapy. The best predictor of bleeding in patients with malignancy is the platelet count (Slichter and Harker, 1974; Belt et al., 1978).

Elevated platelet counts occur in the myeloproliferative disorders (i.e., chronic myelocytic leukemia, polycythemia vera, essential thrombocytosis). Instrinsic platelet functional defects ranging from hyperaggregation to diminished platelet aggregation have been described with these disorders (Wu, 1978). The abnormal platelet function tests in the myeloproliferative disorders have been associated with clinical thrombosis and bleeding problems. Although platelet counts over 400,000/ml may be encountered with metastatic malignancy, complications of thrombosis or bleeding related to platelet dysfunction are not usually encountered.

Defective platelet function has been described in patients with acute leukemia (Cowan and Haut, 1972), but is difficult to document in the face of significant thrombocytopenia. Drug-induced platelet dysfunction is possibly an underestimated cause of bleeding in cancer patients. A wide variety of medications such as aspirin, antihistamines, sedatives, antibiotics (carbenicillin), and cancer drugs can diminish platelet aggregation. Even though aspirin is rapidly cleared from the plasma, the acetylated platelet membrane is unable to undergo the release reaction of ADP and serotonin for the remainder of its life span. Plasma abnormalities have been described in uremia, cirrhosis, dysproteinemic states and with platelet iso-antibodies. When the plasma defects are corrected (dialysis, plasma exchange, chemotherapy), platelet function returns to normal.

The causes of altered coagulability in cancer patients are complex involving both thrombosis and hemorrhage. The clinical setting of the patient may help to clarify the factors that can change the normal hemostatic balance.

Since most of the coagulation factors are synthesized by the liver, impairment of liver function (i.e., metastasis or drug-induced damage) may cause deficiency of factors I, II, V, VII, IX, and X. Qualitatively abnormal fibrinogen has been described in patients with hepatoma and metastatic liver disease (Vander Walt et al., 1977). Vitamin K dependent coagulation factors (II, VII, IX, and X) can be diminished in patients treated with chemotherapy or antibiotics, because of reduced food intake, decreased vitamin K synthesis by bacteria in the intestine or malabsorption (Al-Mondhiry, 1975a).

ACCELERATED COAGULATION

Trousseau (1865) was the first to describe the clinical appearance of deep vein thrombosis in the legs of patients with malignant disease (Sack et al., 1977). Many reports have confirmed this relationship and have further clarified chronic alterations of coagulation in these patients. Bowie and Owen (1977) have described a syndrome of chronic intravascular coagulation seen in patients with cancer showing increased coagulation activity, particularly increased levels of fibrinogen and often increased factor VIII. The level of the platelets or coagulation factors in the circulating blood is a balance between the rate of production and the rate of destruction or utilization. Many different forms of neoplasm have been associated with intravascular coagulation and include leukemia, carcinoma of the lung, prostate, breast, pancreas, stomach, gallbladder, and colon, malignant melanoma, rhabdomyosarcoma, and ovarian epithelioma (Weick, 1978; Gralnick and Abrell, 1973). Most leukemic patients with intravascular clotting have granulocytic forms of leukemia, particularly acute promyelocytic leukemia, since promyelocytes are particularly rich in tissue factor activity (Gralnick and Abrell, 1973).

There is little evidence that elevated levels of coagulation factors by themselves cause an increased risk of thrombosis. These high levels of clotting factors may represent either a nonspecific response to the presence of extensive thrombosis or a response to the underlying malignancy. The factor VIII molecule loses its biologic coagulant activity in serum, but retains its immunologic reactivity (Hirsh, 1977). A fall in factor VIII biologic coagulant activity without change in factor VIII immunologic activity has been observed in overt disseminated intravascular coagulation (Denson, 1977). Factor VIII antigen to coagulant protein ratio and factor VIII Von Willebrand factor to coagulant ratio was significantly higher in cancer patients and correlated with progression of their malignancy (Scialla et al., 1978). Serial observations of factor VIII (vwf/c = Von Willebrand factor/coagulant) activity in a patient with metastatic colon cancer to the liver paralleled his clinical course (Fig. 32.1).

It has been suggested that the entrance of mucus derived from adenocarcinomas into the circulation may activate coagulation. Pineo et al. (1974) have demonstrated that partially purified mucus extracts can activate the coagulation mechanism, both in vitro and in vivo. The action appeared to be via factor X activation. Removal of sialic acid with neuraminidase inactivated the mucus extracts.

ACUTE INTRAVASCULAR COAGULATION AND FIBRINOLYSIS (ICF)

The delicate hemostatic balance of a compensated, chronic ICF syndrome seen in cancer patients may be upset by acute clinical changes in

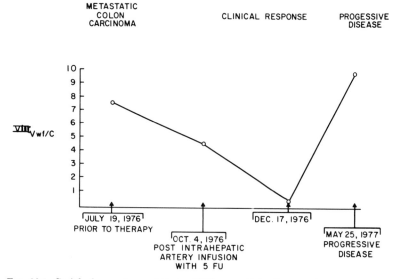

Fig. 32.1. Serial observations of factor VIII$_{vwf/c}$ activity in a patient with metastatic colon cancer to the liver. (vwf/c = Von Willebrand factor/coagulant.)

the patient's condition such as sepsis, liver disease, administration of chemotherapy, or operations that can trigger an acute ICF syndrome and subsequent hemostatic failure. Bleeding occurs in skin, mucous membranes, gastrointestinal tract, genitourinary tract, lung, retina, and the central nervous system. Thromboembolic complications can occur and cause acute renal failure secondary to renal cortical necrosis or neurologic syndromes secondary to multiple blood vessel occlusion in the brain.

The diagnosis of an acute ICF syndrome can be confirmed by the following laboratory tests: (1) significant thrombocytopenia; (2) prolonged clotting times (if they do not correct with normal plasma, this may indicate the presence of circulating inhibitors such as fibrin degradation products); (3) presence of fibrin degradation products and demonstration of a fibrin monomer in plasma; (4) determination of fibrinogen levels (although classically hypofibrinogemia is present, cancer patients may have initially high levels of fibrinogen); and (5) low values of factors V and VIII.

MANAGEMENT OF COAGULATION PROBLEMS

Platelet Transfusion. As noted above, the most common cause of bleeding in cancer patients is drug-induced thrombocytopenia. Platelet transfusions have been effective in reducing the incidence of bleeding due to severe thrombocytopenia. To raise the platelet count by 30,000–40,000/ μl an adult patient of average weight and size would require 4 to 6 units of platelets. Patients with sepsis and fever often respond poorly to platelet transfusions. Patients with qualitative platelet disorders may be thought of as having a functional thrombocytopenia and may be benefited by platelet transfusion (i.e., a patient with hemorrhage and recent ingestion of aspirin). Greater care should be exercised to avoid medications known to inhibit normal platelet function, particularly in the face of incipient or actual thrombocytopenia.

Accelerated Coagulation. Thromboembolism is a common complication in patients with malignancy, especially those who are confined to bed or following major surgery. In these patients, the physician should look for pulmonary embolus with a high index of suspicion. In the absence of a major contraindication to anticoagulant therapy, all patients proven to have deep vein thrombosis and/or pulmonary embolus should receive heparin. Recent data implies that preoperative minidose heparin may be of benefit in prevention of postoperative thrombosis especially in cancer patients.

Acute ICF. Patients with acute ICF should be managed by treating the underlying and precipitating factors. The goal is to try to return the coagulation system to a compensated state. Decisions of treatment should be based on present laboratory parameters of the patient. Correction studies of the patient's plasma will help clarify the feasibility of plasma replacement. With continued bleeding and laboratory signs of ongoing thrombosis (i.e., positive fibrin monomer) a trial of heparin with plasma and platelet replacement can be instituted. The dosage of heparin may vary from 500 to 1000 units per hour depending upon clinical response, liver function, and the platelet count. During heparin therapy patients can be monitored by following changes in fibrinogen levels, fibrin degradation products, presence of fibrin monomer, and change in platelet count. Improvement in fibrinogen levels usually precedes increases in platelet count.

Promyelocytic Leukemia. Goodnight (1974) noted 89 instances of leukemia who had evidence of intravascular coagulation with 76 of these being seen in acute promyelocytic leukemia. Gralnick et al. (1972) have reported on the usefulness of heparin therapy in these patients and a recent report by Drapkin and co-workers (1978) emphasized the potential benefit for remission induction if heparin is used prophylactically in these patients.

EFFECT OF CHEMOTHERAPY

The influence of cytotoxic drugs on hemostasis has yet to be fully clarified. The following chemotherapeutic agents have been described in the literature as having an effect on coagulation and/or platelet function.

Adriamycin. Adriamycin has been reported to activate the fibrinolytic system (Bick et al., 1976). Patients taking Adriamycin were noted to have elevated fibrinogen/fibrin degradation products and in vitro studies demonstrated direct activation of plasminogen by Adriamycin. In addition, a recent report has suggested that Adriamycin may accelerate the increased fibrinolytic activity associated with prostate carcinoma (Case and Carroll, 1978).

L-Asparaginase. L-Asparaginase, an enzyme purified from *Escherichia coli* B, is an effective agent in the treatment of acute lymphocytic leukemia, but patients so treated develop various coagulation abnormalities (Ramsay et al., 1977). Hypofibrinogenenia occurs frequently following L-asparaginase administration and is felt to be associated with decreased synthesis. Other reported findings have included prolongation of the prothrombin time, partial thromboplastin time, and thrombin time (PT, PTT, and TT). In studies, low levels of factor II, V, VII, IX, X, and XI have been reported in isolated cases. Factor VIII was consistently elevated. These coagulation changes improved following discontinuation of the asparaginase even when vincristine and prednisone were continued.

Mithramycin. Mithramycin is useful in the treatment of patients with testicular tumors, but the effectiveness of this agent has been limited due to the frequent appearance of hemorrhage. Previous reports have described abnormalities in platelet function, depression of coagulation factor levels, and enhancement of fibrinolysis in the presence or absence of thrombocytopenia in some patients treated with this agent (Kennedy, 1969; Monto et al., 1969). Ahr and co-workers (1978) have described three patients treated with mithramycin demonstrating the appearance of a cyclic, reversible hemorrhagic diathesis associated with prolongation of the bleeding time, decreased platelet aggregation responses, and depleted platelet stores of ADP in the absence of thrombocytopenia. These findings of early manifestation of mithramycin toxicity were concurrent with a rise in LDH.

Vincristine. Steinherz and co-workers (1976) have studied platelet dysfunction in vincristine-treated patients. Vincristine eliminated second phase aggregation responses to epinephrine and ADP from 1 to 4 weeks after administration. The exact mechanism by which vincristine effects platelet aggregation is uncertain. Since bleeding times were normal and the patients were asymptomatic, the clinical significance is uncertain. Hypofibrinogenemia has been reported by Al-Mondhery (1975b) in four patients receiving vincristine and prednisone. The etiology of this hypofibrinogenemia is unclear, but may be related to subclinical intravascular coagulation. The patients had no bleeding complications and no treatment was required.

HEMOSTASIS AND METASTASIS

Many factors that relate to the establishment of tumor metastases have been recognized (Wood et al., 1961). Significant among these are platelets, fibrin deposition and agents affecting the plasma or platelet coagulation mechanism (Brodsky et al., 1976). Some of the important factors that may play a role include (1) characteristics of the tumor cell surface or substances elaborated or released by the tumor cell(s), (2) the potential of platelet-tumor cell interaction or vascular endothelium-tumor cell interaction, and (3) the requirement of fibrin deposition with the tumor cell for "successful" establishment of a metastasis (Warren, 1974). In experimental systems it can be shown that an early phase of blood-borne tumor metastases are characterized by tumor cell-platelet aggregates (Jones et al., 1971). It certainly is conceivable that the platelet fibrinogen may be the initial source for fibrin necessary for establishment of a tumor metastasis. Gasic and co-workers (1972) have presented data to support the concept that drugs that interfere with the platelet-tumor cell interaction, such as aspirin, might diminish the establishment of tumor metastases following the intravenous injection of tumor cells in mice. Wood and Hilgard (1972) were unable to document this therapeutic effect in a different experimental system.

In view of the observation that clot formation might play an intricate role in the establishment of metastases (Wood, 1958), it is not surprising that a number of investigators have looked at the role of various antico-agulants in preventing the establishment of metastases following the injection of tumor cells in various experimental animal systems. Fisher and Fisher (1961) demonstrated that the duration of anticoagulant treat-ment and the time of beginning administration in relationship to tumor cell injection were both important. Anticoagulant administration 24 hours after tumor cell administration did not protect the animals nearly as well as injection 4 hours prior to tumor cell administration. There was a direct correlation between the degree of protection and the duration of heparin administration, the maximal protection being afforded by 7 days of therapy. These authors also demonstrated a protective effect of activating the fibrinolytic mechanism. The degree of protection was somewhat dose dependent. Again, maximal effect was demonstrated by giving the plas-min prior to tumor cell administration. Agostino and co-workers (1961) demonstrated similar protection against systemic metastases when hep-arin administration (50 units) preceded tumor cell administration by 10 min. Interestingly, tumor cells incubated with heparin and then admin-istered subcutaneously, all showed tumor growth, suggesting no direct cytotoxic effect of heparin (up to 30-min incubation time). The question of a direct cytotoxic versus an anticoagulant effect producing the protec-tion is not answered. Eichbaum (1975) and Leblanc (1977) have reviewed and presented data to support a direct cytotoxic effect. Agostino and co-workers (1966) likewise demonstrated a similar protective effect for orally administered coumadin (given 7 days prior to tumor cell administration and continued until sacrifice). This work was confirmed by Ryan and co-workers (1968) and subsequently the same group (Ketcham and co-workers, 1971) published data to support the concept of a direct inhibitory effect on the growth of primary tumors. The same laboratory has not been able to demonstrate this direct effect on primary tumor growth in subsequent work (Hoover and co-workers, 1976). Some of the protective effects of warfarin in these experimental tumor systems may be due to direct cytotoxicity (Hilgard and Thornes, 1976), but it is probable that at least some of the effect is mediated through their anticoagulant action. A similar protective effect of vitamin K-deficient diet reported by Hilgard (1977) would be consistent with this hypothesis. A combined therapeutic approach to the prevention of metastases in various experimental sys-tems, using heparin plus BCG immunotherapy (Kiricuta and co-workers, 1973), heparin plus nitrogen mustard (Agostino and Cliffton, 1963) and warfarin plus Adriamycin (Hoover and Ketcham, 1975) demonstrated an additional effect over anticoagulants or chemotherapy alone.

The role for anticoagulants in the treatment of human neoplasia remains undefined. Michaels (1964) studied patients who were on long term anticoagulant therapy for diseases other than cancer. In 540 patients he demonstrated that the incidence of cancer was unchanged, but that the death rate due to cancer was reduced to one-eighth of the expected rate. The protective effects of coumadin have been reported in the treatment of several human tumors (Thornes, 1975; Hoover and co-workers, 1978). Elias and Brugarolas (1972) claimed a similar role for heparin in the treatment of lung carcinoma, but this has not been substantiated (Rohwedder and Sagastume, 1977). The role of fibrinolytic agents is incompletely evaluated or anecdotal.

There is good evidence to support a role for both the platelet and plasma coagulation mechanism in the establishment of tumor metastases. There is growing evidence that drugs interfering with either or both of these systems may play a useful role as adjuvant therapy. The role of these agents in established metastatic disease is unknown. The role for these agents when combined with other modalities (chemotherapy or immunotherapy) for the treatment of metastatic disease is only now being defined.

REFERENCES

Agostino, D., and Cliffton, E. E. Decrease in pulmonary metastases; potentiation of nitrogen mustard effect by heparin and fibrinolysin. Ann. Surg., *151*: 400–408, 1963.

Agostino, D., Grossi, C. E., and Cliffton, E. E. Effect of heparin on circulating Walker carcinosarcoma 256 cells. J. Nat. Cancer Inst., *27*: 17–24, 1961.

Agostino, D., and Cliffton, E. E., and Girolami, A. Effect of prolonged coumadin treatment on the production of pulmonary metastases in the rat. Cancer, *19*: 284–288, 1966.

Ahr, D. J., Scialla, S. J., and Kimball, D. B. Acquired platelet dysfunction following mithramycin therapy. Cancer, *41*: 448–454, 1978.

Al-Mondhiry, H. Disorders of hemostasis in acute leukemia; Part II. Clin. Bull. *5*: 51–56, 1975a.

Al-Mondhiry, H. Hypofibrinogenemia associated with vincristine and prednisone therapy in lymphoblastic leukemia. Cancer, *35*: 144—147, 1975b.

Belt, R. J., Leite, C., Haas, C., and Stephens, R. L. Incidence of hemorrhagic complications in patients with cancer. J. A. M. A. *239*: 2571-2574, 1978.

Bick, R. L., Fekete, L. F., and Wilson, W. L. Adriamycin and fibrinolysis. Thromb. Res., *8*: 467-475, 1976.

Bowie, E. J., and Owen, C. A. Hemostatic failure in clinical medicine. Semin. Hematol., *14*: 341-364, 1977.

Brodsky, I., Fuscaldo, A. A. and Fusdaldo, K. E. Hemostasis and cancer. *In* Oncologic Medicine: Clinical Topics and Practical Management, edited by A. Sutnick and P. F. Engstrom, pp. 247–259. University Park Press, Baltimore, 1976.

Case, D. C. Jr., and Carroll, R. J. Adriamycin-accelerated fibrinolysis in disseminated prostate cancer. Proc. Am. Soc. Clin. Oncol., *19*: 311, 1978.

Cowan, D. H., and Haut, M. J.: Platelet function in acute leukemia. J. Lab. Clin. Med., *79*: 893-905, 1972.

Denson, K. W. E. The ratio of factor VIII related antigen and factor VIII biologic activity as an index of hypercoagulability and intravascular clotting. Thromb. Res., *10*: 107- 119, 1977.

Drapkin, R. L., Gee, T. S., Dowling, M. P., Arlin, Z., McKenzie, S., Kempin, S., and Clarkson, B. Prophylactic heparin therapy in acute promyelocytic leukemia. Cancer, *41*: 2484-2490, 1978.

Eichbaum, F. W. Anticoagulants and cancer; a review. Rev. Bras. Pesqui. Med. Biol., 8: 489–496, 1975.

Elias, E. G., and Brugarolas, A. The role of heparin therapy in the chemotherapy of solid tumors; preliminary clinical trial in carcinoma of the lung. Cancer Chem. Rep., 56: 783–785, 1972.

Fisher, B., and Fisher, E. R. Experimental studies of factors which influence hepatic metastases; VIII. Effect of anticoagulants. Surgery, 50: 240–247, 1961.

Gasic, G. J., Gasic, T. B., and Murphy, S. Anti-metastatic effect of aspirin. Lancet, 2: 932–933, 1972.

Goodnight, S. H., Jr. Bleeding and intravascular clotting in malignancy; a review. Ann. N. Y. Acad. Sci., 230: 271–288, 1974.

Gralnick, H. R., and Abrell, E. Acute promyelocytic leukemia; hemorrhagic manifestations and morphologic criteria. Br. J. Haematol., 24: 59–99, 1973.

Gralnick, H. R., Bagley, J., and Abrell, E. Heparin treatment for the hemorrhagic diathesis of acute promyelocytic leukemia. Am. J. Med., 52: 167–174, 1972.

Hilgard, P. Experimental vitamin K deficiency and spontaneous metastases. Br. J. Cancer, 35: 891–892, 1979.

Hilgard, P., and Thornes, R. D. Perspectives in cancer research; anticoagulants in the treatment of cancer. Eur. J Cancer, 12: 755–762, 1976.

Hirsh, J. Hypercoagulability. Semin. Hematol., 14: 409–425, 1977.

Hoover, H. C., Jr., Jones, D., and Ketcham, A. S. The optimal level of anticoagulation for decreasing experimental metastasis. Surgery, 79: 625–630, 1976.

Hoover, H. C., Jr., and Ketcham, A. S. Decreasing experimental metastasis formation with anticoagulation and chemotherapy. Surg. Forum, 26: 173–174, 1975.

Hoover, H. C., Jr., Ketcham, A. S., Millar, R. C., and Gralnick, H. R. Osteosarcoma; improved survival with anticoagulation and amputation. Cancer, 41: 2474–2480, 1978.

Jones, D. S., Wallace, A. C., and Fraser, E. E. Sequence of events in experimental metastases of Walker 256 tumor; light, immunofluorescence and electron microscopic observations. J. Natl. Cancer Inst., 46: 493–504, 1971.

Kennedy, B. J. Metabolic and toxic effects of mithramycin during tumor therapy. Am. J. Med., 49: 494–503, 1969.

Ketcham, A. S., Sugarbaker, E. V., Ryan, J. J., and Orme, S. K. Clotting factors and metastasis formation. A. J. R., and 111: 42–47, 1971.

Kiricuta, I., Todorutiu, C., Muresian, T., and Risca, R. Prophylaxis of metastases formation by unspecific immunologic stimulation associated with heparin therapy. Cancer, 31: 1392–1396, 1973.

Leblanc, P. O. Proteases during the growth of Ehrlich ascites tumor; III. Effect of ε-aminocaproic acid (EACA) and heparin. Eur. J. Cancer, 13: 947–950, 1977.

Lisiewicz, J. Mechanisms of hemorrhage in leukemias. Semin. Thromb. Hemostas., 4: 241–267, 1978.

Merskey, C. Pathogenesis and treatment of altered blood coagulability in patients with malignant tumors. Ann. N. Y. Acad. Sci., 230: 289–293, 1974.

Michaels, L. Cancer incidence and mortality in patients having anticoagulant therapy Lancet, 2: 832–835, 1964.

Monto, R. W., Talley, R. W., Caldwell, M. J., Levin, W. C., and Guest, M. M. Observations in the mechanism of hemorrhagic toxicity in mithramycin (NSC 24559) therapy. Cancer Res., 29: 697–704, 1969.

Pineo, G. F., Brain, M. C., Gallus, A. S., Hirsh, J., Hatton W. C., and Regoeczi, E. Tumors, mucous production, and hypercoagulability. Ann. N. Y. Acad. Sci., 230: 262–270, 1974.

Ramsay, N. K. C., Coccia, P. F., Krivit, W., Nesbit, M. E., and Edson, J. R. The effect of L-asparaginase on plasma coagulation factors in acute lymphoblastic leukemia. Cancer, 40: 1398–1401, 1977.

Rohwedder, J. J., and Sagastume, E. Heparin and polychemotherapy for treatment of lung cancer. Cancer Treat. Rep. *61:* 1399–1401, 1977.

Ryan, J. J., Ketcham, A. S., and Wexler, H. Reduced incidence of spontaneous metastases with long-term coumadin therapy. Ann. Surg., *168:* 163–168, 1968.

Sack, G. H., Jr., Levin, J., and Bell, W. R. Trousseau's syndrome and other manifestations of chronic disseminated coagulopathy in patients with neoplasma; clinical, pathophysiologic and therapeutic features. Medicine, *56:* 1–36, 1977.

Scialla, S. J., Barr, C. F., Waldorf, M. A., and Kimball, D. B. Factor VIII complex in cancer patients. Clin. Res., *26:* 441A, 1978.

Slichter, S. J., and Harker, L.A. Hemostasis in malignancy. Ann. N. Y. Acad. Sci., *230:* 252–261, 1974.

Steinherz, P. G., Miller, D. R., Hilgartner, M. W., and Schmalzer, E. A. Platelet dysfunction in vincristine treated patients. Br. J. Haematol., *32:* 439–450, 1976.

Thornes, R. D. Adjuvant therapy of cancer via the cellular immune mechanism or fibrin by induced fibrinolysis and oral anticoagulants. Cancer, *35:* 91–97, 1975.

Trousseau, A. Phlegmasia Alba Dolens: Clinique Medicale de l'Hotel Dieu de Paris, Ed. 2, Vol. 3. Balhiere, Paris, 1865.

Vander Walt, J. A., Gomperts, E. D., and Keu, M. C. Hemostatic factors in primary hepatocellular cancer. Cancer, *40:* 1593–1603, 1977.

Warren, B. A. Tumor metastasis and thrombosis. Thromb. Diath. Haemorrh. Suppl. *59:* 139–156, 1974.

Weick, J. K. Intravascular coagulation in cancer. Semin. Oncol., *5:* 203–211, 1978.

Wood, S., Jr. Pathogenesis of metastasis formation observed in vivo in the rabbit ear chamber. Arch. Patholo., *66:* 550–568, 1958.

Wood, S., Jr., and Hilgard, P. Aspirin and tumour metastasis. Lancet, *2:* 1416–1417, 1972.

Wood, S., Jr., Holyoke, E. D., and Yardley, J. H. Mechanisms of metastasis production from blood-borne cancer cells. Can. Cancer Conf., *4:* 167–223, 1961.

Wu, K. K. Platelet hyperaggregability and thrombosis in patients with thrombocythemia. Ann. Intern. Med., *88:* 7–11, 1978.

INDEX